Recent Advances in

FORENSIC MEDICINE AND TOXICOLOGY

Recent Advances in
FORENSIC MEDICINE AND TOXICOLOGY

VOLUME 1

Editor

Gautam Biswas MD
Professor and Head
Department of Forensic Medicine and Toxicology
Dayanand Medical College and Hospital
Ludhiana, Punjab, India

Forewords

Padma Bhushan Prof. P Chandra Sekharan
Prof. Anil Aggrawal

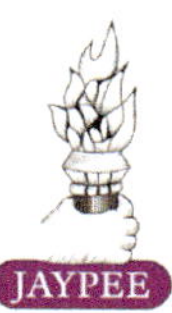

JAYPEE
JAYPEE BROTHERS MEDICAL PUBLISHERS
The Health Sciences Publisher
New Delhi | London

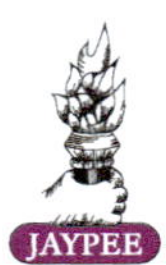

Jaypee Brothers Medical Publishers (P) Ltd

Headquarters
EMCA House
23/23-B, Ansari Road, Daryaganj
New Delhi 110 002, India
Landline: +91-11-23272143, +91-11-23272703
+91-11-23282021, +91-11-23245672
E-mail: jaypee@jaypeebrothers.com

Overseas Office
JP Medical Ltd.
83, Victoria Street, London
SW1H 0HW (UK)
Phone: +44-20 3170 8910
E-mail: info@jpmedpub.com

Corporate Office
Jaypee Brothers Medical Publishers (P) Ltd.
4838/24, Ansari Road, Daryaganj
New Delhi 110 002, India
Phone: +91-11-43574357
Fax: +91-11-43574314
E-mail: jaypee@jaypeebrothers.com

EU GPSR Authorised Representative
Logos Europe, 9 rue Nicolas Poussin
17000, La Rochelle, France
Phone: +33 (0) 6 67 93 73 78
E-mail: Contact@logoseurope.eu

Website: www.jaypeebrothers.com
Website: www.jaypeedigital.com

Inquiries for bulk sales may be solicited at: jaypee@jaypeebrothers.com

Recent Advances in Forensic Medicine and Toxicology (Volume 1)

First Edition: **2015**

Reprint: 2026

ISBN: 978-93-5152-558-5

Printed at Replika Press Pvt. Ltd.

Dedicated to

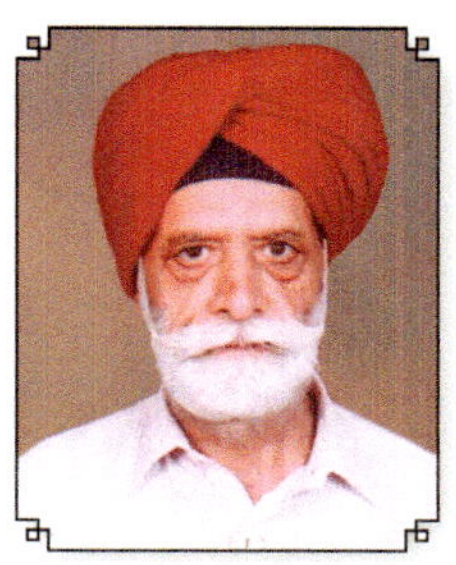

Late Dr (Maj. Gen.) Ajit Singh Philosopher, guide and mentor	Late Mr Gurupada Biswas (Dad) Inspiration and admiration

And

My dear wife Anupama and son Gaurav
for making each moment worth living…

Contributors

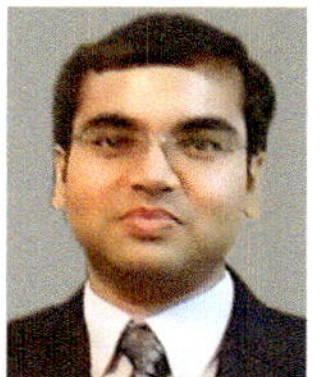

Shouvanik Adhya
Assistant Professor
Department of Forensic Medicine and Toxicology
College of Medicine and JNM Hospital
West Bengal University of Health Sciences
Kalyani, West Bengal, India
shouvanikadhya@gmail.com
Chapter: 21

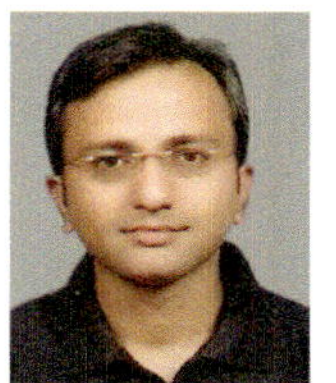

Swapnil S Agarwal
Professor and Head
Department of Forensic Medicine and Toxicology
Pramukhswami Medical College and Shree Krishna Hospital
Anand, Gujarat, India
swapnilagarwal@msn.com
Chapter: 9

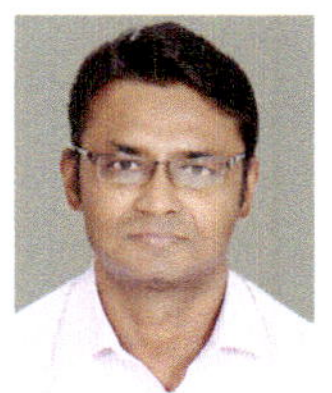

Gautam Biswas
Professor and Head
Department of Forensic Medicine and Toxicology
Dayanand Medical College and Hospital
Ludhiana, Punjab, India
forensicdmc@gmail.com
Chapters: 1, 6, 8, 17

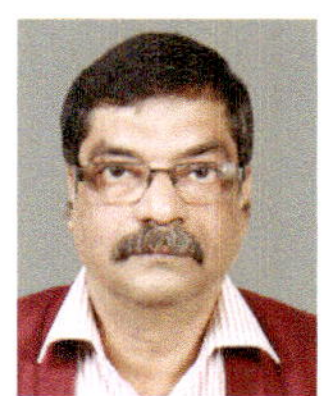

Tapas Kumar Bose
Professor and Head
Department of Forensic Medicine and Toxicology
Calcutta National Medical College
Kolkata, West Bengal, India
drtapasbose@gmail.com
Chapter: 21

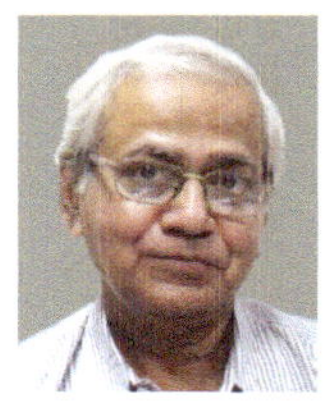

Prabhas Chandra Chakraborty
(Ex) Professor and Head
Department of Forensic Medicine and Toxicology
Nilratan Sircar Medical College
Kolkata, West Bengal, India
prabhasdoc@gmail.com
Chapter: 20

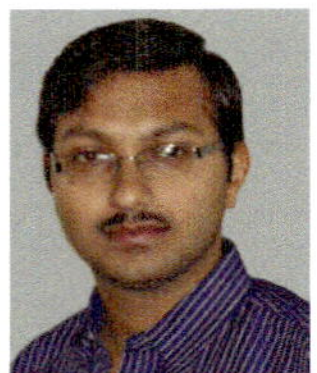

Abhishek Das
Assistant Professor
Sikkim Manipal Institute of Medical Sciences
Gangtok, Sikkim, India
abhishek.das.forensic@gmail.com
Chapter: 20

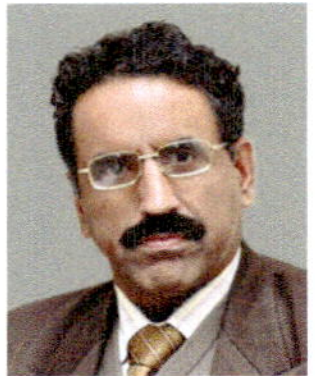

Suresh K Dhattarwal
Professor and Head
Department of Forensic Medicine and Toxicology
Pt. Bhagwat Dayal Sharma
Postgraduate Institute of Medical Sciences
Rohtak, Haryana, India
drskdhattarwal@gmail.com
Chapter: 16

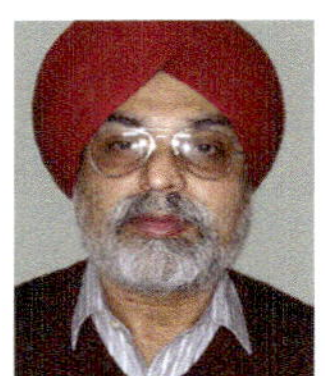

Sarvpreet Singh Grewal
Professor and Head
Department of Neurosurgery
Christian Medical College (CMC) and Brown Hospital
Ludhiana, Punjab, India
sarvpreetgrewal@yahoo.co.in
Chapter: 13

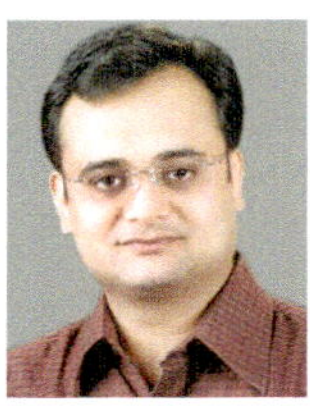

Punit Gupta
Senior Resident
Department of Neurosurgery
Christian Medical College (CMC) and Brown Hospital
Ludhiana, Punjab, India
punitdeepali@gmail.com
Chapter: 13

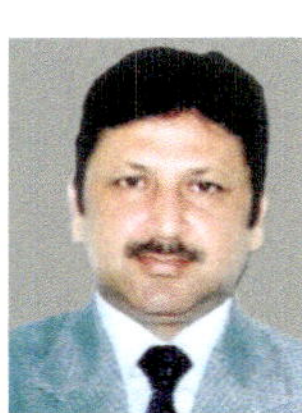

Bhupesh Khajuria
Professor and Head
Department of Forensic Medicine and Toxicology
Government Medical College, Jammu
Jammu and Kashmir, India
bhupeshkhajuria@gmail.com
Chapter: 14

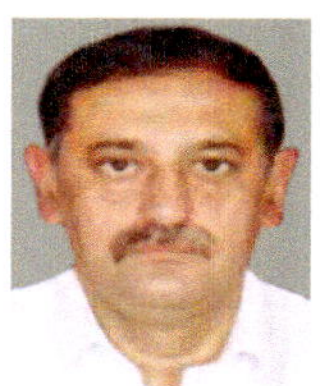

Anil Kohli
Reader
Department of Forensic Medicine and Toxicology
University College of Medical Sciences (UCMS) and
Guru Teg Bahadur (GTB) Hospital
New Delhi, India
anil_kohli@hotmail.com
Chapters: 4, 10

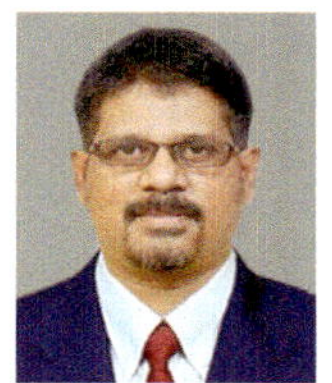

Pradeep Kumar MV
Professor
Department of Forensic Medicine and Toxicology
Rajarajeswari Medical College and Hospital
Bengaluru, Karnataka, India
pradimv@gmail.com
Chapter: 7

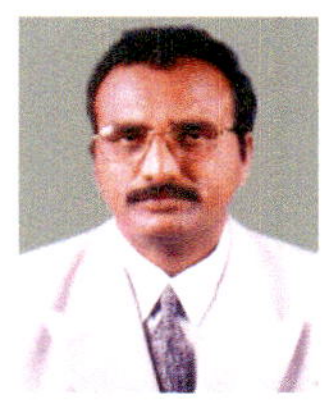

Jagadeesh Narayanareddy
Professor
Department of Forensic Medicine and Toxicology
Vydehi Institute of Medical Sciences and Research Centre
Bengaluru, Karnataka, India
forensicjagadeesh@gmail.com
Chapter: 15

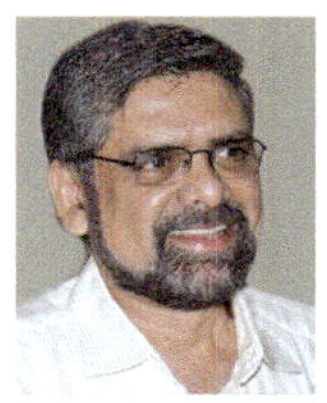

Vijay Vasudev Pillay
Professor
Department of Forensic Medicine and Toxicology
Amrita School of Medicine
Amrita Vishwa Vidyapeetham
Kochi, Kerala, India
toxicology@aims.amrita.edu
Chapter: 3

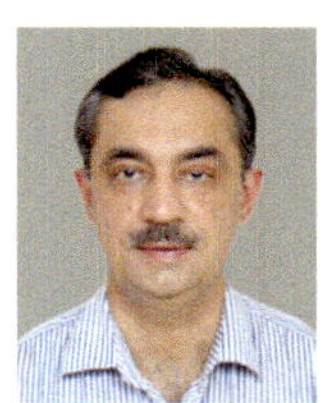

Sandeep Puri
Professor and Head
Department of Medicine
Dayanand Medical College and Hospital
Ludhiana, Punjab, India
drsandeeppuri@yahoo.com
Chapters: 11, 12

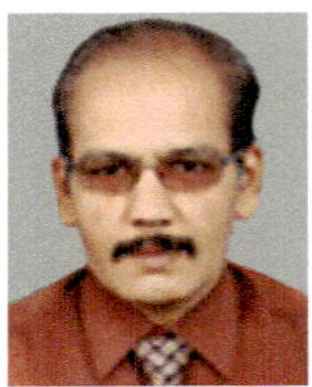

N Srinivasa Ragavan
Professor and Head
Department of Forensic Medicine and Toxicology
Saveetha Medical College and Hospital
Kanchipuram, Tamil Nadu, India
ragavan6464@gmail.com
Chapter: 22

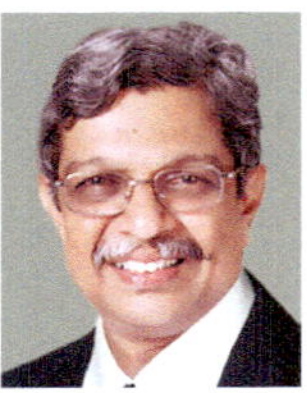

Nageshkumar G Rao
Medicolegal Consultant
Director, Medilegal Point, Manipal
Former Professor, Head and Director
Department of Forensic Medicine
Kasturba Medical College (KMC), Manipal and Mangalore
Manipal University, Manipal, Karnataka
Sikkim Manipal Institute of Medical Sciences (SMIMS)
Sikkim Manipal University, Sikkim
Meenakshi Medical College and Research Institute (MMCRI)
Kanchipuram, Meenakshi University, Chennai, Tamil Nadu
SDM College of Medical Sciences and Hospital, Dharwad
Rajiv Gandhi University of Health Sciences (RGUHS)
Bengaluru, Karnataka, India
prof.nkgr@gmail.com
Chapter: 18

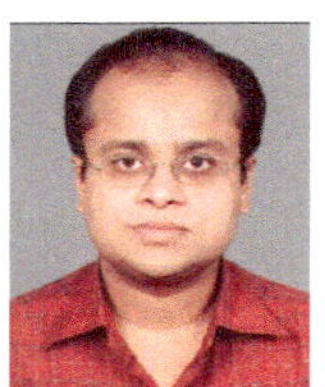

Prateek Rastogi
District Medicolegal Consultant and Associate Professor
Department of Forensic Medicine and Toxicology
Kasturba Medical College
Mangalore (Manipal University), Karnataka, India
rastogiprateek@rediffmail.com
Chapter: 19

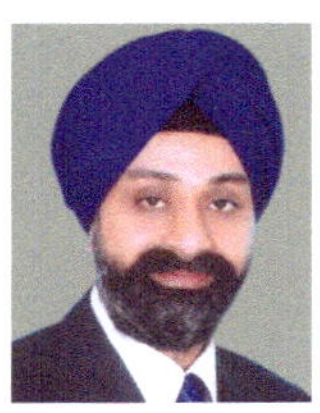

Virendar Pal Singh
Associate Professor
Department of Forensic Medicine and Toxicology
DMC and Hospital
Ludhiana, Punjab, India
singhvp@gmail.com
Chapter: 6

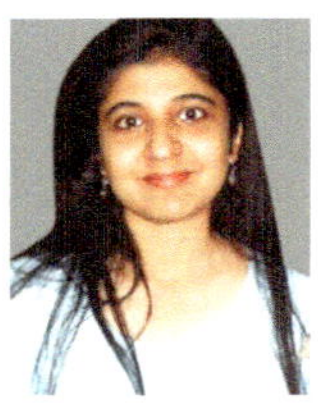

Aditi Verma
Senior Lecturer
Kalka Dental College
Meerut, Uttar Pradesh, India
ver.aditi@gmail.com
Chapter: 5

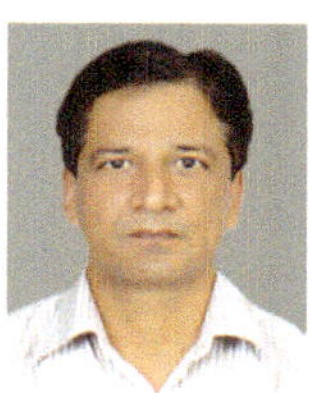

Satish Kumar Verma
Professor
Department of Forensic Medicine and Toxicology
University College of Medical Sciences (UCMS) and
Guru Teg Bahadur (GTB) Hospital
New Delhi, India
vermasatish2003@gmail.com
Chapter: 5

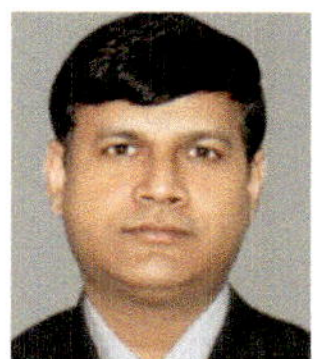

Mukesh Yadav
Professor and Head
Department of Forensic Medicine and Toxicology
School of Medical Sciences and Research
Sharda University, Greater Noida, Uttar Pradesh, India
drmukesh65@yahoo.co.in
Chapter: 2

Foreword

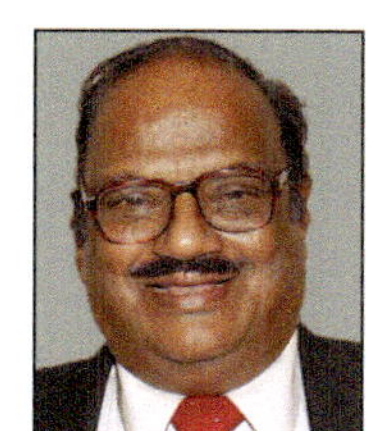

There are not many good and useful books on forensic medicine and toxicology for Indian students, researchers and practitioners of both medicine and law. In this context, Dr Gautam Biswas's *Recent Advances in Forensic Medicine and Toxicology (Volume 1)* is a welcome one.

The book is a compilation of well-written chapters, each chapter bearing an interesting topic and being handled by renowned expert(s) in that field. Vijay Vasudev Pillay's chapter *Euthanasia: Legal, Social and Humanitarian Aspects* ponders on the ethical issues involved in the procedure and the current legal status around the world. Bhupesh Khajuria's chapter *An Approach to a Case of Near-hanging and Attempted Strangulation* deals with the tricky problems of 'homicide or suicide' decisions, and is a necessary update. The treatise on *Dyadic Deaths* by Nageshkumar G Rao is a novel one, not usually dealt with in books on forensic medicine. This is an interesting topic to be read by all those interested in forensics. Grievous hurt which is concerned with opining the nature of injuries has been dealt admirably by Anil Kohli. Some chapters are handled by experienced clinicians while the editor himself has dealt with diverse topics ranging from consent, court room procedures, medical records to judicial hanging. All the chapters are useful and written in lucid technical language along with necessary illustrations and photographs.

Dr Gautam's updated book on *Recent Advances in Forensic Medicine and Toxicology (Volume 1)* is highly commendable and recommended as a guide not only to forensic practitioners in medicine and law but also to students aspiring for higher studies and research in forensic medicine.

Padma Bhushan Prof. P Chandra Sekharan
Consultant-in-Chief, Forensics International
Fellow, American College of Forensic Examiners Institute
Honorary Professor, Dr Ambedkar Law University, Chennai
Guest Faculty, National Law School of India University
Bengaluru, Karnataka, India
[Formerly, Pro-Vice-Chancellor, National Law University, Jodhpur, Rajasthan
Emeritus Fellow, University of Madras
UGC Professor, Faculty Forensic Engineering, Anna University
Professor-Director, Forensic Sciences Department, Government of Tamil Nadu,
Chennai, India]

Foreword

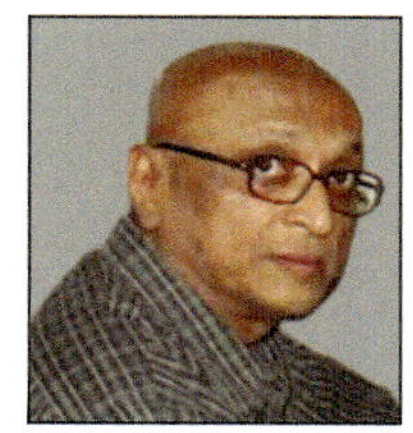

It is a pleasure and an honor to write a foreword for Gautam Biswas's *Recent Advances in Forensic Medicine and Toxicology (Volume 1)*. We all are aware of the stupendous success his textbook *Review of Forensic Medicine and Toxicology* enjoys. I myself refer to his book for my lectures and court work. However, whenever I had an occasion to talk to him, I always goaded him to write a textbook on forensic medicine for postgraduate students. Such a book currently does not exist and our postgraduates have to run from pillar to post in order to get material for their examinations. There are a few excellent books for postgraduates published in the US and UK, but they mainly cater to foreign milieu, and do not deal with Indian situation and law at all. For instance, one would not find an advanced text on forensic medicine, dealing with, say, latest changes in rape law, euthanasia, medical records, age, sex verification, or issues regarding grievous hurt for that matter.

Gautam has been kind enough to send me the proofs of all 22 chapters in his book. Initially, we had mutually decided that I would write an epilogue to each chapter and this idea sounded very attractive to me, because then I would get a chance to express my opinion on each chapter, which was my fond dream. However, due to my own limitations, I could not do that. And thankfully Gautam, magnanimous as he is, did not mind that.

I have gone through each chapter in great detail and find each chapter well written. Each chapter includes, as one would expect in a book of this nature, latest advances in the subject that the chapter deals with. Each chapter is written by a stalwart in his own field—Gautam himself writing as many as four chapters. As I am an inveterate fan of Gautam, I read those chapters first, and immediately came to the conclusion that he has written an instant best seller!

Thanks a ton for fulfilling my wish and the wish of thousands of your fans, including postgraduates in this country and abroad. I have not an iota of doubt in my mind that this text would become a standard reference for our postgraduates as well as faculties. He would keep writing sequels to this volume, where he would keep dealing with advanced and newer topics. Ultimately, after 6–7 volumes, when we will combine all of them together, we will have a true postgraduate encyclopedia of forensic medicine and toxicology. Good luck to you and do not fail our expectations!!

As for our faculty and postgraduates, I can unhesitatingly say, "Go and read this book. You will enter into a journey you will never forget."

Anil Aggrawal
Director-Professor
Forensic Medicine and Toxicology
Maulana Azad Medical College
New Delhi, India

Preface

In recent times, the field of forensic medicine has undergone enormous expansion. There are now several outstanding, up-to-date forensic medicine textbooks available for undergraduate students. However, none of these textbooks have been written specifically for postgraduates, faculty and medical practitioners working in the casuality set-up.

In the year 2010, my first textbook *Review of Forensic Medicine and Toxicology* was published. Soon after publication of that work, Dr Anil Aggrawal, Director-Professor, Forensic Medicine and Toxicology, Maulana Azad Medical College, suggested me to write a book for postgraduates. Keeping this in mind, *Recent Advances in Forensic Medicine and Toxicology* was conceived. I considered bringing out this series with contribution from experts of national and international reputes to cater to the needs of postgraduates, faculty and medical practitioners working in casuality. This book is also meant for those medical professionals who frequently or occasionally interact with forensic specialists for their opinions in medicolegal cases. Since, there are many misconceptions and myths, opinions given by these professionals often face criticism of the judiciary. It is hoped that the book will succeed in serving as a practical guide to the practice of daily forensic pathological and medicolegal routine, as well as providing encouragement and inspiration for future research projects.

Recent Advances in Forensic Medicine and Toxicology (*Volume 1)* is designed to provide up-to-date knowledge on some common and special topics in the field, focusing closely on the dynamic and rapidly growing evolution of medical science and law. An attempt has been made to provide as much information as possible within the book, since the book is meant to be an overview of forensic issues concerned.

The book has been divided into three sections. In this, individual chapters present a problem-oriented approach to a central theme of medical jurisprudence, medical ethics, forensic pathology or toxicology. A comprehensive review of the national and international literature that is otherwise difficult to assimilate, is given in each chapter. It is hoped that the book fills the vacuum for a forensic book needed by those medical and legal professionals who work alongside or interact with forensic experts.

Gautam Biswas

Acknowledgments

It is with immense gratitude that I acknowledge the support of late Dr (Maj. Gen.) Ajit Singh for his mentoring role in writing this book *Recent Advances in Forensic Medicine and Toxicology (Volume 1)*. In my career, I have been exceptionally blessed by knowing, working with, and learning from many outstanding forensic experts. I wish to acknowledge the influences of Dr SK Verma, Dr NK Aggarwal, Dr KK Banerjee, Dr AK Tyagi and Dr Anil Kohli who taught me to inquire, think and persist; and late Dr BBL Aggarwal whose knowledge and humanity inspires me still.

The book is the result of contribution of many experts from different fields coming together to share their knowledge, and I am indebted to them all. I express my deepest gratitude and thanks to my contributors who are well-recognized national and international researchers and pioneers in their particular scientific fields. In spite of their busy schedule, they have made their practical and scientific knowledge accessible to a broad range of readership.

I deeply appreciate the invaluable suggestions of some of the senior reputed professionals with whom I had lengthy academic communications and exchange of views of the technical aspects of major parts of the book, this includes Dr Anil Kohli, Reader, Department of Forensic Medicine, University College of Medical Sciences (UCMS) and Guru Teg Bahadur (GTB) Hospital and Dr Anil Aggrawal, Director-Professor, Department of Forensic Medicine and Toxicology, Maulana Azad Medical College, New Delhi, whose immeasurable help and wisdom can never be appropriately or adequately acknowledged. My colleague, Dr Virendar Pal Singh, deserves special mention for providing constant and friendly support in this venture.

I also express my thanks to Dr Mushtaq Ahmad, Armed Forces Medical College, Dhaka, Bangladesh; Dr JS Dalal, Christian Medical College, Ludhiana, Punjab; Dr Dasari Harish, Government Medical College and Hospital, Chandigarh; Dr Vijay Pal Khanagwal, Postgraduate Institute of Medical Sciences, Rohtak, Haryana; Dr KK Aggarwal and Dr Akash Deep Aggarwal, Government Medical College, Patiala, Punjab; Dr B Khurana, Shri Guru Ram Das Institute of Medical Sciences and Research, Amritsar, Punjab; Dr Rajiv Joshi, Government Medical College, Faridkot, Punjab; Dr Ashok Chanana, Government Medical College, Amritsar, Punjab; Dr Parmod Goel, Adesh Institute of Medical Sciences, Bhatinda, Punjab; Dr RK Bansal, Shri Guru Ram Rai Institute of Medical and Health Sciences, Dehradun, Uttarakhand; Dr Farida Noor, Government Medical College, Srinagar, Jammu and Kashmir; and Dr Anju Gupta, Punjab Institute of Medical Sciences, Jalandhar, Punjab, India, for their valuable suggestions.

I would also like to thank the following for their contributions: Dr Mukul Awasthi, Department of Forensic Medicine, Christian Medical College, Ludhiana, for assistance in the manuscript preparation; Dr Praveen Sobti, Department of Pediatrics, Christian Medical College, Ludhiana, for her help and encouragement, and Mr Ramesh Kumar, for his secretarial assistance.

I cannot find words to express my gratitude to M/s Jaypee Brothers Medical Publishers (P) Ltd, New Delhi, India for their patience, encouragement and professionalism during the entire process. I am especially grateful to Shri Jitendar P Vij (Group Chairman), Mr Ankit Vij (Group President), Mr Tarun Duneja (Director–Publishing), Mr Sunil Kumar Dogra (Production Executive), Mr Neelambar Pant (Production Coordinator), Mr Manoj Pahuja (Senior Graphic Designer) and Mr Chandra Dutt (Typesetter) for shaping up of the book and making all the changes, without any complaints.

This work would not have been possible without the blessings of my family. I would like to thank my parents Mr Gurupada Biswas and Mrs Rina Biswas, my brother Mr Rajib Biswas and my in-laws Dr Amitav Sinha and Mrs Ratna Sinha for their unconditional love, support and encouragement throughout my life. I would like to express my love and thanks to my son Gaurav. I would like to express my earnest gratitude and love for my wife Anupama, for her constant support and encouragement. Finally, I would like to express my thanks to Almighty for giving me the courage to engage in this mammoth work.

Contents

Section I MEDICAL JURISPRUDENCE

Section II CLINICAL FORENSIC MEDICINE

I

MEDICAL JURISPRUDENCE

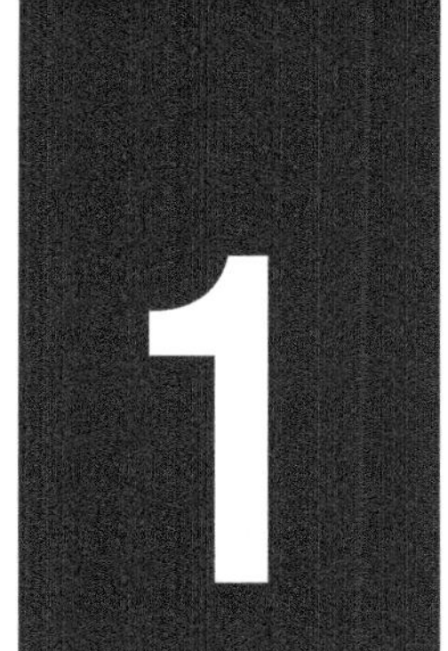

Medicolegal Issues in Consent

Gautam Biswas

'Life is short, art is long; opportunity is fleeting, experiment is dangerous; judgment is difficult. It is not enough for the physician to do what is necessary, the cooperation of the patient and the attendants must be secured, and circumstances must be favorable.'
Hippocrates (Greek physician and father of Western Medicine)

ABSTRACT

According to the standard conception of medical ethics, informed consent is fundamental to ethical practice. It is the mechanism by which patients authorize medical intervention or course of treatment. This also acts a constraint on medical practitioner's power and a curb to their paternalistic impulses. Since the origins of the consent doctrine, physicians have been perturbed by the difficulty of attaining meaningful consents—consents that truly fulfilled the high ideals of the doctrine. The blanket consent taken by most of the hospitals and nursing homes is legally invalid. The consent should be informed one. The basic essentials for valid consent are—voluntary decision, competent patient, sufficient disclosure of the relevant facts, understanding of those facts and then authorization (informed consent) or decline (informed refusal) of the proposed course of treatment are discussed. Exceptions to informed consent, economic or financial consent, rules of consent and consent related to various medicolegal cases have also been discussed.

Keywords: Informed consent, legally valid consent, economic or financial consent, invalid consent, reasons for consent, consent in medicolegal cases.

INTRODUCTION

Medicine nowadays is practiced within an expanding and evolving system of legal rights and obligations, patient protections, health care financing regulation and standards of care. Thus, medical care can involve significant legal issues, including capacity of patients to make health care decisions, confidentiality of medical information and malpractice liability.

The element of consent is perhaps the only principle that runs through all aspects of health care provisions (Box 1.1). It also represents the legal and ethical expression of the basic right to have one's autonomy and self-determination (Article 21 of the Indian Constitution).[1]

In actual practice, this important principle is usually either ignored or only partially accepted, particularly in the Indian context since the scenario is

Box 1.1 Consent in health and practice

- Examination, investigation and treatment
- Examination for medicolegal purposes
- Pathological autopsy
- Organ/tissue retrieval
- Unconscious/unknown patient admitted in hospital

Box 1.2 Reasons for not obtaining consent

- Some doctors feel that informed consent as directly interfering with patient care by wasting their valuable time and sometimes frightening patients into rejecting treatment which may be lifesaving and thus adopt paternalistic attitudes towards the patient.
- Some are of the view that the patients need not be told about their treatment/operation as they are unable to understand the complexities and will forget the salient facts soon.

somewhat different from the West with respect to the doctor-patient relationship. Here, the doctor-patient relationship is governed more by trust wherein doctor is the authoritative figure. Obtaining informed consent is therefore considered to be an unnecessary ritual (Box 1.2).[2] Moreover, it is taught in 2nd Professional MBBS curriculum as a small note during their study in forensic medicine. At that time, the students are not mature enough to understand the intricacies involved in the process of informed consent.

In India, informed consent was practically nonexistent till the Consumer Protection Act was made applicable to the medical profession. Now, both doctors and patients are becoming more aware about this concept, and patients are better informed of their rights.[2,3]

All over India, there are diversities in the way consent are taken and interpreted. The consent practiced in most hospitals in which patients being admitted are asked to sign a form stating that they are willing for any form of treatment, is a *blanket consent* of questionable legal validity. In some cases, patients are presented with complex information that they do not understand, and they duly sign or place their thumb prints on the dotted line.[2,3] At present, legal cases concerning absence of consent are rare. Such cases will increase in the coming years as level of awareness and education of population increases.[4]

The present chapter examines the entire gamut of issues pertaining to consent from the point of view of the legal environment as it exists in India and worldwide as of today.

DEFINITION

Literally, consent [Etymology Latin: *consentire,* to feel with; to agree] means to give assent or permission or compliance.[5,6] 'Consent' as defined under Section 13 of the Indian Contract Act, 1872—'Two or more persons are said to consent when they agree upon the same thing in the same sense'.[6]

Furthermore, there is a stipulation in the contract law stating that consent of any party (in our case it is the patient) that is obtained by coercion, undue influence, mistake, misrepresentation or fraud, will render the agreement invalid.

The relationship between a medical professional and his patient is a contract by parties competent to contract giving rise to contractual obligations. Consent, in the context of medical profession, implies to voluntary permission or authorization by the patient to perform an act on his body, either for diagnosis or therapeutic procedure.[7]

HISTORY

The principle of patient's autonomy is a not a new concept. Documents pertaining to the Egyptian, Greek and Roman civilization show how the medical practitioner's intervention had, in some way, first to be approved by the patient. The procedures and the modes of information which Plato advocated were the principles of the present day informed consent and correlated the practice of information and consensus with the quality and social position of the patient.[8]

The first reported legal case in which surgeons were accused of disuniting a patient's healing fracture without the patient's consent occurred in England during the 18th century (Box 1.3).[9] In another case, the court found that the operation to which the plaintiff did not consent constituted medical battery (Box 1.4). Justice Benjamin Cardozo wrote in the court's opinion:

'*Every human being of adult years and sound mind has a right to determine what shall be done with his own body; and a surgeon who performs an operation without his patient's consent commits an assault for which he is liable in damages.*'[4,7,9-11]

TYPES OF CONSENT

Broadly, consent is of two types: (i) implied or (ii) expressed (Flow chart 1.1).[2,4-6]

I. **Implied consent:** It is the granting of permission for health care without a formal agreement between the patient and the doctor. Usually, the demeanor of the patient implies consent. Consent may be inferred from the general submission by a patient to orders given by a doctor during clinical diagnosis.

   Implied consent is restricted only to history taking, routine examination (inspection, palpation, percussion and auscultation) and prescribing

Box 1.3 Slater vs. Baker and Stapleton, 1767

The physician in this case initially set the patient's femoral fracture in accordance with prevailing practice at that time but, at a follow up visit, rebroke the healing fracture and placed the rebroken bone in a mechanical device with teeth. Physicians called into court to testify reported that physicians usually secured their patients' consent before embarking on a medical intervention. The Judge concluded that obtaining a patient's consent was a custom of physicians, and ruled for the patient that consent should have been obtained.[9,12]

Box 1.4 Schloendorff vs. Society of New York Hospital, 1914

Mary Schloendorff sued New York Hospital alleging that the doctors it employed performed the surgery contrary to her express direction. The plaintiff was admitted to New York Hospital and consented to being examined under ether to determine if a diagnosed fibroid tumor was malignant or not, but withheld consent for removal of the tumor. The physician examined the tumor, found it malignant, then disregarded Schloendorff's wishes and removed the tumor. In the case at hand, the wrong complained of is not merely negligence. It is trespass.[9]

Flow chart 1.1 Types of consent

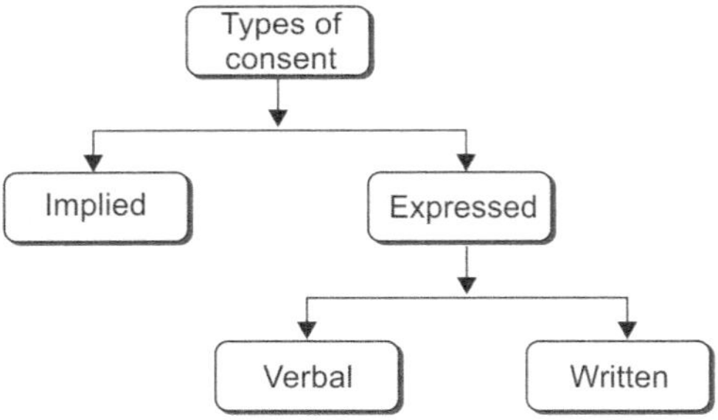

treatment. This does not extend to the performance of intimate examination (such as breast or vaginal examination) or diagnostic procedures.

For interventions considered routine and unlikely to cause harm, implied consent will suffice. For example, patients are presumed to indicate consent to receive certain routine interventions by holding out their arm (routine phlebotomy, placement of an intravenous line), or by opening their mouth for a dental examination. For more invasive or risky interventions, express informed consent is always required.[1,6,7]

II. **Expressed consent:** This may be verbal (oral) or written and should be taken for all procedures beyond routine examination.

a. *Oral:* Oral consents are easily administered, and can aid doctor-patient rapport because of the joint decision making shared by them. Oral consent should be taken in the presence of disinterested third party (for e.g., a near relative of the patient or female police constable) mainly in cases where intimate examination of female is required. Some medical practitioner may take this in presence of a nurse which may not be adequate. She is an employee of the examining physician and not actually an independent party. Tests necessitating removal of body fluids, gynecological examinations, such as, per vaginal examination or radiological examination can be done, after securing oral consent. If, for whatever reason, only oral consent is taken, it is recommended to make an entry in the patient's hospital record. If any action is brought on this count, this entry may afford corroborative evidence to support the defense taken by the medical practitioner concerned. Without such documentation, the burden will be on the doctor to demonstrate legally sufficient reasons for such absence.[5,6,8]

b. *Written:* It is advisable to take written consent in the presence of disinterested third party (this third party is only to attest the signature of the patient). Expressed written consent should be obtained for the following:[5,6]

1. Medicolegal examinations for injury, sexual assault, alcoholism, determining age, potency and virginity.
2. All invasive and major diagnostic procedures like lumbar puncture, ventricular tap, invasive monitoring (for e.g., intracranial pressure), nerve or bone harvesting, putting any foreign body such as implants, coils and devices.
3. Extraction of tooth or restorative procedures by a dentist.
4. General or spinal anesthesia.
5. Surgical operations.

It is to be noted that law demands mere consent and not written consent and does not prescribe such requirement on a mandatory basis. There is no mandate that a doctor should always obtain written consent and failure of which would hold him liable. However, as per the Indian Medical Council (Professional Conduct and Ethics) Regulations 2002, a written consent should be obtained before performing an operation.[5] This would afford documentary evidence that the consent was actually obtained in case of litigation.[1,6]

DOCTRINE OF INFORMED CONSENT

The term 'informed consent' entered American jurisprudence in 1957 and was first used in medical malpractice case by Paul G. Gebhard.[4] The doctrine of informed consent underlines the principle of providing sufficient information to a patient so as to enable him/her make an informed and knowledgeable decision about the course of examination, procedure or treatment. The doctor must ensure that the patient is explained the following as given in Box 1.5.[2,4,6,7,10,13,14]

Informed consent is considered as a process (mutual communication) rather than an event (document signing) (Fig. 1.1). The information provided to patients should be simple, easy to understand and list any possible major complications to enable the patient determine whether to undergo or decline a procedure. The

Box 1.5 Doctrine of informed consent

- Condition of the patient or nature of illness
- Purpose or necessity for further testing
- Natural course of condition and possible complications
- Nature of procedure or treatment proposed
- Risks and benefits of treatment or procedure
- Risks and benefits of alternative treatment or procedure
- Prognosis in the absence of intervention
- Duration and approximate cost of treatment
- Expected outcome and follow-up

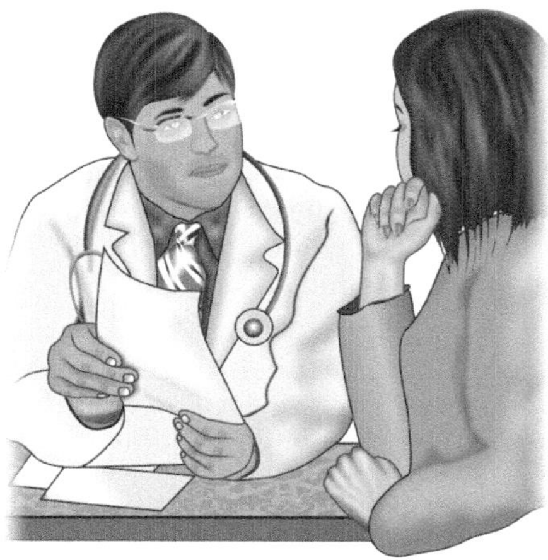

Fig. 1.1 Process of informed consent

knowledge regarding the intervention should be imparted in an understandable language and format so that decision in the form of authorization by patient can be made.[11] The law requires that health care practitioners take reasonable steps to communicate adequately with patients who do not speak English or who have other communication barriers. Patient should be given opportunity to ask questions and clarify all doubts. Video of the procedure, wherever possible and feasible, may be shown to make the patient aware of the details that were discussed earlier.

Impairments to reasoning and judgment which may make it impossible for someone to give informed consent include factors such as basic intellectual or emotional immaturity, high levels of stress such as PTSD, severe mental retardation, senility, severe mental illness, delirious intoxication, severe sleep deprivation, Alzheimer's disease, or being in a coma.[15]

REASONS FOR OBTAINING CONSENT

Legally, consent is obtained for the following reasons:[1,3,6,13,14,16]

i. To examine, treat or operate upon a patient without consent is considered *battery/assault* in law, even if it is beneficial and done in good faith. If a medical practitioner attempts to treat a person without valid consent, then he will be liable under both civil and criminal law. The definition of battery is an act that directly and either intentionally or negligently causes some physical contact with another person without that person's consent. If a person has consented to contact, then there is no battery. The consequences would be payment of compensation (in civil) and imprisonment (in criminal).
ii. If a doctor fails to give the required information to patient before taking consent to a particular procedure/treatment, he may be charged for *negligence* in case of any undesirable side-effects (Box 1.6). The practitioner can cite proof of consent as evidence of disclosure, thereby protecting him from an action based on failure to disclose material facts.
iii. Not taking consent is considered as deficiency in medical services under the Section 2(1) of the Consumer Protection Act.

Legally Valid Consent

The following three separate but correlated elements are the legal requisites to conform to the doctrine of informed consent:[5,7,10,11,13,15,17]

1. Voluntariness—willingness of patient to undergo treatment.
2. Capacity—degree of ability of the patient to understand the nature and consequences of treatment offered. The law presumes that such ability is generally acquired with the attainment of the age of maturity.

Box 1.6 Duty to warn

> In *Salgo vs Stanford University*, the patient's legs were paralyzed following aortography performed to locate an obstruction in his abdominal aorta. Apparently, the treating physician had not warned the patient of the risk inherent with the procedure. In its decision, the court held that 'a physician violates his duty to his patient and subjects himself to liability if he holds any facts which are necessary to form the basis of an intelligent decision by the patient to the proposed treatment.'[4]

3. Knowledge—appropriate and adequate amount of information about the nature and consequence of treatment has been disclosed to patient.

Invalid Consent

Consent is invalid if:[6]

- It is not an informed consent
- Given for committing a crime or an illegal act such as criminal abortion
- Obtained by misrepresentation or fraud
- Given by one who had no legal capacity to give it, for e.g., a minor or an insane person.

Exceptions to Informed Consent

Consent is not required in situations mentioned in Box 1.7.[2,5,6,9,14]

Emergency cases: If a patient is unconscious or in a state of coma and there is an imminent danger to the life of the patient and there is no designated surrogate or the surrogate is unavailable, then the law presumes that consent for treatment has been deemed to be given (implied consent, Sec. 92 IPC). For implied consent to apply, the injured party must require emergency treatment to save life or limb and the treatment rendered must be so limited. Once the emergency treatment is no longer required, the doctrine of implied consent does not govern.[1,5-7,18]

Therapeutic privilege: In case of full disclosure (for e.g., presence of malignancy or unavoidable total results) in patients prone for anxiety or have detrimental effect on the health of the patient, the doctor should use therapeutic privilege in the interest of patient. However, he should disclose full information to the competent relative of the patient.[6]

Therapeutic waiver: A competent person who is aware of being entitled to informed consent may give up his right by waiving it.[6]

Placebo: The doctor may use placebos in certain self-limiting conditions or in patients with high psychological overlay or in those who insist for some particular medication (for e.g., addiction forming drugs). Informed consent may be withheld since there are high chances of benefit to the patient with negligible risk. Revealing the truth to the patient takes away the very purpose of administration of placebo.[14]

Box 1.7 Exceptions to informed consent

- Medical emergencies
- Medical examination requested by a police officer of an arrested accused under Sec. 53 (1) CrPC
- Therapeutic privilege
- Therapeutic waiver
- Medicolegal postmortems (Sec. 174 CrPC)
- Psychiatric examination or treatment by court order
- Use of placebos
- Prisoners (new entrants)
- Person suffering from disease under 'notified' category (to notify the authorities only)
- Treatment of notifiable diseases for greater community interest

Prisoners: Prisoners and persons released on bail can be treated without their consent in the interest of the society. A registered medical practitioner can examine an accused by using reasonable force (force should be applied by police) if the examination is requested by the investigating police officer not below the rank of police subinspector (Sec. 53 CrPC). The obtaining of such evidence is not violative of Article 20(3) of Constitution, which grants protection against self-incrimination, it was held so by High Court of Bombay in Kathi Kalu case.[4]

INFORMED FINANCIAL/ECONOMIC CONSENT

Medical decisions are increasingly shared decisions. In current scenario, where the cost of treatment is exorbitant, the cost of surgical procedure, diagnostic test, biopsy, MRI or any other procedure are not discussed. This may be one of the issues for litigation. The patient may refuse to pay citing no information regarding the cost of the treatment being given during the process of consent. In this regard, the patient should be provided an opportunity for a 'financial or economic informed consent'. Informed consent can only be given by a patient who has had the opportunity to consider a range of reasonable treatment options along with associated fee estimates.

A frank discussion about the treatment costs and charges, and the options available for payment, whether by the patient or insurance company, or shared, should be included in the consent process. Discussion of fees should typically include the cost of the procedure/therapy, any escalation in costs once treatment has started, types of reimbursement accepted (for e.g., cash, checks, credit card payments, direct payment from insurance companies).[19] This information should preferably be provided in writing.

In instances wherein a doctor is unfamiliar with the cost of treatment or the patient's insurance plan, he/she should advise the patient to communicate with the billing section or insurer and discuss coverage and payment options.[19] The patient should enquire whether he/she needs to pay an excess over and above the insurance cover.

Case Report 1

In a case (*Dr. Shailesh Shah vs. Aphraim Jayanand Rathod*), the operation of appendicitis was performed without written consent under the guise of removal of stitches and no explanation was given for the second operation. The National commission found that the doctor was deficient in service and was liable for compensation.[4]

Case Report 2

In another case that came up before Gujarat State Commission where the complainant, a lady, having the son and the daughter, both minors, consulted the doctor while she was carrying 13 weeks pregnancy. She was advised MTP and consent in writing was taken. After the operation, the husband of the complainant was informed that the uterus was removed. The complainant filed a case alleging that no consent for the removal of uterus was obtained either from the patient or from her husband. It was found that an eminent gynecologist had participated in order to save life of the patient and they all were unanimous for removal of the uterus, as there was continuous bleeding and the condition of the patient was deteriorating. Thus, no negligence regarding removal of uterus was found on the part of doctors.[4]

Case Report 3

In *Dr Thomas vs. Smt. Elisa*, the court held that the doctor was guilty of negligence for not operating on a patient with life-threatening peritonitis following a perforated appendix only because the patient was not in a condition to give consent and the relatives were not available. The Judge ruled that "when a medical man advances a plea that the patient did not give his consent for the course of treatment advised by him, the burden is on him to prove that the non-administration of the treatment was on account of the refusal of the patient to give consent thereto. Consent is implicit in the case of a patient who submits to the doctor and the absence of consent must be made out by the patient alleging it".[1,3,4]

Case Report 4

In a recent judgment of Supreme Court (*Samira Kohli vs. Dr Prabha Manchanda, 2008*), it held that no additional procedure can be performed to what had been explained to the patient. The judgment was related to a case where hysterectomy was done as an additional procedure. While the initial consent was obtained for diagnostic laparoscopy, hysterectomy and removal of both ovaries was performed in the same sitting under general anesthesia. The consent for hysterectomy was however obtained from the mother of the patient. The Supreme Court held the doctor liable for malpractice, and opined that additional surgery however beneficial to the patient in saving time, expenses, pain and suffering are no ground for defense. It is contended that it is not only informed consent which is imperative, but the same shall be 'prior informed consent' unless there is imminent threat to the patient's life. In addition, this decision curtails the scope of proxy consent from the person having parental authority or an attendant.[1]

RIGHT TO REFUSE

Although, medical practitioners are ethically bound to provide sufficient information and to encourage decisions judged to be in the patient's best interest, a competent patient still has a right to refuse treatment even if others, including the medical practitioner, believe that the refusal is neither in his/her best interest nor reasonable.

If a patient refuses the treatment/procedure after explanation, his/her understanding should be checked and concerns addressed. If the patient still refuses, the doctor should not proceed further. There should not be a forceful approach, as consent obtained under duress is invalid. The patient's signature should be taken along with witness and document each step of refusal process.[4,12]

There had been instances where the patient has alleged forgery or had claimed signing it under stress or pressure of doctors, without actually understanding the document. It is advisable to have consent from at least two persons—one from the patient and other from spouse, parents or close relatives.[7]

CONSENTING AGE

In India, the age of consent for medical or medicolegal examination is not legally laid down. There are unclear provisions made in Criminal Procedure Code (CrPC), Indian Penal Code (IPC Sec 87 to 90) and Indian Contract Act which refers to the validity of consent, which may occur from any act done in good faith and for individual benefit. These provisions are not specifically directed at medical examination or treatment. When combined, one can conclude that:[1,4-6,13,20,21]

- Majority is achieved at the age of 18 years but a person above the age of 12 years can give valid consent for medical examination (simple physical examination).

- For a person under 12 years of age or of unsound mind, his/her guardian or person in whose lawful custody he/she is, can give consent.
- For any invasive and diagnostic procedures, general anesthesia and surgical operations, age of consent is 18 years and above.

For medicolegal examination, the consent should be signed by the person if he/she is above 12 years of age. Consent must be taken from the guardian/parent if the individual is under the age of 12 years (Department of Health Research guidelines for 'Forensic medical care for Victims of Sexual Assault' and Ministry of Health and Family Welfare 'Guidelines on Sexual Assault Survivors'). However, the author is of the view that a person between 12 and 18 years of age may not be able to understand the intricacies associated with such an examination, and nature and consequences for which he/she is giving consent (invasive examination, appearing in the court, cross-examination, etc). Written consent can also be considered as a contract between the doctor and the patient which has got legal consequences. Hence, the age of consent for such examination should be 18 years.

It is emphasized that persons with mental illness and intellectual disabilities should also be informed of the examination procedure or treatment. Some specific steps may be required while taking consent from such persons. If necessary, they should be:

- Provided the necessary information in a simple language and in a form that makes it easy for them to understand the information.
- Given adequate time to arrive at a decision.
- Provided the assistance of a friend/colleague/caregiver in making the informed consent decision and in conveying their decision to medical personnel.

The decision of the person to either give or refuse consent with the above supports, to the medical examination, should be respected (MOHFW, Guidelines on Sexual Assault Survivors).

In accordance with the Indian Contract Act, a person is generally competent to contract (i) if he has attained the age majority (18 years in India), (ii) is of sound mind, and (iii) is not disqualified by any law to which he is subject to.[4,20]

Global Scenario

In England, Wales and Northern Ireland, the General Medical Council guidelines state that the consenting age is 16 years old. In many respects, they are treated as adults and can give consent for their own surgical and medical treatment. The Department of Health recommends that it is nevertheless good practice to encourage children of this age to involve their families in decisions about their care, unless it would not be in their interests to do so. If a competent child requests that confidentiality be maintained, it is respected, unless the doctor considers that failing to disclose information would result in significant harm to the child. However, a child aged 16–18 years cannot refuse treatment, if it has been agreed by a person with parental responsibility or the court, and it is in their best interests. Therefore, they do not have the same status as adults. If the child is under the age of 16, he/she may have the capacity to decide, depending on his/her ability to understand what is involved.[1,4,5,22]

Most states in the United States allow minors aged 13 through 18 to provide consent for some medical care, including contraception, sexually transmitted diseases, pregnancy, alcohol and drug abuse and psychiatric problems, varying by state.[22] No state explicitly requires parental consent or notification for any of these services. In Alabama, for e.g., minors aged 14 years and older may consent to general medical care; in South Carolina, they may do so at 16 years. However, some states prohibit the use of state funds to provide contraceptive services to minors without parental consent. The one notable exception to the expansion of minors' decision-making authority on health care matters is abortion. Only three states have laws that affirm a minor's ability to obtain an abortion on her own. In contrast, rest of the states requires the involvement of at least one parent in their daughter's abortion decision.

In Australia, according to the Minors (Property and Contracts) Act 1970, a child aged 14 years or over may consent to his/her medical or dental treatment. The Consent to Medical Treatment and Palliative Care Act, 1995 prescribes that an individual of 16 years of age or over can consent to medical and dental treatment 'as validly and effectively as an adult'.[22]

HOW MUCH INFORMATION IS ADEQUATE?

The amount of information that a patient must be given in order to give informed consent is a debatable question. There are three concepts:

a. Reasonable physician standard (*prudent doctor test*): It asserts that a physician has a duty to disclose information (including risks) that any reasonable physician would disclose under similar circumstances.[10]
b. Reasonable patient standard (*prudent patient test*): It asserts that a physician has a duty to disclose information that is material in determining what the reasonable patient would want to know to consent to the proposed treatment.[8,10,14]
c. Subject specific standard: It asserts that the nature of disclosure shall depend upon physical (state of illness) and mental condition (psychological status) and cultural background of the patient.

In the United States, Australia and Canada, a more patient-centered approach is taken which provides the highest respect for the patient's right of self-determination about a particular therapy. Informed consent in these jurisdictions requires that significant risks be disclosed, as well as risks which would be of particular importance to that patient. This approach combines an objective (the reasonable patient) and subjective (this particular patient) approach.[1,3,13,23]

In the United Kingdom, Malaysia and Singapore, informed consent requires proof as to the standard of care to be expected as a recognized standard of acceptable professional practice, that is, what risks would a medical professional usually disclose in the circumstances.[1,13]

There are no clear parameters laid down by the courts about the Indian position regarding the quantum of information. Therefore, it is reasonable information which a doctor deems fit considering best practices. The standard to which physicians are held in negligence suits is that of a 'reasonable physician' dealing with a 'reasonable patient.' The nature and extent of information imparted to a patient is a question of professional judgment and is subject to proof by the testimony of expert witnesses.[1,7,12]

Whatever might be the difference of approach, there is a need to provide adequate information so as to enable the patient make a balanced judgment as to whether he/she should submit himself/herself to a particular procedure or not. But, there is no need to explain the remote or theoretical risks which may frighten the patient resulting in refusal of treatment or opting for fanciful or unnecessary options or resulting in psychological stress of the patient.[14]

Case Report 5

In *Blythe vs. Bloomsbury Health Authority* (1993), the plaintiff complained that the doctor had not disclosed all the risks of Depo Provera. The court held that the doctor is not obliged to explain all possible risks of a treatment in responding to a general inquiry from the patient.[3]

An important issue in informed consent cases deals with whether the complication or side effect suffered by the patient was actually discussed. Most often, a disagreement exists between the doctor, who claims that he/she did advise the patient of the risk, and the patient, who claims that the occurring risk was never mentioned. A significant study, assessing the degree to which patients actually recall the information imparted during the informed consent discussion, found that patients had primary recollection of only about 20% of the information provided. Significantly, the discussion least remembered by patients was the one regarding complications, where only 10% of the patients indicated that the possible complications associated with the operation had been discussed.[24]

GUIDELINES FOR CONSENT

Following are the general and some specific guidelines for consent:[4-6,14,25]

i. Consent should be free, voluntary, clear, intelligent, direct and personal, and only for legal acts. There should be no undue influence, fraud, compulsion, misrepresentation of facts, coercion or other consequences.
ii. During the consent process, the doctor should remain emotionally detached/impartial so as to allow the patient's decision/choice to be made voluntarily. The medical practitioner should politely refuse anyone, even another qualified doctor, from interfering in the consent process.
iii. Mental capacity, physical condition as well as age of the patient should be considered while delivering the information, or else the same information can be passed on to any other authorized person.
iv. Consent should be obtained in the presence of a witness and the same documented in writing to prevent any allegation that the consent was forged or obtained under pressure. Assisting nurse preferably should not be a witness.
v. Written consent should refer to one specific procedure and not blanket permission on admission to hospital. In case alternative procedures have already been contemplated, it is advisable to clearly specify each of these procedures in the consent form. Specific consent for each and every type of anesthesia that is anticipated should be taken.
vi. The consent form should be filled by the concerned doctor, in one sitting, if possible without changing the pen, though counseling the patient may take more than one sitting. It should be prepared in duplicate and a copy handed

over to the patient. In the consent form, the entries should be made at the appropriate spaces. Entries made at the wrong place may raise suspicion.

vii. If the patient withdraws consent during the procedure, it should be stopped and concerns addressed. If the patient does not consent again, the procedure should be discontinued.
viii. Unconscious/unknown patient when admitted in hospital, the medical superintendent/in-charge of hospital can give consent for treatment.
ix. Consent of one's spouse is not necessary for the treatment of other.
x. Husband or wife has no right to refuse consent to any operation, which is required to safeguard the health of the partner.
xi. In prenatal diagnostic procedures, informed written consent of pregnant woman is obtained and a copy of the consent obtained above is given to the woman (as per PCPNDT Act, 1988).
xii. If found under the influence of alcohol, then consent of such person will not be valid, so it is always better to obtain consent from guardian/parents.
xiii. In civil cases, examination should not be done without the consent of the person to be medically examined.
xiv. Informed consent is necessary for photographing a patient for scientific/educational/research purpose. Although efforts should be made not to reveal the identity of the patient in publication, specific consent must be taken in case of the unlikely event where the identity is likely to be revealed.
xv. Informed consent is a must for participation in clinical trials and research projects.
xvi. In case of consent for donation of organ after death, the will of the deceased is enough.
xvii. Pathological autopsy should not be carried out, without the consent of next of kin of the deceased.

INFORMED CONSENT RELATED TO MEDICOLEGAL CASES

In medicolegal cases, following protocol is suggested:

1. In case of conscious patient, he/she should be asked whether he/she wants any medicolegal report (MLR) or not.
2. In case of unconscious/serious patients, accompanying relatives should be asked, whether they want any MLR or not.
3. If there is consent for MLR, a call should be sent in writing/telephone to the concerned doctor on the duty roster.
4. The concerned doctor should come immediately and do the medicolegal examination.
    - The doctor should explain the object of examination to the patient—that the examination conducted will be medicolegal and would culminate in the preparation of a medicolegal injury report.
    - All relevant investigations needed for the said purpose would be done (X-ray, CT, MRI, etc).
    - Patient should be informed that he/she has right to refuse to submit to examination and the result may even go against him/her, if they do not corroborate with the history given. If the patient refuses, he/she cannot be examined.

- The patient must have a clear understanding of the implications of the release of the medical records, laboratory investigations, photographs and related information. The normal expectation of confidentiality between doctor and patient does not exist, or is limited, and the report may be seen by others including the opposite party, lawyer, counsel, Judge, or others. Further, the patient needs to be explained that the doctor/hospital authorities would not be held liable for any claims of injury which may in any manner result from the release of such information.

In case, patient does not want any medicolegal action against the alleged perpetrator(s), the same should be documented in writing in the hospital register/file and signature should be taken from the concerned person(s).

At any given time, the patient may withdraw the consent already given or may even leave the hospital. The doctor has no right to force anything on the patient, even though its a medicolegal case. In all such situations, the doctor should carefully document all the findings in the case file, note the exact moment at which the consent was withdrawn and inform the nearest police station regarding the same, giving reasons for his actions. Hospital file should be stamped on the title page about the status of the case by the emergency medical officer. The following should be documented:

- Police informed
- Medicolegal examination done/refused/deferred.

CONSENT FORM

Consent forms should be clearly worded, comprehensive, and provide doctors with the necessary authority to carry forward the specified examination/ procedure/treatment. The ideal consent form will therefore depend upon the individual case and circumstances (Box 1.8).[2] Nonetheless certain essential ingredients of an ideal consent form shall provide all possible and likely happenings in most of the cases.

Who should obtain consent?

A house surgeon, interns or even a postgraduate (resident) are the ones who obtain the consent. Ideally, the attending doctor who will be actually examining/ treating the patient should obtain the informed consent.[7]

Who should sign the consent form?

Consent has to be signed by the patient, unless minor, unconscious or insane wherein a legal guardian should sign. The form should also be signed by the doctor and an independent witness. Even in emergency, unless patient is unconscious, the consent offered by the parents of major is void and amount to negligence, if the procedure/treatment is not an emergency.[7]

When patients lose their ability to make treatment decisions (*incompetent patient*), some other reasonable person has to take decisions on behalf of the patient. Usually 'next of kin' (legal heir) would be the surrogate decision maker. In India, the typical hierarchy sequence is spouse, eldest child, next child, parent, sibling and lawful guradian.[5,18]

Box 1.8 Model of expressed consent for medicolegal examination (victim of sexual assault)

I hereby agree for a complete physical examination (including examination of genital organs) and the recording of findings, collection of medical and medicolegal specimens as necessary for laboratory analysis, photographic documentation and any other investigations as recommended by the treating doctor, release of a report to the police officials/court of law concerned, and to treatment. This procedure has been fully explained to me.

(Strikeout whichever is not given permission)

- I have not been medicolegally examined earlier for these injuries.
- This information may be used for teaching and research purposes provided no identifying data is released.
- I have been explained that the result may go against me.
- The above has been explained to me in my own language and I have fully understood the same and I am signing this consent by my own free will.

....	....	....
Signature and name of witness Address.................	Signature/thumb impression of patient/parent/guardian Name..................	Signature of Doctor Name and Registration Number...........

Date.....................

Is a signed consent form adequate defense?

A signed consent form of any nature neither guarantees a doctor protection against legal action nor ensures patient satisfaction. It merely demonstrates that some process to exchange information was followed.[3]

Just providing information is not sufficient—a patient needs to have an understanding of the information in order to make an informed decision. Validity depends on whether the patient understood what was on the consent form and had the opportunity to ask questions. If the patient didn't understand it, it is invalid.[12]

Despite the potential shortcomings, written consent forms may nevertheless serve as deterrents to negligence suits alleging failure to obtain informed consent because of the existence of written evidence to disprove this claim. In addition, patients are usually presumed to have read the consent forms they sign, thereby requiring the plaintiff to disprove this presumption.

At some places, the literate patient is asked to write down the salient features of consent in his/her own dialect and handwriting or video recording of the process is done. In this way, chances of subsequent denial of informed consent become negligible.

In spite of taking all necessary precautions, a doctor cannot sit contentedly with the belief that the signed 'informed consent' can certainly avoid legal liability. This is highlighted by one of the observation by the California Supreme Court 'one cannot know with certainty whether a consent is valid until a lawsuit has been filed and resolved'.[14]

COMMON MEDICOLEGAL SITUATIONS

Abortion

Consent of the female is mandatory except when she is minor or mentally ill, where consent of guardian is obtained. Consent of husband is not necessary.

In some states of the United States, informed consent laws require that a woman seeking an elective abortion be given factual information by the doctor about her legal rights, alternatives to abortion (such as adoption), available public and private assistance and medical facts (some of which are disputed—fetal pain), before the abortion is performed (usually 24 hours in advance of the abortion).[15]

Contraception, Pregnancy and Delivery

Written informed consent needs to be taken after explaining reasons and possible consequences. For contraceptive sterilization, consent of both husband and wife should be obtained. It is on the safer side to take the consent of spouse, if the operation destroys or limits sexual functions.

Consent to obstetric procedure should be discussed during the antenatal period. If the medical practitioner finds that the wishes of the pregnant woman are unusual, these should be noted carefully in the antenatal record. It is necessary because the doctor who discussed the matter with the patient may not be on duty when she is admitted in labor.

Case Report 6

In *Devi vs. West Midland Area Health Authority*, the patient was admitted to the hospital for a minor operation on her womb. Without her consent and knowledge the surgeons decided to sterilize her because they feared that if she becomes pregnant again her womb would rupture. She already had four children but her religious belief prohibited sterilization and contraception. Although acting in the patient's interest, there was no immediate urgency to perform the operation without permission. The defendants admitted the liability and damages were awarded.[4]

Case Report 7

In another case, in Canada, the doctor tied the patient's fallopian tubes during a cesarean operation, as he was concerned about the consequences of a second pregnancy. No consent for it had been obtained. It was held that there was no immediate danger and therefore, the liability existed.[4]

Impotence and Sterility

In cases of impotence and sterility, the person is examined only when asked by court or by the police. Informed consent of the person should be taken.

In artificial insemination homologous (AIH), consent is needed from both husband and wife. In artificial insemination donor (AID), consent is needed from husband, wife, donor and donor's wife.[6]

Rape

In alleged rape cases, the written consent of the victim is mandatory and should be obtained in the presence of a witness.[6] It must be 'informed consent', as she must be told that any evidence obtained may be used in court and she will then be exposed to publicity and cross-examination (Box 1.9).

The victim or guardian may refuse to give consent for any part of examination. In this case the doctor should explain the importance of examination and evidence collection; however the refusal should be respected. Such informed refusal for examination and evidence collection must be documented. In case there is informed refusal for police intimation, then that should be documented. At the time of intimation being sent to the police, a clear note stating 'informed refusal for police intimation' should be made (MOHFW, Guidelines on Sexual Assault Survivors).

Sec. 164A (7) CrPC explicitly states the court or the police have no power to compel the victim of sexual assault for medicolegal examination against her consent. It also recognizes her right to consent for partial examination—she may also decide on whether she wants to undergo a physical examination and/or genital examination and allow the collection of bodily evidence.[21]

Consent should be obtained from parents/guardian when examining a child. If a child's legal guardian is not available, the superintendent/in-charge of the hospital can give the necessary permission. In such situations, a female person appointed by the head of the hospital/institution may be called in to be present during the examination. Otherwise, a police officer can apply for legal consent from a Magistrate or the police official in charge of the police station for the child to be examined. These procedures can be followed in cases where the parent or legal guardian is unable to give consent, such as in the following circumstances:

- Cannot be traced or grant consent within a reasonable time
- Is a suspect in the possible rape/sexual abuse case
- Unreasonably refuses to consent to the examination
- Is incompetent due to mental disorder to consent to the examination
- Is deceased.

Box 1.9 Information given to the victim/parents (MOHFW, Guidelines on Sexual Assault Survivors)

- The medicolegal examination is to assist the investigation, arrest and prosecution of those who committed the sexual offence. This may involve an examination of the mouth, breasts, vagina, anus and rectum, as necessary depending on the particular circumstances.
- To assist investigation, forensic evidence may be collected. This may include removing and isolating clothing, scalp hair, foreign substances from the body, saliva, pubic hair, samples taken from the vagina, anus, rectum, mouth and collecting a blood sample.
- The victim/parent/guardian has the right to refuse either a medicolegal examination or collection of evidence or both, but that refusal will not be used to deny treatment.
- The hospital/examining doctor is required/duty bound to inform the police about the incidence. However, if she does not wish to participate in the police investigation, it should not result in denial of treatment.

Rape Accused

In case of accused, consent should be asked for. But if refused, he can be examined and necessary evidence, for e.g., blood and swabs can be collected with application of reasonable degree of force by the accompanying police personnel [Sec. 53 (1) CrPC].[6]

Sodomy

Written informed consent should be obtained in case of nonconsenting victim of sodomy. Consent in case of accused and consensual partner is guided by Sec. 53 (1) CrPC.

Drunkenness

Detained intoxicated person should not be examined and blood, urine or breath should not be collected without his written consent.[6] If unconscious or incapable of giving consent, examination and treatment can be carried out, but the doctor should not disclose any information and wait for his consent till he regains consciousness. At places where Bombay Prohibition Act, 1949 (Mumbai/ Gujarat) is in vogue, the person can be examined and samples can be taken even without consent as per the said act.

Examination of an accused (for e.g., a driver involved in road traffic accident) can be carried out at the request of the police even without his consent and by use of force, if necessary. Such examination may include taking of body fluids [Sec. 53 (1) CrPC].

To examine a person under *Sec. 53 CrPC,* certain criteria need to be fulfilled:

a. The person should have been arrested on charge of committing an offence punishable under law.
b. There are reasonable grounds for believing that an examination of his person will afford evidence as to the commission of the offence.
c. The requisition for medicolegal examination is from an officer of the rank of a sub-inspector of police or above.

Examination under this section may include the examination of blood, blood stains, semen, swabs in case of sexual assault, sputum and sweat, hair samples and fingernail clippings by use of modern techniques including DNA profiling and any other test the medical practitioner thinks necessary in that particular case.[21,26,27]

CONCLUSION

The doctor-patient relationship is a fiduciary one. Respect for patients is a foundational principle for informed consent and renders it a deontological obligation. However, surrogate consents seem more problematic than might be expected. Doctors are willing to override patient wishes at the request of surrogates.

It is also important not to overemphasize the gap between the legal and ethical senses of informed consent. Both seek to establish and protect patients' rights to be informed about the consequences of medical choices and to select the choice that is most consistent with their values and goals.

REFERENCES

1. Nandimath OV. Consent and medical treatment: The legal paradigm in India. *Indian J Urol* 2009; 25: 343-47.
2. Bansal YS, Singh D. Medicolegal aspects of informed consent. *Ind J For Med Toxicol* 2007; 1: 19-23. Available from: http://www.indmedica.com/journals.php?journalid=11...98.
3. Bal A. Informed consent—legal and ethical aspects. A review of the case law. *Ind J Med Ethics* 1999; 7: 56-57. Available from: http://www.issuesinmedicalethics.org/072mi056.html.
4. Murkey PN, Khandekar IL, Tirpude BH, Ninave SV. Consent—Medicolegal aspects. *Medicolegal Update* 2006; 6(4). Available from: http://www.indmedica.com/journals.php? journalid=9...86.
5. Kohli A. Medical consent in India—Ethical and legal issues. Anil Aggrawal's Internet Journal of Forensic Medicine and Toxicology [Internet]. 2007; 8(2). Available from: http://www.anilaggrawal.com/ij/vol_008_no_002/papers/paper004.html.
6. Biswas G. Medical jurisprudence and ethics. Review of forensic medicine and toxicology. 2nd edn, New Delhi: Jaypee brothers; 2012. p. 3-24.
7. Singh D. Informed vs. valid consent: Legislation and responsibilities. *Indian J Neurotrauma* 2008; 5: 105-08.
8. Mallardi V. The origin of informed consent. *Acta Otorhinolaryngol Ital* 2005; 25: 312-27.
9. Brazell NE. The significance and application of informed consent. *AORN Journal* 1997 [Internet]. Available from: http://findarticles.com/p/articles/mi_m0FSL/is_n2_v65/ai_19163364/.
10. Makdessian AS. Informed consent in facial plastic surgery. *Arch Facial Plast Surg* 2004; 6: 26-30.
11. Joffe S, Truog RD. Consent to medical care: the importance of fiduciary context. In: Miller FG, Wertheimer A (eds). The ethics of consent-theory and practice. New York: Oxford university press; 2010. p. 347-74.
12. Saunders N. It's a matter of consent. 2007. Synergy [Internet]. Available from: http://findarticles.com/p/articles/mi_hb5752/is_200707/ai_n32234936/.
13. Sabatino C. Legal and ethical issues. Merck manual online medical dictionary. Available from: http://www.merckmanuals.com/home/sec01/ch009/ch009c.html.
14. Rao KHS. Informed consent: An ethical obligation or legal compulsion? *J Cutan Aesthet Surg* 2008; 1: 33-35.
15. Informed consent. Available from: http://www.en.wikipedia.org/wiki/Informed_consent.
16. Lupton M. Informed consent: can a patient ever be fully informed? *Curr Opin Obstet Gynecol* 2005; 17: 601-04.
17. Chaturvedi A. Consent—its medicolegal aspects. In: Singal RK (ed). Medicine Update. The Association of Physicians of India. 2007. p. 883-87. Available from: http://www.apiindia.org/medicine_update_2007/153.pdf
18. Sundaram ALM. Medicolegal aspects of critical care medicine. *Ind J Anaesth* 2007; 51: 344. Available from: http://www.ijaweb.org/text.asp?2007/51/ 4/344/61163.
19. Lundberg G. Why we need an economic informed consent? Available from: http://www.kevinmd.com/blog/2012/04/economic-informed-consent.html.
20. Indian Contract Act 1872 (act number 9 of 1872).

21. Criminal Procedure Code 1973 (act number 2 of 1974) Govt. of India, New Delhi.
22. Sobti PC, Biswas G. Adolescent health care: Informed consent and confidentiality. In: Gupte S (ed). Recent advances in pediatrics. New Delhi: Jaypee brothers; 2005. p. 375-99.
23. Hassan M. Informed consent and the law—an English legal perspective. *Dig Dis* 2008; 26: 23-7.
24. Trosty RS. Key issues in the litigation of informed consent claims. American Physicians Assurance Corporation.
25. Consent in radiology practice. *Indian J Radiol Imaging* 2009; 19: 21-22. Available from: http://www.ijri.org/text.asp?2009/19/1/21/ 45339.
26. Harish D, Chavali KH. The medicolegal case— should we be afraid of it? Anil Aggrawal's Internet Journal of Forensic Medicine and Toxicology [Internet]. 2007; 8(1). Available from: http://www.anilaggrawal.com/ij/vol_008_ no_001/others/pg/pg001.html.
27. The Criminal Law (Amendment) Act, 2013. Available from: http://indiacode.nic.in/acts-in-pdf/132013.pdf.

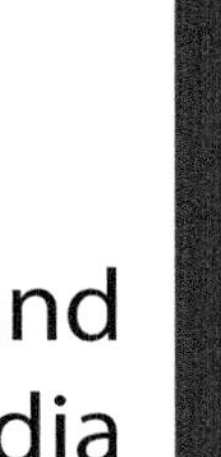

Medical Ethics and Negligence Cases in India

Mukesh Yadav

'Ethics is knowing the difference between what you have a right to do and what is right to do.'
Potter Stewart (Associate Justice, United States Supreme Court)

ABSTRACT

With the awareness in the society and the people in general gathering conscious about their rights, actions for damages in tort are on the rise. Not only civil suits are filed, but with the availability of a forum for grievance redressal under the Consumer Protection Act, 1986 having jurisdiction to hear complaints against medical professionals for 'deficiency in service', which expression is very widely defined in the Act, has given rise to a large number of complaints against professionals, particularly against doctors, being filed by the persons feeling aggrieved.

Criminal complaints are being filed against doctors alleging commission of offences punishable under Sec. 304 A or Secs. 336/337/338 of the IPC alleging rashness or negligence on the part of the doctors resulting in loss of life or injury (of varying degree) to the patient.

This chapter deals with critical review of few recent judgments of the Supreme Court of India and the National Consumer Disputes Redressal Commission (NCDRC) on the issue of medical negligence against medical professionals and administrators of healthcare institution. The aim is to attract attention of all the stakeholders on the relevant issues leading to medical negligence and recommendations to prevent this rising trend in future, in the larger public interest in general and medical practitioner in particular.

Keywords: Res ipsa loquitur, civil negligence, criminal negligence, consent, informed consent, expert opinion, unethical practice, dichotomy, false reporting.

INTRODUCTION

India is recording a whopping 5.2 million injuries each year due to medical errors and adverse events. Of these, biggest sources are mishaps from medications, hospital-acquired infections and blood clots that develops in legs from being immobilized in the hospital. A landmark report by an Indian doctor from Harvard School of Public Health has concluded that more than 43 million people are injured worldwide each year due to unsafe medical care. Approximately 3 million years of healthy life are lost in India each year due to these injuries.[1]

The health ministry was set to launch a national patient safety policy and a national infection control policy to provide patients with a safer healthcare environment. In this regard some initiative was taken at AIIMS, New Delhi, but has not taken shape till date.[2]

This chapter tries to critically review some recent judgments of the Supreme Court of India, the National Consumer Disputes Redressal Commission (NCDRC) and the State Consumer Disputes Redressal Commission (SCDRC) on issues of medical negligence and unethical practices. This is highlighted through three case reports wherein issues like dichotomy, false reporting and non-disclosure of facts were leveled against medical professionals and administrators of healthcare institution. The aim is to attract attention of all the stakeholders on these issues leading to allegation of negligence and unethical practice and recommendations to prevent this rising trend for the larger public interest in general and medical practitioner in particular.

MAGNITUDE OF PROBLEM

About two-thirds of medical injuries occur in low and middle income countries like India.

Fatal Errors[1,2]

- Health care errors is the 8th leading cause of death in the world.
- Globally, 234 million surgeries take place every year, one in every 25 people undergo a surgery at any given time.
- Over 7 million people across the globe suffer from preventable surgical injuries every year.
- Mortality from general anesthesia affected one in 150 patients while infections were reported in 3% of surgeries with the mortality rate being 0.5%.
- Nearly 50% of the adverse effects of surgery were preventable.
- In developing countries, the death rate was nearly 10% for a major surgery.

Death due to Medical Negligence[1]

- *United States:* 98000 deaths every year
- *Canada:* 24000 deaths every year
- *Australia:* 18000 deaths every year

No empirical data are available from India regarding incidence of medical negligence cases at national level or state level.

NEGLIGENCE AS A TORT

The jurisprudential concept of negligence defies any precise definition. Eminent jurists and leading judgments have assigned various meanings to negligence. The concept that has been acceptable to Indian jurisprudential thought is well-stated in the Law of Torts, Ratanlal and Dhirajlal.[3] It is stated as:

'Negligence is the breach of a duty caused by the omission to do something which a reasonable man, guided by those considerations which ordinarily regulate the conduct of human affairs would do, or doing something which a prudent and reasonable man would not do. Actionable negligence consists in the neglect of the use of ordinary care or skill towards a person to whom the defendant owes the duty of observing ordinary care and skill by which neglect, the plaintiff has suffered injury to his person or property. The definition involves three constituents of negligence:

i. A legal duty to exercise due care on the part of the party complained of towards the party complaining, the former's conduct within the scope of the duty.
ii. Breach of the said duty.
iii. Consequential damage.

Cause of action for negligence arises only when damage occurs; for damage is a necessary ingredient of this tort'.

According to Charlesworth and Percy, negligence has three meanings.[4] They are:

i. A state of mind, in which it is opposed to intention.
ii. Careless conduct.
iii. The breach of duty to take care that is imposed by either common or statute law.

All three meanings are applicable in different circumstances, but any one of them does not necessarily exclude the other meanings.[4]

Essential Components of Medical Negligence

The essential components of negligence, as recognized, are three: 'duty', 'breach' and 'resulting damage', that is to say:

i. The existence of a duty to take care, which is owed by the defendant to the complainant.
ii. The failure to attain that standard of care, prescribed by the law, thereby committing a breach of such duty.
iii. Damage, which is both causally connected with such breach and recognized by the law, has been suffered by the complainant.

If the claimant satisfies the court on the evidence that these three ingredients are made out, the defendant should be held liable in negligence.[4]

Negligence as Tort and as Crime

The term 'negligence' is used for the purpose of fastening the defendant with liability under the civil law and, at times, under the criminal law. It is contended on behalf of the respondents that in both the jurisdictions, negligence is negligence, and jurisprudentially no distinction can be drawn between negligence under civil law and negligence under criminal law. The submission so made cannot be countenanced in as much as it is based upon a total departure from the established terrain of thought running ever since the beginning of the emergence of the concept of negligence up to the modern times. Generally speaking, it is the amount of damages incurred which is determinative of the extent of liability in tort; but in criminal law, it is not the amount of damages but the amount and degree of negligence that is determinative of liability. To fasten liability in criminal law, the degree of negligence has to be higher than that of negligence enough to fasten liability for damages in civil law.[5]

MEDICAL LAW AND ETHICS

It is pertinent to mention words of Supreme Court of India in a case of alleged medical negligence: 'Medical negligence plays its game in strange ways. Sometimes it plays with life; sometimes it gifts an 'unwanted child' as in the instant case where the respondent, a poor laborer woman, who already had many children and had opted for sterilization, got pregnant and ultimately gave birth to a female child in spite of sterilization operation which, obviously, had failed' —*Justice S Saghir Ahmad, 2000.*[6]

Cases of medical negligence involve either utter disregard for medical ethics and violation of regulations framed in this regard by the Medical Council of India in 2002[7] or case of criminal negligence involving various sections of Indian Penal Code.

In a recent case from state of Tamil Nadu of alleged death due to negligence of the doctor due to delay in the delivery of a pregnant woman, NCDRC observed that 'it is a fact that in present days the Hippocratic Oath is at stake; and medical ethics being violated by some medical professionals have led to demoralized health services to the poor who lost their precious life..!! In this case, deficiency in service resulted in loss of complainant's wife as well as the newborn baby was deprived of her mother's love and feed from birth'.[7]

The NCDRC mentioned provisions in this regard which was included in the Indian Medical Council (Professional conduct, Etiquette and Ethics) Regulations, 2002, that reads as: *Engagement for an obstetric case*: When a physician who has been engaged to attend an obstetric case is absent and another is sent and delivery accomplished, the acting physician is entitled to his professional fees, but should secure the patient's consent to resign on the arrival of the physician engaged.[7,8]

Issue of Difference of Opinion and Medical Negligence

The issue of medical negligence is now well established by number of judgments of NCDRC and Hon'ble Supreme Court.[9]

The Hon'ble Apex Court observed that 'simply because a patient has not favorably responded to a treatment given by a doctor or a surgery has failed, the doctor cannot be held straightway liable for medical negligence by applying the *doctrine of res ipsa loquitur*. No sensible professional would intentionally commit an act or omission which would result in harm or injury to the patient since the reputation of the professional would be at stake. A single failure may cost him dear in his lapse'.[10]

It also observed that 'medical opinion may differ with regard to course of action to be taken by a doctor treating a patient, but as long as a doctor acts in manner which is acceptable to medical profession and court finds that he has attended on a patient with due care, skill and diligence and if the patient still does not survive or suffer a permanent ailment, it would be difficult to hold doctor to be guilty of negligence'.[11]

In another case it was observed that 'the doctors have acted in accordance with the practice accepted as proper by the authors of medical books cannot be held guilty of negligence'.[12]

CASE REPORT I[13]

Specialty: Orthopedics.

Issues: Denial of treatment, unethical practices, dichotomy practices, record (cash memo of medicines and diagnostic labs), no X-ray was available.

Brief facts of the case: On 5/12/05, Ms Priya Dubey (PD, complainant) attended the OPD of Dr SK Bijpuriya (SKB), a Government medical officer of Sadar Hospital, Deoghar, Jharkhand for acute pain in her left wrist. He examined her and prescribed certain medicines and X-ray without taking any fees, but insisted PD to purchase medicines from Satyanaryana Medical Hall and get the X-ray done from Central X-ray, both private establishments. Further, she was diagnosed with fracture of lower end of radius and advised POP, but the pain did not subside.

On 27/1/06, she consulted another orthopedic surgeon Dr Ajay Kumar (AK), and her pain and swelling was relieved by his treatment. SKB denied of any treatment given to PD and no negligence on his part.

Observations of the District Forum: The district forum dismissed the complaint observing no negligence or deficiency in service by SKB.

Observations of the SCDRC: Aggrieved by the decision of district forum, PD appealed before the State Commission. After considering the prescription slips and evidence on record, SCDRC held SKB to have put POP and prescribed medicines to PD, as alleged. The reports as well as prescription on different dates contradicted him and his counsel failed to explain this. The denial itself is deficiency in service for which the State Commission imposed a fine of ₹ 5000 on SKB.

Observations of the NCDRC: Revision petition was filed by SKB at NCDRC. On perusal of OPD slip and prescriptions, they observed that PD attended the OPD of SKB who advised X-ray and POP from outside. The assertion of SKB that he did not treat or put the POP was not sustained. Moreover, it was also evident that SKB advised POP and asked for required material to be purchased from Satyanarayana Medical Hall vide receipt No. 1331 dated 5/12/05 which clearly mentioned the name of prescribing doctor. Hence, it was impossible for any other than SKB himself to have put POP and prescribed medicines to PD. They held SKB had plastered the left wrist of PD on 5/12/05 and treated her again on 10/1/06, 27/1/06. The POP was removed on 10/1/06 but pain persisted. Thereafter, PD consulted AK for same complaints of pain in her wrist which was treated by him and shown curative results. SKB *claimed falsely that he has not treated* PD nor got the X-ray done from Central X-ray; the reports as well as prescription on different dates contradicted him. They wondered, if it was true, then why the cash memos of Satayanarayana Medical Hall and the X-ray mention SKB's name.

But, to establish medical negligence as alleged by complainant, there was no evidence and her counsel was not able to prove that the treatment was incorrect. In absence of X-ray report or X-ray film it is difficult to held SKB negligent in treatment. Even if SKB found fracture on X-ray, it is an error of judgment and further putting POP does not amount to medical negligence. The complainant did not file any evidence of AK to prove her case. The consultation slip showed that AK diagnosed it as '*De Quervain's tenosynovitis*' where the extensor tendons of thumb were involved and treated PD with steroids and advised wrist brace.

NCDRC did not find any infirmity that even if X-ray did not show fracture, and SKB had put POP which is also one of the preferred lined of treatment in such patients.

Compensation/damages awarded: The denial of treatment itself was deficiency in service. No pharmacy or diagnostic center mentions doctor's name casually. Therefore, such denial itself was deficiency in service for which they upheld the decision of State Commission which has imposed a fine of ₹ 5000 on SKB.

Conclusions: NCDRC agreed with the findings of State Commission that there was no medical negligence as such, but SKB was *liable for the deficiency in service as denial of reality and unethical practices.*

However, the Judges expressed surprise that the Government hospital doctor advised medicines and X-ray from outside. It was not mentioned whether such facilities were not available in the hospital at that time. It appeared to them as unethical indulgence by a Government doctor to refer patients to private X-ray clinics, laboratories and for medicines. It is well-known that there are rampant dichotomy practices, but is difficult to prove. In such cases, the patients are real sufferers.

CASE REPORT II[14]

Specialty: Obstetrics and Gynecology, Anesthesia.

Issues: MTP, family planning operation, sterilization operation, absence of anesthetist, denial of treatment, nondisclosure of events.

Brief facts of the case: On 12/8/92, complainant Mr A Ravi's (AR) wife Shanti was admitted for delivery in Subam Nursing Home run by Dr Usha Rani (UR). Next day, she delivered a baby by normal delivery. UR advised Shanti to undergo family planning operation for which she agreed. The operation was arranged at Anandi clinic of Dr Niraimadi Diwakaran (ND). Before taking discharge, the AR paid ₹ 1500 to UR to cover the fees for delivery and advance for family planning operation. The balance was to be paid after the operation. On 15/8/92, she came to Anandi clinic for operation and AR paid a sum of ₹ 250. At that time, she was in good health and was not suffering from any ailment. During operation, UR, ND and Dr Athilakshmi (Appellant, AL) were inside the operation theatre (OT). But, there was no anesthetist. AR's wife was taken inside the theater, and after 15 minutes, UR opened the doors and rushed to call her husband to bring Dr Shanthinathan (SN), the anesthetist.

Thereafter, AL came out of the OT, got into her car and left the clinic in a hurry. Within few minutes of the departure of AL, UR's husband brought the anesthetist SN into the OT. Simultaneously, ND came out and asked AR to bring a van immediately. Minutes after SN entered the OT, he came out. He recognized Shanti's father-in-law and signaled with his hands indicating that all was over. Soon after that, UR and ND came out of the OT with AR's wife in a stretcher and handed her over without informing about her condition. Under the impression that she was in a serious condition, AR took her in a van to Janki Hospital where she was pronounced dead. On 19/8/92, ND informed the Health Inspector concerned that death was due to cardiac failure.

Dr Usha Rani deposed that the operation was decided to be performed by AL, in the presence of SN (anesthetist) at Anandi clinic. She was present in the OT at the request of the deceased who was her patient. When she went inside, both ND and AL were present. AL performed the operation under local anesthesia. She first took out one fallopian tube and after cutting it, made necessary knots and put it inside. While she tried to take out the other fallopian tube, the patient developed pain and hence she stopped further operation and called for SN. Within few minutes, SN was brought who after analyzing the condition of the patient, opted for general anesthesia. He administered ether and after verifying the condition asked the surgeon to proceed further with the operation. AL took the second fallopian tube, treated and closed the abdomen. SN tried to arouse the patient, but there was no response. Suddenly, the patient got deteriorated and the blood pressure fell. In spite of their best efforts, the patient collapsed. Similarly, ND also contended that AL has performed the operation.

However, AL contended that on 15/8/92 at about 10 AM she received a phone call from Anandi clinic requesting her to get over a critical situation in family planning operation. She rushed to the clinic at 10.30 AM. By the time, SN had arrived. She found that the patient was in a serious state. She, therefore, expressed her inability to do anything and left the clinic immediately. She denied that she had performed the operation and was not responsible for the death of Shanti. It was her contention both UR and ND tried to shift their responsibility on her.

Alleged negligence/deficiency in service: It was the contended that the doctors handed over AR's wife without informing her condition and what was the cause of death. For the deficiency in service, he filed the case of negligence against all the three doctors who performed the family planning operation that resulted in her death.

Observations of the SCDRC: After going through the evidence, the SCDRC, Tamil Nadu arrived at the conclusion that the AL was engaged to do the operation which she performed and due to her negligence the patient died. The State Commission also observed that she was not telling the truth and what had really happened. If she was not at fault, she would have narrated the details of the operation and should have also stated as to how the patient died. The State Commission also relied upon the case sheet which was maintained by ND's husband who is also a doctor. It clearly mentioned that the operation was performed by AL, and SN was called in the middle of the operation. The State Commission directed AL to pay a sum of ₹ 4 lakhs with interest at the rate of 18% p.a. till realization and to pay ₹ 2000 as costs of the proceedings.

Observations of the NCDRC: Aggrieved by the order of SCDRC, AL filed an appeal at NCDRC. Considering the evidence presented before the State Commission, Judges at NCDRC held that AL did perform the operation, and not UR or ND as stated by her.

If the version of the AL was to be believed then it would mean that the operation was performed by the doctors who were not entitled to do so. In that case, she should have informed the police about the misdeeds of UR and ND, since the operation was done by unqualified doctors that resulted in the death of the patient. She neither referred the matter to the Medical Council nor informed the State Medical Council for taking appropriate action against UR and ND.

It appeared to them that the entire story narrated by AL was concocted and not reliable. They did not believe that either UR or ND would operate since they were not entitled to carry out such operations. There was also no reason to disbelieve the evidence of the anesthetist SN who was called subsequently, and has not given any anesthesia at the time of operation. This showed negligence of the concerned doctors in not performing the operation without calling the anesthetist. If UR was to perform the family planning operation, then she would have done that at her clinic when Shanti was admitted during delivery. There was no necessity for UR to tell her to go to the clinic of ND.

It was on record that ND had earlier called AL for carrying out such operations. Further, there was no reason to disbelieve AR's evidence that all the three doctors were in the OT during the operation. They dismissed the appeal.

Compensation/damages awarded: NCDRC directed AL to pay ₹ 4 lakhs as awarded by the State Commission, within a period of 4 weeks from the date of the order. It also directed AL to pay ₹ 20,000 as costs to the complainant.

Conclusion: The bench of NCDRC was aggrieved to note that the noble profession of doctors has gone down to such an extent that they are not prepared to disclose the events correctly.

CASE REPORT III[15]

Specialty: Multispecialty case—Radiology, Gynecology, Internal Medicine, Administration, and Surgery.

Issues: Wrong reporting of gallbladder stones, prolonged stay in the hospital, unethical practices, pseudolithiasis.

Brief facts of the case: On 22/4/09, Ms Neeta Kapoor (NK, complainant) got an ultrasound done from Arun Imaging Center of the lower abdomen. The report showed fibroid with adenomyosis of the uterus; the gallbladder was not subject of this ultrasound. Her second ultrasound was done at the same place on 1/5/09 in which the gallbladder was reported as normal in size with echo-free lumen, CBD normal in caliber.

NK consulted Dr Rekha Sareen on 24/6/09 and was advised hysterectomy. She was admitted for the operation at Pushpanjali Medical Center on 11/5/09 and was operated upon on 12/5/09. On 14/5/09, the ultrasound of the whole abdomen was done at Pushpanjali Medical Center by Dr Mukesh Koshal (MK). He reported that uterus was not seen but there were multiple gallbladder stones. He advised her to undergo another operation for the removal of the stones from the gallbladder. She was shocked as there was nothing abnormal reported in ultrasound dated 1/5/09.

On 17/5/09, she again visited MK since she wanted to satisfy her query as to how the gallstones were seen in the latest ultrasound. MK stood by his opinion. Subsequently, on 20/5/09 she met Dr Gaurav Aggarwal (GA), Director, Pushpanjali Medical Center who also stood by the report of MK. On 10/6/09, she got another ultrasound done at Diwan Chand Satyapal Aggarwal Imaging and Research Center so as to clarify her doubts. This report stated that the gallbladder and bile duct were normal in appearance and no calculi were observed.

In their defense, MK and GA admitted the report of ultrasound taken on 14/5/09, although they denied that they have advised NK to go for removal of the stone in the gallbladder. The ultrasound examination of the gallbladder did show multiple small calculi. This may be due to the third generation antibiotic ceftriaxone which was given to her that may represent 'pseudolithiasis'. This drug combines with calcium bile salts to form a precipitate that can mimic gallstones on sonographic examination. This disappears with the cessation of the therapy. They also denied that the complainant visited MK on 17/5/09 since he did not visit the Pushpanjali Medical Center on that day.

Alleged negligence/deficiency in service: The complainant prayed for restraining MK and GA from unethical practice so as to earn more from suggested operation.

MK and GA have specifically pleaded that third generation antibiotic may react with bile salts to form a precipitate which appear like calculi. As such this cannot be termed as a deficiency or negligence but it may be a case of having a different opinion. They relied upon AIR 2009 SC 2049 Martin F. D'souza vs. Mohd. Ishfaq wherein the Hon'ble Apex Court has ruled that a medical practitioner is not liable to be negligent because things went wrong through an error of judgment in choosing one reasonable course of treatment in preference to the another. They further argued that no expert medical opinion has been obtained before accepting complaint and in so far as the first contention is concerned, the same is not tenable. There was no proof that patient was ever treated for gallstones.

Observations of the District Forum: The matter before district forum was wrong reporting of Dr Mukesh which was supported by Dr Aggarwal. The forum observed that since the complaint was limited to the wrong reporting by MK and when there were specific reports, the medical expert opinion was not at all warranted to be necessary before institution of case or thereafter.

Even if MK formed opinion on the basis of the picture appearing in the ultrasound because of third generation antibiotic which on reaction with the calcium bile salts may create impression of a precipitate that can look gallstone on sonography. But, nowhere in the entire record did Dr Sareen, who treated the patient, suggested any such drug which may be responsible for creating such impression. MK also did not file any affidavit that NK was given any such drug or antibiotic which may react with bile salt and may precipitate and can mimic gallstone on sonographic examination. They also noted that sonography at Diwan Chand was done after 20 days of her discharge from the hospital. MK and GA did not produce any literature in support of their defense that drug induced calculi will disappear after the treatment is stopped.

They held that MK reported presence of the gallstone with an intention to prolong the hospitalization and earn more. GA was also held responsible for causing tension and trauma to NK and equally involved. MK and GA willfully created a document of existence of gallstone which caused mental tension and agony and fear in the mind of NK. In view of the above, the forum held MK and GA guilty of unethical medical practice.

Compensation/damages awarded: The forum directed Pushpanjali Medical Center and its two doctors to pay ₹ 1.5 lakh within 30 days to NK. If not paid within the time period, the complainant will get an interest @ 9% till this amount is finally paid.

Conclusions: District forum observed that there is a general feeling amongst the people that with the advent of corporate culture in the medical profession, the ethics of the medical profession have lost relevance. The doctors work as agent of the corporate hospitals in generating more revenue for hospital by adopting unethical practices at the cost of the patient. Earlier, the doctors were respected as an agent of the God and who provided solace in the hours of pain and sorrow. Nowadays, the doctors are performing surgeries when the patients need none. If a patient is covered by the insurance or he came from the public sector companies, Central Government Health Scheme (CGHS) beneficiaries and got their reimbursement of the amount spent on the treatment, unnecessarily tests and diagnostic procedures are done even in cases where the patient requires no such test. They also suggested the Medical Council of India for restraining such doctors to practice and to take note of the prevailing atmosphere in the medical profession and identify such black sheep who are responsible for creating such wrong impression in the mind of the public. The government should also take steps to restore back faith in the mind of the public and to protect patients from unscrupulous medical practitioners who do not have regard for ethics and the Hippocratic Oath.

Observations of the SCDRC: No appeal has been made before the SCDRC till date.

Observations of MCI: In its response, the Ethics Committee of MCI deliberated and examined the order. The Committee decided to call both the parties, i.e. complainant Mrs Neeta Kapoor, and Dr Mukesh Koshal for personal hearing with all the medical records and supportive documents available with them in the subsequent meeting.

PROPOSED GUIDELINES

Bolam Test (Test of Standard) and its applicability in India: In State of Haryana and Ors. vs. Smt. Santra,[6] Bolam's test has been approved. This case refers to liability for compensation under civil law for failure of sterilization operation performed by a surgeon.

The classical statement of law in Bolam's case has been widely accepted as decisive of the standard of care required both for professional men in general and medical practitioners in particular.[16] It has been invariably cited with approval before courts in India and applied to as touchstone to test the pleas of medical negligence.[5]

In tort, it is enough for the defendant to show that the standard of care and the skill attained was that of the ordinary competent medical practitioner exercising an ordinary degree of professional skill. The fact that a defendant, charged with negligence acted in accordance with the general and approved practice is enough to clear him of the charge.

The NCRDC while disposing of a case on 24/9/13 applied Bolam test and observed that the opposite parties are qualified and adopted the treatment as per standards of medical practice. The method of treatment was also one of preferred choice of nonoperative method. The complainant's sufferings were result of infection caused due to his negligence as he did not follow the instructions of doctor. He has not taken rest for two weeks, but traveled in train.[17]

What constitutes 'medical negligence' is now well established by a plethora of rulings of the Hon'ble Supreme Court of India and by several orders of the NCDRC. The *locus classicus* of the test for the standard of care in law, as required of a doctor, has developed from the landmark case. Mr Justice McNair, in his direction to the jury, said:

[a doctor] *is not guilty of negligence if he has acted in accordance with the practice accepted as proper by a responsible body of medical men skilled in that particular art...Putting it the other way round, a man is not negligent, if he is acting in accordance with such a practice, merely because there is a body of opinion who would take a contrary view.*[13]

In view of above discussions, NCDRC found no illegality or infirmity in order passed by both the fora below, i.e. District and SCDRC, warranting NCDRC interference. The revision petition was accordingly dismissed, with no order as to cost.[17]

In a case, the Supreme Court quoted some of the conclusions arrived at by the learned authors of 'Errors, Medicine and the Law', highlighting the link between moral fault, blame and justice in reference to medical profession and negligence. These are of significance and relevant to the issues discussed. Hence quoted:[18]

- The social efficacy of blame and related sanctions in particular cases of deliberate wrongdoings may be a matter of dispute, but their necessity in principle from a moral point of view has been accepted. Distasteful as punishment may be, the social and possibly moral need to punish people for wrongdoing, occasionally in a severe fashion, cannot be escaped. A society in which blame is overemphasized may become paralyzed. This is not only because such a society will inevitably be backward-looking, but also because fear of blame inhibits the uncluttered exercise of judgment in relations between persons. If we are constantly concerned about whether our actions will be the subject of complaint, and that such complaint is likely to lead to legal action or disciplinary proceedings, a relationship of suspicious formality between persons is inevitable.
- Culpability may attach to the consequence of an error in circumstances where substandard antecedent conduct has been deliberate, and has contributed to the generation of the error or to its outcome. In case of errors, a failure defined in terms of the normative standard of what should have been done. There is a tendency to confuse the reasonable person with the error-free person. While nobody can avoid errors on the basis of simply choosing not to make them, people can choose not to commit violations. A violation is culpable.
- Before the court faced with deciding the cases of professional negligence there are two sets of interests which are at stake: the interests of the plaintiff and the interests of the defendant. A correct balance of these two sets of interests should ensure that tort liability is restricted to those cases where there is a real failure to behave as a reasonably competent practitioner would have behaved. An inappropriate raising of the standard of care threatens this balance. A consequence of encouraging litigation for loss is to persuade the public that all loss encountered in a medical context is the result of the failure of somebody in the system to provide the level of care to which the patient is entitled. The effect is on the distorting doctor-patient relationship and will not be to the benefit of the patient in the long run. It is also unjustified to impose on those engaged in medical treatment an undue degree of additional stress and anxiety in the conduct of their profession. Equally, it would be wrong to impose such stress and anxiety on any other person performing a demanding function in society.

While expectations from the professionals must be realistic and the expected standards attainable, this implies recognition of the nature of ordinary human error and human limitations in the performance of complex tasks.

- Conviction for any substantial criminal offence requires that the accused person should have acted with a morally blameworthy state of mind. Recklessness and deliberate wrong doing are morally blameworthy, but any conduct falling short of that should not be the subject of criminal liability. Common law systems have traditionally only made negligence the subject of criminal sanction when the level of negligence has been high, traditionally described as gross negligence. In fact, negligence at that level is likely to be indistinguishable from recklessness.
- Blame is a powerful weapon. Its inappropriate use distorts tolerant and constructive relations between people. Distinguishing between (a) accidents which are life's misfortune for which nobody is morally responsible, (b) wrongs amounting to culpable conduct and constituting grounds for compensation, and (c) those (i.e. wrongs) calling for punishment on account of being gross or of a very high degree, requires and calls for careful, morally sensitive and scientifically informed analysis; else there would be injustice to the larger interest of the society. Indiscriminate prosecution of medical professionals for criminal negligence is counter-productive and does no service or good to the society.[5]

The Supreme Court in a recent case summed up as under:[19]

- Negligence in the context of medical profession necessarily calls for a treatment with a difference. To infer rashness or negligence on the part of a professional, in particular a doctor, additional considerations should apply. A case of occupational negligence is different from one of professional negligence. A simple lack of care, an error of judgment or an accident, is not proof of negligence on the part of a medical professional. So long as a doctor follows a practice acceptable to the medical profession of that day, he cannot be held liable for negligence merely because a better alternative course or method of treatment was also available, or simply because a more skilled doctor would not have chosen to follow or resort to that practice or procedure which the accused followed. When it comes to the failure of taking precautions what has to be seen is whether those precautions were taken which the ordinary experience of men has found to be sufficient; a failure to use special or extraordinary precautions which might have prevented the particular happening cannot be the standard for judging the alleged negligence. So also, the standard of care, while assessing the practice as adopted, *is judged in the light of knowledge available at the time of the incident, and not at the date of trial.* Similarly, when the charge of negligence arises out of failure to use some particular equipment, the charge would fail if the equipment was not generally available at that particular time (that is, the time of the incident) at which it is suggested it should have been used.
- A professional may be held liable for negligence on one of the two findings: either he was not possessed of the requisite skill which he professed to have possessed, or, he did not exercise, with reasonable competence in the given case, the skill which he did possess. The standard to be applied for judging, whether the person charged has been negligent or not, would be that of an

ordinary competent person exercising ordinary skill in that profession. It is not possible for every professional to possess the highest level of expertise or skills in that branch which he practices. A highly skilled professional may be possessed of better qualities, but that cannot be made the basis or the yardstick for judging the performance of the professional proceeded against on indictment of negligence.

- The test for determining medical negligence as laid down in Bolam's case holds good in its applicability in India.[16]
- The jurisprudential concept of negligence differs in civil and criminal law. What may be negligence in civil law may not necessarily be negligence in criminal law. For negligence to amount to an offence, the element of *mens rea* must be shown to exist. For an act to amount to criminal negligence, the degree of negligence should be much higher, i.e. gross or of a very high degree. Negligence which is neither gross nor of a higher degree may provide a ground for action in civil law but cannot form the basis for prosecution.
- The word 'gross' has not been used in Sec. 304A IPC, yet it is settled that in criminal law negligence or recklessness, to be so held, must be of such a high degree as to be 'gross'. The expression 'rash or negligent act' as occurring in Sec. 304A IPC has to be read as qualified by the word 'grossly'.
- To prosecute a medical professional for negligence under criminal law, it must be shown that the accused did something or failed to do something which in the given facts and circumstances no medical professional in his ordinary senses and prudence would have done or failed to do. The hazard taken by the accused doctor should be of such a nature that the injury which resulted was most likely imminent.
- *Res ipsa loquitur* is only a rule of evidence and operates in the domain of civil law especially in cases of torts and helps in determining the onus of proof in actions relating to negligence. It cannot be pressed in service for determining *per se* the liability for negligence within the domain of criminal law. *Res ipsa loquitur* has, if at all, a limited application in trial on a charge of criminal negligence.

In view of the principles laid down hereinabove and the preceding discussion, the Supreme Court also agreed with the principles of law laid down in Dr Suresh Gupta's case. The Supreme Court clarified that they are affirming the legal principles laid down and the law as stated in Dr Suresh Gupta's case.[20] It further clarified that they may not be understood as having expressed any opinion on the question whether on the facts of that case the accused could or could not have been held guilty of criminal negligence as that question is not before them. The Court also approved of the passage from Errors, Medicine and the Law by Alan Merry and Alexander McCall Smith[18] which has been cited with approval in Dr Suresh Gupta's case.[20]

Guidelines for Prosecuting Medical Professionals for Criminal Negligence Cases

As noticed by the Supreme Court that the cases of doctors (surgeons and physicians) being subjected to criminal prosecutions are on an increase. Sometimes, such prosecutions are filed by private complainants and sometimes by police on an FIR being lodged and cognizance taken. The investigating officer and the private complainant cannot always be supposed to have knowledge of medical science so as to determine whether the act of the accused medical practitioner amounts to rash or negligent act within the domain of criminal law under Sec. 304A IPC. The criminal process once initiated subjects the medical practitioner to serious embarrassment and sometimes harassment. He has to seek bail to escape arrest, which may or may not be granted to him. At the end, he may be exonerated by acquittal or discharge but the loss which he has suffered in his reputation cannot be compensated by any standards.

The Supreme Court clarified that it may not be understood as holding that the doctors can never be prosecuted for an offence of which rashness or negligence is an essential ingredient. All that Court has done was to emphasize the need for care and caution in the interest of society; for, the service which the medical profession renders to human beings is probably the noblest of all, and hence there is a need for protecting doctors from frivolous or unjust prosecutions. Many a complainant prefers recourse to criminal process as a tool for pressurizing the medical professional for extracting uncalled for or unjust compensation. Such malicious proceedings have to be guarded against. Statutory rules or executive instructions incorporating certain guidelines need to be framed and issued by the Government of India and/or the State Governments in consultation with the Medical Council of India. So long as it is not done, they proposed certain guidelines for the future which should govern the prosecution of doctors for offences of which criminal rashness or criminal negligence is an ingredient.

A private complaint may not be entertained unless the complainant has produced prima facie evidence before the court in the form of a credible opinion given by another competent doctor to support the charge of rashness or negligence on the part of the accused doctor. The investigating officer should, before proceeding against the doctor accused of rash or negligent act or omission, obtain an independent and competent medical opinion preferably from a doctor in government service qualified in that branch of medical practice who can normally be expected to give an impartial and unbiased opinion applying Bolam's test to the facts collected in the investigation. A doctor accused of rashness or negligence, may not be arrested in a routine manner (simply because a charge has been leveled against him). Unless his arrest is necessary for furthering the investigation or for collecting evidence or unless the investigation officer feels satisfied that the doctor proceeded against would not make himself available to face the prosecution unless arrested, the arrest may be withheld.[5]

The Supreme Court has summarized rules governing the medical negligence in India as follows:[19]

- Negligence is an essential ingredient of the offence. The negligence to be established by the prosecution must be culpable or gross and not the negligence merely based upon an error of judgment.
- The medical practitioner is expected to bring a reasonable degree of skill and knowledge and must exercise a reasonable degree of care. Neither the very highest nor a very low degree of care and competence judged in the light of the particular circumstances of each case is what the law requires.
- A medical practitioner would be liable only where his conduct fell below that of the standards of a reasonably competent practitioner in his field.

- In the realm of diagnosis and treatment, there is scope for genuine difference of opinion and one medical practitioner is clearly not negligent merely because his conclusion differs from that of another medical practitioner.
- The medical practitioner is often called upon to adopt a procedure which involves higher element of risk, but which he honestly believes as providing greater chances of success for the patient rather than a procedure involving lesser risk but higher chances of failure. Just because a professional looking to the gravity of illness has taken higher element of risk to redeem the patient out of his/her suffering which did not yield the desired result may not amount to negligence.
- Negligence cannot be attributed to a doctor so long as he performs his duties with reasonable skill and competence. Merely because the doctor chooses one course of action in preference to the other one available, he would not be liable if the course of action chosen by him was acceptable to the medical profession.
- It would not be conducive to the efficiency of the medical profession if no doctor could administer medicine without a halter round his neck.
- It is our bounden duty and obligation of the civil society to ensure that the medical professionals are not unnecessarily harassed or humiliated so that they can perform their professional duties without fear and apprehension.
- The medical practitioners at times also have to be saved from such a class of complainants who use criminal process as a tool for pressurizing the medical professionals/hospitals particularly private hospitals or clinics for extracting uncalled for compensation. Such malicious proceedings deserve to be discarded against the medical practitioners.
- The medical professionals are entitled to get protection so long as they perform their duties with reasonable skill and competence and in the interest of the patients. The interest and welfare of the patients have to be paramount for the medical professionals.

CONCLUSION

In conclusion, it is reiterated that there is intense need for doing research to prevent ever increasing number of medical negligence cases in India day by day. Ethical violations should be dealt with stern action in time bound manner may have some deterrent effect on those who are thinking of indulging in unethical practice with impunity.

REFERENCES

1. Jha AK, Larizgoitia I, Audera-Lopez C, Prasopa-Plaizier N, Waters H, Bates DW. The global burden of unsafe medical care: analytic modelling of observational studies. *BMJ Qual Saf* 2013; 22: 809-15.
2. Sinha K. Medical negligence: Govt. to provide cover. The Times of India. 2009 Sept 16.
3. Singh GP (ed). The law of torts. Ratanlal and Dhirajlal, 24th edn. 2002. p. 441-42.
4. Walton C, Cooper R, Wood SE. Charlesworth and Percy on Negligence, 10th edn. London: Sweet and Maxwell; 2001.
5. Jacob Mathew vs. State of Punjab, [(2005) 6 SCC 1]; 2005 AIR 3180, 2005(2) Suppl. SCR307, 2005(6) SCC1, 2005(6) SCALE 130, 2005(6) JT 584.

6. State of Haryana and Ors. vs. Smt. Santra, Date of Judgment: 24/04/2000, Available from: http://judis.nic.in/supremecourt/imgs1.aspx?filename=16386.
7. Dr. S Alagusundarammal vs. V Karuppiah, Revision Petition No. 2737 of 2013 (against order dated 26.06.2012 in First Appeal No. 95 of 2011 of the State Consumer Disputes Redressal Commission, Tamil Nadu, Chennai) with Interim Application No. 5440 of 2013 (Delay). Available from: http://164.100.72.12/ncdrcrep/judgement/001309101 03940501RP27372013.htm.
8. The Indian Medical Council (Professional Conduct, Etiquettes and Ethics) Regulations, 2002.
9. Dr. Naveen Agrohi vs. Shri Parvas, Revision Petition No. 2391 of 2012, (From order dated 19.03.2012 in First Appeal No. 89 of 2007 of the State Consumer Disputes Redressal Commission, Uttarakhand). Available from: http://164.100.72.12/ ncdrcrep/judgement/00130508110839917RP239112.htm.
10. Martin F. D'Souza vs. Mohd. Ishfaq AIR 2009 SC 2049, Civil Appeal No. 3541 of 2002.
11. Gaurav vs. Escorts Medical Center Ltd and Anr. CPR 182 (NC).
12. Dr. Biswanath Das vs. Bijoy Sinha Roy and Ors. 2008 (1) CPR 282 (NC).
13. Dr. Sunil Kumar Bijpuria, vs. Smt. Priya Dubey @ Preetam Mishra, Revision Petition No. 3562 of 2012, (From order dated 19.06.2012 in First Appeal No. 375 of 2009 of the State Consumer Disputes Redressal Commission, Ranchi). Available from: http://164.100.72.12/ncdrcrep/judgement/00130730100157588RP356212.htm.
14. Dr. (Mrs.) A. Athilakshmi vs. A. Ravi and Ors. First Appeal No. 6 of 1999 (From the order dated 24.11.1998 passed in O.P. No. 268 of 1993 of the State Commission, Chennai), dated the 1st February, 2007.
15. NA Zaidi, President, Delhi District Consumer Forum (East Delhi). Mrs. Neeta Kapoor vs. Pushpanjali Medical Center and Ors., Case No-522/09. Available from: http://164.100.72.12/ncdrcrep/judgement/8513041111595233NeetaKapoorVsPush panjaliMedicalCenter.htm.
16. McNair J in Bolam v Friern Hospital Management Committee, [1957] 1 W.L.R. 582, 586.
17. Rajiv Navath vs. Dr. Shajahan Yoosaf Sahib, Revision Petition No. 1311 of 2013 (From order dated 15.11.2012 in First Appeal No. 164 of 2012 of the State Consumer Disputes Redressal Commission, Kerala, Thiruvananthapuram). Available from: http://164.100.72.12/ncdrcrep/judgement/00130924163615305RP13112013.htm.
18. Merry A, Smith AM. Errors, medicine and the law. Cambridge: Cambridge university press; 2001. p. 241-48.
19. Kusum Sharma and Ors. vs. Batra Hospital and Med. Research Center and Ors, Civil Appeal No.1385 of 2001. Available from: http://judis.nic.in/supremecourt/imgs1. aspx?filename=36001.
20. Dr. Suresh Gupta vs. Govt. of NCT of Delhi and Anr. (2004) 6 SCC 422. Available from: http://www.indiankanoon.org/docfragment/650550/?formInput=dr.sureshgupta.

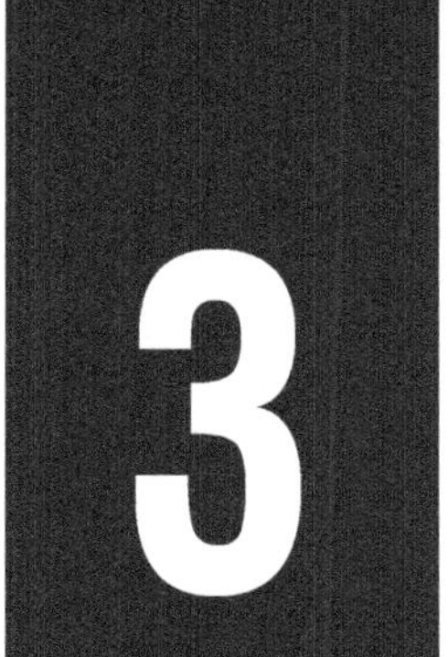

Euthanasia: Legal, Social and Humanitarian Aspects

Vijay Vasudev Pillay

'One has observed life poorly, if one has not also witnessed the hand that mercifully—kills.'
Friedrich Nietzsche (German philologist, philosopher and cultural critic)

ABSTRACT

Euthanasia refers to the practice of intentionally or deliberately causing a painless death of an individual suffering from hopelessly incurable and painful disease. Euthanasia is categorized in different ways, which include voluntary, nonvoluntary or involuntary. Voluntary euthanasia is legal in some countries. Non-voluntary euthanasia is illegal in most countries. Involuntary euthanasia is usually considered murder. Voluntary, nonvoluntary and involuntary euthanasia can all be further divided into passive or active variants. Passive euthanasia entails the withholding of common treatments necessary for the continuance of life. Active euthanasia entails the use of lethal substances or forces, such as administering a lethal injection to kill and is the most controversial means. Physician-assisted suicide (PAS), sometimes shortened to 'assisted suicide' is a new term for euthanasia committed by someone with assistance from a medically qualified person. There are different euthanasia laws in each country. PAS is legal in several countries, including Belgium, Luxembourg, the Netherlands, Switzerland and four American states (Oregon, Washington, Vermont and Montana). The Hippocratic Oath forbids physicians' participation in death, which has been interpreted by many to be a prohibition against PAS, euthanasia and involvement in executions. All forms of euthanasia are generally considered illegal in India, though there have been some recent developments which indicate liberalization of the concept, especially with regard to passive euthanasia.

Keywords: Mercy killing, aid-in-dying, self-deliverance, physician assisted suicide (PAS).

INTRODUCTION

The word 'euthanasia' is derived from the Greek words 'eu' and 'thanotos' which literally means a 'good death', though it has undergone considerable distortion over a period of time to assume its present day meaning of 'mercy killing'.[1] History suggests that the word was used in the 17th century by Francis Bacon to refer to an easy and painless death, since it was the physician's duty and responsibility to alleviate the physical suffering of the patient.[1] Other synonyms include 'aid-in-dying' and 'self-deliverance'.

As far back as 300–400 BC, both Socrates and Plato accorded moral sanction to euthanasia and suggested that it was permissible in certain circumstances. But today, there is a raging controversy all over the world as to its legal standing, aside from the moral and ethical issues involved. It has been at the center of very heated debates for many years and is surrounded by religious, ethical and practical considerations. Euthanasia is the most active area of research in contemporary bioethics. There is paucity of information and confusion prevailing over the medicolegal status and ethical aspects of euthanasia in India and worldwide which led to the compilation of this chapter.

DEFINITIONS

- **Euthanasia:** The infliction of a painless death on an individual suffering from severe, intractable pain or discomfort, arising out of a terminal illness or condition.[2]
- **Physician-assisted suicide:** Physician-assisted suicide (PAS) is the physician prescribing a drug or other action to facilitate a patient taking his/her own life, with the committed action taken by the patient.[3]
- **Terminal illness:** Illness or injury or degeneration of physical or mental condition, causing extreme pain and which, according to medical opinion, will inevitably cause death or has caused persistent and irreversible vegetative condition.[1]
- **Palliative care:** The provision of reasonable medical and nursing procedures for the relief of physical pain, discomfort or emotional and psychological suffering as well as providing food and water.[1]

CLASSIFICATION

Euthanasia can be classified in different ways:[4]

1. *Voluntary euthanasia:* The dying individual consents to the act.
2. *Nonvoluntary euthanasia:* The person cannot make a decision or cannot make his wishes known. This includes cases where the person is:
   a. in a coma
   b. too young (for e.g., an infant)
   c. senile
   d. mentally deficient to a very severe extent
   e. severely brain damaged
   f. mentally disturbed in such a way that he/she should be protected from themselves
3. *Compulsory (involuntary) euthanasia:* Decision by society to terminate the life of an individual.
4. *Active euthanasia:* Inflicting painless death by an act of commission, for e.g., injection of a lethal dose of barbiturates.
5. *Passive euthanasia (negative euthanasia):* Inflicting painless death by an act of omission, i.e. when the patient dies because the medical professionals either do not do something necessary to keep the patient alive, or when they stop doing something that is keeping the patient alive, for e.g.:
   a. Switch off life-support machines
   b. Disconnect a feeding tube

   c. Do not carry out a life-extending operation
   d. Do not give life-extending drugs
6. *Pediatric euthanasia:* Euthanasia administered to seriously sick or deformed infants.

   The *Groningen Protocol* was created in September 2004 by Eduard Verhagen, the medical director of the department of pediatrics at the University Medical Center Groningen (UMCG) in Groningen, the Netherlands.[5] It contains directives with criteria under which physicians can perform 'active ending of life on infants' who are seriously ill or suffer from significant birth defects (for e.g., newborns with spina bifida and hydrocephalus) without the fear of legal prosecution (*child euthanasia*—a form of nonvoluntary euthanasia). The protocol, made up after extensive consultation between physicians, lawyers, parents and the prosecution office, offers procedures and guidelines to achieve the correct decision and performance. The final decision about 'active ending of life of infant' is not in the hands of the physicians but with the parents, with physicians and social workers agreeing to it. Criteria are, amongst others, 'unbearable suffering' and 'unexpected quality of life'. Only the parents can start the procedure. The procedure is reported to be working well.

   However, the Groningen Protocol does not give physicians unassailable legal protection. Case law has so far protected physicians from prosecution as long as they act in accordance with the protocol, but no black-letter law exists in this area.

   Several studies have questioned the basis for the protocol and have recommended abandoning it.[6,7]
7. *Geriatric euthanasia:* Euthanasia administered to seriously sick, aged individuals.
8. *Battlefield euthanasia:* Euthanasia administered to severely wounded or handicapped individual.

HISTORY OF EUTHANASIA

A 20th century chronology of important events relating to voluntary euthanasia and PAS is presented in Table 3.1.[8] Prior to the beginning of the 20th century, the concept of euthanasia was rarely discussed as it was considered taboo and often equated with suicide, and thus deemed illegal.

Table 3.2 lists some of the important personalities around the world who have been campaigning for the legal acceptance and validation of euthanasia.

ARGUMENTS FAVORING EUTHANASIA

According to euthanasia expert Ezekiel Emanuel,[9] proponents of euthanasia invariably present four main arguments:
1. People have a right to self-determination, and thus should be allowed to choose their own fate.
2. Assisting a subject to die might be a better choice than requiring that he/she may continue to suffer.
3. The distinction between passive euthanasia which is often permitted, and active euthanasia which is not substantive (or that the underlying principle—the doctrine of double effect) is unreasonable or unsound.
4. Permitting euthanasia will not necessarily lead to unacceptable consequences.

Table 3.1 Chronology of euthanasia (summary of important events from early 20th century)

Year	Developments
1906	First euthanasia bill drafted in the US (Ohio), but it does not succeed.
1935	World's first euthanasia society is founded in London.
1938	The Euthanasia Society of America is founded in New York.
1967	The first 'living will' is written by American attorney Louis Kutner.
1973	The American Hospital Association creates Patient Bill of Rights, which includes the right to refuse treatment.
1974	The Euthanasia Society in New York is renamed the Society for the Right to Die.
1976	The California Natural Death Act is passed which protects physicians from being sued for failing to treat incurable illnesses. Several other states of the US follow suit with similar legislation.
1976	First international meeting of 'Right to Die' groups.
1978	A Broadway play '*Whose life is it anyway?*' about a quadriplegic wanting to die is staged for the first time. It goes on to become a massive hit and is followed by its movie version in 1982.
1980	Pope John Paul II issues 'Declaration on Euthanasia' opposing mercy killing, but permitting the right to refuse extraordinary means for sustaining life.
1980	Hemlock Society (advocating euthanasia) is founded in California by journalist Derek Humphry.
1980	World Federation of Right to Die Societies is formed in Oxford, England.
1984	The Netherlands Supreme Court approves voluntary euthanasia under certain conditions.
1990	American Medical Association permits physicians to withhold or withdraw treatment from patients who are close to death.
1990	Dr Jack Kevorkian (Michigan, US), assists for the first time, in the death of a patient. Over the next 9 years he assists in a total of 130 deaths. He is tried 4 times before finally being convicted in his 5th trial in April 1999 for 2nd degree murder.
1991	Derek Humphry publishes 'Final Exit', a how-to book on self-deliverance. It quickly tops the US best-seller list and is subsequently translated into 12 languages.
1993	A political action committee Oregon Right to Die is founded to write and subsequently pass the Oregon Death with Dignity Act. The Act is in effect from 5th October 1997, after several unsuccessful attempts to scuttle it.
1996	The Northern Territory of Australia passes voluntary euthanasia law which was drafted the previous year. However, nine months later the Federal Parliament quashes it.
1999	Dr Kevorkian sentenced to 10–25 years in prison for 2nd degree murder of Thomas Youk suffering from motor neuron disease. The videotape of Youk's death had been telecast on national television, provoking public outrage.
2000	The Netherlands becomes the first country in the world to legalize physician-assisted suicide (PAS).

Contd...

Contd...

Year	*Developments*
2000	The Switzerland-based Dignitas, a legal euthanasia center, begins its operations under the lax euthanasia laws of the country. However, a clear-cut law legalizing PAS has so far not been passed in Switzerland.
2002	Belgium becomes the second country to legalize PAS.
2007	Dr Jack Kevorkian is released from prison after serving 8 years.
2008	Luxembourg becomes the third country to legalize PAS.
2008	The Washington Initiative 1000 makes Washington the second US state to legalize PAS.
2009	Luxembourg becomes the third European Union country, after the Netherlands and Belgium, to decriminalize euthanasia.
2010	The Federal Court of Justice of Germany legalizes passive euthanasia with patient's consent.
2011	Kevorkian dies from a thrombosis on 3rd June, eight days after his 83rd birthday at William Beaumont Hospital in Royal Oak, Michigan, US.
2012	World's first mobile euthanasia unit begins to operate in the Netherlands. According to The Daily Mail in London, the units will be dispatched when family doctors refuse to administer lethal drugs on 'ethical' grounds.
2012	International Congress of World Federation of Right-to-Die Societies (WFRtDS), Zürich (Switzerland), hosted by 'EXIT Deutsche Schweiz' on behalf of their sister society ADMD Suisse Romande.
2013	Vermont becomes the first legislature in US to pass a PAS suicide law. Oregon and Washington had earlier passed their laws via citizen initiative vote; subsequently, Montana drafted a law through a court case.

Table 3.2 Some prominent *Right to Die* activists

Country	*Name*
Netherlands	Pieter Admiraal Marion Rookhuizen
Belgium	Wim Distelmans
Scotland	John Beloff
India	Buji Colabawalla
Australia	Lynda Cracknell Philip Nitschke
USA	Derek Humphry Jack Kevorkian
England	Ludovic Kennedy
Switzerland	Jeanne Marchig
Columbia	Clemencia Uribe

Proeuthanasia activists often point to countries like the Netherlands and Belgium, and states like Oregon, where euthanasia has been legalized and is mostly unproblematic.

The medical ethos of the 'sanctity of life' implying the unqualified duty to preserve life at all costs has come under increasing challenge. There is a perceptibly growing movement away from a rigid obligation on the part of a doctor to preserve life 'at all costs', towards a more flexible duty to provide good palliative terminal care. Terminal illness is considered best treated by providing optimum conditions for death rather than by the use of increasingly invasive techniques to prolong some sort of existence. A conscious, dying patient can make his own decision, since patient's autonomy is today considered to be the cornerstone of ethical medical practice. To continue to treat in the face of contrary instructions can attract legal liabilities, though the exact position is still not clear-cut in India (*vide infra*).

In many Western countries, it is generally accepted that there is no moral obligation on the part of a doctor to preserve life at the expense of suffering, and if in the course of good terminal care, the use of drugs inadvertently hastens death, this is ethically acceptable within the concept of '*double effect*', i.e. an ill effect is morally acceptable as long as there is a greater, intended good effect from an action.[10] This concept was first given legal sanction in relation to euthanasia by Justice Devlin in the *Bodkin Adams case* (1957), when he remarked, 'The doctor is entitled to relieve pain and suffering even if the measures he takes may incidentally shorten life' (Box 3.1).[11]

Box 3.1 Case of Bodkin Adams

John Bodkin Adams (21st January 1899–4th July 1983) was an Irish-born British general practitioner (Fig. 3.1). Between the years 1946 and 1956, more than 160 of his patients died under suspicious circumstances. Of these, 132 left him money or items in their will. He was tried and acquitted for the murder of one patient in 1957. Another count of murder was withdrawn by the prosecution in what was later described as 'an abuse of process' by the presiding Judge Patrick Devlin, causing questions to be asked in Parliament about the prosecution's handling of events.

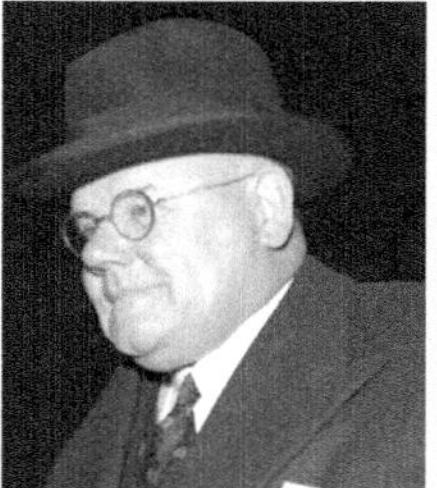

Fig. 3.1 Dr John Bodkin Adams

The trial had several important legal ramifications:

- It established the principle of 'double effect', whereby a doctor giving treatment with the aim of relieving pain may, as an unintentional result, shorten life.
- Secondly, due to the publicity surrounding Adams' committal hearing, the law was changed to allow defendants to ask for such hearings to be held in private.
- Finally, though a defendant had never been required to give evidence in his own defence, the Judge underlined in his summing-up that no prejudice should be attached by the Jury to Adams not doing so.

Adams was found guilty in a subsequent trial of 13 offences of prescription fraud, falsifying cremation forms, obstructing a police search and failing to keep dangerous drugs register. His name was removed from the Medical Register in 1957, but was reinstated in 1961.

The possibility of maintaining 'physiological life', i.e. the continuation of the body functions by artificial means, while the patient remains unconscious over a period of months or years, has introduced a new dimension into the debate—'quality of life'. Clearly, the sustaining of physiological functions with no prospect of recovery of consciousness or contact with the patient's environment has led to considerable debate as to whether or not such support systems should be continued, and who should be responsible for the decision to turn off such systems.

Views vary widely, but there is a substantial proportion of population in countries, such as the US which favors the view that support systems can be switched off by attending doctors with consent from the victim's relatives, in certain cases.

The case of Karen Ann Quinlan (Fig. 3.2) is representative of this. Karen, a 21-year-old girl fell into a coma after imbibing an overdose of alcohol and drugs on 15th April, 1975. She passed into 'persistent vegetative state' from which recovery was extremely remote. Her parents, both devout Roman Catholics, were initially hopeful of a miracle, but as the months passed by they realized that this was only wishful thinking and that their daughter was never going to come back to meaningful existence. They requested that life support systems prolonging the futile ordeal be switched off. The doctors attending on the case refused, and the issue was taken to court. In 1976, the New Jersey Supreme Court delivered a verdict in favor of Karen's parents. However, while the support systems were subsequently switched off, artificial feeding was not stopped and Karen continued to 'live' for nearly 10 years before her heart finally stopped in 1985. The case, however, served to focus attention on a topic that had for decades been considered taboo.[12]

The Terri Schiavo case (another landmark case akin to the Quinlan case) that occurred in the US lasted from 1990-2005.[13] Terri Schiavo (Fig. 3.3) collapsed in her home in Florida due to sudden cardiac arrest, on 25th February 1990. She suffered massive brain damage due to lack of oxygen and after two and a half months in a coma, her diagnosis was changed to 'vegetative state'. For the next

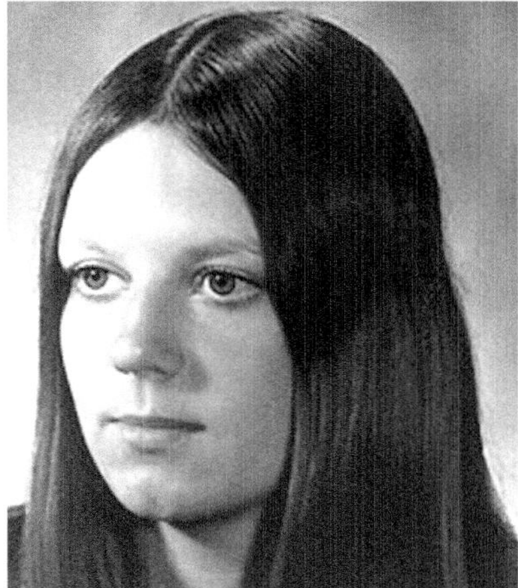

Fig. 3.2 Karen Ann Quinlan

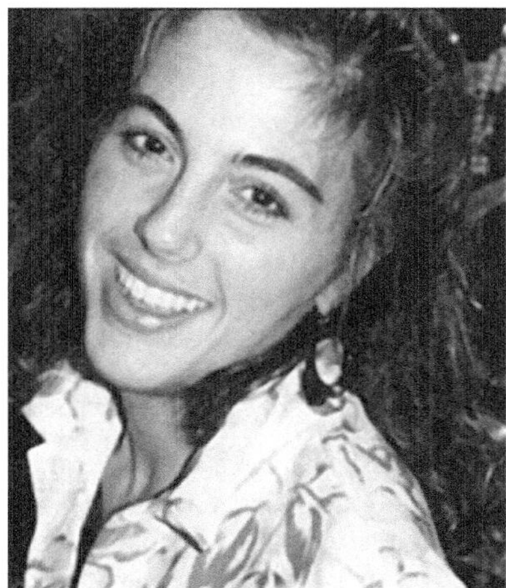

Fig. 3.3 Terry Schiavo

few years, doctors attempted speech and physical therapy and other experimental therapy, hoping to return her to a state of awareness. In 1998, Schiavo's husband, Michael, petitioned the Court of Florida, to remove her feeding tube. He was opposed by Terri's parents, Robert and Mary Schindler, who argued that she was conscious. The court determined that she would not wish to continue life-prolonging measures, and on 24th April 2001, her feeding tube was removed for the first time, only to be reinserted several days later.

On 25th February 2005, a County Judge ordered the removal of Terri Schiavo's feeding tube. Several appeals and federal government intervention followed, which included US President George W Bush returning to Washington DC to sign legislation designed to keep her alive. After appeals through the Federal Court system upheld the original decision to remove the feeding tube, staff at the hospice facility where Terri was being cared for, disconnected the feeding tube on 18th March 2005 and she died on 31st March 2005.

The Schiavo case resulted in a big boost to the activism of prolife movement and disability rights groups. This case differed from the Quinlan case by involving settled law rather than breaking new legal ground on the right-to-die issue.

Today, not only in the case of terminally unconscious patients, but also in conscious patients (who are suffering from an intractable, painful, terminal illness), euthanasia is being increasingly considered as applicable, provided the patient concerned makes the request and he is judged to be of sound and rational mind. Withdrawing treatment and allowing a patient to die (passive euthanasia) is therefore not perceived as repugnant anymore in certain situations. In fact, in several Western countries, adult individuals over a specified age can execute a *living will* or *advance directive* which entitles him to refuse treatment any time in future in the event of a catastrophic accident or natural disease.[14] The usual phraseology in a living will is as follows:

"If I suffer an incurable, irreversible illness, disease or condition and my attending physician determines that my condition is terminal, I direct that life-sustaining measures that would serve only to prolong my dying be withheld or discontinued".

A related document is a specific type of power of attorney or *health care proxy*, in which the person authorizes someone (an agent) to make decisions on their behalf when they are incapacitated.

Similarly, a 'do-not-resuscitate' (DNR) order on a patient's files means that a doctor is required not to resuscitate if the heart stops functioning. DNR can be regarded as a form of passive euthanasia. They are not controversial, unless they are abused, since they are intended to prevent patient's unnecessary suffering.[3]

Other arguments that bolster the cause of euthanasia as an acceptable option in some situations include the high cost of medical treatment in prolonging life in certain terminal illnesses or medical conditions, especially if the 'extra lease of life' is of poor quality or associated with much suffering or pain. The economic and psychological burden on relatives in such cases can be substantial and sometimes debilitating. It is also a fact that medical science is not an infallible science and there are always limitations in curing certain diseases.

While passive euthanasia has been accorded some semblance of acceptance in certain situations by most people, active euthanasia is in the center of a heated (and often bitter) debate, with vociferous sections of the population in India and elsewhere either strongly advocating or condemning its practice. Despite its unresolved status, active euthanasia is being employed without serious legal difficulties in some countries, for e.g., in the US and Sweden.

ARGUMENTS AGAINST EUTHANASIA

Ezekiel Emanuel[9] argues that there are four major arguments presented by opponents of euthanasia:

1. Not all deaths are painful.
2. Alternatives, such as cessation of active treatment, combined with the use of effective pain relief are available.
3. The distinction between active and passive euthanasia is morally significant.
4. Legalizing euthanasia will place society on a slippery slope which will lead to unacceptable consequences.

As applied to the euthanasia debate, the slippery slope argument claims that the acceptance of certain practices, such as PAS or voluntary euthanasia, will invariably lead to the acceptance or practice of concepts which are currently deemed unacceptable, such as non-voluntary or involuntary euthanasia.[15] Thus, it is argued, in order to prevent these undesirable practices from occurring, we need to resist taking the first step.

The opponents of euthanasia (particularly *active euthanasia*) state that there are moral, religious and ethical objections which cannot be ignored. They argue that no one has the right to take away the life of an individual, not even the individual himself. The concept of 'sanctity of life' is inviolable and doctors having taken an oath (the Hippocratic Oath) 'to preserve life at all costs', cannot justify allowing a patient to die either through active or passive means.

It is also true that doctors are not omniscient; there have been several cases where a patient certified as terminally ill, has survived and led a reasonably fulfilling existence for several years with good palliative care.[16] Even if a patient does have only a few months to live, adequate medical care can in most cases serve to make him reasonably comfortable for the remaining period, till natural death supervenes. The emphasis therefore should be on improving palliative care, rather than improving methods of terminating life. Palliative sedation can be used for short periods with the plan to awaken the patient after a given time period, making terminal sedation a less correct term. The patient is sedated while symptom control is attempted, then the patient is awakened to see if symptom control is achieved. In some cases, palliative sedation is begun with the plan to not attempt to reawaken the patient. One such common example is a patient with an enlarging cancer in the throat that compresses the trachea who does not want intubation or a tracheostomy, so that eventually symptom control is impossible. Instead of experiencing death by suffocation, once symptoms are intolerable, some patients will request palliative sedation to ease their symptoms as death approaches. However, while the intent of palliative sedation is to eliminate pain and suffering, a significant minority of patients 'continue to experience pain, dysphoria, or nausea' that is commonly unknown to providers or families. The *Liverpool Care Pathway for the Dying Patient (LCP)* is a UK care pathway (excluding Wales) covering palliative care options for patients in the final days or hours of life.[17] It has been developed to help doctors and nurses provide quality end-of-life care. The LCP was developed by Royal Liverpool University Hospital and Liverpool's Marie Curie Hospice in the late 1990s for the care of terminally ill cancer patients. Since then, the scope of the LCP has been extended to include all patients deemed dying. While initial reception was positive, it was heavily criticized in the media in 2009 and 2012.[18,19] In July 2013, the Department of Health released a statement which stated that the Health Secretary was likely to recommend that the LCP is phased out over the next 6 to 12 months.[20]

The opponents of euthanasia also raise the issue of a possible cure being found over a period of time for illnesses or medical conditions that are considered incurable today. By terminating the life of a person diagnosed with what is deemed an 'incurable' condition, one may deprive that individual's chances of being cured by a new remedy that may be developed within the next few months or years. A disturbing feature that has come to light in those countries where PAS has been accorded legal sanction is the impatience (and sometimes greed) of the relatives of a dying patient who happens to be affluent, in pressing ahead with 'euthanasia' for their own selfish ends. In such cases the patient's 'right to die' is subtly converted to a 'duty to die', pressure being brought on the hapless victim to accede to the infliction of 'painless death'.[21]

RECENT DEVELOPMENTS

Organizations Advocating Legalization of Euthanasia

There are several nongovernmental organizations that have sprung up over a period of time around the world which advocate the legalization of euthanasia. The following are some of the more prominent organizations.

i. **Exit International:** It is an international registered nonprofit organization advocating legalization of euthanasia with offices in Sydney, Adelaide and Queensland. The average age of Exit members is 75 years. It was previously known as the Voluntary Euthanasia Research Foundation (VERF Inc.).[22] Exit International was founded by Dr Philip Nitschke (Fig. 3.4), a 'right to die' activist from Australia in 1997, after the over-turning of the world's first Voluntary Euthanasia law—the Rights of the Terminally Ill (ROTI) Act. During the ROTI Act, Dr Nitschke became the first physician in the world to administer a legal, lethal, voluntary injection. Recently, South Australian Board of the Medical Board of Australia has recommended suspending his medical license.

ii. **Dignitas:** This is a Swiss organization that helps those with terminal illness and severe physical and mental illnesses to die assisted by qualified doctors and nurses.[23] Additionally, they provide assisted suicide for people, provided that they are of sound judgment and submit to an in-depth medical report prepared by a psychiatrist that establishes the patient's condition, as required by Swiss courts.

    Dignitas was founded in 1998 by Ludwig A Minelli, a Swiss lawyer (Fig. 3.5). Swiss laws provide that assistance to suicide is only illegal if it is motivated by self-interest. As a result, Dignitas seeks to ensure that it acts as a neutral party by proving that aside from nonrecurring fees, they have nothing to gain from the deaths of its clients. The person who wishes to die meets several Dignitas personnel, in addition to an independent doctor, for a private consultation. The independent doctor assesses the evidence provided by the patient

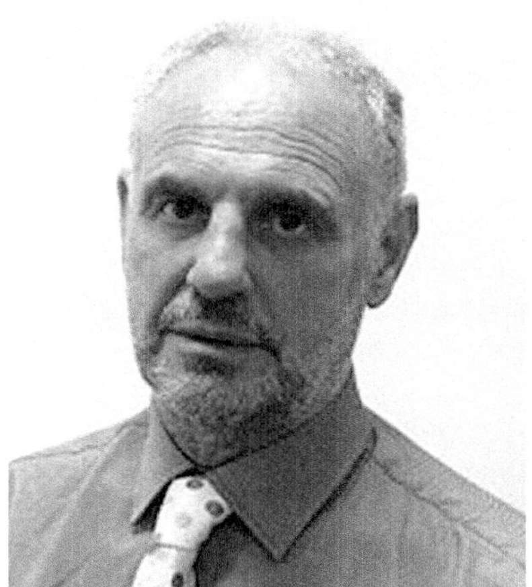

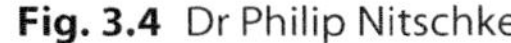

Fig. 3.4 Dr Philip Nitschke

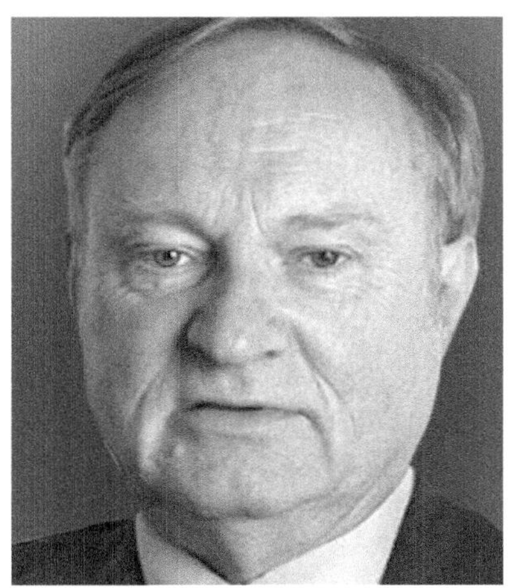

Fig. 3.5 Ludwig A Minelli

and is met on two separate occasions, with a time gap between each of the consultations. Legally admissible proof that the person wishes to die is also created, i.e. a signed affidavit and countersigned by independent witnesses. In cases where a person is physically unable to sign a document, a short video film of the person is made in which they are asked to confirm their identity, that they wish to die and that their decision is made of their own free will, without any form of coercion. This evidence of informed consent remains private and is preserved only for use in any possible legal dispute. Finally, a few minutes before the lethal overdose is provided, the person is once again reminded that taking the overdose will surely kill them. Additionally, they are asked several times whether they want to proceed, or take some time to consider the matter further. This gives the person the opportunity to stop the process. However, if at this point the person states that they are determined to proceed, a lethal overdose is provided.

In general, Dignitas uses the following protocol to assist suicides: an oral dose of an antiemetic drug, followed approximately 1 hour later by a lethal overdose of powdered pentobarbital dissolved in a glass of water or fruit juice. If necessary, the drugs can be ingested via a drinking straw. The pentobarbital overdose depresses the central nervous system, causing the person to become drowsy and fall asleep within 5 minutes of drinking it. Anesthesia progresses to coma as the person's breathing become shallower, followed by respiratory arrest and death which occurs within 30 minutes of ingesting the pentobarbital. In a few cases in 2008, Dignitas used breathing helium gas as a suicide method instead of a pentobarbital overdose. This avoids the need for medical supervision and prescription controlled drugs, and is therefore cheaper.

Even though Dignitas is mainly meant for Swiss individuals, it is open to others from around the world to use its services. This has led to a controversial influx of tourists from other countries such as the UK, resulting in what is referred to by some as '*suicide tourism*'.[24]

Euthanasia Devices

A *euthanasia device* is a machine designed and constructed to allow an individual to die quickly without pain. Early devices to help terminally ill people die without prolonged pain actually consisted of methods of administering lethal doses of drugs, such as barbiturates. These could be operated by the person wishing to die, or by another person, such as a physician. Subsequently, the method of inert gas asphyxiation using nitrogen or some other irrespirable gas via a mask became popular. It was only with the intervention of 'right to die' campaigners such as Dr Jack Kevorkian (Box 3.2)[25] that specialized devices began to be designed and constructed.

i. **Thanatron (Death Machine):** This device (Fig. 3.6) invented by Dr Jack Kevorkian, involved an individual pushing a button that released drugs or chemicals that would end his or her own life.[26] The drugs/chemicals would be delivered mechanically through an intravenous (IV) line. The device (named '*Thanatron*' by Kevorkian after the Greek God of death) had three canisters or bottles mounted on a metal frame, about 6 inches (150 mm) wide by 18 inches (460 mm) high. Each bottle had a syringe that connected to a single IV line in the person's arm. The first bottle contained normal saline, the second, a barbiturate (usually sodium thiopental), and the third a lethal mixture of potassium chloride which immediately stopped the heart, and pancuronium bromide, a muscle relaxant to prevent spasms during the dying process. In the limited number of cases that it was used, the usual procedure was for Kevorkian or an assistant to begin the saline solution flow, while the person who wants to die would have to deliver the barbiturates himself or herself by throwing a switch, pushing a button or pulling a string. After that, either a timer or a mechanical device triggered by the person's falling arm as the drugs take effect starts the lethal drug flowing. The idea is for the deadly chemicals to enter the bloodstream only after the person is asleep. Death usually occurred within 2–3 minutes.

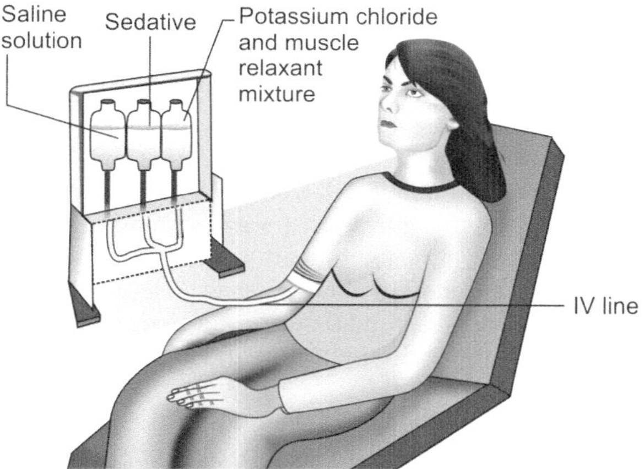

Fig. 3.6 Thanatron

ii. **Mercitron (Mercy Machine):** When Kevorkian found it difficult to continue using Thanatron, mainly because of relative inaccessibility to the drugs/chemicals required, he came up with another device that employed a gas mask fed by a canister of carbon monoxide which he called '*Mercitron*' (Fig. 3.7). This became necessary because Kevorkian's medical license had

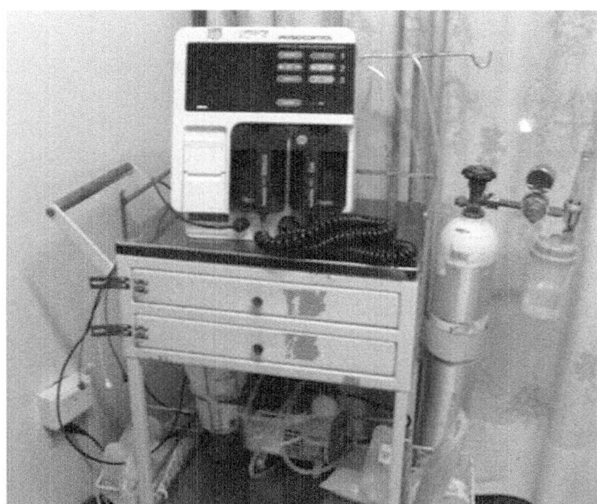

Fig. 3.7 Mercitron

Box 3.2 Jack Kevorkian

Jack Kevorkian (Fig. 3.8) was born in Pontiac, Michigan, US to Armenian immigrants. In 1945, he graduated from Pontiac Central High School with honors at the age of 17. In 1952, he graduated from the University of Michigan Medical School. He completed residency training in anatomical and clinical pathology and briefly conducted research on blood transfusion. Unable to function effectively as a hospital pathologist, Kevorkian left the active practice of medicine and for a time was even homeless.

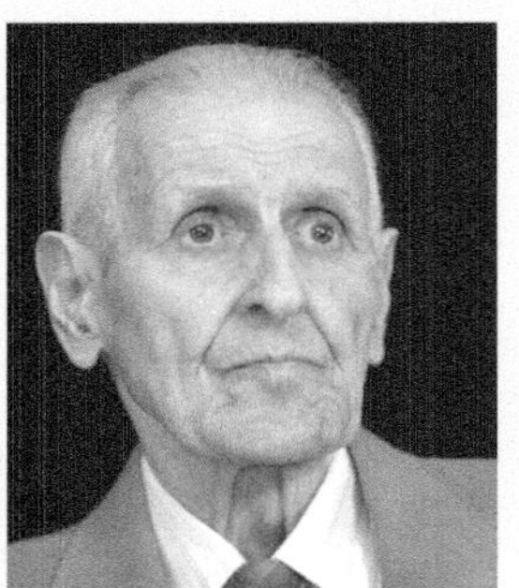

Fig. 3.8 Dr Jack Kevorkian

As a pathologist at Pontiac General Hospital, Kevorkian experimented with transfusing blood from the recently deceased into live patients. He drew blood from dead bodies recently brought into the hospital and transferred it successfully into the bodies of hospital staff members. Kevorkian thought that the US military might be interested in using this technique to help wounded soldiers during a battle, but the Pentagon was not interested.

In the 1980s, Kevorkian wrote a series of articles for the German journal, Medicine and Law that laid out his thinking on the ethics of euthanasia. In 1987, Kevorkian started advertising in Detroit newspapers as a physician consultant for 'death counseling'. His first public assisted suicide of Janet Adkins, a 54-year-old woman diagnosed with Alzheimer's disease took place in 1990. Charges of murder were dropped on 13th December 1990, as there were, at that time, no laws in Michigan regarding assisted suicide. In 1991, however, the State of Michigan revoked Kevorkian's medical license and made it clear that given his actions, he was no longer permitted to practice medicine or to work with patients.

Contd...

Contd...

According to his lawyer Geoffrey Fieger, Kevorkian assisted in the deaths of 130 terminally ill people between 1990 and 1998. In each of these cases, the individuals themselves allegedly took the final action which resulted in their own deaths. Kevorkian allegedly assisted only by attaching the individual to a euthanasia device '*Thanatron*' that he had devised and constructed. The individual then pushed a button which released the drugs or chemicals that would end his or her own life.

In Kevorkian's view, a patient did not have to be terminally ill to be assisted in committing suicide, but did need to be suffering. However, he has said that he declined four out of every five assisted suicide requests, on the grounds that the patient needed more treatment or medical records had to be checked. Kevorkian was tried 4 times for assisting suicides between May 1994 to June 1997. With the assistance of Fieger, he was acquitted 3 times. The 4th trial ended in a mistrial. The trials helped Kevorkian gain public support for his cause. On 22nd November 1998, Kevorkian allowed the airing of a videotape he made on 17th September 1998 which was broadcast on CBS News '60 Minutes'. It depicted the voluntary euthanasia of Thomas Youk, 52, who was in the final stages of amyotrophic lateral sclerosis. After Youk provided his full informed consent, Kevorkian himself administered him a lethal injection. This was highly significant, as all his earlier clients had reportedly completed the process themselves. During the videotape, Kevorkian dared the authorities to try to convict him or stop him from carrying out mercy killings. Youk's family described the lethal injection as humane, not murder.

On 26th March 1999, Kevorkian was charged with second-degree murder and the delivery of a controlled substance. Since Kevorkian's license to practice medicine had been revoked 8 years back, he was not legally allowed to possess the controlled substance. Kevorkian discharged his attorneys and proceeded through the trial representing himself, a decision he later regretted. Inexperienced in law but persisting in his efforts to represent himself, he encountered great difficulty in presenting his evidence and arguments. He was not able to call any witnesses to the stand as the Judge did not deem the testimony of any of his witnesses relevant. After a 2-day trial, the Jury found Kevorkian guilty of second-degree homicide. He was sentenced to 10–25 years in prison and was sent to a prison in Coldwater, Michigan. After his conviction, Kevorkian was denied parole repeatedly until 2007. Reportedly terminally ill with Hepatitis C which he contracted while doing research on blood transfusions, Kevorkian was expected to die within a year in May 2006. After applying for a pardon, he was finally paroled for good behavior on 1st June 2007. He had spent 8 years and 2½ months in prison.

Kevorkian gave a number of lectures upon his release at universities such as the University of Florida, Nova Southeastern University and the University of California and Los Angeles. 'You Don't Know Jack', a film based on Kevorkian's life, premiered in April 2010 on HBO, and at the Ziegfeld Theater in New York City. Kevorkian walked the red carpet alongside Al Pacino, who portrayed him in the film. Pacino received Emmy and Golden Globe awards for his portrayal and personally thanked Kevorkian, who was in the audience, upon receiving both of these awards. Kevorkian stated that both the film and Pacino's performance 'brought tears to my eyes—and I lived through it'.

Kevorkian was hospitalized on 18th May 2011 with kidney problems and pneumonia. His condition grew rapidly worse and he died from thrombosis on 3rd June 2011, eight days after his 83rd birthday at William Beaumont Hospital in Royal Oak, Michigan. There were no artificial attempts to keep him alive and his death was painless. He was buried in White Chapel Memorial Park Cemetery in Troy, Michigan. The epitaph on Kevorkian's tombstone reads, 'He sacrificed himself for everyone's rights'.

been revoked after the first two deaths he had assisted and he could no longer have legal access to the substances required for the '*Thanatron*'. It was a rudimentary device consisting of a canister of carbon monoxide attached to a face mask with a tube. A valve had to be released to start the gas flowing. Depending on the person's disability, a makeshift handle was attached to the valve to make it easier to turn. In a few cases, with the valve in the 'open' position, a clip or clothespin would be clamped on the tubing. Pulling it off would allow the gas to flow. By Kevorkian's estimates, this method took 10 minutes or longer. Sometimes, he encouraged people to take sedatives or muscle relaxants to keep them calm as they breathed deeply of the gas.

iii. **Suicide Bag:** The basic principle of autoeuthanasia by anoxia, using a '*Suicide Bag*' was first described in a book Final Exit by Derek Humphry (Fig. 3.9) in 1991.[27] The original bag was devised using helium, by the NuTech group—engineers, physicians, divers and others, a small number of people first assembled in 1998 under the leadership of three 'right to die' activists—John Hofsess, Philip Nitschke and Derek Humphry. Inhalation of an enclosed inert gas is lethal because it flushes oxygen from the body, but released into the open air, it quickly disperses and hence is safe for others. It is neither flammable nor explosive. Exclusive inhalation of the gas is achieved in Humphry's book by enclosing the head in the suicide bag (nothing but a strong, clear plastic bag of dimensions 36 × 22 inches, secured around the neck by a strap) into which the inert gas is fed by plastic tubing. Later, a product available from the Canadian Right to Die Society called the 'Exit Bag' which has a sewn-in Velcro collar and fastened-in, flexible plastic tubing was substituted in place of the conventional 'suicide bag' (Figs 3.10A and B).[28]

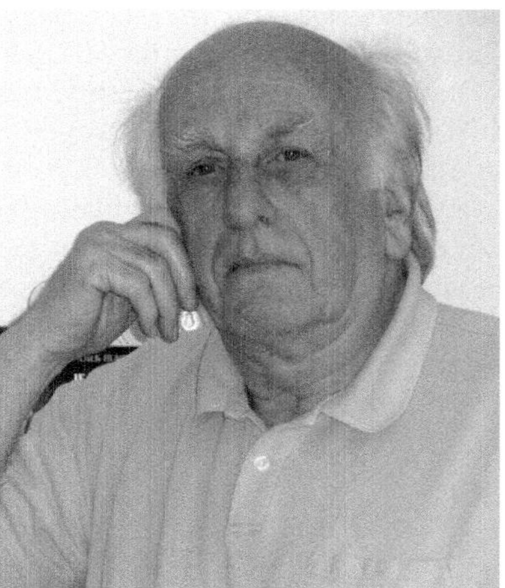

Fig. 3.9 Derek Humphry

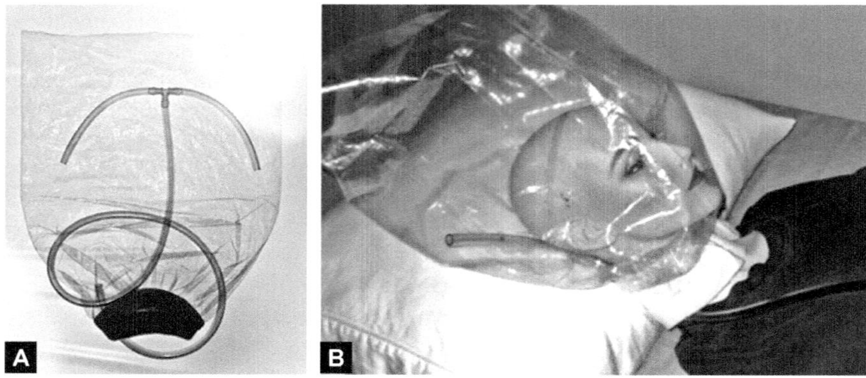

Figs 3.10A and B (A) Exit bag; (B) Exit bag *in situ*

iv. **Deliverance Machine:** This was invented by Dr Philip Nitschke. It consisted of a notebook computer and software titled '*Deliverance*' which would ask the patient a series of questions and automatically administers a lethal injection of barbiturates, if the correct answers are made.[29] Even if it would have been legally possible for a doctor to administer a lethal injection, Dr Nitschke preferred that the patient initiate the process. The machine also allowed a doctor to leave the patient with the family when the button was pushed. The machine was used legally under the Australian Northern Territory's Rights of the Terminally Ill (ROTI) Act 1995, which was later overturned.

v. **Exit International's Euthanasia Device:** The Exit International euthanasia device was invented by Dr Philip Nitschke in 2008. It used an ordinary barbecue gas bottle filled with nitrogen, a plastic suicide bag and some plastic tubing with one end attached to the gas canister and the other fixed inside the bag by a tie held by adhesive tape. In December 2008, Nitschke released details of the euthanasia device to the media. His new device/method was a modification of the 'Exit Bag plus helium' method described in *The Peaceful Pill Handbook*.[30] Instead of using a pre-packaged disposable cylinder of helium, he suggested filling purchased empty LPG cylinders (rated at 3300 kPa) with compressed nitrogen and then regulating this with a jet assembly to give a flow of around 10 liters per minute into the standard plastic 'Exit Bag'. Nitschke called it 'flawless' and 'undetectable', saying the new process uses ordinary household products available from hardware stores. Inhaling the pure nitrogen, patients lose consciousness immediately (in about 12 seconds) and die a few minutes later.

GLOBAL SCENARIO

Some countries have virtually legalized active euthanasia if performed by a physician under strict guidelines *(physician-assisted suicide)*, for e.g., the Netherlands (Holland), Belgium and Luxembourg (Fig. 3.11).[31]

The Netherlands practices physician-assisted suicide (PAS) openly ever since the Royal Dutch Medical Association officially endorsed it in 1984 and the

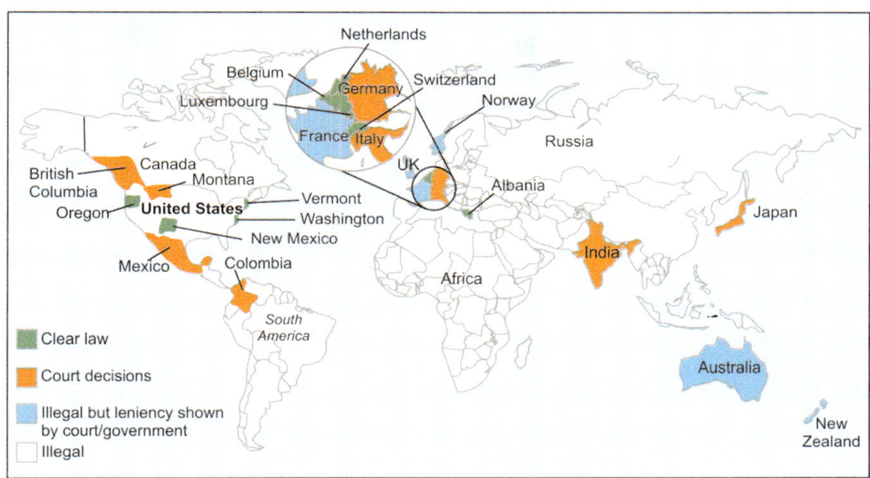

Fig. 3.11 Global status of euthanasia

Parliament approved the practice, provided it was done within a framework of specified guidelines. PAS is legal under specific circumstances and for children over the age of 12 years with parental consent (infants too can be euthanized, and that doctors will not be prosecuted if they act within the guidelines). It also allows doctors to euthanize dementia patients, if they believe the person is experiencing 'unbearable suffering,' although few cases are done practically.[32,33]

In Belgium, PAS is legal for people over the age of 18 years. About 80% of the cases involve terminally ill cancer patients and paraplegic or quadriplegic accident victims. In order to qualify for euthanasia, a patient must suffer from an incurable (not necessarily terminal) condition and experience unbearable physical or psychological pain. In the recent past, several cases of Belgians who were not terminally ill were euthanized—including 43-year-old deaf twins who were going blind, and a patient with childhood abuse and a failed sex-change operation. The government is further considering extending it to seriously ill children and adults with early dementia. Presently, people now can make a written declaration that they wish to be euthanized if their health deteriorates, but the request is only valid for 5 years and they must be in an irreversible coma. The new proposal would abolish the time limit and the requirement the patient be in a coma, whereby someone who is diagnosed with Alzheimer's can be put to death years later in the future.[34]

Elsewhere in Europe, euthanasia is only legal in Luxembourg. Assisted suicide is also allowed in Switzerland. In Mexico, laws allow the terminally ill to refuse further treatment and medication to extend life. France and Canada are also contemplating to legalize PAS for those suffering from an incurable or terminal illness.[32-34]

Some parts of the world have enacted legal statutes, for e.g., The Death with Dignity Act (1994) of the State of Oregon, US, and The Northern Territory of Australia which was however overturned by the Australian Senate in 1997. The state of Oregon accepts assisted suicide requests for residents aged 18 or over with a terminal illness. Initiative 1000 (I-1000) of 2008 established the US state of Washington's Death with Dignity Act which legalizes PAS with certain restrictions. Passage of this initiative made Washington the second US state to permit terminally ill patients to determine the time of their own death. In Montana, a physician can raise a defense of consent if charged with assisting suicide through a trial court ruling on 6th December 2009 in the case of *Baxter vs. Montana*.[35] The Attorney General of the state of Montana sought an appeal from the Montana Supreme Court, but the court, by a decision of five to two affirmed the lower court's ruling on the state law. The court did, however, limit the scope of the decision by not determining if the state's constitution protected the right. In May 2013, the Vermont Legislature passed the Patient Choice and Control at End of Life Act. The Governor signed it into law.[36] The law is based on, but is less restrictive than the Oregon model. In the rest of the US, actions that give the appearance of deliberate euthanasia rather than pain control will lead to criminal prosecution as a homicide, as well as loss of medical license. Some states have outlawed PAS specifically, whereas in others it would be pursued under negligent homicide or a variety of criminal charges.

CURRENT LEGAL STATUS IN INDIA

While euthanasia is not explicitly stated as a criminal offence in the Indian Penal Code (IPC), it is generally accepted that it is covered either under the offence of attempted suicide (Sec. 309 IPC), or abetment of suicide (Sec. 306 IPC).[1,37]

However, judicial opinion acknowledges that euthanasia is a 'gray area' in Indian criminal law. This unsettled status has been brought into stark focus in several past cases, for e.g., *P. Rathinam vs. Union of India* (1994), and *Smt. Gian Kaur vs. State of Punjab* (1996).[38,39] As per the Supreme Court's view, passive voluntary euthanasia can be visualized as a fundamental right protected by Article 21 which assures the right to privacy. Since such right to privacy can be said to encompass the right of a patient to refuse lifesaving medical treatment. In other words, the right to 'personal liberty' as guaranteed by Article 21 of the constitution includes the freedom to die with dignity.

Passive euthanasia is now *legal* in India. On 7th March 2011, the Supreme Court of India legalized passive euthanasia by means of the withdrawal of life support to patients in a permanent vegetative state provided the High Court's permission is obtained in case of incompetent patient. For incompetent patients, the Supreme Court has mandated the High Court to provide sanction after seeking assistance from a committee of three medical experts and consult the close relations or the next friend of the patient and the State. Hence, the role of a High Court is described as that of '*parens patriae*' (Latin, 'parent of the nation').[40] The decision was made as part of the verdict in a case involving Aruna Shanbaug (Box 3.3), who has been in a vegetative state for 37 years at King Edward Memorial Hospital, Mumbai.[41] The Court rejected active euthanasia by means of lethal injection. In the absence of a law regulating euthanasia in India, the court stated that its decision becomes the law of the land until the Indian Parliament enacts a suitable law. Active euthanasia (voluntary or otherwise) is unambiguously viewed as a crime under Sec. 302 (murder) or 304 (culpable homicide not amounting to murder) of the IPC, along with PAS under Sec. 306 IPC, though convictions have

Box 3.3 Case of Aruna Shanbaug

Aruna Shanbaug (Fig. 3.12) from Haldipur, Uttara Kannada, Karnataka was working as a nurse at King Edward Memorial Hospital, Parel, Mumbai. She was planning to get married to a junior doctor in the hospital. On the night of 27th November 1973, she was sexually assaulted by a ward boy while she was changing clothes in the hospital basement. He choked her with a dog chain and sodomized her. The asphyxiation cut off oxygen supply to her brain, resulting in brainstem contusion injury and cervical cord injury apart from leaving her cortically blind. The police case was registered as a case of robbery and attempted murder on account of the concealment of anal intercourse by the doctors under the instructions of the Dean of KEM, perhaps to avoid the social rejection of the victim and her impending marriage. The perpetrator was caught and convicted and served two concurrent 7-year sentences for assault and robbery, neither for rape or sexual molestation, nor for the 'unnatural sexual offence' (which could have got him a 10-year sentence by itself).

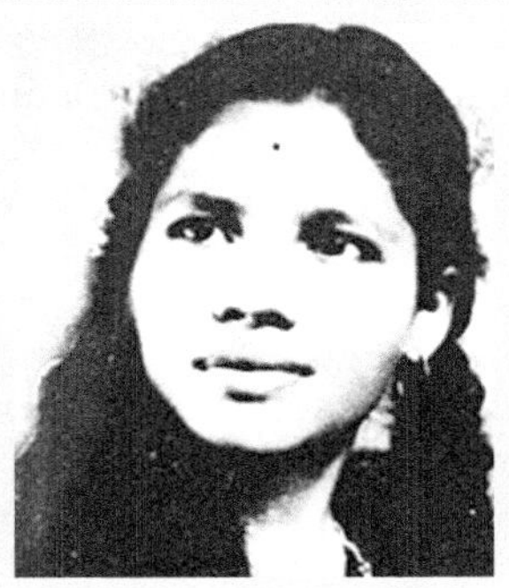

Fig. 3.12 Aruna Shanbaug

Since the assault, she has been in a vegetative state. On 17th December 2010, the Supreme Court of India (SC) while admitting the plea to end the life made by journalist Pinki Virani, sought a report on her medical condition from the hospital in Mumbai and the Government of Maharashtra. On 24th January 2011, after she had been in this status for 37 years, the SC responded to the plea for euthanasia filed by Pinki Virani, by setting up a medical panel to examine her. The three-member medical committee subsequently checked upon Aruna and concluded that she met 'most of the criteria of being in a permanent vegetative state'. On 7th March 2011, the SC in its landmark judgment turned down the mercy killing petition, but allowed passive euthanasia under 'exceptional circumstances' and laid down guidelines for it. According to these guidelines, passive euthanasia involves the withdrawing of treatment or food that would allow the patient to live.

not been brought so far against any individual in India for the commission of such an 'offence'.[1]

The Law Commission made recommendation to the government for a 'separate legislation' to deal with withdrawal of life support to those terminally ill and had the right to refuse treatment. The Commission prepared a draft '*Medical Treatment of Terminally-ill Patients (Protection of Patients and Medical Practitioners) Bill, 2006*' for the government's consideration which has not yet been passed. The Commission is of the view that 'competent' adult patient who can take an informed decision, has the right to insist that there should be no invasive medical treatment by way of artificial life sustaining measures. If a patient communicates his/her decision to the doctor concerned, it would be binding on the doctor. But the doctor has to be satisfied that the patient has taken an informed decision based upon his/her free will. However, if the patient is not in a position to take healthcare decisions due to an irreversible coma or is in a persistent vegetative state, the doctors or relatives should get the clearance from the High Court for withdrawing or withholding the life sustaining treatment. The Commission's proposals also include protection from prosecution for both patient's relatives and their doctors. The Commission said those below 16 years of age are 'incompetent' to take a decision without the permission of an adult next of kin. It suggested provisions for protection of medical practitioners and others who act according to the wishes of the competent patient or the order of the High Court from criminal or civil action. The recommendation is part of the Commission's latest report in which it changed some of the provisions of a draft bill that dealt with this issue.[1,42]

Recently, however, the government dropped plans for the implementation of the Bill because it is not in favor of 'mercy killings'. The government is of the opinion that effective pain management and treatment of patients with cancer and other terminal illnesses is now possible and so is rehabilitation of patients with spinal injuries, hence withdrawal of life support is not required. Suffering is a state of mind that varied from person to person and depended on various environmental and social factors, and therefore it is difficult to quantify. Moreover, it would be impossible for doctors to certify with certainty that the disease was incurable and the patient would remain permanently an invalid.[43]

RECOMMENDATIONS

The following is a list of current trends and some important recommendations:

i. Euthanasia must be considered as a separate and distinct entity, and must never be confused with suicide. The right terminology may be 'end-of-life decisions' and not euthanasia. Terms such as 'physician-assisted suicide' which can be misleading must be substituted with more acceptable terminology, for e.g., physician-assisted euthanasia. In the debate revolving around euthanasia, religion and moral tenets must not be allowed to take center stage. The issue must be debated purely on ethical, psychological and scientific lines.

ii. Euthanasia must, as far as possible, be discussed from the actual sufferer's point of view taking into consideration today's emphasis on patient's rights as being superior to physician's rights or society's beliefs. The person should have the right to die with dignity and to die without suffering, just as people have the right to live with dignity.

iii. The time honored conviction of the importance of preserving life at all costs must make way for the emerging view that 'quality of life' is an issue that must be incorporated in all cases where the life of a person is prolonged indefinitely by artificial means.

iv. To force a patient to be kept alive in a vegetative state when medical opinion is certain that there is no chance of recovery, is cruel both on the patient and on his/her family and friends. The law must, therefore, clearly allow for euthanasia—both active and passive—in such situations. There must, however, be very strict safeguards to ensure that the provision is not misused by people, who may benefit from the death of the patient.

CONCLUSION

Death must be viewed as the inevitable consequence of life and hence there is no point in prolonging it using artificial life-support systems. A competent adult patient should have the right to voice his/her decision for withdrawing of artificial life-sustaining measures/treatment and such decision should be 'informed decision' based on free exercise of his/her will.

Although, the Supreme Court has legalized passive euthanasia—withdrawing or withholding life support in the context of incurable illness, the government is not in favor of legalizing any form of euthanasia, assisted suicide or hastening of death through withdrawal of treatment or life support.

While the debate on euthanasia is bound to rage for some more time, and there will always be proponents and opponents, it is desirable for physicians to understand current concepts and rectify certain well entrenched misconceptions. This is especially true for a country such as India which is composed of diverse religions, communities, traditions, customs and beliefs. It is high time that India legalizes PAS and be a part of the handful of nations that allows euthanasia on grounds of compassion and maintaining the dignity of the individual.

REFERENCES

1. Passive euthanasia - A relook. Available from: http://164.100.47.132/paperlaidfiles/LAWANDJUSTICE/report241.pdf
2. Letellier P. History and definition of a word. Euthanasia. Vol. 1. Strasbourg: Council of Europe publishing; 2003. p. 13-24.
3. Reynolds NC, Reynolds A, Berman SA, Talavera F, Caselli RJ, Benbadis SR. End of life: Medicolegal issues. Medicolegal Neurology, Special issues. Available from: http://www.sonesp.com.br/novo/wp-content/uploads/Medicolegal_neurology2.pdf.
4. Pillay VV. Euthanasia. Textbook of forensic medicine and toxicology, 16th edn. Hyderabad: Paras medical publisher; 2011. p. 42-47.
5. Verhagen E, Sauer PJJ. The Groningen protocol - euthanasia in severely ill newborns. *N Engl J Med* 2005; 352: 959-62.
6. de Jong TH. Deliberate termination of life of newborns with spina bifida, a critical reappraisal. *Childs Nerv Syst* 2008; 24: 13-28.
7. Kon AA. Neonatal euthanasia is unsupportable: the Groningen protocol should be abandoned. *Theor Med Bioeth* 2007; 28: 453-63.
8. Historical timeline - euthanasia. Available from: http://euthanasia.procon.org/view.timeline.php?timelineID=000022.
9. Emanuel EJ, Battin MP. What are the potential cost savings from legalizing physician-assisted suicide? *N Engl J Med* 1998; 339: 167-72.
10. Johnson L. Euthanasia, double effect, and proportionality. *Monash Bioeth Rev* 2002; 21: 23-34.
11. John Bodkin Adams. Available from: http://en.wikipedia.org/wiki/John_Bodkin_Adams.
12. Kinney HC, Korein J, Panigrahy A, Dikkes P, Goode R. Neuropathological findings in the brain of Karen Ann Quinlan - the role of the thalamus in the persistent vegetative state. *N Eng J Med* 1994; 330: 1469-75.
13. Cranford R. Facts, lies, and videotapes: The permanent vegetative state and the sad case of Terri Schiavo. *J Law Med Ethics* 2005. p. 363-71.
14. Damato AN. Advance directives for the elderly: A survey. *NJ Med* 1993; 90: 215-20.
15. Wright W. Historical analogies, slippery slopes, and the question of euthanasia. *J Law Med Ethics* 2000; 28: 176-86.
16. Kennedy BJ. Communicating with patients about advanced cancer. *JAMA* 1998; 280: 1403-04.
17. Wilkinson S, Ellershaw J. Care of the dying: A pathway to excellence. Oxford [Oxfordshire]: Oxford University Press; 2003.
18. Stevens J. A pathway to euthanasia? Family revive father doctors ruled wasn't worth saving. Daily Mail. 2012 Oct 12.

19. Adams S. Hospitals letting patients die to save money. The Daily Telegraph. 2012 July 8.
20. BBC News. Liverpool Care Pathway should be phased out. 2013 July 13.
21. Konishi E, Davis AJ. The right-to-die and the duty-to-die: Perceptions of nurses in the West and in Japan. *Int Nurs Rev* 2001; 48: 17-28.
22. Exit International (Assisted Suicide/ Voluntary Euthanasia). Available from: http://www.exitinternational.net/.
23. Dignitas. Available from: http://www.dignitas.ch/index.php?lang=en.
24. BBC News. More Britons seeking suicide help. 2008 Nov 17.
25. Jack Kevorkian. Available from: http://en.wikipedia.org/wiki/Jack_Kevorkian.
26. Frontline. The Kevorkian Verdict: The Thanatron. 1996 May. Available from: http://www.pbs.org/wgbh/pages/frontline/kevorkian/aboutk/thanatronblurb.html.
27. Humphry D. Final exit: The practicalities of self-deliverance and assisted suicide for the dying. California: Hemlock Society; 1991.
28. Schön CA, Ketterer T. Asphyxial suicide by inhalation of helium inside a plastic bag. *Am J Forensic Med Pathol* 2007; 28: 364-67.
29. Lopez KJ. Euthanasia sets sail. An interview with Philip Nitschke, the other 'Dr. Death.' National Review. 2001 June 5.
30. Nitschke P, Stewart F. The peaceful pill handbook. Michigan, USA: Exit International US Ltd; 2007.
31. Smartt U. Euthanasia and the law. *Crim Law Justice Wkly* 2009; 173: 100.
32. Legality of euthanasia. Available from: http://en.wikipedia.org/wiki/Legality_of_euthanasia
33. Johnson D. Legalized euthanasia. Available from: http://www.infoplease.com/spot/euthanasia1.html.
34. Cheng M. Belgium moves to make euthanasia legal for children, dementia patients. Available from: http://life.nationalpost.com/2013/10/31/belgium-moves-to-make-euthanasia-legal-for-children-dementia-patients/.
35. Johnson K. Montana court to rule on assisted suicide case. The New York Times. 2009 Aug 31.
36. Hallenbeck T. Vermont governor signs end-of-life bill. The Burlington (Vt.) Free Press. 2013 May 20.
37. The Indian Penal Code. Available from: http://mha.nic.in/pdfs/IPC1860.pdf.
38. Jaswal PS, Jaswal N. Human rights and the law. New Delhi: APH Publishing Corpn; 1996.
39. Srivastava L. Law and medicine. New Delhi: Universal Law Publishing Co Pvt Ltd; 2010.
40. The Hindu. India joins select nations in legalizing 'passive euthanasia.' 2011 March 7. Available from: http://www.thehindu.com/news/national/india-joins-select-nations-in-legalising-passive-euthanasia/article1516973.ece
41. Virani P. Aruna's story: The true account of a rape and its aftermath. Bangalore: Penguin Books; 2000.
42. Law Commission favors law on passive euthanasia. 2013 March 14. Available from: http://news.oneindia.in/2013/03/14/law-commission-for-comprehesive-law-on-passive-euthanasia-1171737.html
43. Choudhuri N. Indian government shelves plans for mercy killing law. *BMJ* 2013; 347: f5218.

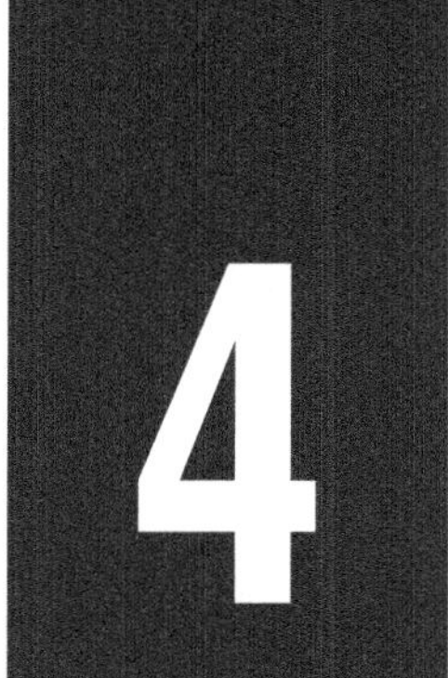

Age of Child: Legal Perspective

Anil Kohli

'There can be no keener revelation of a society's soul than the way it treats its children.'
Nelson Mandela (Nobel laureate, politician and philanthropist)

ABSTRACT

Indian laws (Codes and Acts) which define 'child' with regard to its age are different in many of the existing laws. Gender inequality also exists in some laws with regard to the age of 'child'. The study of the various Indian laws makes it evident that experts may be asked to determine the age of the 'child' not only with regard to 18 years of age but for many varied ages, and experts should be well versed in scientific knowledge for estimating these varied ages. This chapter explains various legal provisions in India defining the age of the child for the purpose of protection and realizing the rights of children.

Keywords: Age, child, laws, Acts, marriage, employment, age of consent, sexual intercourse, medical treatment.

INTRODUCTION

The law, policy and practice of child welfare have undergone significant changes from an historical perspective. In the 18th century, authority and control over the child was important. It was an established common law doctrine that the father had absolute rights over his children. After this, the welfare principle emerged, and finally the concept of children's rights. Today, nearly all cultures share the view that the younger the child, the more physically and psychologically vulnerable he/she becomes. Age limits are now regulating children's activities like when they can give consent, when they can work or when they can marry.[1] Therefore, the definition of child, i.e. the age till the human being would be said to be a child, becomes very important. But the definition of child differs from activity to activity and from country to country.

Laws have fixed ages up to which benefits, concessions or protection should be granted to the child. The age of the child will thus determine whether he/she will be considered to be a 'child' under that particular law. The role of the medicolegal expert will be all the more important because he/she may be asked to determine the age of the child in order for the law to assess whether the child qualifies for benefits or protection under the law. Medicolegal experts need to have knowledge of various laws in India where the age of the child is defined, as they may be required to determine the age of the child in such cases.

The Census of India, (2011) has collected single year age data with regard to the number of children for every year of age. Table 4.1 highlights the number of children in various age groups and their percentage of the total population in India.[2] The number of persons in the age group of 0–18 years is 472.1 million comprising 39% of the population. It is quite evident that children form quite a large and important chunk of the Indian population and their special needs and the support required by them has to be addressed by the lawmakers of India.

DEFINITION OF A CHILD

The Oxford dictionary describes a child as a young human being below the age of puberty or below the legal age of majority.[3] Biologically, childhood is the stage between infancy and adulthood.

The word 'child' has been used in law as a term denoting relationship, as a term indicating capacity and as a term of special protection. Underlying these alternative specifications are very different concepts about the child. Thus, if a child is considered a burden, then he/she needs maintenance and support; if a child has temporary disabilities, then he/she needs special treatment and special discrimination; if a child is considered especially vulnerable, then he/she needs special protection; and if children are considered as resources for the country's development, then they need special nurturing and advancement.[1] Hence, in many laws, though the word 'child' is not present, the law is indirectly specifying the age of 'child' for that particular law.

The Convention on the Rights of the Child (CRC) is the first legally binding international instrument to incorporate the full range of human rights—civil, cultural, economic, political and social rights. In 1989, world leaders decided that children needed a special convention just for them because people under 18-year-old often need special care and protection that adults do not. The convention was adopted by the UN General assembly in 1989 and came into force in 1990. India ratified the CRC in December 1992.

Article 1 of the CRC defines child as 'every human being below the age of 18 years, unless under the law applicable to the child, majority is attained earlier'. The Convention clearly specifies the upper age limit for childhood as 18 years, but recognizes that majority may be obtained at an earlier age under laws applicable to the child. The upper limit on childhood is specified as an age of 'childhood' rather than 'majority', recognizing that in most legal systems, a child can acquire full legal capacity with regard to various matters at different ages. Thus, while

Table 4.1 Number of children in various age groups (Census of India, 2011)

Age group (years)	*Number (millions)*	*Percentage (%) of total population*
0–4	112.8	9.3
5–9	126.9	10.5
10–14	132.7	11
15–18	99.7	8.2

the Convention defines a 'child' as every human being below the age of 18 years, it allows for minimum ages to be set, under different circumstances, balancing the evolving capacities of the child with the State's obligation to provide special protection.[4] Thus individual countries have the discretion to determine by law whether childhood ceases at 12 years, 14 years, 16 years or whatever age found appropriate.

'Age of majority' or legal age pertains solely to the acquisition of control over one's person, decisions and actions, and the correlative termination of the legal authority and responsibility of the parents (or guardians) over the child's person and affairs. One need not have attained the age of majority to have permission to exercise certain rights and responsibilities. Some ages of license to do certain things are actually higher than the age of majority, like purchasing alcohol and minimum age for marriage for boys in India. The age of majority is the threshold of adulthood as it is conceptualized (and recognized or declared) in law. It is the chronological moment when minors cease to legally be considered children and assume control over their persons, actions, and decisions, thereby terminating the legal control and legal responsibilities of their parents or guardian over and for them. Most countries set majority at 18 years of age. But in many countries the age of majority varies from 15 years to 21 years of age, depending on the country.[5] Table 4.2 lists some countries where age of majority is not 18 years.

In the United States, the age of majority is 18 years in most of the states, except for the states of Alabama (19 years), Nebraska (19 years or upon marriage), Pennsylvania (21 years) and Mississippi (21 years).

DISCUSSION

Indian legislation has defined minimum ages under various laws related to the protection of child rights. Article 15(3) of the Indian Constitution permits the State to make special provisions for women and children. Special enactments made for the benefit of children cannot be struck down on the ground of discrimination.

In some cases, the age defining a child is that from the time of its conception, i.e. even before its birth. Indian Succession Act, 1925 under Sec. 20 gives the right to property to a child in the womb whose parent dies before the child is born alive giving such a child the same rights to inherit as if he/she had been born before the death of the parent. Similarly, the Transfer of Property Act, 1882 under Sec. 13 gives similar rights to a child in the womb.

Table 4.2 Countries where age of majority is not 18 years

Age	*Countries*
15 years	Indonesia, Iraq
16 years	Cuba, Guatemala, Bolivia, Colombia, Kyrgyzstan, Uzbekistan
17 years	Tajikistan, Gibraltar, East Timor
19 years	Algeria, Botswana, Canada, South Korea
20 years	Thailand, Tunisia, Taiwan
21 years	Azerbaijan, Bahrain, Chad, Egypt, Honduras, Namibia, Swaziland, Zambia, Kuwait

There are some cases where the age of a child is a recommendation and is not legally binding. According to Article 21(a) of the Indian Constitution, all children between the ages of six to fourteen should be provided with free and compulsory education. According to Article 45 of the Indian Constitution, State should provide early childhood care and education to all children below the age of six. Article 51(k) of the Indian Constitution states that the parents/guardians of children between the ages of six and fourteen should provide them with opportunities for education. The Constitution of India under the 86th Amendment Act 2002, Sec. 2 suggests that the State shall provide free and compulsory education to all children of the age of six to fourteen years in such a manner as the State may by law decide. So, till the States made suitable laws, these rights would not come into existence.

In August 2009, seven years after the 86th Amendment of the Constitution of India, 'The Right of Children to Free and Compulsory Education Act, 2009' was notified in the official gazette and made applicable to the whole of India (except in the State of Jammu and Kashmir). As a result of this consequential legislation, the fundamental right under Article 21(a) of the Indian Constitution got legal sanctity.

Legal ages defined for children in the Indian Penal Code, 1860, Criminal Procedure Code, 1973 and Indian Evidence Act, 1872 are tabulated in Table 4.3.[6] Even though the word 'child' has not been mentioned in some of these laws, these laws are defining 'child' when one takes into consideration the definition of 'child' discussed at the beginning of this chapter.

As is evident from Table 4.3, Indian law recognizes different ages of 'child' for various matters. Hence, for the purpose of criminal liability the law considers a person a 'child' till the age of seven years and holds the view that such a 'child' is not capable of criminal offence. For offences like abandonment or acts done in good faith for benefit of 'child', the age of 'child' is 12 years. In matters like power to compel restoration of abducted female 'child' or abetment of suicide of 'child', the age of 'child' is 18 years. With regard to the age for the male and female child, some Indian laws make a distinction, which goes against the spirit of the CRC where it was felt that gender discrimination as far as the age of the child is concerned should be eliminated. Indian laws for kidnapping from lawful guardianship and kidnapping or maiming a minor for the purpose of begging have different ages defined for the male and female 'child' (16 years for the male 'child' and 18 years for the female 'child').

To keep pace with the changing times and perceptions in society many laws have been enacted by Indian Parliament on matters which were not covered by the Indian Penal Code, 1860 and Criminal Procedure Code, 1973. Many such laws (in the form of Acts) are specifically for the child, and others involve giving rights to a child, and for which the age of child for that particular law has been defined. Some of these Acts were legislated as early as 1875 (when India was under British rule) and some as recently as 2013. The legal ages defined for the 'child' under these Acts have been tabulated in Table 4.4.

The various Acts of India recognize different ages of 'child' for various matters. For the purpose of inheritance, age of 'child' is considered to be from the time of conception when the child is in the womb of the mother. The Right of Children to Free and Compulsory Education Act, 2009 defines a 'child' to be one between six

Table 4.3 Legal ages defined for children in Indian Penal Code (IPC) and Criminal Procedure Code (CrPC)

Matter in question	*Section of law applicable*	*Legal age (in years)*	
		Males	*Females*
Criminal liability - not capable of criminal offence	Sec. 82 IPC	0-7	0-7
Criminal liability - capable of criminal offence if attained sufficient maturity of understanding	Sec. 83 IPC	7-12	7-12
Act done in good faith for benefit of child or insane person or by consent of guardian	Sec. 89 IPC	12	12
Consent	Sec. 90 IPC	12	12
Sale of obscene objects to young person	Sec. 293 IPC	20	20
Abetment of suicide of child or insane person	Sec. 305 IPC	18	18
Abandonment of child	Sec. 317 IPC	12	12
Kidnapping from lawful guardianship	Sec. 361 IPC	16	18
Kidnapping or maiming a minor for purposes of begging	Sec. 363 A IPC	16	18
Procuration of minor girl	Sec. 366 A IPC		18
Importation of girl from foreign country	Sec. 366 B IPC		21
Kidnapping or abducting child with intent to steal from its person	Sec. 369 IPC	10	10
Selling minor for purposes of prostitution	Sec. 372 IPC		18
Buying minor for purposes of prostitution	Sec. 373 IPC		18
Valid consent for sexual intercourse	Sec. 375 IPC Criminal Law (Amendment) Act, 2013		18
Valid consent for sexual intercourse with wife	Sec. 375 IPC Criminal Law (Amendment) Act, 2013		15
Power to compel restoration of abducted female child	Sec. 98 CrPC		18
Boy child to be examined at his residence by police when investigating a case	Sec. 160 CrPC	15	
Testifying in law courts	Indian Evidence Act (Sec. 118), 1872	No age fixed	No age fixed
		Courts to assess the ability of child to understand	

Table 4.4 Legal ages defined for children under various Acts of Parliament

Matter in question	*Act*	*Legal age (in years)*	
		Males	*Females*
Major	Indian Majority Act (Sec. 3), 1875[7]	18	18
Major when under guardianship of courts of law	Indian Majority Act (Sec. 3), 1875[7]	21	21
Inheritance	Hindu Succession Act (Sec. 20), 1956[8] Indian Succession Act (Sec. 27), 1925[9] Transfer of Property Act (Sec. 13), 1882[10]	From when the child is in womb	From when the child is in womb
Child to be in custody of mother	Hindu Minority and Guardianship Act [Sec. 6 (a)],1956[11]	5	5
Child to be in custody of father		5-18	5-18
Age of child for adoption	Hindu Adoptions and Maintenance Act (Sec. 10) , 1956[12]	<15	<15
Employment	Child Labor (Prohibition and Regulation) Act,1986[13]	<14	<14
	Merchant Shipping Act,1958[14]	<15	<15
	Motor Transport Workers Act, 1961[15]	<15	<15
	Apprentices Act, 1961[16]	<14	<14
	Beedi and Cigar Workers Act, 1966[17]	<14	<14
	Plantation Labor Act, 1951[18]	<15	<15
	Factories Act, 1948[19]	<15	<15
	Mines Act,1952[20]	<15 (child) 15–18 (adolescent)	<15 (child) 15–18 (adolescent)
	Delhi Excise Act, 2009[21]	21	21
Child	Women's and Children's Institutions (Licensing) Act, 1956[22]	18	18
Marriage	Prohibition of Child Marriage Act, 2006[23] Hindu Marriage Act [Sec. 5(iii)], 1955[24]	21	18
Restriction on imprisonment of offenders found guilty of an offence punishable with imprisonment less than life	Probation of Offenders Act (Sec. 6), 1958[25]	21	21
Age of consent for MTP	Medical Termination of Pregnancy (MTP) Act, 1971[26]		18

Contd...

Contd...

Matter in question	*Act*	*Legal age (in years)*	
		Males	*Females*
Contract	Indian Contract Act (Sec. 11), 1972[27]	18	18
Child	Immoral Traffic (Prevention) Act, 1986[28]	18	18
Voter	Representation of People Act (Sec. 19), 1950 (Amended by Act 21 of 1989)[29] The Constitution 61st Amendment Act, 1988 (Article 326)	18	18
Restrictions on sale, offer for sale or permitting sale of cigarette/ tobacco products to persons under a certain age	Cigarettes and other Tobacco Products (Prohibition of Advertisement and Regulation of Trade and Commerce, Production, Supply and Distribution) Act (Sec. 6), 2003[30]	18	18
Child	Protection of Women from Domestic Violence Act, 2005[31]	18	18
Child victim in sexual offences	Protection of Children from Sexual Offences Act, 2012[32]	18	18
Juvenile	Juvenile Justice Amendment Act, 2006[33]	18	18
Free education for child	Right of Children to Free and Compulsory Education Act, 2009[34]	6-14	6-14
Age for purchasing drinking alcohol	Different Excise Acts of Indian States	18-25 (depending on State)	18-25 (depending on State)
Driving motor vehicle	Motor Vehicles Act, 1988[35]	18	18
Driving motor cycle without gear		16	16
Driving transport vehicle		21	21

to fourteen years of age. Under the Hindu Minority and Guardianship Act [Sec. 6(a)], 1956, a minor who has not attained the age of 18 years will be under the custody of his/her father, unless the child is less than five years of age when the custody of the child will be with the mother. In this Act, 'child' has been defined as someone up to 5 years of age for a particular protective benefit and 'child' has also been defined as someone up to 18 years of age for other aspects of this Act. With regards to employment, definition of 'child' for employment in various professions is age up to 14 years/15 years. For employment in mines where the definition of 'child' is age up to 15 years and adolescents 15-18 years, children are not allowed to work in any mine, and adolescents are allowed to work below the ground only when they have medical certificates stating that they are fit to do work of adults. Under the Delhi Excise Act 2009, a person less than 21 years of age cannot be employed in a liquor shop. Hence, from Table 4.4 it is quite evident that even with regard to the legislated legal age of 'child' enacted by Parliament, there are variations, with ages ranging from when a child is in womb of mother to 21 years of age.

The Prohibition of Child Marriage Act, 2006 and The Hindu Marriage Act, 1955, have different ages defined for the male and the female child for the purpose of marriage. Under these Acts, the minimum age of marriage for males is 21 years and for females it is 18 years. This glaring instance of gender inequality with regard to the minimum age of marriage in India should be removed. For protecting the right to healthy life of girl child, the minimum age for marriage for females should also be raised up to 21 years to bring it at par with the minimum age for marriage of boys.

The Juvenile Justice Act, 1986 was amended in the year 2000 to rise the age defining the male child so that the male child up to the age of 18 years can be defined as a child or juvenile under this Act. Recently, some concerns have been raised in the Indian society regarding the age of child for it to qualify to be a child or juvenile under this Act, with demands for lowering this age (particularly in relation to the offence of rape). This issue needs a prolonged and thorough debate as lowering the age would go against the spirit of the CRC. The author is of the view that children up to 18 years of age committing crimes need protection as provided for under this Act. However, distinction can be made for crimes involving punishment for life or death, for which the age of the child qualifying it to be a child or juvenile under this Act could be lowered to 16 years (the age in the Act before the amendment in the year 2000).

Another controversial area is with regard to age defining a 'child' for the purpose of employment. In the current scenario, most laws regulating employment define a 'child' as a human of age up to 14 years, except for employment in mines, where the age of employment is from 18 years (Mines Act, 1952). It is felt by many that the age for employment should be 18 years for all occupations and 'child' should be defined as a human of age up to 18 years for all Acts related to employment to protect the child and ensure his/her healthy growth. This will also be in line with the spirit of the CRC. However, the economic status of a section of our population requires children to work in many families in order to ensure the economic survival of the family. To prohibit employment of children below 18 years of age without first ensuring the economic upliftment of this section of society could be counterproductive. These concerns made the government of India place before Parliament 'The Child Labor (Prohibition and Regulation) Amendment Bill, 2012'.[36] It prohibits the engagement of children in all occupations and prohibits the engagement of adolescents in hazardous occupations and processes. In this Bill, 'child' means a person who has not completed his 14th year of age. However, a child can help his/her family after school hours or help his/her family in the fields, home based work and forest gathering. Adolescent in this Bill has been defined as a person who has completed his/her 14th year of age, but not completed his/her 18th year.

Consent by children for medical treatment is an area where there is a great deal of variation in the age defining the child, i.e. age at which child is legally allowed to give consent. In India, there is no separate law defining the age for consent for medical treatment. Most countries use the age of majority as the age for giving valid consent for treatment. In most of the states of the United States, the age for giving consent for medical treatment is 18 years. However, there are some exceptions which are mentioned in Table 4.5.

In the United Kingdom, the age of child for giving consent for medical treatment is 16 years (Family Law Reform Act, 1969, Secs. 8 and 21). In Portugal, the age of child for giving consent for medical treatment is 14 years if the child has the ability to fully understand what is involved in the treatment in question. In the Netherlands, age of child for giving consent for medical treatment is 16 years. In Australia, the age of child for giving consent for medical treatment is 16 years, except for state of New South Wales where it is 14 years.

The age of child for giving consent for sexual intercourse also varies across the world, with ages ranging from 14 years to 21 years. The age of consent for sexual intercourse in some countries is mentioned in Table 4.6.[37-40] In India, it was 16

Table 4.5 Age of child for giving consent for medical treatment in some states of the US

State	Age
Tennessee	14 years to 18 years, if the child is mature enough to understand.
South Carolina	16 years except for surgery. Surgery can only be performed without the parent's consent, if the doctor feels it is essential to do so for the health or life of minor.
Alabama	18 years, but 14 years, if married. Child of 12 years of age can give consent for treatment of sexually transmitted diseases or pregnancy.
Kansas	16 years, if married.
Oregon	15 years.
Rhode Island	16 years.

Table 4.6 Age of child for giving consent for sexual intercourse

Age	Countries
12 years	Angola
13 years	Niger, Japan, Spain, Argentina (18 under some circumstances)
14 years	Chad, Democratic Republic of Congo, Madagascar, Malawi, Bangladesh, China, Albania, Austria, Bosnia, Herzegovina, Bulgaria, Germany, Hungary, Portugal, Serbia, Brazil, Colombia, Ecuador, Paraguay, Chile (18 under some circumstances)
15 years	Cambodia, North Korea, Syria, Thailand, Croatia, Denmark, Greece, Poland, Romania, Sweden, Costa Rica, Honduras, Uruguay
16 years	Algeria, Botswana, Cameroon, Ghana, Kenya, Lesotho, Mauritius, Mozambique, Namibia, Senegal, South Africa, Zambia, Armenia, Indonesia, Israel, Malaysia, Russia, Sri Lanka, Belgium, Cyprus, Finland, Netherlands, Norway, United Kingdom, Canada, Cuba, Venezuela, Australia, New Zealand
17 years	Ireland, Grenada
18 years	India, Central African Republic, Egypt, Ethiopia, Gabon, Gambia, Panama, Liberia, Morocco, Nigeria, Tanzania, Uganda, Iraq, Jordan, Nicaragua, Peru, Republic of Congo, Benin
20 years	Tunisia
21 years	Bahrain

years till 2013, and after the Criminal Law (Amendment) Act, 2013, the age of child for giving consent for sexual intercourse has been raised to 18 years. In the US, the age of child for giving consent for sexual intercourse varies across the different States. It is 16 years in 30 states, 17 years in 9 states and 18 years in 12 states.

In most cases, the Indian laws are in conformity with the CRC with regard to the definition of 'child' who is defined as a person up to 18 years of age. Exceptions are there where the 'child' is not defined as someone up to 18 years of age. These can be corrected in some cases after suitably amending the concerned laws. However, some laws may need to have a lower age for the definition of 'child' because of socioeconomic factors peculiar to India. Laws like competency to appear as witness require a flexible definition of 'child'.

There is no separate law in India for medical consent unlike many other countries. Section 90 of the IPC gives age of child able to give consent as 12 years and above, whereas under the Indian Contract Act 1972, the age for doctor-patient contract is 18 years and above. This anomaly needs to be rectified and a legal definition of 'child' for the purpose of medical consent should be legislated.

CONCLUSION

For all protective purposes, the age of the child should be uniformly 18 years. Whether this should also be the case for defining the age of child for all types of employment in the Indian scenario is a matter for debate. However, 'The Child Labor (Prohibition and Regulation) Amendment Bill, 2012' when passed by Parliament could to some extent bring more clarity on this issue.

For the purposes of protecting the right to healthy life of girl child, the minimum age for marriage should also be raised to 21 years, at par with the male child, as young girls in this country require more protective cover or at least equal protective cover. There is no separate law in India defining age for giving valid consent for medical treatment, leading to a lot of confusion in this regard. Hence, there is a need for a law in India defining age of child for giving consent for medical examination, procedures and treatment.

The medicolegal expert has to determine the age of a person in both civil and criminal cases wherever there is no satisfactory documentary proof of the person's age. This is especially true for countries like India where because of illiteracy and lack of adequate healthcare in rural areas, there is no proper documentation of the age of the child, either at birth or in the school. A study of the various Indian laws makes it evident that experts may be asked to determine the age of the 'child' not only for 18 years of age but for many varied ages like 5 years, 7 years, 10 years, 14 years, etc. Experts should be well versed in scientific knowledge for estimating these varied ages.

REFERENCES

1. Infochangeindia.org [homepage on the internet]. India: Centre for Communication and Development Studies; 2007 [cited 2013 October 08]. Available from: http://infochangeindia.org/agenda/child-rights-in-india/who-is-a-child.html

2. Censusindia.gov.in [database on the internet]. New Delhi: The Registrar General and Census Commissioner, India; 2013 [cited 2013 October 08]. Available from: http://www.censusindia.gov.in/2011census/Age_level_data/Age_level_data.html
3. Oxforddictionaries.com [homepage on the internet]. Britain: The Oxford university press, 2013 [cited 2013 September 08]. Available from: http://oxforddictionaries.com/definition/english/child?q=child
4. United Nations Children's Fund. Implementation handbook for the convention on the rights of the child. 3rd ed. Geneva: United Nations Children's Fund; 2007. p.1-5
5. En.wikipedia.org [homepage on the internet]. San Francisco: Wikimedia foundation Inc, 2013 [cited 2013 September 08]. Available from: http://en.wikipedia.org/wiki/Age_of_majority
6. Universal's Criminal Manual. New Delhi: Universal Law Publishing Company Pvt. Ltd.; 1996.
7. Theindianlawyer.in [homepage on the internet]. New Delhi: The Indian Lawyer [cited 2013 October 11]. Available from: http://theindianlawyer.in/statutesnbareacts/acts/i27.html
8. Theindianlawyer.in [homepage on the internet]. New Delhi: The Indian Lawyer [cited 2013 October 11]. Available from: http://www.theindianlawyer.in/statutesnbareacts/acts/h22.html
9. Theindianlawyer.in [homepage on the internet]. New Delhi: The Indian Lawyer [cited 2013 October 11]. Available from: http://www.theindianlawyer.in/statutesnbareacts/acts/i50.html
10. Theindianlawyer.in [homepage on the internet]. New Delhi: The Indian Lawyer [cited 2013 October 11]. Available from: http://www.theindianlawyer.in/statutesnbareacts/acts/t27.html
11. Theindianlawyer.in [homepage on the internet]. New Delhi: The Indian Lawyer [cited 2013 October 11]. Available from: http://www.theindianlawyer.in/statutesnbareacts/acts/h21.html
12. Theindianlawyer.in [homepage on the internet]. New Delhi: The Indian Lawyer [cited 2013 October 11]. Available from: http://www.theindianlawyer.in/statutesnbareacts/acts/h15.html
13. Theindianlawyer.in [homepage on the internet]. New Delhi: The Indian Lawyer [cited 2013 October 11]. Available from: http://www.theindianlawyer.in/statutesnbareacts/acts/c43.html
14. Theindianlawyer.in [homepage on the internet]. New Delhi: The Indian Lawyer [cited 2013 October 11]. Available from: http://www.theindianlawyer.in/statutesnbareacts/acts/m32.html
15. Theindianlawyer.in [homepage on the internet]. New Delhi: The Indian Lawyer [cited 2013 October 11]. Available from: http://www.theindianlawyer.in/statutesnbareacts/acts/m46.html
16. Theindianlawyer.in [homepage on the internet]. New Delhi: The Indian Lawyer [cited 2013 October 11]. Available from: http://www.theindianlawyer.in/statutesnbareacts/acts/a50.html
17. Theindianlawyer.in [homepage on the internet]. New Delhi: The Indian Lawyer [cited 2013 October 11]. Available from: http://www.theindianlawyer.in/statutesnbareacts/acts/b13.html
18. Theindianlawyer.in [homepage on the internet]. New Delhi: The Indian Lawyer [cited 2013 October 11]. Available from: http://www.theindianlawyer.in/statutesnbareacts/acts/p25.html
19. Theindianlawyer.in [homepage on the internet]. New Delhi: The Indian Lawyer [cited 2013 October 11]. Available from: http://www.theindianlawyer.in/statutesnbareacts/acts/f1.html

20. Theindianlawyer.in [homepage on the internet]. New Delhi: The Indian Lawyer [cited 2013 October 11]. Available from: http://www.theindianlawyer.in/statutesnbareacts/acts/m40.html
21. delhi.gov.in [homepage on the internet]. New Delhi: Government of the national capital territory of Delhi [cited 2013 October 11]. Available from: http://delhi.gov.in/wps/wcm/connect/55759700448c4e46ad1dbd12ff2aa0bf/Delhi+Excise+Act+2009_softcopy.pdf?MOD= AJPERES&mod=-180562011
22. wcddel.in[homepage on the internet]. New Delhi: Department of women and child development, Government of the national capital territory of Delhi [cited 2013 October 11]. Available from: http://wcddel.in/ila1956.html
23. wcddel.in[homepage on the internet]. New Delhi: Ministry of women and child development, Government of India [cited 2013 October 11]. Available from: http://wcd.nic.in/cma2006.pdf
24. Vakilno.1.com [homepage on the internet]. India: Vakilno.1.com [cited 2013 October 11]. Available from: http://www.vakilno1.com/bareacts/hindumarriageact/hindumarriageact.html
25. Theindianlawyer.in [homepage on the internet]. New Delhi: The Indian Lawyer [cited 2013 October 11]. Available from: http://www.theindianlawyer.in/statutesnbareacts/acts/p66.html
26. Theindianlawyer.in [homepage on the internet]. New Delhi: The Indian Lawyer [cited 2013 October 11]. Available from: http://www.theindianlawyer.in/statutesnbareacts/acts/m29.html
27. Theindianlawyer.in [homepage on the internet]. New Delhi: The Indian Lawyer [cited 2013 October 11]. Available from: http://www.theindianlawyer.in/statutesn-bareacts/acts/c91.html
28. childlineindia.org.in [homepage on the internet]. India: Childline India foundation [cited 2013 October 11]. Available from: http://www.childlineindia.org.in/CP-CR-Downloads/ImmoralTrafficPreventionact1956.pdf
29. indiakanoon.org [homepage on the internet] [cited 2013 October 11]. Available from: http://indiankanoon.org/doc/320017/
30. health.bih.nic.in [homepage on the internet]. Patna: Health Department, Government of Bihar [cited 2013 October 11]. Available from: http://health.bih.nic.in/Rules/Tobacco-Control-Act-2003.pdf
31. lawyersCollective.org [homepage on the internet]. New Delhi: Lawyers collective [cited 2013 October 11]. Available from: http://www.lawyerscollective.org/files/protection_of_women_from_domestic_violence_act_2005.pdf
32. wcd.nic.in [homepage on the internet]. New Delhi: Ministry of women and child development, Government of India [cited 2013 October 11]. Available from: http://wcd.nic.in/childact/childprotection31072012.pdf
33. wcd.nic.in [homepage on the internet]. New Delhi: Ministry of women and child development, Government of India [cited 2013 October 11]. Available from: http://wcd.nic.in/childprot/jjactamedment.pdf
34. mhrd.gov.in [homepage on the internet]. New Delhi: Ministry of human resource and development, Department of school education and literacy, Government of India [cited 2013 October 11]. Available from: http://mhrd.gov.in/sites/upload_files/mhrd/files/rte.pdf
35. Theindianlawyer.in [homepage on the internet]. New Delhi: The Indian Lawyer [cited 2013 October 11]. Available from: http://www.theindianlawyer.in/statutesnbareacts/acts/m47.html#_Toc39392213
36. Prsindia.org [homepage on the internet].New Delhi: Prs legislative research[cited 2013 October 13]. Available from: http://www.prsindia.org/uploads/media/ChildLabour/ChildLabour(ProhibitionandRegulation)(A)Bill,2012.pdf

37. En.wikipedia.org [homepage on the internet]. San Francisco: Wikimedia foundation Inc, 2013[cited 2013 October 08]. Available from: http://en.wikipedia.org/wiki/Ages_of_consent_in_Africa
38. En.wikipedia.org [homepage on the internet]. San Francisco: Wikimedia foundation Inc, 2013[cited 2013 October 08]. Available from: http://en.wikipedia.org/wiki/Ages_of_consent_in_Asia
39. En.wikipedia.org [homepage on the internet]. San Francisco: Wikimedia foundation Inc, 2013[cited 2013 October 08]. Available from: http://en.wikipedia.org/wiki/Ages_of_consent_in_North_America
40. En.wikipedia.org [homepage on the internet]. San Francisco: Wikimedia foundation Inc, 2013[cited 2013 October 08]. Available from: http://en.wikipedia.org/wiki/Ages_of_consent_in_South_America

Recent Changes in Sexual Assault and Rape Laws

Satish Kumar Verma, Aditi Verma

'I just want to sleep. A coma would be nice. Or amnesia. Anything, just to get rid of this, these thoughts, whispers in my mind. Did he rape my head, too?'
Laurie Halse Anderson (American author)

ABSTRACT

Aftermath the rape on a 16-year-old physiotherapy intern in south Delhi, Delhi witnessed one of the massive agitation involving the common man, demanding changes in the laws and punishment in relation to the sexual assault and rape cases. It made all stakeholders (governmental and nongovernmental) to ponder over these criminal acts and tighten the laxities wherever possible. Recently, several amendments have been made in the criminal laws related to deal with the cases of sexual assaults pertaining to women and children and making them more stringent. The medicolegal examination of the victim and accused involved in these cases is one of the areas that concern all medical professionals. And, it is their duty to perform this examination with utmost care, devotion and impartiality so that justice can be dispensed with. Such examination is now becoming more and more objective and finding description in the rule books of the country and legal pronouncements. This chapter is an attempt to sensitize medical professional, and more precisely gynecologist and forensic expert on these recent changes brought up in the laws and medicolegal examination pertinent to a doctor.

Keywords: Delhi gang rape, consent for sexual intercourse, Criminal Law (Amendment) Act, penetration, Sec. 164A CrPC, sexual assault kit, medical examination of rape victim, two finger test.

INTRODUCTION

Case of Interest

Delhi Gang Rape, 2012

The Delhi gang rape case[1] involved a rape and murder that occurred on 16th December 2012 in Munirka, a neighborhood located in the southern part of New Delhi, when a 23-year-old female physiotherapy intern[2] was beaten and gang raped in a bus in which she was traveling with her male companion. There were six others in the bus, including the driver, all of whom raped the woman. The woman died from her injuries thirteen days later while undergoing emergency treatment in Singapore.[3]

HISTORY OF SEXUAL VIOLENCE

Understanding the history of sexual violence, and the social and political functions that it serves can go a long way in helping us facilitate dealing with individuals and inform our work in public education and systems change. This is particularly critical when working with people of Indian descent.

The sexual assault has an old history as far as India is concerned. India was a highly patriarchal society. Marriages are for the most part arranged, and a majority of young men has never been on a date with a woman or have a framework for interacting with strangers of the opposite sex. Since, a high value is placed on a bride's virginity, especially in traditional settings, and the dangers to a girl's future if there is a taint on her honor, rape is often not reported, and the men who rape are counting on this silence to go public.[4]

In all the ancient civilizations of the west (and in many others) women were the property of their fathers, and later in life, of their husbands. Marriage was often a monetary transaction, with the suitor or his family paying the 'bride-price' to the father/owner. While bride capture still occurred, it went on with regard to other tribes or peoples who were enemies in war or conquered by a stronger people. When women were property, the right of ownership passed from the father to the husband in marriage. The woman literally belonged to her husband; damage to his property was a direct offense against the husband. If an unmarried woman was raped, her bride-price was lower, for she was 'damaged goods'. Thus, in some ancient societies, rapists paid the traditional bride-price or some variation of it to the father, whose economic interest was harmed by the rape. Under these societies, the woman had few personal rights; her feelings and experiences were discounted.

The practice of treating women as property to uphold the class status of white males became a part of the history of those countries where slavery was prevalent. An African-American woman's body belonged to her master. She had no legal protection and no right to refuse. Women were exchanged or bought in slavery, where their sexual services were part of their labor and where their children were also the property of their masters. Slave children were expected to work as soon as they were able to. Class for white men was determined by the steady production of slaves, and those who owned more slaves could dominate those who did not. The forced exploitation of African-American women by white men was totally acceptable and sanctioned as a means by which white men gained power, and economic and social status.

The problem of rape is in part the problem of a highly unequal society, where women are of low status and are often segregated and disadvantaged. Economist Amartya Sen estimated that because girls are less valued and less well taken care of when ill, there are girls who died from relative neglect compared to what their brothers got. There is also a growing problem of families aborting daughters, once the sex of the embryo is known via ultrasound. In India, typically the bride's family must provide the groom with many expensive gifts, so that marrying off the girls of the family is extremely expensive, and poor fathers and mothers would like to have high-valued sons instead.[5]

Rape at Times of War

In most times and places, rape has been a weapon of war, or the prerogative of the victorious soldiers over a conquered people. Indeed, the city of Rome was founded and created with the rape of Sabine women. During the attack of Troy, women were raped by the victors. At other times in western history, the massive use of rape occurred during war. In 1453, when Constantinople fell, the city's women and young girls were raped by Ottoman's troops. During the Indian massacres by whites, troops committed atrocities against Indian women. In 1864, at the Sand Creek massacre, Indian women were raped and sexually mutilated. In 1937, when Nanking fell to Japanese troops, the women of the city were raped. During the Vietnam war, the rape of Vietnamese women by United States troops was common.

Today, rape is a criminal act of war under the international war laws. Despite this, it continues to be an act of war.

Virgin Rape

In ancient times, a virgin was often believed to possess religious powers by virtue of her chastity. Some thought that she possessed God-given powers to ward off evil spirits, cause fields to be fertile, and ensure divine blessings on her community. Her chastity was often revered and protected for religious reasons, as well as for economic ones. Hence, among some ancient peoples, the rape of a virgin was both an economic loss and a possible risk of the wrath of the Gods.

Babylonians and Assyrians considered raping a virgin to be particularly sinful. If the rapist was married, he was put to death. If he was unmarried, he paid the father three times her marriage price and married his victim without any right to divorce her in his lifetime. The marriage of an unbetrothed rape victim to her assailant was also considered a fair punishment among the ancient Hebrews.

Origin of Word 'Rape'

The English word 'rape' is derived from the Latin '*rapere*' which means to steal, seize or carry away. This was a very old means by which a man 'seized' or 'stole' a wife in ancient western societies. In reality, it constituted enforced marriage, since a man simply took whichever woman he wanted, raped her and brought her into his tribe or nation. Rape was thus conducted under the guise of respectable behavior, rewarding the rapists for the misuse and abuse of women. To a certain extent, this attitude has not changed.[6]

EPIDEMIOLOGY

One in three women in the United States will be a victim of sexual assault sometime in her life; 7–10% of rape victims are male.[7] One in four women will experience rape or attempted rape during her college years. Large population-based surveys indicate a lifetime prevalence of 13–39% among women and 3% among men.[8,9] Only 10–15% all sexual assaults are reported to police. Rape victims are less likely to report assault when the assailant is known to them.

Sexual assaults that are facilitated by the use of alcohol and drugs which in some cases are voluntarily ingested by the victim, are increasingly recognized and are more common than classic forcible assaults among college students.[10,11]

Crimes under the Indian Penal Code (IPC)

i. Rape (Sec. 376 IPC).
ii. Kidnapping and abduction for specified purposes (Sec. 363-373 IPC).
iii. Homicide for dowry, dowry deaths or their attempts (Sec. 302/304B IPC).
iv. Torture—both mental and physical (Sec. 498A IPC).
v. Assault on women with intent to outrage her modesty (Sec. 354 IPC).
vi. Insult to the modesty of women (Sec. 509 IPC).
vii. Importation of a girl up to 21 years of age from foreign country for illicit intercourse with another person (Sec. 366B IPC).

Crimes under the Special and Local Laws (SLL)

i. Immoral Traffic (Prevention) Act, 1956.
ii. Dowry Prohibition Act, 1961.
iii. Indecent Representation of Women (Prohibition) Act, 1986.
iv. Commission of Sati Prevention Act, 1987.

Statistics on Crime Against Women and Children in India

As per the National Crime Records Bureau, a total of 3,09,546 incidents of crime against women were reported in 2013 (both under IPC and SLL).[12]

These crimes have continuously increased during 2006–2013 with 1,64,765 cases in 2006, 1,85,312 cases in 2007, 1,95,856 cases in 2008, 2,03,804 cases in 2009 and 2,13,585 cases in 2010. Andhra Pradesh (32,809 cases, 10.6%), Uttar Pradesh (32,546 cases, 10.5%), West Bengal (29,826 cases, 9.6%), Rajasthan (27,933 cases, 9%) and Maharashtra (24,895 cases, 8%) accounted for nearly 50% of total crime against women in 2013.[12]

An increasing trend in cases of rape has been observed during 2006–2008. A mixed trend in the incidence of rape has been observed during 2008–2010. These cases reported an increase of 7.2% in 2007 over 2006, an increase of 3.5% in 2008 over 2007, a decline of 0.3% in 2009 over 2008 and an increase of 3.6% in 2010 over 2009. In 2013, the number of rape cases reported was 33,707 (rate of crime being 5.7%). *Madhya Pradesh has reported the highest number of rape cases (4335) accounting for 12.9% of total such cases reported in the country.*[12]

Crime against children includes:

1. Crimes against children punishable under the Indian Penal Code (IPC) are:
   a. *Murder:* Sec. 302 IPC.
   b. *Feticide* (crime against a fetus): Sec. 315 and 316 IPC.
   c. *Infanticide* (crime against newborn child) *(0–1 year):* Sec. 315 IPC.
   d. *Abetment to suicide* (abetment by other persons for commitment of suicide by children): Sec. 305 IPC.
   e. *Exposure and abandonment* (crime against children by parents or others to expose or to leave them with the intention of abandonment): Sec. 317 IPC.
   f. *Kidnapping and abduction:* Sec. 360-369 IPC.

g. *Procuration of minor girls* (for inducement to force or seduce to illicit intercourse): Sec. 366A IPC.
h. *Selling of girls for prostitution:* Sec. 372 IPC.
i. *Buying of girls for prostitution:* Sec. 373 IPC.
j. *Rape:* Sec. 376 IPC.
k. *Unnatural offences:* Sec. 377 IPC.

2. Crime against children punishable under SLL:
   a. Immoral Traffic Prevention Act, 1956 (where minors are abused in prostitution).
   b. Child Labor (Prevention and Regulation) Act, 1986.

A total of 58,224 cases of crimes against children were reported in the country during 2013 as compared to 26,694 cases during 2010. Among IPC crimes, number of cases under Procuration of Minor Girls increased from 679 in 2010 to 1224 in 2013. Cases of exposure and abandonment remained nearly same (857 cases in 2010 and 869 cases in 2013). Cases of kidnapping and abduction registered maximum in Uttar Pradesh (6002 cases, 21.3%) and Delhi (5809 cases, 20.6%).Uttar Pradesh (9857), Madhya Pradesh (8247), Delhi (7199) and Maharashtra (6410) have accounted for 16.9%, 14.2%, 12.4% and 11% of total crimes respectively against children at the national level.[12]

RAPE AND SEXUAL ASSAULT

Sexual assault is defined as any sexual act performed by one (or more) person(s) on another without consent. It may include the use or threat of force. In some cases, the person cannot give consent to sex because he/she is unconscious or otherwise incapacitated. A person may be raped by a stranger, an acquaintance or date or a family member. Rape is a legal term, and in the United States it refers to any penetration of a body orifice (mouth, vagina or anus) involving force or the threat of force or incapacity (i.e. associated with young or old age, cognitive or physical disability, or drug or alcohol intoxication) without consent.

Indian context: The statutory definition of the offence of 'rape' is found under Sec. 375 IPC. Till, *2nd February 2013*, it was read as:

Sec. 375 IPC (Rape): A man is said to commit 'rape' who, except in the case hereinafter excepted, has sexual intercourse with a woman under circumstances falling under any of the six following descriptions:

- *First:* Against her will.
- *Secondly:* Without her consent.
- *Thirdly:* With her consent, when her consent has been obtained by putting her or any person in whom she is interested in fear of death or of hurt.
- *Fourthly:* With her consent, when the man knows that he is not her husband and that her consent is given because she believes that he is another man to whom she is or believes herself to be lawfully married.
- *Fifthly:* With her consent, when, at the time of giving such consent, by reason of unsoundness of mind or intoxication or the administration by him personally or through another, of any stupefying or unwholesome substance, she is unable to understand the nature and consequences of that, to which she gives consent.
- *Sixthly:* With or without her consent, when she is under sixteen years of age.

Explanation: Penetration is sufficient to constitute the sexual intercourse necessary to the offence of rape.

Exception: Sexual intercourse by a man with his own wife, the wife not being under fifteen years of age, is not rape.[13]

However, from 3rd February 2013, this definition of rape stands modified as: According to the Criminal Law (Amendment) Act 2013 of Sec. 375 of the IPC, a man is said to commit 'rape' if he:

a. Penetrates his penis, to any extent, into the vagina, mouth, urethra or anus of a woman or makes her to do so with him or any other person; or
b. Inserts, to any extent, any object or a part of the body, not being the penis, into the vagina, the urethra or anus of a woman or makes her to do so with him or any other person; or
c. Manipulates any part of the body of a woman so as to cause penetration into the vagina, urethra, anus or any part of body of such woman or makes her to do so with him or any other person; or
d. Applies his mouth to the vagina, anus, urethra of a woman or makes her to do so with him or any other person, under the circumstances falling under any of the following seven descriptions:
   - *First:* Against her will.
   - *Secondly:* Without her consent.
   - *Thirdly:* With her consent, when her consent has been obtained by putting her or any person in whom she is interested in fear of death or of hurt.
   - *Fourthly:* With her consent, when the man knows that he is not her husband and that her consent is given because she believes that he is another man to whom she is or believes herself to be lawfully married.
   - *Fifthly:* With her consent, when, at the time of giving such consent, by reason of unsoundness of mind or intoxication or the administration by him personally or through another of any stupefying or unwholesome substance, she is unable to understand the nature and consequences of that, to which she gives consent.
   - *Sixthly:* With or without her consent, when she is under eighteen years of age.
   - *Seventhly:* When she is unable to communicate consent.

Explanation 1: For the purpose of this section, 'vagina' shall also include labia majora.

Explanation 2: Consent means an unequivocal voluntary agreement when the woman by words, gestures or any other form of verbal or nonverbal communication, communicates willingness to participate in the specific sexual act; provided that a woman who does not physically resist to the act of penetration shall not by the reason only of that fact, be regarded as consenting to the sexual activity.

Exception 1: A medical procedure or intervention shall not constitute rape.

Exception 2: Sexual intercourse or sexual acts by a man with his own wife, the wife not being under fifteen years of age, is not a rape.[14]

Simply put, the offence of rape is 'ravishment of a woman' without her consent or against her will by force, fear or fraud and also includes the 'carnal knowledge' of a woman. 'Carnal knowledge' means penetration to any slightest degree. This ingredient of rape has been statutory incorporated under the explanation to Sec. 375 IPC.

INGREDIENTS OF THE OFFENCE

Consent

In order to bring home the charge of rape against a man, it is necessary to establish that the 'sexual intercourse' complained of was either against the will or without her consent. Where the consent is obtained under the circumstances enumerated under clauses firstly to sixthly, the same would also amount to rape. In Dileep Singh vs. State of Bihar, the Supreme Court observed that 'though will and consent often interlace and an act done against the will of the person can be said to be an act done without consent, the Indian Penal Code categorizes these two expressions under separate heads in order to as comprehensive as possible'.[15]

The difference between the two expressions was brought out by the Supreme Court in State of UP vs. Chottey Lal in the following words:[16]

"Be that as it may, in our view, clause sixthly of Sec. 375 IPC is not attracted since the prosecutrix has been found to be above 16 years (although below 18 years). In the facts of the case what is crucial to be considered is whether clause firstly or clause secondly of Sec. 375 IPC is attracted. The expressions 'against her will' and 'without her consent' may overlap sometimes but surely the two expressions in clause firstly and clause secondly have different connotation and dimension. The expression 'against her will' would ordinarily mean that the intercourse was done by a man with a woman despite her resistance and opposition. On the other hand, the expression 'without her consent' would comprehend an act of reason accompanied by deliberation." It must be noted that the courts have followed the tests laid down under Sec. 90 of the IPC for establishing 'consent'.

Section 90 IPC reads thus: 'Consent known to be given under fear or misconception: A consent is not such a consent as is intended by any section of this Code, if the consent is given by a person under fear of injury, or under a misconception of fact, and if the person doing the act knows, or has reason to believe that the consent was given in consequence of such fear or misconception; or (consent of insane person) if the consent is given by a person who, from unsoundness of mind, or intoxication, is unable to understand the nature and consequence of that to which he gives his consent; or (consent of child) unless the contrary appears from the context, if the consent is given by a person who is under 12 years of age.'

In this context, the decision of Supreme Court in State of HP vs. Mango Ram is noteworthy.[17] The court observed as follows:

".........The evidence as a whole indicates that there was resistance by the prosecutrix and there was no voluntary participation by her for the sexual act. Submission of the body under the fear of terror cannot be construed as a consented sexual act. Consent for the purpose of Sec. 375 IPC requires voluntary participation not only after the exercise of intelligence based on the knowledge of the significance and moral quality of the act, but after having fully exercised the choice between resistance and assent. Whether there was consent or not, is to be ascertained only on a careful study of all relevant circumstances. From the evidence on record, it cannot be said that the prosecutrix had given consent and thereafter she turned round and acted against the interest of the accused. There is clear credible evidence that she resisted the onslaught and made all possible efforts to prevent the accused from committing rape on her. Therefore, the finding entered by the learned Sessions Judge that there was consent on the part of the prosecutrix is without any basis."

The United Nations handbook points out that the definitions of rape and sexual assault have evolved over time, from requiring use of force or violence to requiring a lack of positive consent.

The United Nations recommends that the definition of rape should require the existence of 'unequivocal and voluntary agreement' as well as proof by the accused of steps taken to ascertain whether the complainant was consenting. This has the advantage of shifting the burden to the defence to prove that such steps were taken.[18]

Similarly, under Canadian law, the accused cannot argue that there was belief in consent, if the accused did not take reasonable steps to ascertain that there was consent to the specific sexual activity. It is not enough that the accused subjectively believed there was consent. He must also demonstrate that he took reasonable steps to ascertain it.

Under the law of England and Wales, a person consents, if he/she 'agrees by choice and has the freedom and capacity to make that choice'. There are certain statutory presumptions regarding consent. For example, lack of consent is assumed if violence was used or threatened or the accused had induced a fear of violence; the complainant was unlawfully detained, asleep or unconscious; or the accused had administered a substance capable of causing the complainant to be stupefied or overpowered. Lack of consent is conclusively proved, if the defendant intentionally deceived the complainant as to the nature or purpose of the relevant act, or induced consent by impersonating a person known to the complainant.[19] The underlying principle is that consent to sexual activity 'requires a conscious, operating mind, capable of granting, revoking or withholding consent to each and every sexual act. There are some similar presumptions in the Indian statute. We have defined consent keeping the above in mind.

Penetration

The section further clarifies that mere penetration is sufficient to constitute the offence of rape.

In Koppula Venkatrao vs. State of AP, the Supreme Court held as follows:[20]

"The *sine qua non* of the offence of rape is penetration, and not ejaculation. Ejaculation without penetration constitutes an attempt to commit rape and not actual rape. Definition of 'rape' as contained in Sec. 375 IPC refers to 'sexual intercourse' and the explanation appended to the section provides that penetration is sufficient to constitute the sexual intercourse necessary to the offence of rape. Intercourse means sexual connection."

Pursuant to the aforesaid observation, the offence of 'attempt to commit rape' also need elaboration. Sec. 376 read with Sec. 511 of IPC penalizes the offence of 'attempt to rape'.

Evidence and Proof

It is well settled that the evidence of the victim of rape is on the same footing as the evidence of an injured complainant or witness. Her testimony alone is sufficient for conviction. In prosecutions of rape, the law does not require corroboration. It is only by way of abundant caution that the court may look for some corroboration so as to satisfy its conscience, and rule out any false accusation.

However, the above principle of presumption while prosecuting rape cases emerged in the aforesaid background.

In Tukaram vs. State of Maharashtra, the Supreme Court had disbelieved the statement of the victim of rape, on the ground that the circumstantial evidence did not lead to the inference of guilt and 'in fact derogates in no uncertain measure from the inference drawn by it'.[21]

The facts were these—Mathura was a young laborer girl of 14–16 years. She along with her brother were brought to the local police station to record their statements in respect of a complaint lodged by her brother. While at the police station, Mathura was raped by head constable Tukaram and constable Ganpat, a fact which she reported to a crowd that had gathered outside the police station. Mathura was then examined by a doctor, who advised her to file a police complaint which was registered by the police after some hesitation and protests from the crowd. Mathura's medical examination revealed no injuries and evidence of prior intercourse. Presence of semen was detected on her clothes and the pyjama of Ganpat. The trial court, however, refused to convict the accused. The High Court reversed the finding and sentenced Tukaram to rigorous imprisonment for one year and Ganpat for five years. The High Court held that both these 'gentlemen' were perfect strangers to Mathura and that it was unlikely that 'she would make any overtures and invite the accused to satisfy her sexual desires'. The High Court came to the conclusion that Mathura did not consent to intercourse. The Supreme Court reversed the High Court verdict and held that as there were no injuries shown by the medical report, the story of 'stiff resistance having been put up by the girl is all false' and the alleged intercourse was a peaceful affair. The court further held that crimes and alarms were a concoction on her part, and under Sec. 375 IPC only the 'fear of death or hurt' could vitiate consent for sexual intercourse.

Following this verdict, a nationwide protest was launched for inclusion of custodial rape within the legislative provision. The Supreme Court's judgment was criticized by eminent law teachers who posed the following questions in an open letter to the Supreme Court:[18]

i. Was this not a decision which violated human rights of women under the law and the Constitution?
ii. The judgment provided no cogent analysis as to why the factors which weighed with the High Court were insufficient to justify conviction for rape?
iii. The fact remains that Mathura was asked to remain in the police station even after her statement was recorded and her friends and relations were asked to leave. Why?
iv. Why were the lights put off and the doors shut?

The decision of Tukaram vs. State of Maharashtra is a relevant case to show how public opinion and various organizations have espoused the rights of women.

Accordingly, the Criminal Law (Amendment) Act, 1983 was passed which included situation of 'aggravated rape' under Sec. 376A to E. Further, the India Evidence Act, 1872 was also amended by the Criminal Law (Amendment) Act, 1983 and Sec. 114A was incorporated which imposed the burden of proving 'consent' upon the accused in the aforesaid cases of aggravated rape. This was an exception of the general rule of presumption of innocence of the accused.

However, even before the above amendments came into force, in the case of Bharvada Gohinbhai Hirjibhai vs. State of Gujarat, the Supreme Court reversed the trend and came to a conclusion that it was open to the court to rely upon the evidence of a complainant even without seeking corroboration, if corroboration by medical evidence is available.[22] We also notice that the said judgment seems to have stereotyped Indian and western women in a somewhat unorthodox way:

"In the Indian setting, refusal to act on the testimony of a victim of sexual assault in the absence of corroboration as a rule is adding insult to injury. Why should the evidence of the girl or the woman who complains of rape or sexual molestation be viewed with the aid of spectacles fitted with lenses tinged with doubt, disbelief or suspicion? To do so is to justify the charge of male chauvinism in a male dominated society. We must analyze the argument in support of the need for corroboration and subject it to relentless and remorseless cross-examination. And we must do so with a logical and not an opinionated eye, in the light of probabilities with our feet firmly planted on the soil of India and with our eyes focused on the Indian horizon."

"We must not be swept off the feet by the approach made in the western world which has its own social milieu, its own social mores, its own permissive values and its own code of life. Corroboration may be considered essential to establish a sexual offence in the backdrop of the social ecology of the western world. It is wholly unnecessary to import the said concept on a turn-key basis and to translate it on the Indian soil regardless of the altogether different atmosphere, attitudes, mores, responses of the Indian society and its profile. The identities of the two worlds are different. The solution of problems cannot, therefore, be identical. It is conceivable in the western society that a female may level false accusation as regards sexual molestation against a male for several reasons such as:

a. The female may be a 'gold digger' and may well have an economic motive to extract money by holding out the gun of prosecution or public exposure.
b. She may be suffering from psychological neurosis and may seek an escape from the neurotic prison by fantasizing or imagining a situation where she is desired, wanted and chased by males.
c. She may want to wreak vengeance on the male for real or imaginary wrongs. She may have a grudge against a particular male or males in general, and may have the design to square the account.
d. She may have been induced to do so in consideration of economic rewards, by a person interested in placing the accused in a compromising or embarrassing position, on account of personal or political vendetta.
e. She may do so to gain notoriety or publicity or to appease her own ego or to satisfy her feeling of self-importance in the context of her inferiority complex.
f. She may do so on account of jealousy.
g. She may do so to win sympathy of others.
h. She may do so upon being repulsed."[18]

MEDICOLEGAL EXAMINATION OF THE VICTIM

1. It is recommended that when a call is made to the sexual assault helpline, police personnel and a designated unmarked ambulance attached to a 'Sexual Assault Crisis Center' (hereinafter referred to as 'the Center', SACC) should reach the location and, as soon as possible, transport the survivor to the Center. Other injured people, if any, should be taken to the nearest hospital.
2. The Center should have a specifically and exclusively designated space within the premises of a hospital, and should be a reclusive and inconspicuous space. The hospital in question could either be a government or a private hospital. There should be adequate security provided at the place. There should be at least three rooms—a waiting room, a medical examination room and a counseling/consultation room. The examination room should preferably have access to a toilet and a shower. The surroundings should also be child friendly. They should be non-threatening, sanitized and well-lit.
3. It goes without saying that the life of the victim is to be preserved before legal formalities are met. In an eventuality that the life of a victim will be better protected by taking him/her to the nearest hospital rather than SACC, this option will have to be adopted as an emergency measure. Justice Verma committee emphasized that this should be resorted to only in extreme emergencies.
4. The Supreme Court in the case of Parmanand Katara vs. Union of India[23] has emphasized the paramount, absolute and total obligation of doctors, whether in private or government service to extend his/her services with due expertise for protecting the life of the victim without interference from laws. This duty needs no support from any code of ethics or rule of law. The said decision also casts a duty on the state machinery to abstain from unduly harassing doctors who will have to be witnesses in such cases. The court directed that this duty be duly published through visual, audio and print media.

   However, we observe that these directions have not been adequately complied with and doctors, especially in private hospitals, are extremely wary to deal with cases of this nature. In our opinion, the duty of the medical profession to extend unqualified services to victims of such heinous offences should be duly publicized, and medical professionals and hospitals who abstain from performing the same ought to be punished in accordance with law.
5. The Center should be private, discreet and should at all times have all the facilities required to preserve the life of the victim and for her recovery. In particular, it should have a female gynecologist and a professionally qualified counselor (who is trained to handle medicolegal cases and is also female as far as feasible) available on the premises. The counselor should be professionally qualified to deal with victims with disabilities also. The Center should have a sanitized medical examination room with a 'Sexual Assault Investigation Kit' available on the premises. Proper refrigeration and storage facilities for preserving forensic evidence including DNA should be available at the Center.

6. Subject to her physical health and choice, the first interaction of the victim should be with the counselor, and thereafter, with the doctor and the police. At the very outset, the counselor must inform the victim about the procedure to ensue and also make her aware of her rights. There will also be a readily available set of names and telephone numbers of lawyers at the Center, and a lawyer from the list will be contacted by the counselor to render assistance during recording of her statement by the police.
7. The issue of whether sexual assault occurred is a legal issue and not a medical diagnosis. Consequently, doctors should not, on the basis of the medical examination conclude whether rape had occurred or not. Only findings, both positive and negative, should be recorded in the medical report.
8. It is crucial to underscore that the size of the vaginal introitus has no bearing on a case of sexual assault, and therefore, a test to ascertain the laxity of the vaginal muscles which is commonly referred to as the *two-finger test must not be conducted.* On the basis of this test, observations/conclusions such as 'habituated to sexual intercourse' should not be made and this is forbidden by law.
9. Routinely, there is a lot of attention given to the status of hymen. The 'two-finger test' is also conducted to note the distensibility of the hymen. However it is largely irrelevant because the hymen can be torn due to several reasons. An intact hymen does not rule out sexual assault, and a torn hymen does not prove previous sexual intercourse. Hymen should therefore be treated like any other part of the genitals while documenting examination findings in cases of sexual assault. Only those that are relevant to the episode of assault (findings such as fresh tears, bleeding or edema) are to be documented.

   Recently, in case of Lillu @Rajesh and anr vs. State of Haryana,[24] apex court of the country in a judgment said, "In view of International Covenant on Economic, Social and Cultural Rights 1966; United Nations Declaration of Basic Principles of Justice for Victims of Crime and Abuse of Power 1985, rape survivors are entitled to legal recourse that does not retraumatize them or violate their physical or mental integrity and dignity. They are also entitled to medical procedures conducted in a manner that respects their right to consent. Medical procedures should not be carried out in a manner that constitutes cruel, inhuman or degrading treatment, and health should be of paramount consideration while dealing with gender-based violence. The State is under an obligation to make such services available to survivors of sexual violence. Proper measures should be taken to ensure their safety and there should be no arbitrary or unlawful interference with her privacy.

   Thus, in view of the above, undoubtedly, the 'two finger test' and its interpretation violate the right of rape survivors to privacy, physical and mental integrity and dignity. Thus, this test, even if the report is affirmative, cannot *ipso facto*, be given rise to presumption of consent".
10. We also are of the opinion that the medicolegal examination report should note the date and time of examination, and be sent without delay to the concerned investigating officer (IO). To avoid unnecessary delays, the report must be transmitted to the IO by way of e-mail (as a secure PDF file—digitally signed where possible), in addition to sending by way of regular government post. It is in this background that Sec. 164A was introduced to the CrPC. The

Law Commission, in its 84th Report,[18] recommended the insertion of Sec. 164A in the following terms:

'In many cases, the report of the medical examiner as to the examination of the female victim is also found to be somewhat cursory and does not give adequate information about the material particulars which are necessary for an adjudication as to the various ingredients of Sec. 375. Further, it is sometimes noticed that the medical examination report is not sent promptly to the IO. As a result, the possibility of tampering with the report remains. In our opinion, the report of the examination of the rape victim should (besides containing the usual formal particulars) deal specifically with:

i. The age of the victim.
ii. The question whether the victim was previously used to sexual intercourse.
iii. Injuries on the body of the victim.
iv. General mental condition of the victim.
v. Other material particulars in reasonable detail.

It is also necessary that the report should note the time of examination and be sent without delay to the IO. It is very important that the report should state reasons for the conclusions recorded'.

11. Parliament enacted the said section, twenty-five years later which is as follows:

Sec. 164A CrPC: Medical examination of the victim of rape.

a. Where, during the stage when an offence of committing rape or attempt to commit rape is under investigation, it is proposed to get the person of the woman with whom rape is alleged or attempted to have been committed or attempted, examined by a medical expert, such examination shall be conducted by a registered medical practitioner employed in a hospital run by the Government or a local authority and in the absence of a such a practitioner, by any other registered medical practitioner, with the consent of such woman or of a person competent to give such consent on her behalf and such woman shall be sent to such registered medical practitioner within twenty-four hours from the time of receiving the information relating to the commission of such offence.
b. The registered medical practitioner, to whom such woman is sent shall, without delay, examine her and prepare a report giving the following particulars, namely:
   i. The name and address of the woman and of the person by whom she was brought.
   ii. The age of the woman.
   iii. The description of material taken from the person of the woman for DNA profiling.
   iv. Marks of injury, if any, on the person of the woman.
   v. General mental condition of the woman.
   vi. Other material particulars in reasonable detail.
c. The report shall state precisely the reasons for each conclusion arrived at.
d. The report shall specifically record that the consent of the woman or of the person competent to give such consent on her behalf to such examination, had been obtained.

e. The exact time of commencement and completion of the examination shall also be noted in the report.
f. The registered medical practitioner shall, without delay forward the report to the investigation officer who shall forward it to the Magistrate referred to in Sec. 173 CrPC as part of the documents referred to in clause (a) of subsection (5) of that section.
g. Nothing in this section shall be construed as rendering lawful any examination without the consent of the woman or of any person competent to give such consent on her behalf.

Explanation: For the purposes of this section, 'examination' and 'registered medical practitioner' shall have the same meanings as in Sec. 53 CrPC.

12. Thus, we note that Parliament has acted in alignment with modern understanding that previous sexual intercourse of woman would be irrelevant.
13. We are also of the opinion that the medical examination of a rape/sexual assault victim must necessarily take place under the supervision of a senior female obstetrician/ gynecologist. In the event an obstetrician/gynecologist is not available, it shall be a senior female doctor who will examine a rape victim. We also recommend that in order to ensure that there is a consensus of opinion on the medical examination, a board of three doctors must examine a rape/sexual assault victim. We believe it is important that the deliberations of the said board of doctors be recorded as an audio recording which must be later made available to a court to satisfy itself that there has been a fair consensus building in relation to the opinion formation as far as the victim is concerned.

As per directions of High Courts of Punjab and Haryana, and Andhra Pradesh, it is mandatory for the victim to be examined by a female registered medical practitioner only (wherever female doctor is available).

14. We are of the opinion that the medical examination of a victim of sexual assault/rape ought to be conducted in the following minimum conditions:
    a. The equipment used in the examination must be adequate for the purpose and must, to the extent possible, conform to international standards.
    b. The examination room must be well ventilated and well lit with fixed lighting.
    c. It is better, unless the victim is an adult woman of mature years, to take the history from the mother or older relative with whom the victim is accompanied. The circumstances in which the offence is alleged to have been committed shall be ascertained from such relative.
    d. In any event, a trained same-sex support person or trained health worker should be present during the course of the examination.
    e. The examining doctor, with the help of the victim's relatives/health worker, must explain to the victim each step of the examination and why each such step is important to the examination.
    f. The victim must be assured that she is in control of the pace, timing and components of the examination and that she will not be forced to undergo any particular step(s) of the examination, if she is uncomfortable with the same.

g. In the event the victim does not consent to the whole or part of the medical examination, the medical examiner should refrain from making any adverse remarks in this regard.
h. The victim must be reassured that the examination findings will be kept confidential.
i. The victim must be shown a copy of the report and the contents of the same must be explained to her.

We have examined various protocols issued from time to time relating to medical examination of rape/victims of sexual offences by the WHO, and we have also discussed the matter at length with doctors and experts working in this field.

We have perused the order dated 23rd April 2009 passed by the Delhi High Court in Delhi Commission for Women vs. Delhi Police WP (Crl) No. 696 of 2008. The said order contains a set of comprehensive guidelines to police, hospitals/ doctors, Committees, Sessions Courts, Magistrate Courts, prosecutors and other concerned authorities in order to tackle cases of sexual offences. The said guidelines have comprehensively laid down protocols and procedures to be followed for medical examination of the victim. In our opinion, these guidelines which are extracted below, ought to be the starting point for arriving at a standardized protocol for medical examination which adheres to international standards. The orders read as:

a. 'Crises Intervention Center' (CIC) means a recognized agency, appointed by the Delhi Police and the Delhi Commission for Women for responding to calls of sexual assault at the police station to provide counseling and other support services to victims of rape.
b. 'Expert' means a person who is qualified and has experience in dealing with cases of sexual violence.
c. 'Guardian' includes besides the natural guardian, support person or any person appointed by the Child Welfare Committee for a specified period to take case of the victim during the pendency of trial.
d. 'Rape Crises Cell' means a cell established under the Delhi Commission for Women to provide legal assistance in the cases of sexual assault who would coordinate the CICs and provide legal support to the victim and her family.
e. 'Support person' means a person working in the capacity of a counselor working with a recognized and registered CICs, approved by the Delhi Commission for Women.
f. The expression 'offence' for the purpose of these guidelines shall mean and include offences of rape, attempt to rape and unnatural offences.

Instructions for Doctors/ Hospitals/Health Department

a. Special rooms to be set up in all Government hospitals for victims to be examined and questioned in privacy.
b. A sexual assault evidence collection kit or sexual assault forensic evidence (SAFE) kit consisting of a set of items used by medical personnel for gathering and preserving physical evidence following a sexual assault should be available with all the Government hospitals. A sexual assault evidence collection kit should contain commonly available examination tools as given in Box 5.1. Other items needed for a forensic/medical examination and treatment that may be included in the kit are given in Box 5.2. Some of the items of the SAFE kit developed by IMA (HQ) are shown in Figures 5.1 to 5.3.

c. A detailed description of 'assault/abuse history' should be mentioned by the attending doctors on the MLR of victim. The doctor must ensure that the complete narration of the history of the case detailed by the victim and her escort is recorded.
d. After the examination is complete, the victim should be permitted to wash up using toiletries provided by the hospital. The hospital should also have clothing to put on, if her own clothing is taken as evidence.

Box 5.1 Sexual assault evidence kit

Detailed instructions for the examiner	Large sheet of paper for patient to undress over
Forms for documentation	Paper bags for clothing collection
Tube for blood sample	Urine sample container
Glass slides	Sterile water
Wooden stick for fingernail scrapings	Unwaxed dental floss
Cotton swabs for biological evidence collection	Envelopes or boxes for individual evidence samples and labels

Box 5.2 Other items needed for examination

Woods lamp	Toluidine blue dye
Drying rack for wet swabs and/or clothing	Patient gown, cover sheet, blanket, pillow
Needles/syringes for blood drawing	Speculums
Post—it notes used to collect trace evidence	Colposcope
Camera (35 mm, digital or polaroid), film batteries	Clean clothing and shower/ hygiene items (for the victim's use after the examination)
Microscope	Acetic acid diluted spray
Surgilube	Medications

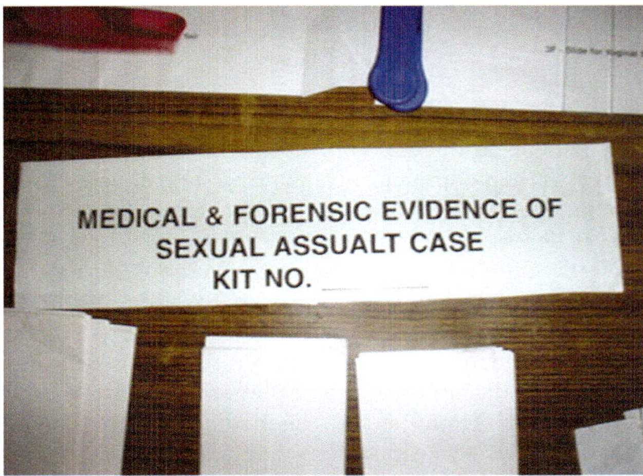

Fig. 5.1 Different envelopes

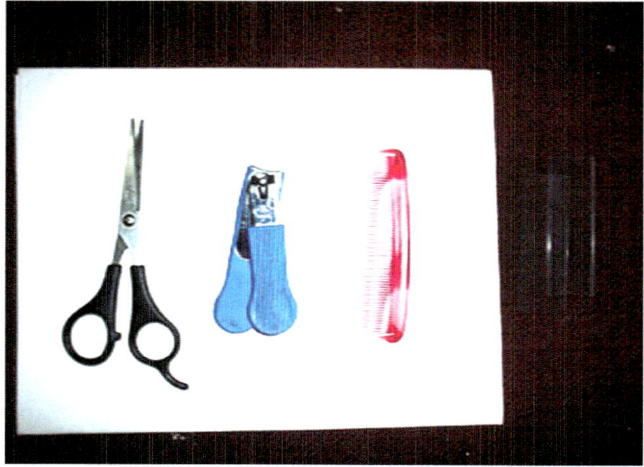

Fig. 5.2 Scissors, clippers, comb and glass slides

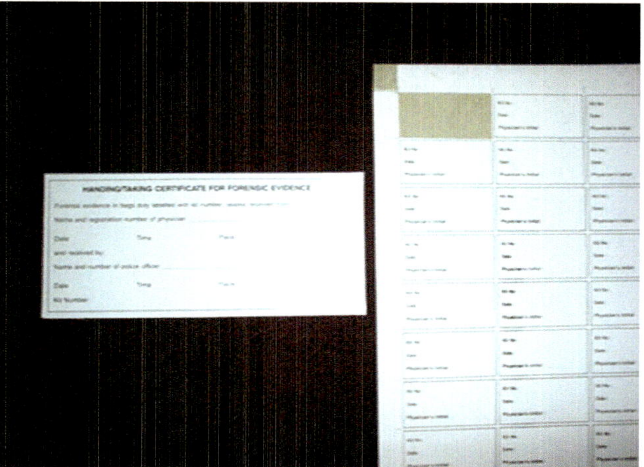

Fig. 5.3 Labels

e. All hospitals should co-operate with the police and preserve the samples likely to putrefy in their pathological facility, till such time the police is able to complete their paper work for dispatch to forensic lab test including DNA.

We are also of the opinion that the medical examination report must be prepared, preferably immediately after the examination, but most certainly on the same date as the examination and must be forwarded to the investigating agency forthwith without delay. The DNA and other samples should be sent to the concerned Forensic Science Labs or DNA Profiling Centers within two days of the incident. We are also of the opinion that any dereliction of duty on part of the examining doctor(s) to undertake the medical examination properly and forwarding the report to the IO without any delay, and any dereliction of duty on the part of the investigating agency in collecting the report or causing the victim to be taken to the nearest hospital for examination should be punishable as offences (in respect of the investigating agency) and by way of disciplinary proceedings (in respect of the examining doctor).

Judgment of the Delhi High Court dated 29th September 2009 in Criminal Appeal No. 121 of 2009, suggested guidelines in relation to medical examination to be implemented immediately in Delhi are worth to be noted at this stage:

Medical Examination

i. Orientation should be given to the doctors, who prepare MLRs or conduct postmortems to ensure that the MLRs as well as PMRs are up to the mark and stand judicial scrutiny in courts.
ii. While conducting medical examination, child victim should be first made comfortable as it is difficult to make her understand as to why she is being subjected to a medical examination.
iii. In case of a girl child victim, the medical examination shall be conducted preferably by a female doctor.
iv. In so far as it may be practical, psychiatric help be made available to the child victim before medical examination at the hospital itself.
v. The report should be prepared expeditiously and signed by the doctor conducting the examination, and a copy of medical report be provided to the parents/guardian of the child victim.
vi. In the event, results of examination are likely to be delayed, the same should be clearly mentioned in the medical report.
vii. The parents/guardian/person in whom child have trust should be allowed to be present during the medical examination.
viii. Emergency medical treatment, wherever necessary, should be provided to the child victim.
ix. The child victim shall be afforded prophylactic medical treatment against STDs.
x. In the event, the child victim is brought to a private/nursing home, the child shall be afforded immediate medical attention and the matter be reported to the nearest police station.

SEXUAL ASSAULT AGAINST CHILDREN

The Protection of Children from Sexual Offences Act, 2012[25]

An Act to protect children from offences of sexual assault, sexual harassment and pornography, and provide for establishment of Special Courts for trial of such offences and for matters connected therewith or incidental thereto.

The Protection of Children from Sexual Offences Act, 2012 defines a child as any person below the age of 18 years and provides protection to all children under the age of 18 years from the offences of sexual assault, sexual harassment and pornography. These offences have been clearly defined for the first time in law. The Act provides for stringent punishments which have been graded as per the gravity of the offence. The punishments range from simple to rigorous imprisonment of varying periods. There is also provision for fine which is to be decided by the court.

Section 3 of the Act defines 'penetrative sexual assault' as a person is said to commit 'penetrative sexual assault' if:

a. He penetrates his penis, to any extent, into the vagina, mouth, urethra or anus of a child or makes the child to do so with him or any other person, or
b. He inserts, to any extent, any object or part of the body, not being the penis into vagina, the urethra or anus of the child or makes the child to do so with him or any other person, or
c. He manipulates any part of the body of the child so as to cause penetration into the vagina, urethra, anus or any part of the body of the child or makes the child to do so with him or any other person, or
d. He applies his mouth to the penis, vagina, urethra of the child or makes the child to so to such person or any other person.

Reporting of the cases under this Act is given in Sec. 19(1) as—Notwithstanding anything contained in the Code of Criminal Procedure, 1973, any person (including the child), who has apprehension that an offence under this Act is likely to be committed or has knowledge that such an offence has been committed, he shall provide such information to:

(a) The Special Juvenile Police Unit, or
(b) The local police.

Section 27 deals with medical examination of such cases and states:

i. The medical examination of a child in respect of whom any offence has been committed under this Act shall, notwithstanding that a FIR or complaint has not been registered for the offences under the this Act, be conducted in accordance with Sec. 164A of the Code of Criminal Procedure,1973.
ii. In case the victim is a girl child, the medical examination shall be conducted by a woman doctor.
iii. The medical examination shall be conducted in presence of the parent of the child or any other person in whom the child reposes trust or confidence.
iv. Where, in case the parent of the child or other person referred to in subsection (3) cannot be present, for any reason, during the medical examination of the child, the medical examination shall be conducted in presence of a woman nominated by the head of the medical institution.

Medical care is usually provided by a doctor and/or a sexual assault nurse examiner (SANE) in a hospital emergency department or medical clinic. Evidence collection may occur up to 120 hours from the assault, and occurs with the consent of the patient.

A sexual assault examiner is a specially trained professional who will provide needed care, document the details of the assault and collect evidence. The professional can recommend treatment for sexually transmitted infections and pregnancy prevention, if needed. In addition, she/he is available to testify in court.[26]

Reporting sexual assault to the police: Only 16–38% of rape victims report to law enforcement, and only 17–43% present for medical evaluation after rape; one-third of victims of rape never report the assault to their primary care doctor.[27] It is recommended that all victims should seek medical evaluation.

The best chance of collecting accurate information and evidence is within the first 24 hours of the sexual assault, although many states allow evidence to be collected up to 7 days later. Changing clothes, showering or bathing, eating, douching, going to the bathroom and brushing hair or teeth should be delayed until evidence is collected, if possible.

Preventive treatments: There is a small risk of becoming infected or pregnant as a result of sexual assault. The risk that a woman will become infected with HIV after a single episode of consensual vaginal intercourse (not sexual assault) with an HIV infected man is estimated at 0.1%, and from a single episode of consensual anal intercourse at 2%. The risk of developing HIV from a sexual assault may be higher, especially, if the skin is torn or cut, if there is bleeding or if there are multiple assailants.

The Centers for Disease Control and Prevention (CDC) and other expert groups recommends preventive treatment if mouth, vagina, anus or nonintact skin (for e.g., a cut) is exposed to the assailant's blood or bodily fluids.

Follow-up care: Most experts recommend for a follow-up visit with a healthcare provider within two weeks of the assault. Testing for pregnancy, gonorrhea, chlamydia, trichomonas and bacterial vaginosis is recommended after the assault. Testing for HIV is usually repeated at six weeks, three months and six months after the assault. This schedule of testing is recommended because, in some cases, it takes up to six months for the blood test to become positive.

Counseling or psychotherapy: Counseling or psychotherapy can be helpful in dealing with the events of the assault itself, as well as the anger, fear, depression or anxiety that many people feel afterwards. Several types of healthcare providers provide counseling, including social workers, psychologists, nurses and psychiatrists. Some people prefer to meet one-on-one with a counselor while others prefer to meet in a group setting with other people who have had similar experiences.

Recently, in March 2014, Ministry of Health and Family Welfare, Government of India issued a comprehensive guidelines and examinations proforma for medicolegal cases of victims of sexual violence. While incorporating most of the above mentioned recommendations in preparing the protocol and guidelines, the committee deliberated various issues and took cognizance of the lack of uniform protocols and gaps in existing provision of medicolegal care to survivors/victims of sexual violence, recommendations of the Justice Verma Committee, the Criminal Law (Amendment) Act, 2013 and Protection of Children from Sexual Offences Act, 2012. While doing so, international standards especially the WHO guidelines on medicolegal care (2003) and Clinical and Policy Guidelines for responding to Intimate Partner Violence (IPV) and Sexual Assault (2013) were referred to.

Besides the general guidelines for the victim of rape and sexual violence, the document also highlight the issues concerning the transgender and intersex persons as well as person with disability, and have given detailed guidelines in examination of such a victim.

These guidelines for health workers are aimed at providing an appropriate understanding of sexual violence and the needs and rights of survivors/victims of sexual violence, and to highlight the medical and forensic responsibilities of health professionals. The detailed document can be accessed at: **www.mohfw.nic**

CONCLUSION

In last few years, new laws/amendments have been made pertaining to sexual assault and rape. It is quite evident that the courts and society expects a lot from doctors while dealing with the cases of violent crime against women and children, and thus the importance of medicolegal examination in cases of sexual assaults cannot be over-emphasized. Slowly, but steadily efforts are being made to objective the medicolegal examination in cases of victims of sexual assaults. Thus, it is the duty of the doctors to refine their skills in accordance with the changing milieu of the medicolegal examination of these cases in order to protect themselves from any legal complications latter on, as well as, to help the victims of these crimes.

REFERENCES

1. "IAP condoles death of Delhi gang-rape victim". New Delhi: Zee News. Press Trust of India [Internet]. 2012 Dec 29. Available from: http://zeenews.india.com/news/delhi/iap-condoles-death-of-delhi-gang-rape-victim_819606.html.
2. Mandhana N, Trivedi A. Indians outraged by account of gang rape on a bus. The New York Times [Internet]. 2012 Dec 30. Available from: http://india.blogs.nytimes.com/2012/12/18/outrage-in-delhi-after-latest-gang-rape-case/.
3. 2012 Delhi gang rape case. Available from: http://en.wikipedia.org/wiki/2012_Delhi_gang_rape.
4. Cole J. Rape in India, and the low status of women. Informed consent. Available from: http://www.juancole.com/2012/12/india-status-women.html.
5. Leeming C. Fifty million Indian women missing. Street News Service. 2008; 15(39). Available from: www.realchangenews.org/index.php/site/archives/719.
6. Macnamara D. History of sexual violence. Clairmont B, County R, Warner CG (eds). Sexual assault interactive theatre. Available from: http://www.interactivetheatre.org/resc/history.html.
7. Koss MP. The women's mental health research agenda. Violence against women. *Am Psychol* 1990; 45: 374-80.
8. National Center for Victims of Crime and Crime Victims Research and Treatment Center. Rape in America: A report to the nation. Arlington, VA, 1992.
9. Tjaden PG, Thoennes N. Extent, nature, and consequences of rape victimization: findings from the national violence against women survey. Washington, DC: National Institute of Justice; 2006. (NCJ 210346).
10. Krebs CP, Lindquist CH, Warner TD, Fisher BS, Martin SL. College women's experiences with physically forced, alcohol- or other drug-enabled, and drug-facilitated sexual assault before and since entering college. *J Am Coll Health* 2009; 57: 639-47.
11. Lawyer S, Resnick H, Bakanic V, Burkett T, Kilpatrick D. Forcible, drug-facilitated, and incapacitated rape and sexual assault among undergraduate women. *J Am Coll Health* 2010; 58: 453-60.
12. Crime in India-2013. National Crime Record Bureau, Ministry of Home Affairs, Govt. of India; 2014. Available from: http://ncrb.gov.in.
13. Indian Penal Code, 1976. Section 375.
14. The Criminal Law (Amendment) Act, 2013. No. 13 of 2013.Gazette of India, 2 April, 2013.
15. Dileep Singh vs. State of Bihar (2005) 1 SCC 88.
16. State of UP vs. Chottey Lal (2011) 2 SCC 550.
17. State of HP vs. Mango Ram (2000) 7 SCC 224.
18. Report of the Committee on Amendments to Criminal Law. JS Verma, Leila Seth, Gopal Subhramanium. 23 January, 2013. Available from: http://www.prsindia.org/parliamenttrack/report-summaries/justice-verma-committee-report-summary-2628/.
19. Sexual Offences Act, 2003 (UK). Section 74-76.
20. Koppula Venkatrao vs. State of AP (2004) 3SCC 602.

21. Tukaram vs. State of Maharashtra (1979) 2 SCC 143.
22. Bharvada Gohinbhai Hirjibhai vs. State of Gujarat (1983) 3SCC 217.
23. Parmanand Katara vs. Union of India (1989) 4 SCC 286.
24. Lillu @ Rajesh vs. State of Haryana, Cr. Appeal No. 1226/2011, Judgment dated April 9, 2013.
25. The Protection of Children from Sexual Offences Act, 2012.
26. Linden JA. Clinical practice. Care of the adult patient after sexual assault. *N Engl J Med* 2011; 365: 834-41.
27. Feldhaus KM, Houry D, Kaminsky R. Lifetime sexual assault prevalence rates and reporting practices in an emergency department population. *Ann Emerg Med* 2000; 36: 23-27.

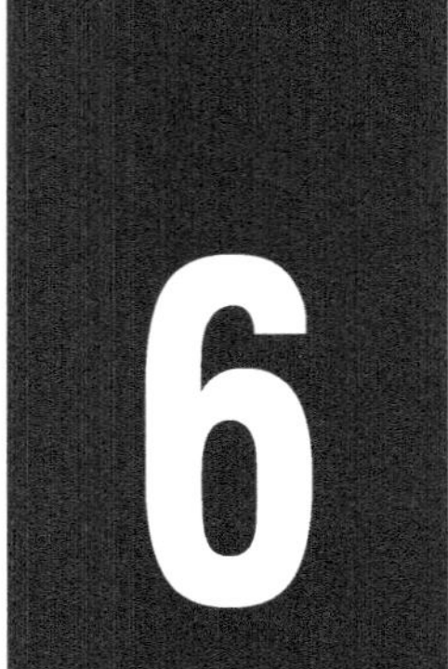

Court Room Procedures

Gautam Biswas, Virendar Pal Singh

'Success in the court room and life itself comes from a combination of character, competence and commitment.'

Anonymous

ABSTRACT

Expert medical evidence has become a central component of the civil and criminal justice system. Scholarly examination of how this is used to inform and shape legal decision-making is very limited. Often the medical practitioner is asked to give evidence about the factual information related to care and management of the patient, and to give opinion on issues related to standard of care and nature of injury in trauma/assault cases. An experienced practitioner may be called to testify as expert witness regarding matters outside the normal scope of knowledge and experience of the Judge. A medical professional must be aware of his/her duty to the court to provide his/her expert opinion objectively and not to skew it to help the case of the party who has asked for the opinion. The purpose of this chapter is to expose the medical professionals to the common legal terminology, existing legal system, court room proceedings, admissibility of evidence, and role of an expert medical witness in court cases.

Keywords: Evidence, burden of proof, deposition, cross-examination techniques, hostile witness.

INTRODUCTION

Medical practitioners are required to testify before a court or a tribunal or before a disciplinary committee at some point of their professional career. Court comes to the conclusion about the facts of the case and pronounces judgments thereupon based on the evidence provided by them. The Criminal Procedure Code (CrPC) contains elaborate details about the procedure to be adopted in every investigation, inquiry and trail, concerned with every offence that is defined under Indian Penal Code (IPC) or under any other law.

The interface between medical practitioner and the legal system is not always an easy one, since both medicine and law are complex fields and neither is an exact science. Most medical practitioners are ignorant of the obligatory penal law; they are fearful and overcautious of interacting with the legal world. There is a tendency to avoid medicolegal cases and subsequent appearances in the court. They have little or no exposure to court room procedures and are ignorant of basic proceedings and formalities. Moreover, doctors consider this as an unpleasant job to stand in the witness box, where his/her credibility is questioned in cross-examination. A good working knowledge of the law coupled with a thorough understanding of the correct method of deposition will help him/her testify confidently in the court of law. This chapter discusses some of the common practical issues associated with court room proceedings.

DEFINITIONS

Given below are short definitions of some of the terms related to court proceedings which a medical practitioner ought to be familiar with.[1,2]

- **Adversarial system:** A system of justice in which two opposing sides contend against each other and puts arguments to an impartial and disinterested Judge for a result favorable to themselves.
- **Inquisitorial system:** A system of justice in which the Judge does not sit as an independent arbiter but acts as an investigator in search of the truth.
- **Amendment:** Alteration of a law or resolution.
- **Common law (case law):** A system in which crimes and punishments are dictated by a contemporary interpretation of prior court decisions passed down through history.
- **Crime or offence:** Any act or omission which is contrary and made punishable by any law or statute for the time being in force.
- **Presumption of innocence:** Law presumes that a person is innocent till his guilt is proved. The onus of proof is on prosecution.
- **Civil trial:** A trial in which a party seeks money or some other remedy that may arise due to the occurrence of events such as a contractual breach or an act of alleged negligence; a suit.
- **Criminal trial:** A type of trial that may arise from the commission of, and subsequent detection of, a crime or alleged crime.
- **Torts:** Wrongful acts that cause or lead to the infringement of an individual's rights and result in legal liability.
- **Liability:** In civil disputes, the measure of responsibility that a group or individual incurs for any harm that has been caused.
- **Appeal:** A request that a case be removed from a lower court to a higher court in order for the case to be reviewed.
- **Judicial proceeding:** It includes any proceeding in the course of which evidence is or may be legally taken on oath.
- **Local jurisdiction:** The local area within which the court or Magistrate may exercise all or any of its or his powers and such local area may comprise the whole of the State, or any part of the State, as the State Government may, by notification, specify.
- **Inquiry:** Every inquiry, other than a trial, conducted by a Magistrate or court.
- **Investigation:** It includes all the proceedings for the collection of evidence conducted by a police officer or by any person (other than a Magistrate) who is authorized by a Magistrate in this behalf.
- **Lawyer:** A person learned in the law; as an attorney, counsel or solicitor; a person who is practicing law.

- **Public prosecutor:** A law officer who conducts criminal proceedings on behalf of the government or in the public interest.
- **Petition:** A written document filed in the court, initiating the case and requesting a decision in a matter described therein.
- **Complaint:** Any allegation made orally or in writing to a Magistrate, with a view to his taking action, that some person, whether known or unknown, has committed an offence. It is the initial written pleading on the part of the plaintiff of a civil case.
- **Plaintiff (claimant or pursuer):** The party that initiates a lawsuit; the party claiming to have been wronged and/or injured in civil cases.
- **Defendant (respondent):** The person accused of committing a crime in criminal cases and/or the person accused of causing harm in civil cases.
- **Prosecution:** The lawyer(s) representing the state who are responsible for bringing criminal charges against defendants based on the investigations of complaints conducted by law enforcement agencies.
- **Expert:** Someone deemed an expert by virtue of his or her knowledge, skill, experience, training or education.
- **Hypothesis:** An educated estimate regarding the possible answer to a question or problem.
- **Scientific method:** An approach to knowledge building and problem solving employed by scientists in which how or why something works or how something happened is investigated through the development of hypotheses and subsequent attempts at falsification through testing and other accepted means.
- **Scientific fact:** Information and events that have been established based on a broad factual record to a reasonable degree of scientific certainty by scientists using the scientific method.
- **Warrant:** An order issued by the court, magistrate or a competent judicial authority, directing a police officer to make arrest, seize or search or to do any other work incidental to administration of justice.
- **Warrant cases** are related to an offence punishable with death, life imprisonment or imprisonment for more than 2 years. For example, if a doctor helps a pregnant woman in getting rid of the child or to cause its death after its birth.
- **Summons cases:** Cases other than warrant cases are *summons cases,* i.e. those cases where the punishment is 2 years or less. For example, a doctor acts negligently by using infected syringe or instrument resulting in an infection in an uninfected patient.
- **Cognizable offences** are those in which a police officer may arrest without warrant from the Magistrate, according of Schedule I of Criminal Procedure Code (CrPC) or any other law for the time being in force. These offences include rape, dowry deaths, ragging, death due to rash or negligent act (negligence), etc.
- **Noncognizable offences** are those in which a police officer has 'no authority' to arrest without a warrant from a Magistrate, for e.g., a doctor knowingly disobeying a quarantine rule is liable to be punished with imprisonment up to 6 months or fine.

Just because the allegations made by somebody constitute a cognizable offence, it does not automatically empower the police to arrest the accused/suspect. In this context, Sec. 157 CrPC states that after receiving information about a cognizable offence, the police officer should proceed to the spot to investigate the facts and circumstances of the case and, if necessary, take measure for the arrest of the offender. Thus, an arrest becomes necessary only if evidence of offence cannot be collected, except by interrogating the accused in police custody or if the offence is heinous.

- **Bailable offences** are those in which bail can be granted by any law for the time being in force. In such cases, bail is matter of right. The court cannot refuse bail and the police have no right to keep the doctor in custody, for e.g., offences under Sec. 304A IPC (criminal negligence). If any police officer puts a doctor in detention in such cases, he is liable for the offense of wrongful confinement under Sec. 340-342 of IPC.
- **Nonbailable offences** are offences other than the bailable or an offence in which bail cannot be granted. These are the serious offences in which a person may be convicted and imprisoned for term extending more than ten years. For example, offences under Sec. 304 IPC or PCPNDT Act 2002.
- **Mistake of law:** *'Ignorentia juris non excusat',* means ignorance of law or mistake of law (existence or mistaken understanding) is not excusable. All persons are presumed to know and understand the law, except minors, persons who lack mental capacity to contract with others; and in criminal cases, persons who are insane. For example, if a doctor carries out prenatal test intended to abort a female fetus, he/she cannot avoid prosecution by saying that he was unaware of any law which punishes such act.
- **Mistake of fact** is a situation where a person not intending to do unlawful act, does so because of wrong conclusion or understanding of fact. The guilty mind was never there while doing the act. The person may not be held responsible in such cases.
- **Res Ipsa Loquitur** (things speak for itself) is a situation of gross negligence and there is no need for any proof of negligence in such cases (mostly in relation to civil cases). Common examples include giving blood transfusion to wrong patient, or operating on wrong side of the body or wrong patient.
- **Common knowledge:** Judges are assumed to possess knowledge and experience of general fields of human endeavor and experience. Experts may not provide evidence regarding matters of 'common knowledge'. There are several areas of medicine which intersect with day to day life, and therefore, invoke the common knowledge rule.
- **Res Judicata:** This doctrine of law means 'the things have been decided'. According to this principle, once the case is completed between two parties and finally decided by competent court, it cannot be tried again between the same parties. Suppose a patient sues a hospital for any wrong, damages or malpractice and the things are decided; he cannot subsequently sue the doctor again separately for the same negligence.

HISTORY OF LAW OF EVIDENCE

Currently, there are two basics of evidence upon which rules and judgment of the court is formulated. One rule is that only the facts bearing importance to the matter being heard, and second that all facts that will help the court to reach a decision. Among others from ancient Hindu period, Vasistha recognized the following kinds of evidence:[3]

i. Lekhya (Documentary evidence)
ii. Sakshi (Witnesses)
iii. Bukhti (Possession)
iv. Divya (Ordeals)

Though the concept of justice in Islam is that of divine disposition, the Mohammedan law givers have dealt with evidence in various forms as indicated by:

i. Oral that may be direct hearsay
ii. Documentary (less preferred than oral)

Initially, at many places and in many beliefs, the parties to litigation would fight each other and it was believed that divine help will come to the rightful party. Trial by battle has been abrogated only in 1817. The trials by ordeal included putting a person on bed of hot coals or putting one's hand in boiling water. Anyone who suffered injury was held to be guilty. Though it was believed that fate will not let harm come to the innocent, often it was the priests who manipulated the tests so that certain people could go scot-free.[3]

A man was held responsible for the crime and punished for the same when the accused is made to touch a corpse and if it shows a reaction. Refusal to touch a corpse by a guilty man was considered as the acceptance of his guilt.

Witch-hunts and witch-craft were the most cruel evidence law that existed in Europe. The suspected woman used to be tied up and thrown into a pond. If she floated to the surface, she was a witch and was burned alive at stake. If the woman sank to the bottom, she was not a witch. Regrettably, she would be dead by then, but nonetheless innocent in the eyes of law and people.[3]

Evolution of Indian Evidence Act

Britishers first gave the existing facts of the 'law of evidence'. In 1837, an Act was a passed, where a convicted person was also allowed to give evidence. Subsequently, parties to litigation could bring witnesses for their respective sides. Between 1835 and 1855, there were eleven Acts which were all consolidated and touched upon the subject of law of evidence.

In 1856, Sir Henry Summer Maine, the then law member of the Governor General's Council was asked to prepare the Indian Evidence Act. His draft was found unsuitable for the Indian conditions. Sir James Fitzjames Stephan in 1871 formulated the Indian Evidence Act. His draft bill was approved and came into being as the Indian Evidence Act, 1872 and came into force from 1st September 1872. Before independence, many states accepted this as the law in their respective state.[3] After independence, the Indian Evidence Act was held to be the law for all Indian courts.

EVIDENCE

The word 'evidence' has been derived from the Latin word '*evidere*' which implies to show distinctly, to make clear to view or sight, to discover clearly, to make plainly certain, to certain, to ascertain, to prove.[4]

a. Black's law dictionary defines evidence as 'which demonstrates that a fact is so, testimony, proof, witness-to make evident, to prove'.[5]
b. Taylor defines evidence as 'all legal means, exclusive of mere argument which tend to prove or disprove any matter of fact; the truth of which is submitted to judicial investigation'. This definition includes methods of proof and excludes 'actual facts proved'.
c. McKelvey states 'evidence is any matter of fact from which an inference may be drawn as to another matter of fact, the former fact is called the evidential fact; the latter, the ultimate, main or principal'.
d. Nokes' define evidence as 'judicial evidence consisting of facts which are legally admissible and the legal means of attempting to prove such facts'.
e. According to Philpson, evidence means 'testimony, whether oral, documentary or real which may be legally received in order to prove or disprove some facts in dispute'.

The truth is that the court may be satisfied by oral or documentary or real evidence or by a combination of any of them or all of them together. Phipson's definition is restricted to oral, documentary and real evidence.[6]

As per the Indian Evidence Act, 'evidence' means and includes:[7]

i. All statements which the court permits or requires to be made before it by witnesses in relation to matters of fact under enquiry—such statements is called *oral evidence.*
ii. All documents including electronic records produced for the inspection of the court—such documents are called *documentary evidence.*

Medical Evidence

The term 'evidence' has different meanings in law and medicine. In law, as discussed above, evidence is material or testimony which is admissible to the court. In medicine, it refers to data obtained through scientific investigation. The quality of such evidence is defined by the scientific methodology employed in the investigation. In law, complex rules restrict the type of evidence that may be presented to the court. These rules aim to exclude evidence which may be unreliable, irrelevant or misleading and include evidence which has the maximum probability of being the truth.[8]

Before going further in the subject matter, it is important to know about 'fact'. Sec. 3 of IEA defines 'fact' as:[7]

i. Anything, state of things or relation of things capable of being perceived by the senses.
ii. Any mental condition of which any person is conscious.

One fact is said to be related with other when it is shown to be connected in any of the ways referred to in the provisions of this act relating to the relevancy of facts. The law of evidence rest upon two aspects:[8]

1. *Quid probandum,* i.e. thing to be proved.
2. *Modus probandi,* i.e. mode of proving.

Fact is said to be 'proved', when, after considering the matter in issue, the court either believes it that it exist or believes its existence so probable that a prudent man ought to act upon the supposition that it exists. A fact is said to be 'disproved', when after considering the matter before it, the court either believes that it does not exist or considers its non-existence so probable that a prudent man ought to act upon the supposition that it does not exist. A fact is said to be 'not proved' when it is neither proved nor disproved.[8]

Proof is attempted by:
a. Oral deposition
b. Document production
c. Material objects
d. Marshalling probabilities
e. Highlighting surrounding circumstances
f. Relying on admissions and presumptions

The burden of proof as to any particular fact lies on that person who wishes the court to believe in its existence, unless it is provided by any law that the proof of that fact shall be on a particular person. Under Sec. 101 of IEA, the burden of proof lies on the party who asserts the affirmative of the issue, while Sec. 103 of the Act provides for the proof of a particular fact.

'Presumption' is an inference of fact, drawn from other known or proved facts. There are two classes of presumptions:[7]

1. *Presumption of fact* is inferences which the human mind naturally and logically draws from facts and they are rebuttable unless they are conclusive. Sec. 86-88, 90, 113A and 114 of IEA relate to presumption of facts.
2. *Presumption of law* is arbitrary consequences expressly annexed by law to particular facts and may either be conclusive or rebuttable. Sec. 41, 79-85, 89, 105, 107-113, 113B and 114 A of IEA relate to presumption of law.

THE LEGAL SYSTEM

The two prevailing legal systems in the world are the adversarial and the inquisitorial systems. In common law countries (such as India, United States, Australia and the United Kingdom), all criminal courts operate under the adversarial system. In civil law jurisdictions (such as France and other mainland European countries), the inquisitorial system is followed.[9,10]

The adversarial system being followed is based on the philosophy that the true facts of a given situation and hence justice will emerge, if the parties act as adversaries rather than cooperative participants. Each side vigorously advances its own version of the facts and an impartial Judge will sort through the truth.[9]

Most court rooms, whether operating under the adversarial or inquisitorial systems, have several common features in the physical layout. The Judge(s) have a clearly delineated area, usually sits at a higher platform with a clear view of the witness box or stand (that will invariably face toward the Judge) and from where the expert and other witnesses give their evidence.

Courts in India (Flow chart 6.1)

The Supreme Court of India is the highest judicial tribunal of the country. It has power of supervision over all courts and the law declared by it is binding on all courts. The High Courts are the highest judicial tribunal for the states. These are the courts of appeal. Sessions Courts are the highest judicial tribunal of the districts and can pass any sentence. The lower courts are the Magistrate Courts. There are also special courts like the Fast Track Courts.[1,8]

Flow chart 6.1 Criminal courts in India

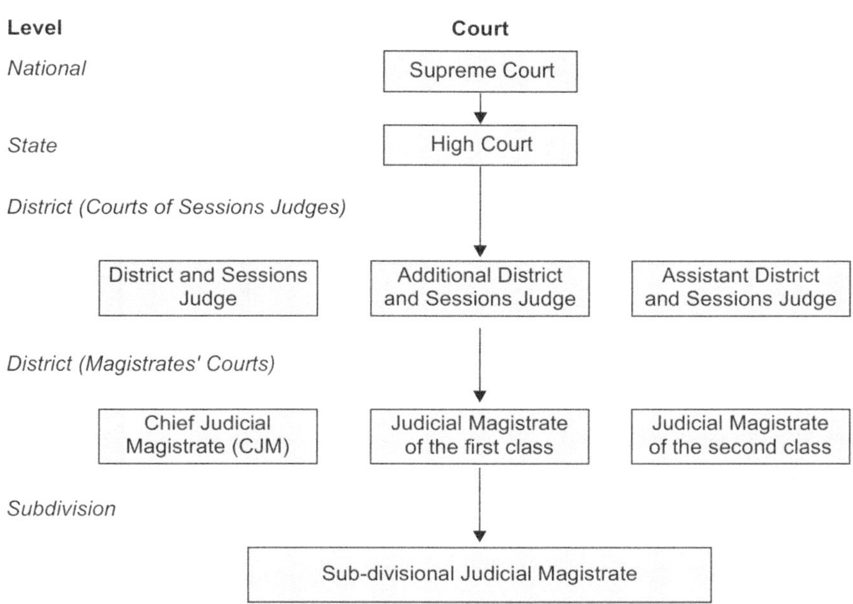

Special Magistrates: They could be either Judicial or Executive Magistrates and may be appointed for a special purpose, for e.g., to try cases of rioting.

Juvenile Courts: A juvenile court (or young offender's court) is a tribunal having special authority to try and pass judgments for crimes committed by children or adolescents who have not attained the age of majority. In the year 2000, the Juvenile Justice Act was passed comprehensively based on the United Nations Convention on the Rights of the Child (CRC), defining children as persons up to the age of 18 years [Sec. 2(k) of the Act defines a child 'as a person who has not completed 18 years of age]. Trial against a juvenile will be done by a Juvenile Justice Board which consist of a Metropolitan Magistrate or a Judicial Magistrate of the first class, as the case may be, and two social workers of whom at least one should be a woman, forming a Bench and every such Bench have the powers conferred by the Code of Criminal Procedure, 1973 (2 of 1974), on a Metropolitan Magistrate or, as the case may be, a Judicial Magistrate of the first class and the Magistrate on the Board should be designated as the Principal Magistrate.[8]

WITNESS

Definition

A witness is a person who gives sworn testimony (evidence) in a court of law as regards facts and/or inferences that can be drawn from those facts.

Types

i. *Common, ordinary or lay witness:* Common witness is a person who has seen or observed the facts. It has to be proved that he/she was capable of perceiving the facts or has actually seen the facts. This principle is known as 'first hand knowledge rule'.[1,9]

   Section 118 IEA deals about the person who may testify as witness in court of law. It states that all persons are competent to testify, unless the court considers that they are prevented from understanding the questions put to them, or from giving rational answers to those questions as a result of tender age, extreme old age, disease of mind or body or any other cause of the same kind. Even a mentally ill person is not incompetent to testify unless he is prevented by his illness from understanding the questions put to him.[7]

ii. *Expert or skilled witness:* They are not only medical experts, but can be experts in other subjects. Such persons because of their professional training and experience are capable of drawing a conclusion on the facts observed by them or by others.[1,9-11]

Hostile Witness

Hostile witness is one who purposefully makes statements contrary to the fact or has some interest or motive for concealing truth.[1] During examination-in-chief, if the examining lawyer who has called the witness finds his/her testimony as antagonistic or contrary to the legal position of his client, the lawyer may request the Judge to declare the witness as hostile. Once the request is accepted, the lawyer may proceed to ask the witness leading questions. Criminal consequences of witnesses turning hostile are given in Sec. 191, 192, 193, 199, 503 and 506 of the IPC.

Recently, the Supreme Court held that the law permits the court to take into consideration the deposition of a hostile witness, to the extent that the same is in consonance with the case of the prosecution and found to be reliable under careful judicial scrutiny. Evidence tendered by a prosecution witness would not get entirely erased merely because the prosecution has chosen to treat him as hostile.

EXPERT WITNESS

The earliest known use of an expert witness in English law came in the 1782, when a court that was hearing litigation relating to the silting-up of Wells harbor in Norfolk accepted evidence from a leading civil engineer, John Smeaton. The need for professionals to testify in medical litigation has its origins in English Common Law. In 1767, in the case of Slater vs. Baker and Stapleton, the concept of professional standard was established; physicians and surgeons were to be judged by 'the usage and law of surgeons...the rule of the profession as testified to by surgeons themselves'.[12]

Section 45 IEA deals with opinion of expert witness. When the court has to form an opinion upon a point of foreign law, science or art, or identity of hand writing or fingerprints, the opinion of persons especially skilled in such foreign law, science, art, handwriting or fingerprints are relevant facts. Such persons are called *experts*.[7] For example:

i. The question is, whether the death of A was caused by poison. The opinions of experts as to the symptoms produced by the poison by which A is supposed to have died are relevant.
ii. The question is whether A, at the time of doing a certain act, was by reason of unsoundness of mind, incapable of knowing the nature of the act or that he was doing what was either wrong or contrary to law. The opinions of experts upon the question whether the symptoms exhibited by A commonly show unsoundness of mind and whether such unsoundness of mind usually renders persons incapable of knowing the nature of the acts which they do, or knowing that what they do is either wrong or contrary to law are relevant.

Doctors are not necessarily expert witnesses. Medical practitioners are considered '*professional witnesses*' akin to witnesses of fact when he/she is providing factual medical evidence. They can be testifying about events that they themselves have observed, for e.g., the doctor may confirm the physical examination findings in case of accident or a diagnosis made after investigation or may report the findings of an X-ray or treatment given to the patient. The medical practitioner is not giving comment or opinion on any report based on the medical facts.[9,10]

An expert witness expresses an opinion about medical facts. The difference between a 'professional witness' and an 'expert witness' is that experts can offer opinions beyond the facts of what they have personally witnessed and can respond to questions about hypothetical situations posed to them.[9] Although experts can testify in any case in which their expertise is relevant, criminal cases are more likely to use forensic specialists. However, senior attending physicians in India, United Kingdom, Ireland and the United States are routinely summoned in both the civil and criminal courts for their expert evidence.

Non-testifying experts: In the United States, a party can hire experts to help him/her evaluate the case. For example, an ECG machine manufacturer may hire an experienced engineer to decide if its machines were built to specification. This kind of expert opinion will be protected from discovery. If the expert finds something that is against its client, the opposite party will not know it.

Testifying experts: If the witness needs to testify in the court, the privilege is no longer protected. The expert witness's identity and nearly all documents used to prepare the testimony will become discoverable.

ROLE OF AN EXPERT MEDICAL WITNESS

A medical witness called in as an expert to assist the court is not a witness of fact and the evidence given by the doctor is essentially of an advisory nature given on the basis of the signs and symptoms found during examination. Sometimes, a medical practitioner may also be called to testify about cases in which he or she played no preceding role. The witness is expected to put before the court all materials inclusive of the data which convinced him to come to the conclusion and enlighten the court on the technical aspects of the case by explaining the medical terms. The court may then form its own judgment on those materials, after giving due regard to the expert's opinion because once the opinion is accepted, it is not the opinion of the doctor but of the court.[8]

Typically, in a malpractice suit, a plaintiff hires a medical expert to show both a breach of the standard of care and causation, and a defendant hires an opposing expert to show the doctor's conduct met the standard of care and/or the breach did not directly or proximately cause injury to the plaintiff. In such cases, witnesses of fact must restrict their testimony to the facts of the case at issue.[12] The expert witness is allowed to describe the applicable standards of care relevant to the given case and interpret whether the evidence indicates a deviation (breach) from the standard of care. The witness also provides an opinion (within a reasonable degree of medical certainty) as to whether that breach in care is the most likely cause of the patient's injury. In addition, the expert may be needed to testify about the current clinical state of a patient to assist the process of determining damages. Expert witnesses may rely on their observations and experiences in their practice, medical literature, training, laboratory and radiological examinations, histories, physical examination and the like, to formulate their opinions. Hypothetical questions may also be posed to an expert.[12-14]

Without the expert's explanation of the range of acceptable treatment modalities within the standard of care and interpretation of medical facts, the Judge would not have the technical expertise needed to distinguish malpractice (caused by negligent care) from maloccurrence (caused by 'bad outcome'). Moreover, whenever a medical intervention is undertaken, several outcomes can occur—the patient's condition can improve, stay the same, or deteriorate. A negative outcome alone is not sufficient to indicate professional negligence.[13,14]

In some malpractice cases, expert testimony may not be required where negligence is obvious and within the common knowledge of a Judge, such as operating on the wrong limb or leaving surgical instruments or sponges within the body.

Inadequate performance by an expert may damage the proper conduct and outcome of a trial and may lead to criticism by the Judge, or the referral of the expert to a relevant professional body such as the State Medical Council or MCI for disciplinary action.[12]

The expert has a heavy responsibility and perjury by an expert is a severely punished crime in most countries. The use of expert witnesses is sometimes criticized in the United States because in civil trials, they are often used by both sides to advocate differing positions, and it is left up to a Jury to decide which expert witness to believe.[13,14] The reader is directed to read more about expert witness in the chapter 'Expert Medical Evidence'.

ADMISSIBILITY OF EVIDENCE AND TESTIMONY

When the witness qualifies as an expert, he or she does not possess complete discretion to express any opinion within the area of expertise. The courts also suggest that testimony must be based on scientifically reliable information. An expert's opinion based on assumption of fact without evidentiary support or on speculative or conjectural factors has no evidentiary value, and it is likely that that information will not be relied upon and may be excluded from evidence.[8]

Rules of evidence: One of the principal rules relevant to the admissibility of evidence requires that any evidence presented in a trial be 'relevant' and if such testimony is likely to be helpful. Two rules, called the 'general acceptance' test and the 'Daubert test' give trial Judges authority to exclude expert testimony based on faulty reasoning.[12,14-17]

Legal Doctrines

The 'general acceptance' test was established in Frye vs. United States in 1923. The case held that expert witness testimony is deemed reliable if deduced from a well-recognized scientific principle or discovery and the deduction made must have gained 'general acceptance' in the particular field in which it belongs.

The case of Daubert vs. Merrell Dow Pharmaceuticals, Inc. established that for scientific evidence to be admissible in court, trial Judges can consider the following:

a. Whether the expert's opinion has been peer reviewed?
b. Whether the theory can be and has been tested?
c. The known or potential error rate of the theory.
d. The general acceptance of the theory in the relevant scientific community.

Trial Judges are to focus on the reasoning or scientific validity of the methodology, not the expert's conclusion.

The Frye test advocates that in order to be classified as an area of expertise, the area must be sufficiently established to have gained general acceptance in the particular field to which it belongs. The Daubert ruling has further specified the criteria to determine the admissibility of scientific evidence. The expert must be able to clearly justify his opinion on the basis of facts using his expertise, describing how he was able to reach at the opinion using any documents, books and photos. Challenges to questionable testimony are to be contested via cross-examination and the presentation of contrary evidence.

The law also requires that a medical expert give an opinion based only upon 'reasonable medical certainty' or 'reasonable medical probability'. The legal definition of the two phrases is that the doctor must believe or feel that the opinion is *more likely than not accurate.* For example, if the doctor is asked, based upon the reasonable medical certainty, whether the injuries were the result of the accident, the doctor need to believe that the accident was 'more likely than not' the cause of the injury claimed in order to answer 'Yes'.

The law makes a legal distinction between 'possibility' and 'probability'. Opinions based upon possibility are *not* necessarily admissible. Therefore, if the doctor uses any of the following phrases in connection with his/her opinion, such testimony may not be accepted by the Judge: it 'might be' true, it 'is possible', it 'might have' that effect, it 'could have' that effect.

While there must be more than a bare possibility, the law does recognize that a degree of uncertainty is present in almost every medical opinion.

BURDEN AND STANDARD OF PROOF

The burden of proof is the obligation to prove a fact in issue. The burden generally rests with the party bringing the case. It is also known as the legal or persuasive burden. The standard of proof is the probative effect required to persuade the court, and measures the quality of the evidence. The probative effects of evidence in civil and criminal cases differ. In civil court, a fact may be regarded as proved, but evidence may not be sufficient enough to convict in a criminal case.[9,13]

In civil cases, the standard is the 'balance of probabilities' or 'weight of evidence'; the court must conclude the facts asserted are more probable than not to accept them. The plaintiff bears the burden of proof and must convince the Judge by a preponderance of the evidence that its case is more plausible. A preponderance of the evidence is at least 51%. The plaintiff and defense lawyers will present their respective experts, each side hoping their witnesses will appear more knowledgeable, objective and credible than their counterparts. That means that Judge in a medical negligence case must be persuaded that the evidence presented by the plaintiff is more plausible as the proximate cause of the injury than any counterargument offered by the defendant.[17-21]

In criminal cases, the prosecution must prove their case 'beyond reasonable doubt'. The prosecution bears this—the accused is innocent until proved guilty, and the prosecution must prove the case against him/her.[17-21]

Law relating to burden of proof deals with the question, by whom and in what manner evidence must be produced and by which party any fact is to be proved.

GOING TO THE COURT

Court Proceedings

The procedure is quite similar for civil and criminal courts (Flow chart 6.2).[11] The petitioner in a civil cases or the prosecution in a criminal trial will put their

Flow chart 6.2 Proceedings of a criminal court

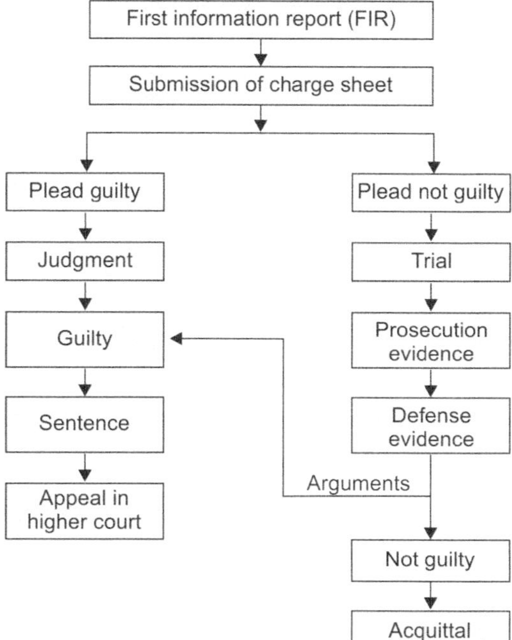

case first. Their witnesses will give evidence and be cross-examined. Following this, the other side will respond. Subsequently, after the evidence has been heard, both parties will make closing speeches and the Judge will sum up the evidence.

In a civil case, the Judge will decide on the basis of the law and the evidence presented, whether to rule in favor of the petitioner or the defendant and the amount of compensation that should be paid. In a criminal case, based on the facts and the law applied, the Judge will give the verdict.

Subpoena/Summons

Subpoena is a document compelling the attendance of a witness in a court of law under penalty, on a particular day, time and place for the purpose of giving evidence. It can be of two types:[1,9]

i. *Subpoena duces tecum* require the person to bring certain documents or other evidence to the court (for e.g., postmortem or the medicolegal report) specified in the subpoena.
ii. *Subpoena ad testificandum* require the individual to testify before the court.

The subpoena has its source in English Common Law and it is now used almost with universal application throughout the Anglo-American Common Law world. However, for civil proceedings in England and Wales, the term has been replaced by *witness summons* or *claim form,* as part of reforms to replace Latin terms with easier to understand English terms and to simplify legal terminology. In ancient Persian law, if one failed to answer the summons of the King, the punishment was death. The United States Congress also has the power to issue subpoenas and can punish individuals who fail to comply by contempt of Congress, which is similar to contempt of court.[9,11]

A witness subpoena legally requires an individual to appear in court to give evidence or testimony. Subpoena is often issued in cases when a witness may not voluntarily come forward to testify. It is important to ensure that the subpoena is served legally, otherwise the witness may be dismissed or his evidence and testimony could be rendered inadmissible. Summons is issued by the court in writing, in duplicate and signed by the Presiding Officer of the court and bears the seal of the court. The provisions regarding summons are dealt in the Sec. 61 to 69 CrPC. It is served on the witness by a police officer, by an officer of the court or other public servant. The witness retains one copy (original) and returns the other one duly signed by him on the back in acknowledgement of its receipt. According to Sec. 66 CrPC, if the witness is a government servant, the summons can be sent to the head of the office in duplicate, and the head in turn serves it to the concerned person.[1]

It may also require the witness to bring with him any books, documents or other things under his control which he is bound by law to produce in evidence. The witness should not leave the court without the permission of the Presiding Officer. When summons are issued to produce a document or any other article required for investigation or trial (Sec. 91 CrPC), the person in possession of the said document or article may send it, instead of attending the court personally.[11]

Summons is issued in both civil and criminal cases. It must be obeyed and honored. If the medical practitioner is not in a position to attend the court on the appointed date for some valid reason, the court should be informed in writing, requesting for an adjournment of the case. The witness may be excused from attending the court, if he has valid and urgent reason. If the witness fails to attend the court after receiving the summons, he will be liable to pay damages in civil cases. In criminal cases, the court may issue notice under Sec. 350 CrPC and after hearing the witness, if it finds that the witness neglected to attend the court without justification, may sentence him to a fine (not exceeding ₹ 100), or the court may issue bailable or non-bailable warrants to secure the presence of witness (Sec. 172-174 IPC and Sec. 87 CrPC). If a witness is summoned by two courts on the same day, one criminal and other civil, he should attend the criminal court—criminal courts have priority over civil courts. Higher court has priority over the lower. If summoned to two courts on the same day, either civil or criminal, he must first attend the higher court. When the witness receives the summons from two courts of equal cadre, then he must first attend the court from which he received the summons first and intimate the other court about his attendance to the court which has served the summons first.[1]

A subpoena does not necessarily overrule the obligation towards a patient. If the medical practitioner believes that the information is confidential and the patient does not want it revealed, and/or that some information in the record is irrelevant or harmful, it is the obligation of the doctor to argue to the court through a motion to quash the subpoena, that the record should not be submitted. In making these determinations, it is also important to remember that any document turned over to the court will be turned over to all parties, including the accused.

Conduct Money

Conduct money is the fee offered or paid to a witness *in civil cases*, at the time of serving the summons to meet the expenses towards attending the court. This fee may be paid in the court also. If fee is not paid or if he feels that the amount is less, the doctor can bring this fact to the notice of the Judge.[1] The Judge will decide the amount to be paid.

In criminal cases, no fee is paid to the witness at the time of serving the summons. He must attend the court and give evidence because of the interest of the State in securing justice, otherwise he will be charged with contempt of court.[1] However, conveyance charges and daily allowance are paid according to government rules. This is sometimes paid by the institute/hospital where the medical practitioner works.

Deposition

A deposition is testimony of a witness. It is given under oath on being questioned by lawyers for the parties in the case. The words spoken by the witness are treated as court room testimony and the proceeding is conducted in accordance with the applicable court rules.[13] A deposition is a discovery device—lawyers gather information on what factual and expert witnesses says orally and assess the relative effectiveness of their testimony. The purpose of discovery is to identify all the facts related to the case.[14]

After receiving summons or subpoena, the expert witness must appear before the court at the appointed time with the relevant documents. Unlike ordinary witnesses to fact, experts can sit in court prior to giving evidence and hear other witnesses' evidence of fact.

GIVING EVIDENCE

The evidence is presented in a systematic order (Sec. 138 IEA):[1,8-11,14]

i. Oath (Sec. 51 IPC)
ii. Examination-in-chief (direct examination, Sec. 137 IEA)
iii. Cross-examination (Sec. 141-146 IEA)
iv. Re-examination (Re-direct examination, Sec. 138 IEA)
v. Court questions (questions by Judge, Sec. 165 IEA, Sec. 311 CrPC)

Witness is first examined-in-chief, then (if the adverse party so desires) cross-examined, then (if the party calling him so desires) re-examined.

The Oath

It is compulsory for the witness to take an oath in the witness box before he gives his evidence. The main aim is that the witness must tell the truth during the evidence.

Procedure: The witness stands in the witness box and takes the oath by holding the Gita/Bible in right hand (not in left hand with the right hand upraised). He/she is required to swear by Almighty God to tell the truth, the whole truth and nothing but the truth. If the witness is an atheist, he/she makes a solemn affirmation in same terms, instead of swearing by God.

The oath is administered by the Presiding Officer in all courts, other than High Courts and Supreme Courts. In cases where the witness appears before a bench of Judges or Magistrates, one of the Judges or the Magistrate can administer the oath (Indian Oath Act 44 of 1969). The provision is incorporated in Sec. 51 IPC. The word 'oath' includes a solemn affirmation substituted by law for an oath and any declaration required or authorized by law to be made before a public servant or to be used for the purpose of proof, whether in a court of justice or not.

Perjury: A witness who after taking oath or making a solemn affirmation, willfully makes a false statement which he knows or believes to be the false (Sec. 191 IPC and Sec. 344 CrPC) is liable to be prosecuted for perjury under **Sec. 193 IPC** with imprisonment of up to 7 years and fine.

Sec. 191 IPC states that whoever, being legally bound by an oath or by an express provision of law to state the truth or being bound by a law to make a declaration upon any subject, makes any statement which is false and which he either knows or believes to be false or does not believe to be true, is said to give false evidence. The common, as well as expert witnesses can be hostile.

Punishment for false evidence as per Sec. 193 IPC: Whoever intentionally gives false evidence in any stage of judicial proceedings, or fabricates false evidence for the purpose of its being used in any stage of judicial proceeding shall be punished with imprisonment of either description for a term which may extend to 7 years, and shall also be liable to be fined.

Review of Credentials

In some places, after being sworn or affirmed, the credentials of the expert witness is reviewed before the Judge pronounces that he or she can testify as a witness.

It would also highlight the important accomplishments of the expert's professional career and experience in litigation.

Examination-in-chief

The witness is then examined by the lawyer of the party that has called him. It is also known as direct examination. It is realm of a party by whom the witness is called for, and the purpose is to of elicit all the material facts within his knowledge which tend to prove the party's case. In criminal cases, the State becomes a party so the burden of proof is always on the prosecution and the public prosecutor commences this examination. In the adversarial system of our country, it becomes a tool of extracting truth from the facts. Usually, *no leading questions are allowed*, except in those cases in which the Judge is satisfied that a witness is hostile (Sec. 142 of the IEA).

Objectives: The main objectives are to place before the court all the facts that bear on the case, and if the witness is an expert, his interpretation of these facts.

Major Objectives

i. The evidence must be admissible.
ii. The witness needs to be convincing and credible.
iii. Each and every element of the offence must be proven beyond a reasonable doubt through the witnesses' oral evidence and exhibits.

Minor Objectives

i. Present a logical, complete and coherent theory of the offence.
ii. Present each witness in the best possible light.
iii. Knitting all witnesses' evidence together in a coherent fashion in order to prove all the elements of the offence beyond a reasonable doubt.
iv. Fill in gaps in the evidence and attempt to explain any inconsistencies.
v. Shut down potential cross-examination thereby limiting the exposure of witnesses.
vi. Allow the defense as little room to move as possible by minimizing the possibilities of a defense being supported through cross-examination of witnesses.

Before giving the evidence, the doctor should always go through the relevant documents and previously prepared report (if any). If needed, he can meet the public prosecutor and go through the files and other records. The expert should help the lawyer prepare a series of questions so that proper facts are elicited. The more effective technique is free narrative where the lawyer asks basic questions and gives the expert some flexibility in answers. During testimony, the Judge needs to understand the details of the circumstances, and hence, the expert should start at the beginning and go through until the end.

The medical witness is usually asked questions as to when he saw the patient and started the medicolegal examination. In assault cases, the question pertaining to description of the injuries, duration of injuries and possible weapon of offence is also asked during examination-in-chief. With medical procedures, first describe them, then tell what the outcome or interpretive result is.

Sec. 141 IEA: *Leading question:* Any question suggesting the answer which the person putting it wishes or expects to receive. It includes a material fact and admits of a conclusive answer by a simple 'Yes' or 'No'. For example, "Was the length of the knife 15 cm?" Instead, question should be "What was the length of the knife?"
Sec. 142 IEA: *When they must not be asked:* Leading questions must not, if objected to by the adverse party, be asked in an examination-in-chief or in re-examination, except with the permission of the court.
Sec. 143 IEA: *When they must be asked:* Leading questions may be asked in cross-examination.

Cross-examination

During the cross-examination, the lawyer of the adverse party (defense lawyer) examines the witness. The main objectives are:

i. To elicit facts favorable to his case.
ii. To test the accuracy of the statements made by the witness.
iii. To modify or explain what has been said.
iv. To develop new or old facts.
v. To discredit the witness.
vi. To remove any overemphasis which may have been given to any fact in direct examination.

The lawyer tries to weaken the evidence of the witness by showing that his/her details of the report given are inaccurate, conflicting, contradictory, untrustworthy and biased one. It is not necessary that the question should be confined to the facts told in examination-in-chief (Sec. 143 IEA). The defense lawyer may even ask questions pertaining to the qualifications or experience, especially in the type of the case in question. During this time, the court observes whether a particular question should be answered or not. The court has power to disallow a question, if it indecent and scandalous (Sec. 151 IEA) or if it is intended to insult or harass the witness (Sec. 152 IEA), but if it is relevant to the case, the court cannot disallow. The witness has to answer the question that relates to the case, even if it is harmful to the witness or it exposes his fault or negligence (Sec. 146 IEA). If a witness is forced to answer that goes against him, he cannot be arrested or prosecuted or cannot be taken as proof against him for any criminal proceedings.

Unlike in direct examination, leading questions designed to elicit a particular response are allowed in cross-examination. Cross-examination has no time limit, may last for hours or even days.

Re-examination

The examination of a witness, subsequent to the cross-examination by the party who called him is called re-examination. After the cross-examination, the lawyer who has called the witness to testify might have further questions, but these can only be about information that arose in the cross-examination. There can be further questioning by the adverse party (re-cross) but only about information that arose in the re-direct examination. The examinations, therefore, become shorter and shorter.

Questions by the Judge

Judge may ask any question to the witness at any stage of the trial to clear or clarify any doubts in the evidences. The court is also empowered to recall and re-examine any witness already examined, if it is essential to arrive at a decision (Sec. 165 IEA and Sec. 311 CrPC).

All the time the witness is speaking, the typist goes on typing that is a word by word account of all that is said in the deposition. In some countries, an audio-recording or video-recording may be produced as well.

Expert medical witnesses are often clear and coherent and straightforward during the stage of examination-in-chief itself, so they are not cross-examined very much. Most of the time, the opposite lawyer asks no questions and the recording of evidence ends here. The typist types the heading 'Cross-examination', and then types beneath it 'Nil, opportunity given', which means that no cross examination was done, despite having been given the opportunity to do so.

After the recording of evidence is over, the typist types ROAC (Read Over and Corrected) below the typed statement. The deposition of the witness is handed over to him. The witness must read the whole written transcript carefully and thoroughly. Any mistakes in the deposition should be brought to the notice of the court and then he can correct it with his initials (Sec. 278 CrPC). It is not an opportunity to change an answer. He is required to sign at the bottom of each page and on the last page immediately below the last paragraph.

The medical witness should not leave the court without prior permission. When there are no further questions to be asked, the Judge permits him to leave. Before exiting through the court doors, the witness should turn and face the Judge and bow slightly before leaving.

CROSS-EXAMINATION TECHNIQUES

Cross-examination by its nature usually involves direct challenge of the witness and may at times be quite an aggressive process with direct personal attack not uncommon. This sort of combative approach to problem solving is obviously unfamiliar to most doctors, some of whom would be rarely challenged, let alone attacked in the course of their professional career. The medical witness should understand that the opposing lawyer has a job to do and it is his/her obligation to test your testimony through the adversarial process.

Most lawyers have their own style but vary it depending on the witness. Marshall described defense lawyers and tactics they use during the deposition in an interesting but still useful way:[14]

- The 'pal' defense lawyer dresses casually and holds the deposition in a rather informal setting. Although the expert is a guest in the court, the lawyers may know each other. The lawyer may joke with each other in an attempt to convince the expert that the deposition itself is informal, so there is no need to be careful about what is said before the deposition. The witness should recognize this tactic for what it is and, keeping in mind the formal and serious nature of the deposition should avoid entering into any chit-chat and avoid joking during the entirety of the deposition process.

- The 'freight train' defense lawyer begins asking questions in a rapid-fire manner in an attempt to 'run over' the expert, resulting in confused, unimaginable and quick answers. If this occurs, the expert witness should remain calm and answer each question one at a time, unhurriedly, in complete sentences to break the rapid-fire rhythm of the questions. This tactic will not have any success with an experienced expert, but may work if the witness shows signs of being unsure, hesitant or timid.
- The 'butterfly' defense lawyer moves from one line of questioning to another, back and forth, confusingly, in an attempt to elicit conflicting statements. The expert should recognize and ignore this tactic and focus on answering out-of-order and repetitive question consistently.
- The 'time bomb' defense lawyer saves the most difficult, contentious and complicated questions until the end of the deposition, when fatigue increases the risk of inconsistent or incorrect responses. If fatigued, the expert should ask for a short break and then remain attentive through the next phase of the cross-examination.
- The 'ignoramus' defense lawyer appears ignorant during the deposition. In an attempt to get the expert to volunteer information, the lawyer may leave time after an answer, and use body language, to prompt him/her to add more to an answer than the question required. He/she should recognize this tactic and just respond to the question asked and no more.

SHORTCOMINGS

When the expert is giving evidence within a court room setting, his/her methods and opinions are exposed to the highest level of scrutiny. Although, it is interesting and professionally challenging, there is still an unnecessarily adversarial environment in the court. In a court room, the language, values, customs, dress and traditions are intimidating, unfamiliar and unhelpful.

Some perceive the purpose of cross-examination as being to impugn their professional integrity by a personal attack on their credibility. The expert may be challenged to the extent of his/her expertise, or forced to defend the validity of his/her chosen field of study against attacks that it is merely guesswork or irrelevant. The attack may not only extend to that of the expert's profession: salvos on his/her personal credibility may be launched with the expert forced to explain matters within his/her personal life, or historical indiscretions. Hence, members of the medical profession, wary of interaction with the legal system may think that the risk to reputation is too great and may be reluctant to help.[22]

Sometimes, the lawyers do not comprehend the specific ideology that the expert medical witness brings to the court. Expert witnesses may only be permitted to present part of their evidence and this may result in an incomplete or distorted version of the truth as they see it. The expert witness is often expected to provide clear 'yes or no' unambiguous answers to questions where there is profound uncertainty within the field of inquiry. This approach to problem solving is alien to most medical practitioners. The medical witness may find the process an intensely frustrating, confusing and unrewarding experience.[22]

Moreover, a lot of time and effort is required to record evidence. Therefore, by and large, members of the medical profession do not like to be involved in medicolegal cases. Some of the possible reasons put forward are undue time consumption, repeated adjournments and lack of work culture. But, the medical practitioner should not fear this situation but rise to the challenge, seeking to educate and explain the frequently complex situations that arise.

CONCLUSION

There is inherent fear to avoid medicolegal cases which may lead to trouble in a court of law. However, if the medical practitioner acquires a minimum level of understanding of the legal system, observes and analyze the cases judiciously and acts patiently, then most of the problems can be solved. It is hoped that the above discussions will help the medical practitioner against procedural lapses in court rooms.

The expert medical practitioner's role is that of an impartial professional—giving detailed consideration of the case and formulating a balanced opinion based on his/her findings irrespective of interest of the patient or the authority requesting the report. The objective of the expert witness is to support the proper administration of justice and the early resolution of dispute through fair and unbiased expert evidence.

ACKNOWLEDGMENT

The authors deeply acknowledge the suggestions made by Dr Pardeep Kumar MV, Professor, Department of FMT, RajaRajeswari Medical College and Hospital, Bengaluru.

REFERENCES

1. Biswas G. Legal procedures. Review of forensic medicine and toxicology. New Delhi: Jaypee Brothers Medical Publishers (P) Ltd.; 2012. p. 34-44.
2. Tiwari SK, Baldwa M. Doctors and criminal law. *Indian Pediatr* 2002; 39: 1119-25.
3. Kanwar N. Introduction to Indian Evidence Act. Available from: http://kanwarn.wordpress.com/2008/12/20/introduction-to-indian-evidence-act/.
4. Kumar S. Different kinds of evidences & witnesses under the Indian Evidence Act; 2012. Available from: http://www.legalindia.in/different-kinds-of-evidences-witnesses-under-the-indian-evidence-act.
5. Black HC. Black's Law Dictionary. 5th edn. 1983.
6. Law of evidence. Available from: http://www.nou.edu.ng/noun/NOUN_OCL/pdf/Laws/LAW445 Law of evidence.pdf.
7. Indian Evidence Act, 1872. Available from: http://indiankanoon.org/doc/1953529/.
8. Aggarwal AD, Singh H, Gorea RK. Medical witness and the Indian courts. *JPAFMAT* 2007; 7: 21-26.
9. Shephard R. The doctor and the law. Simspon's forensic medicine. 12th edn. London: Arnold; 2003. p. 1-7.
10. Franklin PJ. The doctor in court. In: McLay WDS (ed). Clinical forensic medicine. 3rd edn. Cambridge: Cambridge university press; 2009. p. 45-50.
11. Giving evidence; 2013. Available from: http://www.medicalprotection.org/uk/northern-ireland-factsheets/giving-evidence.
12. Bal BS. The expert medical witness in medical malpractice litigation. *Clin Orthop Relat Res* 2009; 467: 383-91.

13. American Academy of Pediatrics. Guidelines for expert witness testimony in medical malpractice litigation. *Pediatrics* 2002; 109: 974-78.
14. Allen TC. Medico-legal issues in pathology. *Arch Pathol Lab Med* 2008; 132: 186-91.
15. Annas GJ. Scientific evidence in courtroom. The death of the frye rule. *N Engl J Med* 1994; 330: 1018-21.
16. Botash AS. Child abuse evaluation and treatment. Available from: http://www.childabusemd.com/law/legal-overview.shtml.
17. Satiani B. Expert witness testimony: rules of engagement. *Vasc Endovascular Surg* 2006; 40: 223-27.
18. Horn C, Caldwell DH, Osborn DC. Law for physicians: an overview of medical legal issues. American Medical Association; 2000. p. 1-4.
19. Mackauf SH. Neurologic malpractice: the perspective of a patient's lawyer. *Neurol Clin* 1999; 17: 345-53.
20. Jasanoff S. Science at the bar: law science and technology in America. Cambridge MA: Harvard university press; 1995.
21. Neufeld PJ, Colman N. When science takes the witness stand. *Sci Am* 1990; 262: 46-53.
22. Johnston RG, Oswald JD. Academic dishonesty: revoking academic credentials. *J Marshall L Rev* 1998; 32: 67.

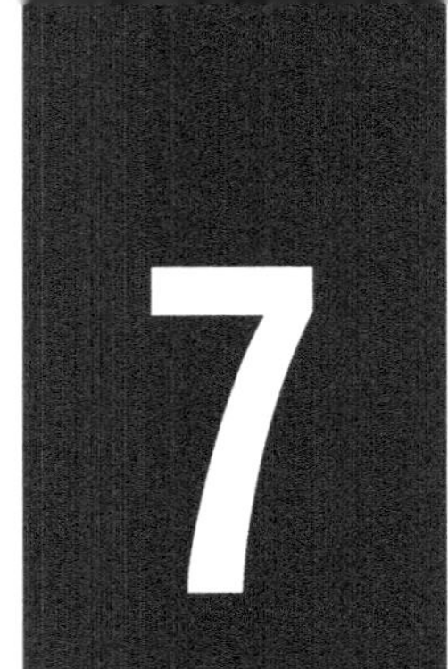

Expert Medical Evidence

Pradeep Kumar MV

'If the law makes you (the medical practitioner) a witness, remain a man of science; you have no victim to avenge, no guilty or innocent person to convict or save. You must bear testimony within the limits of science.'

Paul CH Brouardel (French forensic pathologist)

ABSTRACT

Law of evidence allows a person who is a witness, to state the facts related to either the fact in issue or a relevant fact, but not his inference. It applies to both criminal law and civil law. Expert witness is an exception to this general rule as he is allowed to draw an inference from the facts observed by him. While officers of the court (Judges and counsels for instance) are trained participants, witnesses who are called to court to give evidence are not. As such during direct examinations, which mark the start of the process of evidence taking, witnesses are usually led by counsels through the questioning process to build a foundation of their narrative.

Doctors are called to the court, either as an ordinary witness when he speaks about the facts seen or as an expert witness when he is allowed to draw an inference from the facts observed by him. The opinions of medical men are regularly admitted in matters related to time of death, age of the parties, cause of death, possibility of the weapons used, disease, injury, sanity and insanity of the parties so on and so forth. The Judge is not expected to be an expert in all the fields—especially where the subject matters involves technical knowledge. He is not capable of drawing inference from the facts which are highly technical. In these circumstances, he needs the help of an expert—who is supposed to have superior knowledge or experience in relation to the subject matter. In this respect, it is imminent for the medical man to be well acquitted with the law of evidence and it's functioning to give appropriate evidence.

Keywords: Expert witness, admissibility of evidence, direct evidence, oral evidence.

INTRODUCTION

In this modern era, science should expect to find a warm welcome, perhaps a permanent home in court rooms. The legal disputes are showing an increase in the involvement of the principles and tools of science. Proper resolution of these disputes are essential for those who live in technologically complex society and whom the law serve. Court decisions during the last decade of the 20th century mandated to examine the scientific basis of expert testimony to ensure that it meets the same rigorous standard employed by researchers and practitioners outside the court room. Needless to say, this requirement places a demand on Judges not only to comprehend the complexities of modern science but to adjudicate between parties' differing interpretations of scientific evidence. Methods change, new fields are born, new tests are introduced and fresh approaches to the interpretation of causal relations evolve.[1]

Expert testimony, by negating the power of myth, clears the way for fact-finders to deliberate regarding the actual facts of the case and the logical conclusions that flow from such facts, rather than focusing upon the falsehoods created when viewed through the distorting lens of myth.[2] The role of an expert witness is to assist the court on technical matters within their expertise that will help clarify the actual events. Their role in providing sound opinions and their ability to express their opinions with clarity to petitioner and to the legal profession is critical. Medical evidence helps the courts to draw logical conclusions from the facts presented by the experts.

PURPOSE AND SCOPE OF EXPERT TESTIMONY

There are many types of court cases and trials where the evidence of an expert medical witness might be necessary. Often medical practitioners are asked to give evidence as the attending doctor who has first-hand factual information about the care and management of the patient. If the practitioner is called to give evidence as an expert witness as in the case of personal injury or medical malpractice, the testimony will be expected to include an opinion on issues relating to the case. Some instances where an expert witness is called for an opinion is given in Table 7.1.

Medical practitioners appearing as an expert witness play a significant role in the evidence component of the justice process. For example, in rape cases, medical practitioners can provide important evidence that can be used to prove or disprove necessary elements of a crime. Their testimony can serve to corroborate the woman's history of rape and to enhance her credibility. Moreover, their explanations aid the Judge to understand the forensic evidence. A forensic expert may provide expert testimony to explain how sexually abused child could have normal physical findings upon examination.

Table 7.1 Issues requiring expert opinion in criminal and civil court

Criminal court	*Civil court*
Homicide, suicide or accident	Compensation claims following injury or neglect
Assault (including sexual assault)	Medical negligence and failure of duty of care
Unlawful abortion	Professional competence
Alcoholism (drunken driving)	Reports for juvenile courts
Criminal responsibility of defendant	Other litigations
Insanity	
Infanticide	
Diminished responsibility	
Effects of drugs or medication	
Fitness to appear in court, give reliable evidence or plead and stand trial	

This chapter describes the various types of evidence and outlines responsible practices that medical practitioners should follow to safeguard their objectivity in presenting expert witness testimony.

Medical Evidence

Medical evidence may be defined as the legal means to prove or disprove any medicolegal issue in question.[3] Medical evidence can be used in civil, criminal and consumer trials. Evidence given by doctors plays a significant role in assisting the court to decide, whether a person is liable or not in civil cases, and whether accused person is guilty or not guilty in criminal cases. Medical practitioners find themselves giving evidence as:

a. A defendant in a civil case or an accused in a criminal action (for e.g., in a case of the negligent death of a patient).
b. A witness of fact (for e.g., as a witness to a motor vehicle accident).
c. As a professional witness.
d. As an expert witness.

The medical evidence adduced by prosecution has great corroborative value. It proves that the injuries found on the body could have been caused in the manner as alleged and the death could have been caused by the injuries so that the prosecution case being consistent with matters verifiable by medical science. The use, which the defense can make of medical evidence, is to prove by that the injuries noted over the body could not possibly have been caused as alleged, or death could not possibly have been caused in the manner as alleged by the prosecution. In this endeavor, if it can do so, it discredits the eyewitnesses. It has to be remembered that medical opinion by itself, however, does not prove or disprove the prosecution case, it is merely of an advisory character.

The main purpose of the law of evidence is the establishment of facts in issue by legal system that the court is satisfied with and which is done by production of evidence.[4] Medical evidence is only 'opinion evidence'. In legal sense, it is the statement of an inference by the witness as to the existence or non-existence of a fact in issue, based upon other facts presented directly to the sense of the witness. No doubt, all testimony as to matters of fact is 'opinion evidence' in the sense that it is a conclusion formed from mental impressions of observed phenomena.[5]

Courts have said that the opinions or beliefs of witnesses concerning facts are irrelevant because witnesses should give evidence as to the facts, and the court should form an opinion based on the facts presented by the witnesses. Exception to this rule is evidence of expert witness. The most modern approach, however, is that opinion evidence should be regarded as relevant and can be considered, if it can assist the court to form an opinion, for e.g., where the witness is better qualified to form an opinion than the court.

Expert Witness

Lawson defines an 'expert' as a person who has knowledge and skill in a particular thing to which the enquiry relates.[6]

According to Sec. 45 of IEA, when the court has to form an opinion upon a point of foreign law or of science or art, or as to the identity of handwriting (or finger impressions), the opinions upon that point of persons skilled in such foreign law, science or art, (or in questions as to identity of handwriting or finger impressions) are relevant facts. Such persons are called 'experts'.[7] An expert witness should have the following qualities:

- A sound knowledge and practical experience of the subject matter in dispute.
- The ability to communicate findings and opinions clearly, concisely and in terms adapted to the court or tribunal before which evidence is being given.
- Flexibility of mind and self-confidence to modify opinions in the light of fresh evidence or counter-arguments.
- The ability to 'think on one's feet', needed in order to cope with appearances in court.
- A demeanor that is likely to express and command confidence, particularly in court appearances.

The competency to depose as an expert within the meaning of the section is thus restricted by two limitations, i) the subject matter under inquiry and ii) skill in it. In order to bring the evidence of a witness as that of an expert, it has to be shown that he has made the special study of the subject or acquired special experience therein. In other words, he is skilled and has adequate knowledge about that particular subject. It is the duty of the Judge to decide, whether the skill of that person in the subject under consideration on which evidence of his opinion is offered is sufficient to entitle him to be considered as an expert.

In most of the western countries, before an expert is allowed to give evidence in a court of law, a preliminary analysis is required to ascertain the qualification and competency of the expert about to depose. An expert's testimony is not admissible in the court without making due regard to what claims he has to the character of an expert.

No exact test is laid down by which one can determine with mathematical precision how much skill or experience a witness should possess to qualify him/her to testify as an expert in the court of law. That question rests with the court, whose duty it is to determine whether the experience or study of the witness has been such as to make his opinion of any value so that the court can form an opinion from his testimony.

In India, there is no test to determine the competency of an expert. It is enough if, in his 'examination-in-chief', the competency of the expert is shown. To render his opinion evidence admissible, and for this purpose, he should be examined as to his opportunities and means of knowledge. An expert, in order to be competent as an expert witness, need not have obtained his knowledge professionally; it is sufficient, if he shows to the court that he has made a special study of the subject or has obtained a special experience in the subject under issue. It is enough if he has made the subject matter of inquiry, the object of his particular attention or study.

Prior preliminary questions relating to the technical qualification and experience of the witness before he is permitted to give opinion testimony are legally necessary, though opposing counsel admits the expert qualification of the witness.

Doctors are experts in their own right and when they examine the person and give an opinion. When a doctor states his opinion, as well as, the facts which he noticed and on which his opinion is formed, his statement as to his opinion is pure expert testimony, but his statement as to the facts on which that opinion is based, is not expert testimony but the testimony of an ordinary witness. A medical man who has done a postmortem examination is not deposing as an expert in describing the injuries, but in expressing his opinion as to the cause of death and/or the nature of the weapon used, he is deposing as an expert.

Expert evidence consists of two parts:

1. Data evidence
2. Opinion evidence

The expert witness is expected to put before the court all materials inclusive of the data which induced him to come to the conclusion and enlighten the court on the technical aspect of the case by explaining the term of science so that the court although, not an expert, may judge on those material facts after giving due regard to the expert opinion because once the expert opinion is accepted, it is not the opinion of the medical person, but opinion of the court.[8] 'Data evidence' cannot ordinarily be rejected whereas 'opinion evidence' may or may not be accepted. While it is undoubtedly true that data evidence cannot be rejected, if it is inconsistent to oral evidence, yet, so far as opinion evidence is concerned, it is only an inference drawn from the data and that evidence would not get precedence over the direct eye witness testimony unless, of course, the inconsistency between the two is so great as to falsify the evidence of eyewitness.

Section 60 of IEA says that in all cases wherever it refers to an opinion or to the grounds on which that opinion is held, it must be the evidence of the person who holds that opinion on those grounds.

ADMISSIBILITY OF EXPERT EVIDENCE

An expert witness speaks on a matter of a particular subject, practice or observation, and will have a special experience on the subject. In order to bring evidence of a witness as that of an expert, it has to be shown that he has adequate knowledge of the subject in issue. Where there is no evidence about the nature of the training received by the witness examined as an expert and he had not given evidence about his qualification, and he had not furnished any data from which he had reached his conclusion and furnished his opinion, his evidence will be inadmissible. Where expert evidence is given, it is the duty of the experts 'to furnish the Judge with the necessary scientific criteria for testing the accuracy of their conclusions so as to enable the Judge to form his own independent judgment by the application of these criteria to the facts proved in evidence'. It is for the counsel who examines the person as an expert to bring out necessary data in his evidence.[9]

Expert may testify apart to his own opinion of facts observed by him

a. *Proved aliunde:* When a doctor has not examined the patient and his evidence as an expert is based on probabilities, still he, as an expert is entitled to answer all hypothetical questions put to him. The only safeguard which must be applied is that the hypotheses are correctly set to the expert. If it is required to determine whether a man died of any particular disease, the doctor may be called upon to give his opinion about the disease of which the person died, symptoms having been proved by other witnesses at the trial. That is, the doctor may give his opinion as founded upon the signs thus *proved aliunde*, although he may not have personally attended on the patient and observed the signs for himself, and in fact may never have seen the patient.

b. *Grounds on which the opinion is formed are also admissible:* This is a necessary corollary to the rule admitting opinion evidence. In fact, the admitted opinion of an expert loses its value, unless the grounds on which the opinion is based are permitted to be accepted in evidence, except in the case of the opinions of experts expressed in treatises whose authors are dead.
c. *Professional treatises of accredited authority in support to form an opinion:* Certain opinion is fact which can be canvassed by an expert by citing passages from their treatises in support of his opinion, provided that the conditions of the proviso Sec. 60 are satisfied in respect to the unavailability of the said authors as witnesses. When a party's counsel is allowed to cite passages from such treatises in support of, or in conflict with a particular opinion, there is no reason why an expert witness may not do the same in support of his own opinion.

It has been repeatedly held by the Supreme Court that a particular view taken by authors of the book of Medical Jurisprudence, the said view must be put to the doctor in order to assess how far the view taken by the experts apply to the details of the particular case.[10] However, exceptional cases referred to in the textbooks of Medical Jurisprudence cannot be relied against positive and clear evidence of the case before the court.[11]

Where conflicting views have been expressed in different books on Medical Jurisprudence, the conflict can be resolved by preferring the most specialized book on the subject.[9] In assessing the scientific validity of expert evidence, the court must be careful to distinguish between that and assessing the validity of the literature being offered by a party. The court in an appraisal of medical evidence has power to refer to articles, journals and books by authors acquainted with such matters.[12] The expert may also state facts relating to the causes bearing similarity to the case under inquiry, in order to support his opinion. Certain opinion can be considered by an expert by citing similarity to the case that is under inquiry with the cases which he has already seen or familiar with.

Matters to which an expert is not allowed to testify[9]

a. The opinion of an expert as to the existence of the facts on which his opinion is given is irrelevant, unless he perceived them himself.
b. The expert ought not to answer purely speculative or hypothetical questions having no foundation in the evidence.
c. A witness called in purely as an expert and not as a witness to facts should confine his opinion to the facts submitted to him; it is not open to him to give his opinion by reference to facts collected independently by him.

TYPES OF EVIDENCE

Several authors have classified 'evidence' in different ways.

a. Gross and Williams classified evidence into:[13]
   - Direct and Circumstantial
   - Primary and Secondary
   - Insufficient, Prima facie and Conclusive

b. Nwadialo's classified evidence into:[14]
   - Direct and Circumstantial
   - Direct and Hearsay
   - Oral and Documentary
   - Real evidence
   - Primary and Secondary

Other classifications are:
   - Direct and Circumstantial
   - Direct and Hearsay or Original and Hearsay
   - Oral and Documentary
   - Primary and Secondary
   - Prima facie and Conclusive
   - Personal and Real
   - Pre-appointed and Casual
   - Best evidence
   - Direct and Indirect

No single classification is better than the other. In a conflict situation, it is incumbent to (whether consciously or not) determine the nature of the evidence, whether or not the piece of evidence belongs to any of the categories classified.

In Indian context, the medical man should be well versed with following types of evidence:

Oral Evidence

Oral evidence includes all statements which the court permits or which are required to be made before it by the witness in relation to matters of fact under enquiry. Oral evidence is *more relevant* than documentary evidence as it permits cross-examination. Documentary evidence is accepted by court only on oral testimony by person concerned.

Secion 59 IEA says that all facts, except the contents of documents or electronic records may be proved by oral evidence.

Section 60 IEA prescribed the provision of recording oral evidence.[15] All those statements which the court permits or expects the witnesses to make in his presence regarding the truth of the facts are called oral evidence. Oral evidence is that evidence which the witness has personally seen or heard. Oral evidence must always be direct or positive. Evidence is direct when it goes straight to establish the main fact in issue.[16] Oral evidence is much less satisfactory medium of proof than documentary proof. But justice can never be administered in the most cases without resorting to oral evidence.[17] In the present system of jurisprudence, there is a presumption against perjury. The oral evidence has to be judged with reference to the conduct of the parties, and the presumptions and probabilities legitimately arising in the case.[18] Another way is to find whether the evidence is consistent with the general knowledge of mankind, with the usual course of nature and human conduct, and with well known principles of human action.

Oral evidence should be accepted with caution. The court must assess the evidence, accept the truth and discard the rest. The credibility of the witness should be decided on the following important points:

i. Whether the witness has the means of gaining the right information.

ii. Whether there is any interest in concealing the truth.
iii. Whether they agree in their testimony.

The real test to accept or reject evidence is how consistent is the story in itself, how does it stands of cross-examination and how far does it fit it with the rest of the evidence and circumstances of the case. According to Information Technology Act 2000, every other point, except contents of an electronic record or any document, can be proved by oral evidence.[19]

Falsus in uno, falsus in omnibus: This means that 'false in one, false in all'. This principle is somewhat dangerous maxim. There is always a fringe of embroidery by exaggerating the events to the story. Though, the main story may be true and when it is found that the falsehood is merely an embroidery, then it would not be enough to discredit the whole of the witness's evidence. Whereas, the falsehood relates to a major or material point, then it is enough to discredit the witness evidence.

Exceptions to Oral Evidence[3]

i. *Dying declaration*: It is accepted in court as evidence in the event of victim's death.
ii. *Expert opinions expressed in the treatise:* Expert opinions printed in books are accepted as evidence without oral evidence of the author.
iii. *Deposition of a medical witness taken in the lower court:* It is accepted as evidence in a higher court when it has been recorded and attested by a Magistrate in the presence of the accused who had the opportunity to cross-examine the witness.
iv. *Reports of certain state scientific experts:* They are admitted as evidence without their oral examination, for e.g., reports of Chemical Examiner or Assistant Chemical Examiner, Chief Controller of Explosives, Director of Finger Print Bureau, Director of Haffkeine Institute Mumbai, Director, Deputy Director, Assistant Director of Central or State FSL, Serologist to Government or any other Government scientific expert specified by notification of the Central Government.
v. *Evidence given by a witness in previous legal proceeding:* It is admitted in a subsequent legal proceeding when the witness is dead or cannot be found or is incapable of giving evidence or cannot be called without unreasonable delay or expense to the court.
vi. *Public records:* Birth, death certificates, certificates of marriage.
vii. *Hospital records:* Routine entries such as date of admission, discharge, pulse and temperature are admissible without oral evidence.

Documentary Evidence

Section 3 of IEA says that all those documents which are presented in the court for inspection are documentary evidences.[19] The documentary evidence shows the actual attitude of the parties and their consciousness regarding the custom which is more important than any oral evidence.[20] It has been said that the word 'document' as used in the law of evidence 'should not be construed restrictively'. Etymologically, the word means something which shows or teaches and is evidential or informative in its character. Where the statement of parties containing the terms of a compromise were recorded by a court and duly signed, it was to be held to be a document.[21] The contents of a document may be proved either by primary or secondary evidence. The best evidence rule is to produce the primary evidence, and secondary evidence is not admissible, unless the original is proved to be lost.

The subject of documentary evidence can be divided into three parts:

1. How the contents of the document are to be proved? (Sec. 61-66 IEA).
2. How the document is to be proved to be genuine? (Sec. 67-90 IEA).
3. In what cases the oral evidence is excluded by documentary evidence? (Sec. 91-100 IEA).
   a. **Primary Evidence:** Section 62 of IEA says 'primary evidence' is the best class of evidence. Accordingly, 'primary evidence' means the document itself produced for the inspection of the court. If the document is executed in several parts, each part is primary evidence of the document. If the document is executed in counterparts, each counterpart being executed by one or some of the parties only, each counterpart is primary evidence as against the parties executing it. Where a number of documents are all made by one uniform process, as in the case of printing, lithography or photography, each is primary evidence of the contents of the rest, but where they are all copies of a common original, they are not primary evidence of the contents of the original. The original document is the first permanent record of the transaction. It is first hand evidence and presumptively the most reliable. The notes prepared by the autopsy surgeon at the time of conducting the postmortem examination carries more weightage than the postmortem report prepared leisurely in his chamber by noting the findings from the records. The contents of every paper are, according to the ordinary well established rules of evidence, to be proved by the paper itself, and by that alone, if the paper is in existence. Where the writer of the letter was not examined as a witness, and no opportunity was given to the opposite party to cross-examine him, the letter was held as 'not reliable' evidence by the Supreme Court.[22] The truth of the contents of a document can, however, be proved by any other evidence and not necessarily by the evidence of the author of the document.[23] If the author of the postmortem report is not found, then the person who was working with the author of the report at that material time will be called to depose so as to verify the authenticity of the paper.
   b. **Secondary Evidence:** Section 63 of IEA says 'secondary evidence' is the inferior evidence as compared with primary evidence. It occupies a secondary position. It is such evidence that on the presentation of which it is felt that superior evidence yet remains to be produced. It is the evidence which is produced in the absence of the primary evidence, therefore, it is known as secondary evidence.[23] If in place of primary evidence, secondary evidence is admitted without any objection, then the parties are precluded from raising the question that the document has not been proved by primary evidence but by secondary evidence. But where there is no secondary evidence as contemplated by Sec. 66 IEA, then the document cannot be said to have been proved either by primary evidence or secondary evidence.[24] The most remarkable among the types of secondary evidence is the oral or parol evidence of the contents of the document. The conditions

in which secondary evidence can be given (as listed in Sec. 65 IEA) should exist so as to enable the party to give secondary evidence of a document in question. The second condition is that the oral account of the contents of the document must be that of a person who has himself seen it.

Printouts taken from the computer/servers by mechanical process and certified by an officer in his official capacity can be led in evidence through a witness who can identify the signatures of the certifying officer or otherwise speak of the facts based on his personal experience. Electronic form of evidence means any information of probative value that is either stored or transmitted in electronic form and includes computer evidence, digital audio, digital video, cell phones, digital fax machines. According to IT Amendment Bill 2008 (passed by both houses of Indian Parliament and yet to be enforced), Sec. 79A empowers the central government to appoint any department, body or agency as examiner of electronic evidence for providing expert opinion on electronic form evidence before any court or authority.[25] In Sec. 85B IEA, there is a presumption as to the authenticity of electronic records in case of secure electronic records (i.e. records digitally signed as per Sec. 14 of the IT Act, 2000).[23] The admissibility of electronic records in the form of SMS, MMS and e-mail in India is well demonstrated under the law and the interpretation is provided in various cases. Specific criteria have been made in the IEA for admissibility of electronic records to satisfy authenticity or reliability, and new techniques of security being introduced by advancing technologies.[26]

The important differences between primary and secondary evidence are highlighted in Table 7.2.

Varieties of Documentary Evidence

Documentary evidence is of the following:[3]

i. **Medical certificate:** Medical certificate is regarded as the simple form of documentary evidence. It is issued by a registered medical practitioner in respect of ill health, age and mental condition. It is accepted in the court of law as a piece of evidence as to the facts stated in the medical certificate. The doctor who has issued it may be summoned to the court of law to testify the contents of the certificate on oath, and if needed, cross-examination can be made. So, the medical practitioner must exercise due care and skill in issuing such certificate. The certificate must state the exact nature of the disease and

Table 7.2 Difference between primary evidence and secondary evidence

Primary evidence	*Secondary evidence*
Original document.	Copy of the original document.
Best evidence in all conditions.	Not the best evidence. Admitted in exceptional circumstances.
Giving primary evidence is general rule.	It is an exception to the general rule.
No notice is required before giving primary evidence.	Notice is required to be given before giving secondary evidence.
The value of primary evidence is highest.	The value of secondary evidence is not as that of primary evidence.

should include doctor's opinion in clear language. In the case of ill health, the doctor should write the exact nature of an illness, the duration of disease and probable period of absence in cases of employed persons. The signature of the patient should be at the bottom with the date indicating that he attended the clinic and the doctor has examined him while issuing the certificate. The signature is to be verified by the doctor. Issuing a false certificate under Sec. 197 IPC is punishable under Sec. 193 IPC with imprisonment extending up to 7 years and also fine.

ii. **Death certificate:** It is essential that identification and cause of death should be determined for the lawful disposal of the dead body. It is a vital document, may be needed during cremation, transportation outside state and certain claims. The doctor must inspect the body and satisfy that the person is dead. He is legally bound to issue a certificate, if he has attended the patient during his last illness indicating the cause of death. According to the recommendation of Brodrick committee, a doctor should not issue a death certificate unless he has attended the deceased at least once during seven days preceding death. He cannot charge any fee for issuing a death certificate. He cannot delay or refuse to issue a certificate. He may subsequently sue the legal heirs for his pending dues. He must refuse to give a certificate on the following grounds: (a) If he is not sure about the cause of death. (b) Any suspicion of foul play. (c) Death by violent and unnatural cause, drugs or poisoning. If he is not sure regarding the cause of death and suspects some foul play, he should not issue a death certificate; instead he should notify the police.

The doctor may certify death in doubtful cases but must not give a cause of death and he should notify the police. Failure to do so may result in doctor being prosecuted under Sec. 39 CrPC. Under Sec. 17 (1)(b) of Registration of Births and Deaths Act 1969, any person may obtain an extract from the Registrar relating to any death after paying the requisite fee, though it will not disclose particulars regarding the cause of death as entered in the register. This confidentiality can be overridden in the public interest.

iii. **Medicolegal Report:** These are the legal documents prepared by the doctor. These reports are produced in the court of law. The doctor who has made the report should attend the court to testify under oath and then only they are taken as evidence.

There are two basic categories of physical evidence that may be presented in court: real evidence and demonstrative evidence. Real evidence is a form of physical evidence, though it is different from demonstrative physical evidence that may be used in a hearing.

Real Evidence

'Real evidence' means real or material evidence. Real evidence is the fact that is brought to the knowledge of the court by inspection of a physical object. Real evidence is a type of evidence often used in court hearings or trials which can be presented in both criminal and civil cases. This type of evidence usually consists of objects that were physically present at the scene of a crime or civil violation. They have a direct link or impact on the case itself. Such evidence is in contrast to testimonial evidence that typically consists of the testimony of someone who was involved in or a witness to events related to the case. Real evidence may be authenticated in three ways—by identification of a different object, by identification of an object that has been *made* different and by establishing a chain of custody.

Real evidence consists of objects that are directly related to the case being discussed during a hearing or trial. For example, in a murder trial, the prosecution may wish to present a weapon that was used to kill the victim, photographs of the crime scene, images of wounds on the victim and a wristwatch that was left behind by the perpetrator of the crime.[27]

Demonstrative Evidence

'Demonstrative evidence' is just what the name implies—it demonstrates or illustrates the testimony of a witness. It will be admissible when, with accuracy sufficient for the task at hand, it fairly and accurately reflects that statement and is otherwise unobjectionable. Typical examples of demonstrative evidence are maps, diagrams of the scene of the occurrence, animations and the like. Since, its purpose is to illustrate testimony, demonstrative evidence is authenticated by the witness whose testimony is being illustrated. That witness will usually identify salient features of the exhibit and testify that it fairly and accurately reflects what he saw or heard on a particular occasion, such as the location of people or things on a diagram.

Hearsay Evidence

'Hearsay evidence' is very weak evidence. It is the evidence which the witness has neither personally seen nor heard or perceived through his senses and has come to know about it through some other person.[19] Sometimes, it implies the witness saying of something which the witness has heard others say. For example, during the trial 'A' stated that 'B' had told him that he has seen 'C' driving the car and running over the victim. Here 'A' is giving the hearsay evidence. There is no bar for hearsay evidence given that it has reasonable nexus and credibility.[28] Hearsay evidence, whether or not to be excluded in the case in which its use comes in for question, is governed by the Indian Evidence Act.[29]

Exceptions to hearsay

- Res Gestae [Sec. 6 IEA]
- Admissions and confessions
- Statement relevant under Sec. 32 IEA
- Statements in public documents
- Evidence in former proceedings
- Statements of experts in treatises (Sec. 60, proviso).

Judicial Evidence

Evidence received by court of justice in proof or disproof of facts before them is called legal evidence. The confession made by the accused in the court is also involved in legal evidence. Statements of witnesses and documentary evidence and facts for the study by the court are also judicial evidence.

Non-Judicial Evidence

Any confession made by the accused outside the court in the presence of any person or the admission of a party are called non-judicial evidence, if proved in court, 'in the form of judicial evidence'.

Direct Evidence

Evidence is either direct or indirect. Direct evidence is that evidence which is very important for the decision of the matter in issue. It is the evidence of a person who actually witnessed the crime being committed, or a thing which link the crime and thus describes the offence. The statement before the police is called circumstantial evidence of complicity and not direct evidence in the strict sense.[30]

The evidence is direct if it is based on the personal experience or observation and if true to be believed, proves a fact out of inference or presumptions. It a testimony of:

- What you hear with your ears
- What you see with your eyes
- What you smell with your nose
- What you touch with your hand or body
- What you taste with your mouth or tongue

The term 'direct' relates to the source of the information being deposed to. It is also called 'positive evidence'. For example, when it refers to the fact that could be seen/heard/perceived, it must be the evidence of that person who saw/heard/perceived it. If it refers to an opinion or to the grounds on which that opinion is held, the evidence must confirm to the matters in issue, for e.g., a knife that caused stab injury or a medical prescription that resulted in the ill effects to the patient.

Circumstantial Evidence or Indirect Evidence

There is no difference between circumstantial evidence and indirect evidence. Circumstantial evidence attempts to prove the facts in issue by providing other facts and affords an example as to its existence. It relates to a series of other facts than the point in issue, but by experience have been found so associated with the point in issue in relation of cause and effect that it leads to a satisfactory conclusion. For example, 'A' committed murder of 'B' with knife at a particular place, date and time. Here 'C' will depose that he saw 'A' on that day, date and time with a knife in hand just before the murder. This evidence of 'C' has a bearing to the fact.

In Hanumant vs. State of Madhya Pradesh,[31] the Hon'ble Supreme Court observed, 'In dealing with circumstantial evidence, there is always the danger that suspicion may take the place of legal evidence. It is well to remember that in cases where the evidence is of a circumstantial nature, the conditions from which the conclusion of guilt is to be drawn should in the first instance be fully established, and all the facts so established should be consistent only with the hypothesis of the guilt of the accused. In other words, there can be a chain of evidence so far complete as not to leave any reasonable ground for a conclusion consistent with the innocence of the accused, and it must be such as to show that within all human probability, the act must have been made by the accused'.

In the case of Ashok Kumar vs. State of Madhya Pradesh,[32] the Hon'ble Supreme Court held:

a. The circumstances from which an inference of guilt is sought to be drawn must be cogent and firmly established.
b. Those conditions should be of a definite tendency unerringly pointing towards the guilt of accused.
c. The events, taken cumulatively, should form a chain so full that there is no escape from the conclusion that, within all human probability, the crime was committed by the accused and none else.
d. The circumstantial evidence in order to sustain the conviction must be complete and incapable of explanation on any other hypothesis than that of the guilt of the accused, and such evidence should not only be consistent with the guilt of the accused but should be inconsistent with his innocence.

Direct evidence vs Circumstantial evidence

The debate that among the two, which evidence is excellent is going from a long time, as the Judges differ in their views. Some Judges hold that direct evidence is excellent evidence. When a particular person says that he had seen a particular event happening, then undoubtedly his evidence is excellent. But even relying on direct evidence at once is also hazardous because a witness can make a completely false statement. Especially, the manner in which the court draws inferences from events, they can be wrong and thus conditions also become false.

In the case of Kallu vs. State of Uttar Pradesh,[33] the accused was tried for the murder of the deceased by shooting him with a country made pistol. A cartridge was found near the bed of the deceased. The accused was arrested at a distance of 14 miles from the village which was the place of the event. He produced a pistol from his house which indicated that he could have alone had known of its existence there. The firearms expert proved that it was the same pistol from which the shot was fired and deceased was killed. The Hon'ble Supreme Court while convicting the accused held 'circumstantial evidence has found that the death of the deceased was caused by the accused and no one else'.

Scientific Evidence

It is the evidence which serves to either support or counter a scientific theorem or hypothesis. Such evidence is expected to be empirical and properly documented in accordance with the scientific method as appropriate to the particular field of inquiry. Standards for evidence may vary according to whether the field of inquiry is among the natural sciences or social sciences.[34] Scientific evidence is demonstrative evidence. Unlike oral testimony which depends on the deposition of a witness, scientific evidence is obtained by using the scientific method. Scientific evidence which is admitted in the trial must not only be relevant but also trustworthy. An expert witness is called to testify about the reliability of the scientific evidence sought to be presented at trial.[35] This is highlighted by the following example.

Foot Prints: Foot print identification is reliable. Our bare feet contain friction ridge patterns which are unique. Hence, the fingerprints and foot prints found at the scene of offence can be used to help identify the offender. They can be used for identifying the victim as well. The validity of the scientific method used for fingerprinting and foot printing is accepted by the courts. In Pritam Singh vs. State of Punjab,[36] foot prints found in blood near a dead body and the bathroom were compared with those of the accused taken in printer's ink. The expert gave evidence giving points of nine similarities in respect of the right foot and ten in respect of the left foot, and three dissimilarities only in each case. He explained the dissimilarities with reference to the different densities of blood and ink. It was held that the comparison stood the test well, and under the circumstances, these foot impressions in blood near the area of the incident were proved to be those of the accused.

Digital Evidence

Electronic records come under the ambit of 'document' as per the Information Technology Act, 2000. All facts except the content of the electronic record can be proved by oral evidence. Tape-recorded statements, voice-mail recordings and closed-circuit television footage are often used in litigation. Video recordings of bank robberies and audio recordings of life threats are presented in court rooms by electronic expert witnesses.

Conclusive Evidence

It is also called irrebuttable presumption of law, when the law forbids the evidence to be contrary. Conclusive evidence or conclusive proof is that evidence which is so strong as to oblige the court to come to a particular conclusion or to overbear any other evidence to the contrary, even though it is not irrebuttable, like prima facie evidence. A conclusive evidence is the sum total of the evidence adduced by a party indicating that it has met the requirements of the law and the burden of proof as required of him or her.

GUIDELINES FOR EXPERT MEDICAL WITNESS

A deposition is an adversarial proceeding and should not be considered in any manner 'routine' to the lawsuit. Moreover, cross-examination is the aspect of testifying that all expert witnesses fear most since the plan is to impeach the witness. Questions in cross-examination are just like chess moves. They are not isolated but strung together and usually headed toward a final question of some importance.

Before the deposition, the medical practitioner should be well rested; this will make him or her easier to stay in control and be attentive. Most experts are very good at seeing the weaknesses in their own cases and preparing answers to potential questions.

It has been found that two factors influence the Judges besides the level of expertise of the expert witness: dynamism and trustworthiness.

i. Dynamism refers to the style of delivery that is bold, active, energetic, friendly, frank and empathetic.
ii. Trustworthiness is credited to people who are perceived to be honest, objective, unselfish and just.

There are things to be followed and things not to be followed at the time of deposition. These rules are not exhaustive and do not replace the advice from prosecution; however, these are good rules of thumb to consider in anticipation of a deposition.

a. **Meeting the lawyer who has called you before testifying:** It is necessary to meet the lawyer who has called you to testify, as a lawyer can explain his/her overview of the case to you and what he/she sees as the value of your testimony. A pretrial conference provides the experts with some understanding of how the case will proceed while they are testifying. When the lawyers do not meet you, it may be because they feel uncomfortable with the subject matter or believe you know much better what to say.

b. **Impartial testimony:** Medical practitioners serving as experts should provide accurate, thorough, reliable, knowledgeable, objective, unbiased, fair and truthful analysis of facts of the case. The expert should not knowingly provide statement that is false.

   The evidence should not be biased based upon any individual's age, color, caste, culture, disability, ethnic or national origin, gender, lifestyle, marital or parental status, religion or beliefs, sexual orientation or social or economic status.

c. **Credibility:** The credibility of the expert witness is one of the most important features of any case. Credibility comes from a combination of factors: appearance, demeanor, attitude, consistency and content, to name a few.

   The expert should be well dressed and always appear polite, modest and calm. Although one may be emotionally tested during the deposition, it is necessary to keep one's emotions in check.

   He/she should stand up straight. Be pleasant, courteous and respectful to the court. Being courteous is one of the best ways to make a good impression on the court and the Judge. When addressing the lawyers use 'Yes, sir or madam' and 'No, sir or madam' and to address the Judge as 'Your honor.'

   Do not try to 'stretch' the facts. Experts who know their limits and occasionally say, 'I don't know' raise their credibility. If unsure of an answer, only state, 'I don't know' or 'I don't remember'.

   Do not sigh, mop your brow or look dejected and sneak out of the court room.

   Do not look at your lawyer for help. It will create a bad impression on the Judge if the expert looks at the prosecuting lawyer when a question is asked on cross-examination or for approval after answering a question. Neither the lawyer nor the Judge will help; the expert is on his/her own.

d. **Good communication skills:** Speak slowly, distinctly and audibly, using positive and direct answers to each question. Speak with assurance and be confident, but not over-confident or arrogant. The witness should use language and terminology that will be readily understood by the court and explain any abbreviations and medical or other technical terminology that is used.

   Avoid using 'always' or 'never' or any other such absolute term. Avoid saying 'To be honest' or 'Honestly..' or other such terms or phrases that suggest that prior answers were not truthful.

Avoid superlatives and exaggerations, for e.g., unusually large bruise, savage blow, agonizing pain, etc.

e. **Eye contact:** In giving testimony, answer should be directed towards the Judge. The proper court room etiquette is to turn and look at the Judge when responding to a question. This gives the impression of honesty and also helps to establish a connection with the Judge.

f. **Subject matter knowledge:** The expert witness must keep up to date in the specialized area of practice. He/she should be well prepared with the details of the evidence before entering the witness box; anticipate certain possible questions on it and be prepared answer these in advance. Express an opinion from your own knowledge and experience. Say, 'In my opinion.., 'do not use a phrase such as 'I think..' or 'I imagine..'.

g. **Testifying within expertise:** The witness should provide evidence or testify only in matters in which he/she has relevant clinical experience and knowledge in the areas of medicine that are the subject of the proceeding. He/she should express opinions that fall within the limits of professional competence. Sometimes, the opposing lawyer or the Judge may ask questions related to the testimony but falls outside the area of expertise. In such cases, the witness should resist testifying beyond the limits of expertise. For example, a general practitioner is not qualified to give evidence on the pathology of development of a tumor following assault or accident at a particular site, or blood group inheritance. It is also inappropriate for an obstetrician to provide an opinion as to whether the events of labor caused a child's neurological disability. In such cases, he/she should explain that this is not a matter in which he/she has particular experience and that he/she is not qualified to answer.

If ordered by the court to answer such a question, he/she should answer to the best of his/her ability but make clear that the subject is beyond your competence.

It is difficult for many to say 'I don't know' or 'That is beyond my area of expertise.' Giving a professional opinion beyond one's area of expertise is a clear violation of professional ethics.

h. **Saying 'I don't know' on the witness box:** It is believed that the experts will understand the scientific basis of the testing that was done. However, even the most educated and experienced persons have gaps in their experience. Saying 'I don't know' in answering to the questions that you do not know have effect on the outcome of the trial. The exception to this is if you accept you are not familiar with certain basic process or fact that is an essential part of your area of expertise.

i. **Refreshing memory:** The expert should never try to memorize. During the deposition, he/she can refresh by referring to any writing made by him/her, or may use a copy of the document or refer to professional treatises (Sec. 159 IEA).

The expert witness should take all record and relevant reports that may have to be quoted in the box, for e.g., original records, medicolegal report, photographs, X-rays, CT-scan, MRI scan, toxicology and blood group reports, diagrams, special reports on swabs or smear culture studies, serology and various receipts to prove the chain of custody of the items of evidence.

Do not fumble in referring to case notes or records. The less you fumble, the more the Judge is likely to be impressed.

j. **Understand the question before answering:** During deposition, listen carefully to every question and wait until the question is completed. Make sure the question is clear before answering. The expert cannot possibly give a truthful and accurate answer unless the question is understood. It is appropriate to show that he/she does not understand a question by respectfully asking the lawyer to repeat it or rephrase it.

k. **Stop and think before answering:** Do not be over enthusiastic in answering to the question. Pause for a moment before answering. Be aware of critical questions during cross-examination. It is proper to show that you need a moment to consider the response and shows that the answer is carefully considered. If a question seems inappropriate, pausing before answering may also give the prosecution time to object. If an objection is raised, stop testifying until the Judge decides on the objection. If you understand the question is unfair or indecent or that the defense lawyer is annoying you, look at your lawyer before answering. If he fails to object, turn to the Judge and ask whether you should answer the question.

If multiple questions are asked, separate them in the answer. If the defense lawyer asks a 'yes' or 'no' question that cannot be answered by 'yes' or 'no', say so. If you need to give a complete answer, say so. The court usually rules that the doctor may explain his reply. Keep a sharp lookout for questions with double meaning. The answer to each part of a double question may be different. Do not accept as part of a question a summary of details, if there is any question about the accuracy of those facts. He/she should also state that the assumed facts are not necessarily true. Look out for questions that assume the expert has testified to the fact when that is not the case.

l. **Scientific literature:** Some lawyers may use medical books or articles in an attempt to contradict the testimony of the expert witness. The approach is to ask whether the witness agrees with the statement found in some prestigious medical literature (books/journals) which contradicts the previous statement of the witness.

The medical expert has the right to see it before commenting and must recognize the literature as authoritative in its field or a standard text in the medical field. If you recognize the book or article as authoritative in the field, then admit it. If the medical expert does not recognize it, the cross-examining lawyer may not read from it. If unfamiliar with the literature, be honest about it by simply saying, 'I do not recognize that article (or book) as authoritative.' If you do not 'recognize' the text, the article cannot be entered in testimony. A thorough knowledge of the literature will help show that the publication is misrepresented, obscured or inconsistent with prevailing opinions.

Even so, the medical expert has the privilege of disagreeing with the opinions of the most eminent specialists, particularly where the witness is referring to a specific patient about whom the witness has a great deal of information and the book or article is speaking in generalities.

m. **Correcting the fact or conclusion that has been misstated by the lawyer:** Some defense lawyers will misstate your statement or conclusions hoping to catch you in a contradiction or to provide information to support their case. Usually, however, these errors are not intentional and may be misspeak or misunderstood information. The best solution is to be straightforward. Restate the premise correctly.

n. **Avoid volunteering:** The witness box is not an opportunity to talk about on the latest medical theories. When replying to a question, keep it simple. It is generally advised to avoid speculation or volunteering information, and answer 'Yes' or 'No' when appropriate, or to answer questions in short sentences. Do not nod your head to indicate 'Yes' or 'No'. Volunteered information is often not well prepared and is liable to cross-examination. However, expert medical witness may volunteer a statement, if he thinks that the injustice will result, if he fails to make a statement.

o. **The system is adversarial—do not take it personally:** Defense lawyer may irritate the witness by unfair questions, abuse and unfair remarks. The expert should remain calm and cool and avoid losing temper no matter how hard he/she is pressed. The opposing lawyer has the right to question the expert. He/she should not be rude or sarcastic with the lawyer regardless of the vigor with which questions are asked.

   If the expert witness gets angry he/she is going to lose professional demeanor and the effectiveness of his/her testimony is diminished or destroyed. Do not argue, just disagree if you do not agree; disagree firmly and repeatedly.

p. **Hypothetical questions:** The law requires that an expert who does not have personal knowledge regarding the patient or the occurrence must give his/her opinions by hypothetical questions. A hypothetical question is one that asks the expert witness to assume particular hypothetical facts and express an opinion based upon those facts contained in the question without specifically referring to a particular patient. The law requires, with regard to answering hypothetical questions, that the witness base his/her answer on the facts contained in the hypothetical question.

q. **Information security and disclosure:** The expert should take reasonable steps to access all relevant evidence materials and maintain their integrity and security whilst in possession.

   He/she should not disclose confidential information other than to the parties to proceedings unless the subject consents, obliged to do so by law, ordered by a court, overriding duty to the court and the administration of justice demands disclosure of information.

   A medical witness has no professional privilege and therefore he must answer any question. But, he should first obtain a permission from the Judge, and if directed to do so, he must answer without further delay.

r. **Be well versed with the common tactics used by the lawyers to discredit a witness:** There are several ways by which the lawyers try to impeach a witness. Impeaching a witness using prior statements or testimony is often used, if the witness has provided an interpretation of the facts or findings in a way different from previous testimony in the current or past cases. There may be a reasonable explanation for this difference, but as an expert you must be aware of these contradictory statements and explain to the court why the current case differs from previous conditions. If you cannot give an account, the court will consider your statement biased and may even believe you as untruthful. Both are disastrous for the expert witness.

s. **Conflicts of interest:** If there is any matter that gives rise to a potential conflict of interest, such as any prior involvement with one of the parties or a personal interest (a patient of many years standing or patient's bill has not been paid), then the expert should avoid testifying.

Conflict between opinions of two experts: Opinion of one expert witness is contradicted by another expert witness of equal caliber in forming an opinion. In such cases, court is of the view that the opinion of the expert which supports the direct evidence in the case should be accepted.[37]

Also, court is of the opinion that the opinion of the doctor holding postmortem examination is to be preferred to the expert opinion.[38]

Conflict between expert opinions with that of eye witness: The medical evidence is opinion evidence. By itself, it does not prove or disprove the prosecution case; it is merely of the advisory character. Medical expert's opinion is not always final and binding. When there is inconsistency between the direct evidence and expert evidence in respect to the prosecution case, thereby causing a defect in the prosecution case which unless reasonably explained, the entire prosecution case will be discredited. Since, the witnesses are the eyes and ears of justice, the oral evidence of an eyewitness is superior over medical evidence. If the oral testimony of the witnesses is found reliable, creditworthy and inspires confidence, the oral evidence has to be believed, it cannot be rejected on hypothetical medical evidence.[5]

Exception to this general rule is when the medical evidence completely rules out the prosecution story; the oral evidence if proved unreliable and untrustworthy, can be rejected.

CONCLUSION

The medical evidence is assigned with great importance. However, this system is not based on the concept of 'absolute truth' in a scientific sense but rather on satisfaction 'beyond reasonable doubt' that the legal elements of a crime have been found. Opposing medical expert witnesses may have minor points of disagreement which may be construed as major differences of opinion when this is not the case. There are many instances where court decisions contrary to expert opinion on issues like fracture, rape, burns, age, consent, dying declaration and compos mentis have been delivered.

Moreover, experts should be careful in offering opinions and should not think that they are there to make or imply a decision on the ultimate question before the court, since the responsibility for the judgment rests solely with the Judge.

REFERENCES

1. Kassirer JP, Kessler G. Reference manual on scientific evidence. 3rd edn. Washington DC: National academic press; 2011.
2. Dempsey MM. The use of expert witness testimony in the prosecution of domestic violence. Available from: http://www.cps.gov.uk/publications/docs/expertwitnessdv.pdf.
3. Vij K. Introduction to forensic medicine and Indian legal system. Text book of forensic medicine and toxicology. 5th edn. New Delhi: Elsevier; 2011. p. 3-16.
4. Murugesan D. Appreciation of evidence. 2012. Available from: http://www.hcmadras.tn.nic.in/jacademy/articles/AppreciationofEviDMJ.pdf.
5. Rao YR. Expert evidence medical and non medical. 4th edn. Nagpur: Lexis Nexis Butterworths; 2010.
6. Lawson JD. The law of expert and opinion evidence. Chicago: Flood TH; 1900. Available from: http://www.acera.unimelb.edu.au/materials/endorsed/0611.pdf.

7. Watts P. A reliable witness: how to give credible mental health evidence in court. Canning Bridge, WA: Ogilvie Publishing; 2004.
8. Mohapatra D. State of Himachal Pradesh vs. Jai Lal (AIR 1999 SC 3318, 1999 (2) ALD Cri 855). Available from: http://indiankanoon.org/doc/1652872/.
9. Dayal R. Mahendra Manilal Nanavati vs. Sushila Mahendra Nanavati, Equivalent citations: 1965 AIR 364, 1964 SCR (7) 267. Available from: http://indiankanoon.org/doc/146960/.
10. Singhal ML. Medical evidence and its use in trial of cases *JTRI Journal*; 1995: 1-8. Available from: http://ijtr.nic.in/articles/art28.pdf.
11. Tulzapurkar VD. Baldev Raj vs. Smt. Urmila Kumari Miglani, Equivalent citation: AIR 1979 SC 879, (1979) 3 SCC 782, 1979 (11) UJ 188 SC. Available from: http://www.indiankanoon.org/doc/1278895/.
12. Anand SS. How sacrosanct is the medical examination report of a rape victim in a criminal trial? Available from: http://www.ksnonline.org/forum/topics/how-sacrosact-is-the-medical-examination-report-of-a-rape-victim.
13. Cross R, Wilkins N. An outline of the law of evidence. 3rd edn. London: Butterworth; 1971.
14. Nwadialo F. Modern Nigerian law of evidence 2nd edn. Lagos: University of Lagos press; 1999.
15. Indian Evidence Act. Ratanlal and Dhirajlal. 21st edn. Nagpur: Lexis Nexis Butterworths.
16. Sinha D. Dr. JJ Irani @ Jamshed J. Irani ... vs. State Of Jharkhand and Anr., Equivalent citations: 2006 (4) JCR 117 Jhr. Available from: http://indiankanoon.org/doc/1838649/.
17. Monir M. Textbook on the law of evidence. 8th edn. New Delhi: Universal law publishing co.; 2011. p. 238.
18. Anwar. Oral and documentary evidence [Internet]. Available from: http://mynation.net/docs/oral-documentary-evidence/.
19. Information Technology Act, 2000. Available from: http://cactusblog.files.wordpress.com/ 2010/01/it_act_2008.pdf.
20. Alagiriswami A. Harihar Prasad Singh and Ors vs. Balmiki Prasad Singh and Ors, Equivalent citations: 1975 AIR 733, 1975 SCR (2) 932. Available from: http://indiankanoon.org/doc/1354608/.
21. Singh P. Raksha Rai vs. Ram Lal. Equivalent citations: AIR 1987 P H 60. Available from: http://indiankanoon.org/doc/1414526/.
22. Ranganath M. Vinod Chaturvedi vs. State of M.P., Equivalent citations: 1984 AIR 911, 1984 SCR (3) 93. Available from: http://indiankanoon.org/doc/736162/.
23. Desai DA. Ramji Dayawala vs. Invest Import, Equivalent citations: 1981 AIR 2085, 1981 SCR (1) 899. Available from: http://indiankanoon.org/doc/1666610/.
24. Shetty KJ. Kalyan Singh, London Trained vs Smt. Chhoti and Ors, Equivalent citations: 1990 AIR 396, 1989 SCR Supl. (2) 356. Available from: http://indiankanoon.org/doc/1599568/.
25. IT amendment Bill 2008. Available from: http://cactusblog.files.wordpress.com/2010/01/it_act_2008.pdf.
26. Seth K, Mukherjee HM. Evidentiary value of SMS, MMS and E-mail. Available from: http://www.sethassociates.com/electronic-evidence-sms-mmse-mails.html.
27. Wiesen G. What is real evidence? Available from: http://www.wisegeek.com/what-is-real-evidence.html.
28. Panchal J. Hasmukhlal V. Shah vs. Bank of India and Ors, Equivalent citations: (1997) 3 GLR 1891. Available from: http://www.indiankanoon.org/doc/706645/.
29. Koshal A. K.P. Abdul Kareem Hajee and Anr. vs. Director, Enforcement, Equivalent citations: (1977) 2 MLJ 47. Available from: http://indiankanoon.org/doc/1082503/.
30. Sinha BP. Tahsildar Singh and another vs. The State of Uttar Pradesh, Equivalent citations: 1959 AIR 1012, 1959 SCR Supl. (2) 875. Available from: http://indiankanoon.org/doc/56195/.

31. Mahajan. Hanumant vs. State of Madhya Pradesh. Equivalent citations: AIR 1952 SC 343, 1953 CriLJ 129, 1952 1 SCR 1091. Available from: http://indiankanoon.org/doc/204632/.
32. Pandian SR. Ashok Kumar vs. State of Madhya Pradesh. Equivalent citations: AIR 1989 SC 1890, 1989 CriLJ 2124. Available from: http://indiankanoon.org/doc/425869/?type=print.
33. Kallu vs. State of UP and ORS [1989] RD-SC 317 (24 October 1989).
34. Scientific evidence. Available from: http://en.wikipedia.org/wiki/Scientific_evidence.
35. Kumari AK. Evidentiary value of expert opinion under Indian Evidence Act. 2007. Available from: http://share.pdfonline.com/95bef09dbb3a447789ce53b7cbb6d61e/IEA1.htm.
36. Bhagwati. Pritam Singh and Anr. vs. The State Of Punjab. Equivalent citations: AIR 1956 SC 415, 1956 CriLJ 805. Available from: http://www.indiankanoon.org/doc/1283903/.
37. Krishnaiyer VR. Piara Singh and Ors vs. State Of Punjab. Equivalent citations: 1977 AIR 2274, 1978 SCR (1) 597. Available from: http://indiankanoon.org/doc/1891900/.
38. Ray G, Nanavati G. Tanviben Pankaj Kumar Diveti vs. State of Gujarat, (1977). Available from: http://indiankanoon.org/doc/10878/.

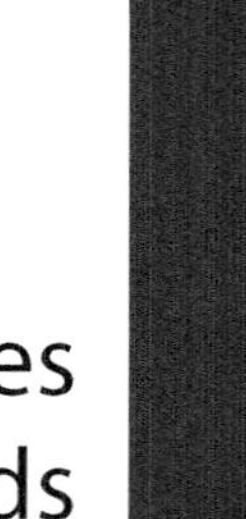

Legal and Ethical Issues of Medical Records

Gautam Biswas

'In God we trust; all others bring data.'

William Edwards Deming (American professor, statistician and author)

ABSTRACT

In India, medical record keeping in hospitals/nursing homes has not developed to the same extent as that in developed countries. In 1946, Bhore Committee first stressed the importance of keeping adequate medical records but still many doctors and institutions do not follow proper documentation of medical records.[1] In fact, many of them do not realize the importance of documenting their records thoroughly, thereby exposing them to frivolous charges of malpractice. When a doctor is confronted by a charge of negligence, the courts are able to judge the correctness of the treatment only by the availability of documentary evidence. The traditional method of keeping the records in most hospitals is the manual method involving papers and files. It is legally more acceptable as documentary evidence since it is difficult to tamper it without detection. Records and documents properly kept can become defense shields for the doctors in the court of law. Hence proper maintenance of such records should form an essential element of good practice. This chapter seeks to impress upon the importance of proper medical documentation and its medicolegal significance.

Keywords: Documentary evidence, ownership of records, confidentiality, retention policy, spoliation.

INTRODUCTION

Medical practitioners are required, both medically and legally, to maintain a current and adequate record for each patient. It is essential that medical records are clear, legible, contemporaneous, accurate, comprehensive and available when needed. The maintenance of record is advantageous to both the hospital and the patient. However, the duration of preservation of records has long been a contentious issue.

In our country, many doctors have not realized the importance of maintaining proper case records. It is common to come across improperly or incompletely written case notes—whether they are treatment notes or medicolegal reports. The most caring and dedicated doctor may be defenseless in a court of law when he/she is accompanied by a chart which is illegible or lacking in good documentation. In litigation, a medical practitioner's care is only as good as his/

her charting. The patient's memory of events will usually prevail over that of the doctor. But if the doctor has the event in question documented in the chart, then his/her case is strengthened considerably.[2-4] If vital information is missing, it may be evidence of negligence on the part of the doctor or health care worker.[1]

Moreover, alteration of notes should never be done, since the question of doctor is innocent or guilty of malpractice quickly becomes a side issue when it is discovered that he has tampered with the evidence, thereby attempting to commit a fraud upon the court.[3]

The chapter discusses the purpose and objectives of medical records, ownership and retention policy, and confidentiality issues regarding the records.

DEFINITIONS

- **Record** can be defined as a documentary evidence of any fact or an event.[5]
- **Medical records** pertains to documents containing a chronological written account of a patient's examination and treatment that includes the patient's medical history and complaints including past and present illness(es), physical findings, results of diagnostic tests and procedures, medications, therapeutic procedures and day-wise progress recorded by a medical or other health practitioner, either personally or at his/her instructions.[6,7]
- **Spoliation** is defined as the intentional destruction, mutilation, alteration or concealment of evidence. This may include any type of records—medical, financial, billing, pharmacy or any procedures.[8,9]

DOCUMENTS CONSTITUTING MEDICAL RECORDS

The following documents can be regarded as the essential components of a health record depending on the nature of the individual case:[7,10]

i. Hand-written contemporaneous notes made by the attending doctor or health care worker including a discharge summary.
ii. Pre-anesthetic and operatives notes.
iii. Notes and histories taken by previous attending doctors or health care workers.
iv. Referral letters to and from other health care practitioners.
v. Laboratory reports and other laboratory evidence such as histology sections, cytology slides and printouts from automated analyzers, X-ray films, CT scans, ECG and EEG.
vi. Audiovisual records such as photographs, videos and tape-recordings.
vii. Clinical research forms and clinical trial data.
viii. Other forms completed during the health interaction such as consent forms, insurance forms, disability assessments and documentation of injuries.
ix. Medicolegal report, death certificates and autopsy reports.
x. Hospital expenditure and bills.

REQUIREMENTS OF MEDICAL RECORDS

The primary purpose of medical record is to provide good continuity of care. The secondary purpose is to provide evidence of care given to the patients.[6] Some important information that is to be included in the record is given in Box 8.1.[2,5,11]

Box 8.1 Information recorded in medical record

- **History:** Present condition and relevant past history including co-existing illnesses, medications and allergies.
- **Examination of the patient:** Positive and relevant negative findings, and all significant observations and measurements (for e.g. pulse, temperature, condition of pupils and blood pressure).
- **Consent:** Details of discussions regarding risk-benefit, treatment plan, prognosis and potential complications (side-effects).
- **Diagnosis:** Clear and concise, justifying how the diagnosis was reached and any differential diagnosis.
- **Investigations:** Lab results and imaging such as X-rays or CT/MRI scans.
- **Management:** Drugs prescribed and administered with dosage, and other treatments, such as physiotherapy.
- **Follow-up and referral:** Details of follow-up tests, future appointments and referrals.

All medical records must be maintained in a standard format with entries and forms filed in chronological order with the most recent on top. Every patient encounter deserves a thoughtful evaluation and notation, no matter how trivial the event may be.

Forensically, good patient records should answer the following fundamental questions:[2]

- Who? The record should clearly identify the patient (name, age, sex, hospital admission number and address), and identify the doctor making the notes, along with his/her signature and name to verify this.
- When? The date and time when a patient was seen or when a test or other procedure/operation was done, or a treatment given should be mentioned. It should also specify when the actual note was made, if there has been a significant time lapse (hours or days-in which case, detail the reasons for delay).
- What? The clinical observations and system examined, investigations done, treatment and instructions given.
- Why? It is important to justify in the notes decisions taken with regard to patient care.

The traditional method of keeping records that is followed in most of the hospitals across India is the manual method involving papers. There are serious limitations of manual record keeping including the need for large storage areas and difficulties in the retrieval of records. However, it is legally more acceptable as documentary evidence, since it is difficult to tamper the records without detection.[7,10]

PURPOSES AND OBJECTIVES OF MEDICAL RECORDS

Medical records may be needed for a variety of reasons—medical, administrative or legal purposes.[2,3,5,7,9,11-15]

Medical

i. **Support patient care:** Record helps in following up patient's progress and response to treatment.

ii. **Communicate between attending doctors:** It documents communication between the attending doctor and other health care professionals dealing with the patient. To ensure good continuity of care, they should clearly communicate this information to anyone who might have future contact with the patient.
iii. **Information for review, study, and evaluation of care given to patients:** The medical record of the patient is anonymized, i.e. the identifying data is removed which may serve as a document to educate medical students/ resident physicians, to provide data for internal hospital auditing and quality assurance, and to provide data for medical research and statistics.
iv. It helps the community to maintain **epidemiological data** thereby assists in improving the health prospects of future generations.

Medicolegal

Medical records are also important in workman's compensation cases, insurance claims, malpractice suits, personal injury cases, criminal cases and even in physician disciplinary hearings as well as collection of bills.

i. **Documentary evidence:** It serves as a documentary evidence of the patient's illness, treatment and response to treatment. It provides written evidence that can be used to protect the legal interests of the patient, hospital and/or health care provider(s). It also provides supporting documentation for the reimbursement of services provided to the patient.
ii. **Claims of the insurances and compensations:** The medical record is used as evidence to show the date of injury, the type, extent and severity of injury, the treatment rendered, duration of the care required and the patient's expected recovery.
    - *Insurance cases:* Frequent requests come from the life insurance corporations regarding details of the hospitalization of a patient including duration of illness and the cause of death.
    - *Workmen's compensation cases:* In labor courts, a person injured in the course of his/her duties and while acting in the scope of his/her employment is entitled to compensation for bodily injury and disability (as per the Workmen's Compensation Act, 1923).
    - *Personal injury suits:* Medical records are used more frequently in this type of cases than in all other cases combined. In this, the claim is made by the individual for damages sustained as the result of injuries, which were due to the fault or neglect of another. For example, in road traffic accident cases under the Motor Accident Claims Tribunal Act for deciding on the amount of compensation.
iii. **Malpractice suits:** An action for malpractice may be brought against the hospital and its employee in a civil or criminal court. In this type of case, the plaintiff (the patient or his relatives) claims damages from the health care professional or hospital for negligence in rendering care or giving improper treatment. Good and accurate record keeping may prove invaluable in responding to and defending against such a complaint or claim. Contemporaneous records of all decisions made about a patient's care and the justifications behind those decisions are essential. Often accurate, legible and complete notes and other records are the only defense. Good

notes corroborate evidence given in court and will enhance the medical practitioner's credibility.

iv. **Execution of will:** The patient may have made a will during his hospital stay. Question of mental competency may arise after the death of the patient and the relatives may try to make it redundant. Medical records may then be used as evidence in proving the mental competency of the patient.

v. **Criminal cases:** Cases which are tried in criminal courts are generally limited to the medicolegal report and postmortem examination report. In such cases, the injured patient may receive medical or surgical care as a hospitalized case. In such situations, clinical sheets are required to decide the nature of injury. The most frequently used include cases like assault cases (including sexual assault) and road traffic accident cases.

OWNERSHIP OF MEDICAL RECORDS

The relationship between doctors and patients has changed over the years and the concept of personal autonomy has become an important aspect of healthcare delivery. The current widely accepted theory about medical records is that the medical practitioner or hospital owns the records, but the patient has the right to the information included in the record and cannot be released without the consent of the patient. In other words, records are the property of the hospital and the personal data contained in the medical record is considered confidential information and the property of the patient.

The doctor is liable for the proper maintenance, custody and storage of the record for the required statutory period. Records should not be taken from the facility except by court order. This does not preclude the routing of copies of the patient's records or portions thereof, including X-ray film, to doctors for consultation. Following guidelines are suggested:[5-7,9,11,12,15,16]

- In the case of government institutions, where records are the property of the institution, original records and images should be retained by the institution. Copies may be made available to the patient (or referring doctor) on request, for which a reasonable fee may be charged.
- In cases where patients are required to pay for records and images (for e.g., private patients or patients in private hospitals) such patients may be allowed to retain such records—unless the health care practitioners deem it necessary to retain such records for purpose of monitoring treatment for a given period. If the patient requires the records and/or images to further protect an interest (for e.g., such as consulting with another practitioner) he/she must be allowed to obtain the originals for these purposes.
- If any request is made for medical records either by the patient/authorized attendant/legal authorities involved, the same may be duly acknowledged and documents shall be issued within a period of 72 hours. The reasonable costs of reproducing copies of written or typed documents or reports may be taken (as per the regulation 1.3.2 of MCI guidelines).
- Not providing medical records to the patient prevents the complainant from seeking an expert opinion. This requires a formal application to the hospital requesting for the records after the hospital bills have been cleared and necessary processing fees has been paid. These documents include copies of inpatient files, records of diagnostic tests, operation notes, videos, medical

certificates and duplicate copies for lost documents (which should be marked properly as 'duplicate'). It is not unusual for an unscrupulous patient to use it for multiple insurance claims without the knowledge of the doctor. However, such information should not be given in original, a photocopy of the same may be handed over to the patient and signature taken in specific format.

- The outpatient file, inpatient file and files of medicolegal cases including the autopsy reports should not be handed over to the patient or relatives without the direction of the court. Original hospital record/file of the medicolegal case (MLC) including X-ray/CT/MRI films should not be handed over to the police. However, if the investigating officer requests, a photocopy of the record (bed-head-ticket/bed-chart) may be supplied and a receipt of the same must be obtained. Patients can get a copy of the medical record only when he is referred to another doctor. However, X-rays are given only after a written undertaking by the patient or relatives that these will be produced in the court as and when required. Original copies of all medicolegal documents should be produced whenever asked for in a court of law.

However, certain records must be given to all patients including patients who leave against medical advice without any charge—discharge summary, referral notes and death summary (in case if natural death). Moreover, the above documents cannot be legally refused even when the hospital bill has not been paid.

In an alleged case where a detailed discharge summary was given to the patient, the National Commission had ruled that there is no question of negligence on part of the hospital. Question arises when there is failure to supply the medical records to patient, if there is a legal duty on the hospital to give records.[1]

CONFIDENTIALITY OF MEDICAL RECORDS

The information contained in the medical record belongs to the patient and is a confidential communication between the medical practitioner and the patient. Medical records should be safeguarded against any unauthorized use. They should be stored in a secure area, and there should be detailed policies regarding confidentiality and the release of patient information.[10,11]

These records frequently contain sensitive and vital information related to a person's physical and mental condition that could be extremely personal which if shared without the patient's consent, could have disastrous effect on the physical, mental, social and economic well-being of the person. Therefore, disclosures of information will be a breach of the confidentiality rule which may result in the doctor being sued for invasion of privacy, defamation or breach of contract.[12,17]

It is professional misconduct to give information concerning the condition of a patient or any services rendered to a patient to any other person except with the consent of the patient. It should only be revealed to another person with the consent of the patient or the patient's authorized representative. Determining who the authorized representative is may sometimes be difficult (for e.g., the patient is deceased or the patient is a minor whose parents are separated). When in doubt about a valid authorization, advice should be taken from the legal advisor of the hospital.[10,12,18]

If a patient is under the age of 18 years or otherwise subject to a guardianship order, any consent for access to information should be given in writing by the patient's parents or legal guardian. In the case of a patient who has died, the written consent to access information from the patient's medical record should be provided by the next of kin shown on the medical records or by the administrator of the patient's estate. If the patient lacks the capacity to provide genuine consent then the written consent must be obtained from the person's legal guardian.[12,17,18]

However, it is sometimes necessary for doctors to breach confidentiality. They should familiarize themselves with the existing laws governing the disclosure of certain kinds of information without the patient's authorization. Whenever possible, any breach of confidentiality should be discussed with the patient beforehand. There are some instances in which health care practitioner are required to disclose personal health information without patient consent:[7,9,11,12,18]

i. The medical records may be needed by other health professionals for the continuing care of the patient.
ii. It may be used for research and health care statistics, as long as the patient is not identified.
iii. There is legislative authority for the production of patient information, i.e. where a court orders the records to be handed to the third party.
iv. The third party is a medical practitioner who is being sued by a patient and needs access to the records to mount a defense.
v. The third party is a medical practitioner who has had disciplinary proceedings instituted against him/her by the State Medical Council and requires access to the records to defend him or her.
vi. The health care practitioner is under a statutory obligation to disclose certain medical facts, (for e.g., reporting a case of suspected child abuse). Any sexually transmitted disease in a girl under 18 years of age should be reported to the local health department as a possible sexual abuse case.
vii. The non-disclosure of the medical information about the patient would represent a serious threat to public health.

Requests for information by the police or a government department where the patient has not authorized access to information from his/her medical records should be dealt with by the attending doctor or senior health care professional. Except in circumstances where the police can confirm that they seek information essential to the execution of the police officer's duty, the information supplied should be limited to confirmation of identity and address. Any other information may only be divulged on production of a search warrant.[12]

Patient information regarding STDs, mental health and drug and alcohol abuse are considered privileged information and must be specifically authorized in the written release signed by the patient or legal guardian prior to the release of these records. When releasing the medical record, entries related to STDs, HIV/AIDS, alcohol and drug abuse or psychological/mental problems are omitted from the record, unless specifically authorized in the written release signed by the patient or guardian. Not maintaining the confidentiality of HIV status of a patient was held as negligence.[1]

Doctors preparing reports for third parties should inform the patient of the purpose of the examination and the way it will be conducted. The patient must be advised in advance that the prepared report will be disclosed to the third party requesting the report. A doctor who discovers, during the third party examination, a significant medical condition requiring treatment is responsible for ensuring that this is disclosed to the patient with a recommendation to seek treatment.

Doctor may refuse a request for access to information from a third party where he/she believes that disclosure of certain information is likely to cause substantial harm to the physical or mental well-being of the patient or to a third party, he/she may withhold the information. While examining a minor whom a medical provider believes may have been a victim of a child abuse, parental permission for release of records is not required. When the parent is accused of an offence, the parent's decision may be based on his/her own protection rather than on the best interests of the child. If an accused parent wants of copy of the child patient's record, law allows a provider to deny a patient (or patient's parent) access to patient records.[18,19]

CUSTODY OF MEDICAL RECORDS

Medical records should be stored in a safe and secure environment to safeguard their physical integrity and confidentiality. Medical practitioner should take reasonable steps to ensure that records are protected from theft, loss and unauthorized use or disclosure, including photocopying, modification or disposal.

It should be kept in restricted access areas or locked in filing cabinets and organizational measures should be in place to ensure that only those who need access to the records for a legitimate purpose are able to see them. Doctors need to consider that nonmedical staff, such as maintenance staff, may have access to records, and should ensure that steps are taken to ensure that access to the records is limited or those who have access to the records are bound by an appropriate confidentiality agreement.[17]

In medicolegal cases, all investigation forms, X-rays, CT/MRI scans and case file should bear the label 'MLC' on the top, so that necessary precautions can be taken by all concerned. X-ray and CT/MRI scan plates also need to be preserved carefully. All such plates must be properly labeled. MLC number of the case is to be mentioned on the X-ray and scans along with the date and time.[17] The medicolegal register should be in the safe custody of the doctor who examines the patient and finalizes the report. He must ensure that it is not tampered at any stage and no one else has access to it. When the register has been fully utilized, the same should be sent to medical record section in hospitals where such facility is available.

Responsibility of Medical Record Department

The medical record department (MRD) is responsible for proper storage, retrieval and maintenance of confidentiality and security of the record. It is important that the record officer is aware of the need to maintain confidentiality and the patient's right to privacy. As the person in-charge of the MRD he/she is responsible for seeing that unauthorized persons do not have access to the medical record and that information is not given out without the patient's written consent.[15]

Medical records should be kept under adequate security and only removed from the hospital or health care center upon receipt of a subpoena, statutory authority or court order. The officer or the clerk issuing the record to any doctor should ensure that it is properly numbered and a certificate regarding the same (the number of forms, X-rays and CT/MRI scans contained there-in) should be given by him. Medicolegal correspondence must follow the principle of the maintenance of the 'chain of custody'. That means the handing over of a particular document or an article must be properly recorded at every step.[21] On return from court, the medical record is checked to ensure that all pages (forms) are present. In many places, when an original medical record leaves the hospital for legal purposes, a photocopy of the medical record is made beforehand and kept in the hospital, until the original is returned. The copy is subsequently destroyed. Similarly, medicolegal documents are considered as strictly confidential records and should be stored under safe custody to avoid tampering. In case any record is issued to any designate individual as per the retrieval policy, the same is recorded in the outgoing patient record entry register for accountability. The record should not be is issued to in any form or to any person without proper authorization from the designated authorities.[15]

A medical record subpoenaed for a legal case should be filed in a secure place until the case is terminated to prevent altering, tampering, or removing the record or any of its contents. A change made in the record after a suit has been filed in the court indicates some foul play. To prevent such untoward event it is suggested that:[15]

- Each page of the record should be numbered.
- A copy of the record should be made.
- The original and the copy is locked in a secure place.
- The original record should be viewed only under proper supervision or the copy of the record may be used for viewing by appropriate parties instead of the original/first copy that will be sent to court.

In case of loss or tampering of patient's medical record data, the medical record clerk should immediately inform the Medical Superintendent (MS) who is responsible for taking appropriate action. The MS should inform the external agencies as applicable, and would hold an internal enquiry for investigating the cause for such event. In case the internal committee confirms any sort of negligence/mischief on part of any hospital employee, the MS should inform the same to higher authorities for further action.

ISSUING OF MEDICOLEGAL REPORT

Medicolegal reports (MLR) should not be issued to third parties by the hospital authorities. Medicolegal cases, because of its sensitive nature, disclosure of information or issue of records to the parties involved in the cases, can very well be withheld by the medical practitioner or the hospital, as this would be obligatory on the part of the hospital, matter being subjudice. Such information is also exempt under RTI Act, and has been upheld by CIC.[20-22]

MLR including the postmortem report (PMR) belongs to the requestor, i.e. the police and the same is held by the doctor in fiduciary relationship (holding in trust or faith). Even the person who was examined has no authority to demand the copy of the medicolegal report directly from the doctor/hospital authority, if the report was prepared by the doctor at the requisition of a police officer or Magistrate. MLR is handed over only to the authorized police official (after getting receipt of the same).[10,20]

If affected party is asking for a record in road traffic accidents or where some issues of compensation or claim is there, then attested photocopy of the MLR may be handed over to the patient or his/her relative, as per prevailing rules of the hospital/State and after the requisite fee has been paid by applicant. The following are required along with the patient's or his/her next of kin's application:[23]

i. A notarized affidavit in the name of the applicant stating his relationship with the patient (if the applicant is not the patient himself/herself) and the particular purpose for which the copy of the MLR is needed and the number of copies needed.
ii. Submitting the requisite fees, as decided by the competent authority with receipt of the same enclosed with the application.
iii. In case, it is a case of alleged physical and/or sexual assault, a 'No Objection Certificate' (NOC) from the concerned police station (investigating the case) should also be produced clearly stating that the issue of copy of MLR will not hinder the investigation. In such cases, where injuries are produced as part of criminal offence, unauthorized leakage of information before police file a *challan* in the court of law is not warranted.

Once these three documents (as the case may be) are submitted to the concerned medical practitioner, attested photocopies of the medicolegal report should be issued.

- A MLR or PMR is a confidential report prepared by an expert and not a public document as has been held by the various courts of India. As such, an accused/third party is not entitled to get a copy of the same during the investigation stage of the case. In has been held that an accused is not entitled to certified copies of the inquest report, statements recorded under Sec. 174 of the IPC, postmortem report, requisition given by the police officers to the medical officer for conducting postmortem and medically treating the injured, rough sketch of the scene place and observation *mahazar* prepared by the investigating officer, before the final report is forwarded to the Magistrate.[20,21]
- Punjab Medical Manual and Punjab Police Rules also prohibit supply of copy of MLR/PMR to an accused.
- Sec. 54 CrPC has been amended to provide that a copy of the report of the medical examination of the arrested person by the registered medical practitioner to the arrested person or his nominee, after his medical examination has been conducted.[24]
- Request for supply of copy of MLR or PMR under the RTI Act are not maintainable [Section 8(1) (e) & Section 8(1) (h)]. In a significant judgment by Delhi High Court, a bench comprising Chief Justice AP Shah and Justices S Muralidhar and Vikramjeet Sen decided that medical records do not fall under the purview of Section 8(1)(j) of Right To Information (RTI) Act, 2005 'unless public interest is attached'. They quoted an American writer 'One man's freedom of information is another man's invasion of privacy'. In this case, the Jaiprakash Narayan Apex Trauma Centre of AIIMS has turned down the request to provide information about the PMR saying that the case was related to medicolegal records. They refused to provide information under Sections 8(1)b and 8(1)h of the RTI to the petitioner.[20-22]
- The Central Information Commission (CIC) also denied a man access to information about his fiancée's health and the treatment she had undergone at a psychiatric center, claiming that a doctor-patient relationship was based on trust, which could not be breached. In that case, the petitioner had filed a RTI petition seeking access to the medical records of his fiancée, from IHBAS, Shahdara.[22]

Section 8 (1) of RTI Act states:[25]

b. Information which has been expressly forbidden to be published by any court of law or tribunal or the disclosure of which may constitute contempt of court cannot be provided to a RTI petitioner.

e. Information available to a person in his fiduciary relationship, unless the competent authority is satisfied that the larger public interest warrants the disclosure of such information.

h. Information cannot be provided about matters which would impede the process of investigation or apprehension or prosecution of the offenders.

j. Information cannot be provided which relates to personal information, the disclosure of which has no relationship to any public activity or interest or which would cause unwarranted invasion of the privacy of the individual unless the Central Public Information Officer or the State Public Information Officer or the appellate authority, as the case may be, is satisfied that the larger public interest justifies the disclosure of such information.

RETENTION OF MEDICAL RECORDS

Medical records should be kept by the hospital as long as required under the Statute of Limitations (retention for legal requirements). However, as per Indian law, there is no specified time limit after which the records including MLR's can be destroyed. Some guidelines have been framed by DGHS, MCI and various courts which refer to minimum periods for which records must be retained, but there may be occasions on which records need to be retained for longer period. Most hospitals have a policy of maintaining all medical records for variable periods.

There are limitation periods for many types of civil cases. There are exceptions too. But there is no limitation period for criminal cases. So, if such proceedings are expected, the relevant records must be kept until such time as it may reasonably be thought that no proceedings or further proceedings would arise. Once a case commences in the court, there is no time limit within which it is going to be concluded. All original copies of certificates and reports issued for medicolegal purposes are to be preserved till the finalization of the case.[13] In one study, the mean lag period between registration of first information report and time to appear before the court of law to give evidence by a medical witness has been found to be more than two years.

Indian Regulations

The following are some of the guidelines for retention of medical records that have been issued by various regulatory bodies:[2,10,15-17]

i. As per regulation 1.3.1 of the Medical Council of India, a doctor should maintain the medical records pertaining to his/her indoor patients for a period of 3 years from the date of commencement of the treatment in a standard proforma laid down by the Medical Council of India. This regulation applies to a doctor in his private capacity in case of indoor patients whom he/she might be treating/operating in hospitals/nursing homes.

ii. Under the Consumer Protection Act 1986, the consumer can file a complaint till 2 years after the service was provided. This is usually extended to mean "....till 2 years after the defect in service comes to notice..." So, there is provision which allows condoning the delay in appropriate cases for which the records may be needed even after 2 years.

iii. Under the PNDT Act 1994, all documents (records, charts, forms, reports and consent letters) are required to be maintained for a period of 2 years or until the disposal of any criminal or other proceedings are instituted against the center/hospital.

iv. Under the Directorate General of Health Services guidelines applicable to government hospitals, the responsibility of hospital to keep medical records is up to 5 years for outpatient department, and inpatient medical record (case sheets of MLC and non MLC) is up to 10 years. These directives are also there in the 'Hospital Manual' published by it.

v. As per Punjab Medical Manual (1934), the medicolegal record is to be preserved for 12 years.

vi. The Maharashtra Government had issued a resolution which states that OPD papers should be kept for 3 years, indoor case papers for 5 years and MLC records for 30 years.

International Guidelines

- In the United States, legal requirements for retention of medical records range from 7 years in some states to perpetuity in others. In Washington, a hospital needs to preserve all medical records of a patient for a period of not less than 10 years following the most recent discharge of the patient; except the records of minors which need to be retained for a period of not less than 3 years following attainment of the age of 18 years, or 10 years following discharge, whichever is longer. In Pennsylvania, the medical records whether original, reproductions or microfilm, should be kept on file for a minimum of 7 years following the discharge of a patient. If the patient is a minor, records are to be kept on file until his majority, and then for 7 years or as long as the records of adult patients are maintained.[7,26]
- In United Kingdom, minimum retention period for hospital records is 8 years after conclusion of treatment or death. For postmortem registers and homicide/serious untoward incident records, retention period of 30 years is recommended. Postmortem reports are to be held in the patient's health record for 8 years after the patient's death. Once litigation has been notified (or a formal complaint received) images (X-ray, CT, MRI scans) should be stored until 10 years after the file has been closed. Maternity records are to be preserved for 25 years. For children and young people, until the patient's 25th birthday, or 26th if the young person was aged 17 at conclusion of treatment. For mentally disordered persons, 20 years after no further treatment considered necessary or 8 years after the patient's death, if the patient died while still receiving treatment.[2,7,10,11]
- According to the Dutch Medical Treatment Act (WGBO), patient data must be retained for at least 10 years or as much longer as required. In practice, patient data are often destroyed after 10 years. A committee of the Health Council of the Netherlands proposed a longer retention period by extending it by 5 years.[27]
- As per the guidelines of College of Physicians and Surgeons, Nova Scotia, for adult patients, records should be retained for a minimum of 10 years from

the date of the last entry in the record. For patients who are children, doctors should keep the record until 10 years after the day on which the patient reached the age of 19 years (the age of majority in Nova Scotia).[28]

- The South African Medical Association recommends that medical records are to be kept from 6 to 9 years. As a general rule, most legal actions start within 10 years and it makes good sense to keep general medical records and medical specimens for at least 10 years.[11]
- The Singapore Medical Association recommended that most medical records can be safely destroyed when 10 years have elapsed since the patient was last treated or since the patient's death. However, if the records related to a minor or are maternity records, they should be kept until the patient reaches 25 unless he/she is brain-damaged, in which case the records should be kept until 10 years after his/her death.[6]
- In West Malaysia, for medical negligence claims against private hospitals and doctors in private practice, the limitation period is six years running from the date that the right to sue arises, which is usually no later than the date of the occurrence of the injury complained of. In East Malaysia, for private hospitals and doctors in private practice, the limitation period is usually three to six years, running from the date that the right to sue arises.[13]
- As per the Health Authority, Abu Dhabi, the medical records (of UAE nationals only) and medicolegal records including medicolegal registers (for all nationality) are to be preserved indefinitely and should not be destroyed. For expatriates, the records (excluding medicolegal cases) should be preserved for 7 years.[29]

In view of the multitude of cases against the doctors under the Consumer Protection Act and the slow process of judicial proceedings wherein the cases come at trial stage after a period of 10-15 years, the medical records needs to be preserved for a longer duration. Till the time the records are not submitted or called for evidence, they cannot be disposed off as such. However, a balance must be reached between the costs of retention of records (in terms of space, manpower and equipment) and the occasional case where the practitioners' defense of a case of negligence is handicapped by the absence of records. The hospital and the doctor were held guilty of negligence when the plea of destroying the medical records as per the hospital policy was cited in the court which was considered as an attempt to suppress certain facts. The value of the record for academic or research purposes, and the risks resulting from the handling or complications of the case are additional considerations.

In considering the above facts, the records should be preserved as recommended in Box 8.2.[9,14,30]

As a matter of good practice, after expiry of the requisite retention period, all these records may be disposed off only after getting a 'No Objection Certificate' from concerned police station (a cumbersome process). However, an account of the records to be destroyed should to be made.

CORRECTION OF MEDICAL RECORDS

During the preparation of medical reports, including medicolegal report, it is preferable not to make any deletion of words or sentences by cutting or erasing. Sometimes, it becomes necessary for the health care providers to correct

Box 8.2 Recommendation for retention of medical records

- Out-patient records need to be preserved for a minimum period of 5 years.
- In-patient records should to be preserved for 10 years.
- Where there is chance of litigation arising out of negligence of the medical practitioner, record should be preserved for at least 25 years.
- In medicolegal cases, the medical records including the medicolegal registers' should be preserved for 30 years.
- Postmortem reports and registers should be preserved for 30 years.
- In the case of minors and those patients who are mentally incompetent, health care practitioners should keep the records for a longer period (there are no formal guidelines in this context):
  - If the patient is less than 18 years of age on his/her last date of consultation, the record should be kept until he/she reaches age 18 plus 5 years or 10 years whichever is the longer time period.
  - If the patient is 18 years of age or older on his/her last date of consultation, the record must be kept for 10 years.
  - For mentally incompetent patients, the record should be kept for the duration of the patient's lifetime.

errors in medical records. Where necessary to ensure accuracy of the medical record, it should be corrected promptly once detected. Deliberately altering the medical record may be considered professional misconduct. To prevent the appearance of spoliation, errors should be corrected or edited only by using the proper methodology. Correcting an error or omission in a medical record can be devastating in a medical negligence case, if the Judge believes that the changes were made to cover up improper care or to include something that was never done. Moreover, the omission of essential details from the notes may also cast a doubt on the truthfulness of the witness.

Following guidelines are suggested:[4,6,9,11,12,14]

1. The proper method is for the doctor to draw a single line through the incorrect information without obliterating it. Then the correct information is recorded above, below or beside the original incorrect data, and is initialed and dated. It is important that it should be readable what has been edited or changed in the clinic or hospital records.
2. It is inappropriate to delete recorded information with correction fluid. Erasing, blotting out or adding information at a different time than the original note was made are not appropriate ways to correct a record. Attempting to obliterate the erroneous entry by applying a whitener or scratching through the entry in such a way that a person cannot determine what was originally written raises the suspicion of someone looking for negligent or inappropriate care.
3. Entries in a medical record should be made on every line. Skipping lines leaves room for tampering the record, a practice not in the best interest of the patient or doctor.
4. Entries that have been erased and not initialed or signed should be returned to the doctor for his/her signature, as without such a signature the legal value of the medical record will be decreased.
5. Correcting of personal identification data of the patient like: name, father/husband name, age, sex, address should only be done on the basis of affidavit by notary or 1st Class Magistrate.

6. Additional entries added at a later date must be dated and signed in full. The reason for an amendment or error should also be explained on the record.

Tampering with medical records can be both costly to the reputation of the doctor and the hospital, resulting in large malpractice awards even when there has been no negligence.[3] Common types of spoliation include:[8,27]

- Adding some notes to an existing record at some later date.
- Intentional placement of inaccurate medical information in the records.
- Absence of information regarding the exact time of patient treatment by nurses.
- Recording of the same or constant vital signs (so-called 'perfect vital signs syndrome').
- Recording of treatment provided at a date after the patient has been discharged or transferred to another hospital.
- Omission of significant medical information or 'fraudulent concealment'.
- Dating a record as if it were written at a previous date.
- Complete rewriting or retyping of part of the medical record (for e.g., discharge summary).
- Hiding or destroying the medical record.

The State Commission had held negligence where the records appeared to be manipulated. It also stated that such cases require detailed examination in civil court rather than in consumer court.[1]

SUBPOENA OF MEDICAL RECORDS

A subpoena or summons to produce medical and medicolegal records is a form of court order and the person who fails to comply is in contempt of court and may be punished. Medical records are acceptable as evidence as per the Indian Evidence Act, 1872 by the court, since the documentation of facts during the course of treatment of patient is considered authentic and unbiased. A medical practitioner is usually summoned as a witness to testify and bring with him the necessary documents to verify his evidence.[10] It is the duty of the medical practitioner to produce the medical records in the court for scrutiny and adverse inference could be drawn for not producing the same.[1] Failure to deliver X-ray films had been held deficiency in service.[1] Whether or not the records are to be admitted as evidence is a matter for the discretion of the court. However, any correspondence not written at the time the patient was in hospital should be removed as it is considered 'hearsay' and not permissible as evidence.

In court, medical records may undergo detailed scrutiny to judge the correctness of the treatment by the available documentary evidence. Their quality tends to be seen as a reflection of the standard of care provided by the medical practitioner. Properly maintained case notes are important defense of the doctor in any case against him. Well-documented medical records may eliminate or reduce the time required to spend in legal activities. Medical record itself can sometime, determine whether or not a malpractice claim will survive beyond counsel's initial review of case.[10]

Doctors may be required to disclose personal health information in the course of proceedings. He/she should read the subpoena carefully and do everything it requires but no more than it requires. For example, a summons may require a doctor to attend a court at a particular time and take a specific patient chart. That summons does not authorize the doctor to discuss the patient's care or show the record to anyone in advance of the court appearance. Medical records which are subpoenaed are to be made over to the court and not to the lawyers who sought the subpoena.[10,12]

There are few instances when a court will allow the restriction of relevant and material evidence, particularly a medical record, to be protected from discovery (for e.g., rape or child abuse cases). In cases where there is a dispute as to whether a record should be turned over, the court may choose to review the record in chambers and make a determination regarding what, if any, information should be submitted. This *in camera* review is prior to turning the records over to the parties.[19]

If the court demands X-rays/CT scan/MRI films, bed-head tickets or any other record of the case, these should be deposited in the court and a receipt of the same should be obtained.[21]

In some circumstances, the MRO is served the summons and he/she is required to produce the medical record in the court on the prescribed day and time. The MRO should notify the attending doctor and hospital administration that a subpoena has been received for the release of medical record to the court. He/she should check that all necessary information, as specified in the subpoena, is in the medical record and that it is complete. He/she may be required to testify that the medical record has been kept as a normal business of the hospital and to the best of his/her knowledge has not been tampered with by unauthorized persons.[12]

DESTRUCTION OF MEDICAL RECORDS

Medical practitioner should not dispose off the record of the patient, unless their obligation to retain the record has come to an end. Hospital management and doctors should identify the cases which have gone to the court or have the potential for litigation when deciding which records to destroy and which to preserve. If a particular record is the subject matter of litigation, the hospital should preserve the record even beyond the limits suggested above during the pendency of the litigation.

At the end of the designated retention period, the medical record clerk should seek written approval from the MS for destruction of the medical records. Only after obtaining written permission from the designated hospital authority, the medical records should be destructed by the department staff. The time frame for the destruction of patient medical records begins from the date of discharge or from the date of outpatient/ancillary services rendered or the last date of patient encounter. However, as a good practice, the hospitals should publish an advertisement in the newspapers for the concerned to take claim of their records.

The purpose of disposal or destruction is to permanently remove records from active use with no possibility of reconstructing the information. In many countries, when medical records are destroyed after the required retention period, a record destruction log is made, individually listing all medical records to be destroyed. That log book should include:[12]

- Patient's full name, age, sex, address and medical record number.
- Admission and discharge dates.
- Name(s) of the attending doctor(s).

- Diagnosis and operations performed (if any).
- Discharge summary for each admission, if more than one.
- Date of destruction of the record.
- Signature(s) of individuals witnessing destruction.
- Method of destruction.

Record destruction logs must be maintained/retained and secured permanently for tracking purposes. In addition, a note should be included with the retained documents stating that the records have been destroyed according to the retention policy.

To ensure that the medical records are completely destroyed, the MRO should supervise their destruction. The records should be destroyed in a way that is in keeping with the obligation of maintaining confidentiality of the patient. Disposing of records in the trash does not provide adequate protection and could lead to allegations of breach of confidentiality. The methods of destruction such as burning and burial are not reliable. It is recommended that records which are approved for destruction after completing the retention period be destroyed by methods of shredding, trammeling or pulping.

Electronic health records (EHR) should be permanently deleted from all hard drives as well as other storage mechanisms. It may not be possible to permanently delete records from a computer's hard drive. In most cases, it is preferable to destroy the hard drive altogether.

ALTERNATIVES TO PAPER RECORD

Medical record department of a hospital faces numerous problems of which lack of planning in storage of inactive records and determination of records retention period being the foremost. That is why there is a need of effective storage and control of inactive records and determination of records retention period.

The problem of storage of records for a long time has been eased by the availability of electronic means of preserving records. Medical records may be archived on microfilm, microfiche or magnetic data files. Scanned copies can be maintained on the computer, even after physical records are destroyed. Care must be taken to preserve the integrity of medical records, whether computerized or otherwise. Further, with the acceptance of electronic records by the courts, the medical records including the MLC/PM reports which are to be destroyed after their retention period may first be scanned and preserved permanently so that even after that process, if any query arises, the record can easily be retrieved.[2,11]

The introduction of the electronic medical record (hospital information system) is an attempt to solve this issue by making the record available on all hospital terminals. The electronic health record is accessible over networks and allows exchange of information both within the institution and across its borders. Efforts have been made to draft ethical code for informatics as fundamental principles according to which data protection and access to official information could be reconciled. It is indeed very essential to maintain confidentiality of these records while still facilitating patient care.[7,18,30,31]

During the transition from paper to electronic medical records, doctors must consider their stewardship responsibilities as a top priority. Management of patient information must be heightened to ensure integrity and security. Potential threats may include: breakdown of service as a result of viruses, power failures, loss of data due to corruption of computer hardware and theft of data due to intrusion.[7,18]

Electronic Medical Record: The electronic record of health related information on an individual that is created, gathered, managed and consulted by licensed clinicians and staff from a single organization who are involved in the individual's health and care. Electronic medical record (EMR) is a record of single diagnosis or treatment which is maintained in separate compartments to be used by specialist concerned with the single disease. There is substantial evidence that the use of EMR can reduce the costs associated with tort claims and malpractice judgments.[4,6,7]

Electronic Health Record: The aggregate electronic record of health-related information on an individual that is created and gathered cumulatively across more than one health care organization and is managed and consulted by licensed clinicians and staff involved in the individual's health and care. Electronic health record (EHR) provides a comprehensive view of the patient's health history, clinical findings that have been collected over time and is more of a comprehensive collection of medical data.[7]

However, some states in the United States expressly prohibit the use of computerized records systems by requiring that orders be written in ink, or by mandating that health record storage be restricted to original paper or microfilm.[7,28]

Records can be digitized and summarized and can be imprinted on a 'smart card'. As concern about breaches in internet security occupies more of the public and legislative agenda, 'smart cards' are being considered a possible solution. The low cost of the cards, their increasing storage capacity and the fact that patients carry their card to the point of care make smart cards an attractive option either as identification token or as a data container.[28]

Micro Filming of Records

In a complex organization, microfilming of records can help in space saving, safe preservation, clean and easy handling. Besides, these reduce the risk of fire hazards and chances of loosing documents. Documents including patient's file, X-rays, CT scans and index cards can be microfilmed as per the record retention schedule or the standing instructions issued by the hospital, health ministry or the state government.[9,13]

CONCLUSION

The patient's record is both a medical and legal document. They are the only authentic, reliable and documented records of the events associated with a patient during the course of his illness and its outcome that may include death. The chief value of medical records as evidence is that they contain unbiased statements in as much as the doctors, nurses and other concerned in making the medical record at the time of the patient's hospitalization had no interest in any subsequent litigation. It is the only written documented evidence that is acceptable in the courts of law and other competent authorities.

In creating and maintaining patient records, doctors and hospitals have several legal duties, including the duty to do so adequately, to safeguard the records' physical existence and to prevent such use of the records as would violate the patient's right to confidentiality. No information should be released without the patient's consent, including the fact that the person is a patient. Where there are legal requirement that prescribe the period for which patient records should be retained, a medical practitioner must comply with these obligations.

REFERENCES

1. Medical record services. Chapter XII. Available from: http://mohfw.nic.in/hmcheck/12Ch.XII MeicalRecord.pdf.
2. Medicolegal aspects of the medical records. Available from: http://www.scribd.com/Legal-Aspects/d/32303807.
3. McCaman B, Hirsh HL. Medical records-legal perspectives. *Prim Care* 1979; 6: 81-91.
4. Heath SW. The medical record: Documentation of care provided. Risk management and medical liability: a manual for Indian health service and tribal health care professionals. 2nd edn. 1996. p. 25-28.
5. Menon A, Rastogi P. Documentation in medical practice. *Ind Internet J For Med Toxicol.* 2007; 5(3). Available from: http://www.indianjournals.com/ijor.aspx?target=ijor:iijfmt&volume=5&issue=3&article=002.
6. Medical records: making and retaining them. Singapore Medical Association. Available from: http://www.sma.org.sg/UploadedImg/files/PositionsStatements/medical_records.pdf.
7. Medical record. Available from: http://en.wikipedia.org/wiki/Medical_record.
8. Hoffman AC, Sanbar SS. Spoliation: Record retention, destruction and alteration. In: Sanbar SS (ed). The medical practice survival handbook. American College of Legal Medicine. Philadelphia: Mosby, Elsevier Inc; 2007. p. 45-53.
9. Singh S, Sinha US, Sharma NK. Preservation of medical records—an essential part of health care delivery. *Ind Internet J For Med Toxicol* 2005; 3(4) [Internet]. Available from: http://www.icfmt.org/vol3no4.
10. Thomas J. Medical records and issues in negligence. *Indian J Urol* 2009; 25: 384-8.
11. Guidelines on the keeping of patient records. Guidelines for good practice in the health care professions. Health professions council of South Africa. Booklet 14, Pretoria 2008. Available from: http://www.hpcsa.co.za/downloads/conduct_ethics/rules/generic_ethical_rules/booklet_14_keeping_of_patience_records.pdf.
12. Medical records manual: A guide for developing countries. World Health Organization. Available from: http://www.wpro.who.int/publications/docs/MedicalRecordsManual.pdf.
13. Ranjan PS. Medical records: preservation and matters of evidence. Medicolegal Updates. Medical Defence Malaysia Berhad. Available from: http://www.mdm.org.my/archived_articles. php?newsID=2&archived=yes.
14. Vijayanath V. Factuals of medical records. *JPAFMAT* 2007; 7: 36-37.
15. Manual of operations medical records department. Quality operating process. Dr. Ram Manohar Lohia Combined Hospital, Lucknow, 2008. Available from: http://www.scribd.com/doc/143715457/Emergency-Department-Policy
16. Hirsh HL. Medical records-their medico-legal significance. *J Fam Pract* 1975; 2: 213-16.
17. Guidelines for preservation of Medicolegal documents. Available at: http://indianarmy.nic.in/writereaddata/Documents/medico_legal.pdf.
18. Soudarssanane MB, Asthana S, Viranjini G. Doctor patient confidentiality-changing scenario. *Ind J Community Med* 2002; 27: 91-93.

19. Botash AS. Medical records. Child abuse evaluation & treatment. Available from: http://childabusemd.com/law/medical-records.shtml.
20. Haryana Medico Legal Manual, 2012. Available from: http://www.haryanahealth.nic.in/userfiles/file/pdf/PMBranch/MedicoLegalManual/2.HaryanaMedicolegalManual201231.1.2012.pdf.
21. Medical records not under RTI: court. 2010 Feb 04. Available from: http://www.doctorsandlaw.com/2010/02/medical-records-not-under-rti-court.html.
22. Cannot access medical records through RTI: information panel. Available from: http://indiarti.blogspot.in/2009_08_01_archive.html.
23. Guidelines for issue of copies of PMR and MLR. Government Medical College & Hospital, Sector-32. Chandigarh. 2009.
24. The Code of Criminal Procedure (Amendment) Act, 2008. Available from: http://www.allindiareporter.in/addons/news/index.php?news=688.
25. Section 8. The Right To Information Act, 2005. Available from: http://indiankanoon.org/doc/758550/.
26. Washington State legislature revised code of Washington (RCW) RCW 70.41.190. Medical records of patients—Retention and preservation. Available from: http://apps.leg.wa.gov/rcw/default.aspx?cite=70.02&full=true.
27. Dondorp WJ, Legemaate J, van de Klippe CJ. Retention period for patient data: the health council of the Netherlands pleads for a change in the law. *Ned Tijdschr Geneeskd* 2004; 148: 743-47.
28. Guidelines for medical record-keeping. Council of Physicians and Surgeons of Nova Scotia 2008. Available from: http://www.cpsns.ns.ca/portals/0/guidelines-policies/2008-medical-record.pdf.
29. Medical record/health information retention and disposal policy. Health authority - Abu Dhabi. 2009. Available from: http://www.haad.ae/HAAD/LinkClick.aspx?fileticket=jRbMRgq1pms%3D&tabid=820.
30. Bhaskaran VP, Satyashankar P, Tarun Koshy Abraham TK, Pera NK. A study of the storage problems of medical records in tertiary hospital. *J Acad Hospital Administration* 2002; 14: 23-26.
31. Mann R, Williams J. Standards in medical record keeping. *Clin Med* 2003; 3: 329-32.

CLINICAL FORENSIC MEDICINE

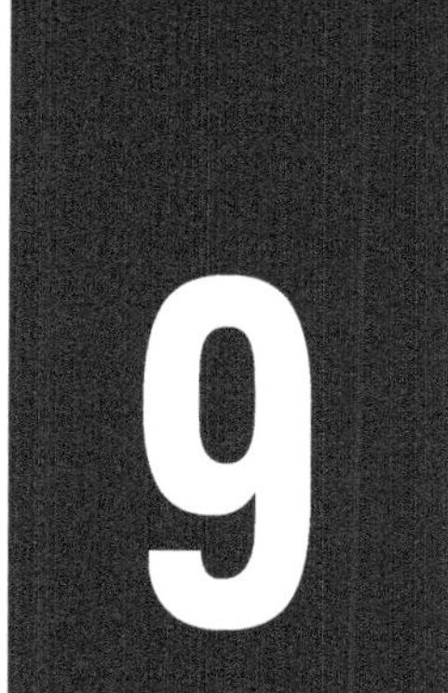

Medicolegal Examination and Certification of a Case of Injury

Swapnil S Agarwal

'In this work, when it shall be found that much is omitted, let it not be forgotten that much is likewise performed.'
Samuel Johnson (Biographer, poet, lexicographer and literary critic)

ABSTRACT

An accurate description and interpretation of injuries is one of the most important function for any registered medical practitioner who comes across cases of injuries. He must be able to record injuries accurately, be aware of their medicolegal significance and be able to give a useful opinion on how they may have been caused. The current scenario is exactly opposite to this. The medical practitioners are following what has been in practice for decades without bothering for validity or reliability of the procedure being followed. Also, most of our books give theoretical knowledge about the injuries without bothering about the practical aspects. An effort has been made to highlight the practical aspects of examination of a case of injuries and its recording to stand a valid scrutiny in the court of law. After going through the chapter, the reader would be able to recognize different types of injuries with proper nomenclature and be able to prepare an authentic medicolegal injury report.

Keywords: Injury, medicolegal report, rulings, law.

INTRODUCTION

There is a vast discrepancy in the way an injured person is examined and certified for medicolegal purposes. The procedure to examine and certify differs from place to place with no uniformity seen in identical set ups too. The registered medical practitioner (RMP) tends to follow what has been in practice for decades without bothering for validity or reliability of the procedure being followed. An accurate description and interpretation of injuries is one of the important duty for any RMP. He should be able to record injuries accurately, be aware of their medicolegal significance and be able to give a useful opinion on how they may have been caused.[1]

Any person who is qualified in modern medicine and has his name enrolled with any State Medical Council (within the meaning of the IMC Act, 1956), is authorized to examine a case of injury and prepare a medicolegal injury report.

During his practice, any such medical practitioner can receive a case of injury in a variety of instances. These can be:

a. Directly from the site of incident.
b. Being referred from other medical facility.
c. Brought by police for medicolegal examination of injuries from site of incident.
d. Referred by court for medicolegal examination of injuries, in case of dispute regarding nature of injuries.

The procedure to be followed varies in different settings. There is no law which states that only RMPs of government hospitals are to examine medicolegal cases and not the RMPs in private practice/working in private institutions. In government setup, concerned police station should be informed of each and every such case. A private RMP is bound to inform the police every case of suspected homicide. In suicidal cases, he is not bound by the law to inform the police of the case, whereas in cases of accidental injury, he should use his discretion to rule out any foul play; if no foul play is suspected, one is not bound to inform the police. To be on a safer side, it is always better to inform the police regarding all the cases as any case may turn out to be a case of legal inquiry at a later date [Sec. 39 CrPC].[2] All details should be entered in the medicolegal register kept separately in each clinic/hospital for all potential medicolegal cases.

DIRECTLY FROM SITE OF INCIDENT

a. *In life-threatening injuries, first duty is to safeguard life with emergency treatment followed by general care. If it is a medicolegal case, preparation of an injury report follows to help the judiciary, once the condition of patient is stable.*

   As per the Supreme Court ruling (Parmananda Katara vs. Union of India),[3] a doctor should not refuse to treat a patient in emergency. In the same case, the MCI filed an affidavit stating that 'the MCI expects that all registered medical practitioners must attend to the sick and the injured immediately, and it is the duty of the medical practitioner to make immediate and timely medical care available to every injured person, whether he is injured in an accident or otherwise.....Life of a person is far more important than the legal formalities.' However, in such cases, the doctor-patient relationship is not established till the patient is in a position to give consent for further treatment and/or medicolegal examination. *All legal formalities stand suspended till the patient's life is out of danger.* The duty of the doctor to provide medical aid, even in medicolegal cases, has been extended to the private doctors also, as exemplified by the High Court of Andhra Pradesh in Pattipati Venkaiah vs. State of AP.[4]

   The matter is straight forward when such a case is attended by a private RMP. He not only treats the patient first to stabilize his condition, but also prepares the MLR based on his observations with regards to the injuries suffered.

   In hospital setups, private or government, usually a Casualty Medical Officer (CMO) receives a case in emergency. He takes the history, examines the case and initiates necessary steps to stabilize the patient's condition, and depending upon the type of injuries over the body, refers the case to concerned specialist, for e.g. surgeon, neurosurgeon, ophthalmologist or orthopedician for expert management. In such situations, the concerned specialist should note down details of the injuries for medicolegal purposes when the condition of the patient is stabilized, and later issue a MLR. This is because he is in total control over the patient's condition. He has the history, bodily findings, treatment rendered and can opine over the outcome of the injuries suffered. Only he has the first-hand knowledge about the issues to be opined for the help of judiciary, rather than the CMO who first attended the case.

[*Present practice at many places is that, for medicolegal purposes, the CMO is supposed to examine the person for injuries and prepares the medicolegal injury report as he was the first person who attended to the patient. Practically, either he delays the treatment for medicolegal examination of injuries or prepares the report after going through the patient treatment records.*]

Consent for the treatment is implied, which includes examination of the injuries too. Making a note of the examination findings and treatment given is the duty of a RMP. Based on his clinical records, the RMP is duty bound to prepare a MLR, if required by law or consent is given.

[*Present practice at some places is that, a patient is being treated for injuries by one RMP. Another RMP is entrusted to examine the patient for preparation of MLR. On approaching the patient, the patient refuses to get the injuries examined for medicolegal purposes. In such a situation, either a negative consent is taken or a report is prepared while going through the patient treatment records. Even when the patient agrees to get himself examined for preparation of MLR, all his wounds are re-exposed for examination for medicolegal purposes only which itself is unethical.*]

The report issued by the doctor who examined the injury of the victim and then prepared the report is considered more reliable than the report from the doctor who opined by seeing the injury and X-ray report [Tanviben Pankaj Kumar Divetia vs. State of Gujarat, AIR, 1997, SC 2193].[5]

b. *In non-life threatening injuries, first duty is to provide first-aid. If it is a medicolegal case, again preparation of an injury report follows next to help the judiciary.*

Many a times, injured persons with non-life threatening injuries come up/ are brought by relatives/police for first aid as well as medicolegal examination of injuries. In such cases, the RMP who receives the case, examines the person and provides the required care, should also prepare the MLR depending upon the case. If the RMP who has thus examined and prepared the MLR, feels that an expert opinion is required not only for investigations and treatment (for e.g., ENT, ophthalmology, orthopedics or gynecology) but also for medicolegal opinion of the injuries, he can keep his opinion pending for arrival of opinion of the concerned specialist medical practitioner. There is no such rule that a MLR has to be issued with opinion on the day of arrival of the patient. A preliminary report can always be issued on the first day with opinion kept pending for arrival of investigation/specialist's report, and separate report can then be issued later on (sample given later).

If for any reason, a person is not ready to get his injuries examined, he cannot be forced and negative consent for the same must be recorded. However, for all purposes the case should be treated as medicolegal case and all the formalities should be done accordingly. The injuries should be mentioned in the treatment file in detail (as done in MLR) and all the samples and specimens should be preserved, since subsequent requisition for MLR may come from legal authorities.

REFERRED FROM OTHER MEDICAL FACILITY

a. *Patient may be referred for expert management with regards to treatment of injuries*

Routinely, injured patients are transferred to higher centers for management of the injuries on account of expert medical professionals and better health facilities. In such situations, the referring RMP should mandatorily send a referral note along with the patient. Such referral note should clearly mention whether the case has been notified to the local police station (from where the case is being referred) as MLC (medicolegal case) and a MLR has been prepared or not. If already notified and report prepared, no separate report needs to be prepared at the referred center. The concerned police station should be informed about arrival of the case by the specialist at the referred center. Apart from treatment, if an opinion is sought by an investigating officer from the treating specialist, it must be complied and investigative findings should be conveyed to the referring RMP. The final opinion regarding the nature of injuries and type of weapon should be given by the RMP who actually prepared the medicolegal report. On discharge/death of the patient, the same police station must be informed again about it.

b. *If it is a medicolegal case, preparation of an injury report depends upon whether or not the case has been already notified/injury report has been prepared by the referring doctor*

If no information regarding intimation to the police station is available from the referral center, it is specialist medical practitioner's duty to inform to his concerned police station about arrival of the case. He should note down all the findings related to injury over the person on the clinical case sheet and if required (and if consent is given), prepare a MLR to help the investigating agencies as per his findings.

[*Present practice at some places is to send the patient back to the referral RMP to get the medicolegal injury report prepared. It is again unwarranted and unethical.*]

BROUGHT DIRECTLY BY POLICE

Many a time, injured persons are brought by police along with a requisition for treatment and preparation of MLR. The case is automatically a medicolegal case. In such cases, no separate consent is required for preparation of MLR (except in cases of alleged victim of rape).

[Present practice at some places is that negative consent is taken for preparation of MLR mentioning that the patient wants to get only treated and does not want a MLR of his injuries to be prepared.]

REFERRED BY COURT

Court can always ask any RMP to examine an injured person, fresh or remote, for providing an expert opinion to help the judiciary. No RMP can refuse for the same. The court can also order for re-evaluation, in case of dispute regarding nature of injuries. It is already a medicolegal case and there is no role of consent in such cases.

It is preferable to have the injury report kept ready and issued to the investigating officer whenever he asks for the same (preferably within 24 hours of the request). No information is to be divulged regarding the medicolegal examination of an injury case, unless asked for by competent judicial and investigating authorities.

INJURY REPORT

An injury report consists of eight columns that describe full details of an injury. There is no set rule that injuries should be reported in above mentioned proforma but it is preferable to do so, as one does not miss out on any important aspect of examination and reporting. It is always better to issue 'injury report' in an injury report proforma, not on a plain paper [Ammine and Ors vs. State of Kerala, AIR, 1998, SC 260—where the injury report was cancelled on the ground that the report was given on a plain paper].[5] A sample is provided below (Proforma 9.1). In cases where opinion with regards to extent or nature of injury cannot be opined at first instance and needs to be kept pending for an investigation or specialist's opinion, sample proformas for referrals too are provided below (Proforma 9.2 and 9.3). A separate proforma for final opinion based on the investigation/specialist's opinion too is given (Proforma 9.4).

Cutting/overwriting should be avoided as much as possible and all corrections should be properly initialed. It should be corrected legibly by lining out with a single line, initializing with date.

The report is usually addressed to the police and the lawyers who are not themselves experts in medical field. Medical terms not in common usage should be avoided or alternatively should be explained so that it can be easily understood, for e.g., 'swelling' is preferable to 'edema', 'nose bleed' to 'epistaxis' and 'pin point bruising' to 'petechiae'. Abbreviations should be avoided—all the entries including the medical terms should be written in a full form. Symbol '#' used to denote a fracture in medical notes should not be used in MLRs.

EXAMINATION AND PREPARATION OF INJURY REPORT

Any MLR consists of three sections: preliminary data, observations and opinion based on those observations. Same applies for an injury report too.

Preliminary Data

While preparing an injury report, the preliminary data must be accurately filled taking special precaution to note down the date, time and place of examination. An injury case can be brought by police or by relatives/friends/passers-by. If the case is brought by police constable, his name, buckle number and police station should be written. If any relative/friend/passer-by bring the case, their name, address and phone numbers must be noted and passed on to the investigating officer. In case of injured female patient being examined by a male registered medical practitioner, a female attendant must be present during the examination process. It is always better to take signatures of the persons whose names have

Proforma 9.1 Injury report

EXAMINATION AND CERTIFICATION OF A CASE OF INJURY

MLC No.:_____ Name:__________ Age:___ [years] Sex:________ Occupation:_______
Address:____ Requested by:______________
Brought by:______________________ Examined in presence of:_____________________
Date, place and time of examination:____
Consent:____
Signature:____
Identification marks:____
Brief history of the case: [Name of the person giving history ___________________]

Sr. No. (1)	Type of injury (2)	Site of injury (3)	Size of injury (4)	Nature of injury (5)	Nature of inflicting weapon (6)	Age of injury (7)	Remarks (8)

Signature:

Signature/left thumb impression of the examinee Name and Designation:

Proforma 9.2 Investigation

[NAME OF THE HOSPITAL/INSTITUTION]
REQUISITION FORM

MLC No.:____ Date:______________
Name of examinee:_________________________________ Age:______ Sex:________
Police Station:____________________ Address:______________________________
Outdoor No.:___________________________ Indoor No.:_______________________
Marks of identification:
1. ____
2. ____

Investigation/opinion desired:
1. ____
2. ____

Brief history
Date: Signature of the Medical Practitioner

Proforma 9.3 Report of specialist

REPORT

MLC Report No. [of the concerned X-ray dept./lab./other dept.]:__________ Date:______

With respect to the above-mentioned investigation/opinion asked, my/our opinion for ______________________________ [name of the examinee], brought by ___________________________ [name of police constable] bearing above-mentioned identification marks is:

1. ____
2. ____

Date: Signature of the Medical Practitioner

Proforma 9.4 Supplementary report

NAME OF THE INSTITUTION/HOSPITAL
Certificate of Final Opinion

To
The Investigating Officer,
__________________ Police Station,
__________________[District].

Date:

Reference: 1. Radiology report no. ________________ dated __________.
2. Pathology/Microbiology/Biochemistry report no. _______ dated ______.
3. ____________ department no. _____________ dated __________.

The final opinion regarding the injuries mentioned in injury certificate no. __________ dated ____________ for ______________________ [name of the examinee] is that injuries no. ________________ are simple in nature and injuries no. ________________ are grievous in nature.

Signature of the Medical Practitioner

Received by:

been entered in the MLR (for e.g., police constable, relative/passerby, or female attendant).

Consent

With regards to consent, if the person is ≥ 12 years, his consent and if he is below 12 years or mentally ill of any age, consent of the nearest relative or nearest guardian is required. It should be an informed consent.

Identification Marks

At least two visible identification marks should be noted. These marks should always be mentioned on investigation requisition forms/expert opinion requisitions so that they can be verified by respective personnel/s in order to avoid an investigation/examination been done on a wrong patient. If this precaution is not taken, an incorrect opinion based on these reports may be formed. For example, a patient is sent to radiology department for getting X-ray done to rule out fracture that would help in deciding whether injury is simple or grievous. The original patient who does not have a fracture gets an X-ray done on a person with fracture so as to increase the gravity of offence based on the report showing presence of a fracture. Such instances are possible where treating RMP is different and RMP preparing a medicolegal injury report is different. In some instances, the modality of treatment does not differ, whether there is a fracture reported or not.

History

Brief 'alleged' history of the incident should be elicited preferably from the examinee himself (making a note of the same by writing the name) and noted down. Many a times it happens that patient is either unconscious or disoriented because of serious injuries. In such cases, if the history is given by somebody else, his full name and relation with the patient should be mentioned. The injured/the relative may or may not give a correct version regarding the cause and manner of injury. Keeping the history given in mind, the medical practitioner should satisfy himself whether the injuries could have been produced in the manner alleged. In case of any suspicion of foul play, the nearest police station must be informed of the case, if not already informed. It may happen that history is given for an accident which later turns out to be a case of homicide. In such cases, proper documentation, if done, would come to the rescue of RMP (doctor's duty is to treat the patient and not to become an investigating officer to find out the veracity of the history provided. Similarly, one should not get biased by the history provided. All conclusions must be based on examination findings).

General Examination

In this, one should always mention the state of consciousness and orientation of the patient. Glasgow Coma Score (in head injury cases), pulse, temperature, blood pressure, reaction of pupils to light should be noted.

Reporting about build, height and weight gives an idea of the relative capacity of the victim to defend himself/herself in cases of assault.

Following general physical examination, next comes the recording of the injuries. The examination should preferably be made in good light; in practice however, conditions are not that ideal. A few basic items are also essential prior to examination: a hand lens, measuring scale and a torch (Fig. 9.1). Body charts are invaluable for recording of injuries. A portable ultraviolet torch may help to highlight faint bruises. If feasible, photographs too can be taken with a suitable scale included beside the wound.[1]

REPORT

As mentioned earlier, an injury report usually consists of eight columns that describe full detail of an injury. Details on how to fill these columns are given next.

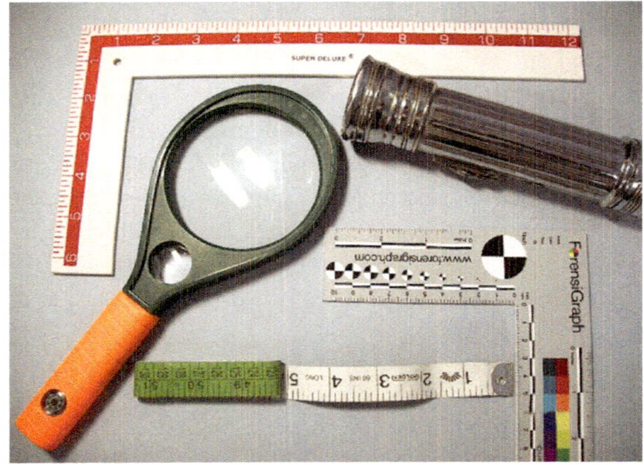

Fig. 9.1 Basic requirements for examination of injuries

Column No. 1 [Sr. No.]

This column is for the serial number of injuries. A look at this column informs about total number of injuries over the body.

Column No. 2 [Type of Injury]

This column is for recording the type of injury. Different types of injuries can be classified depending upon their causation (Table 9.1).

This column is to serially enter any of the injuries mentioned in Table 9.1 one by one. It is essential, especially for medicolegal purposes, that a standard nomenclature is used while describing the wounds.

A brief description regarding all the common injuries is provided below. This would help the reader in better understanding of the injuries, and help in reporting and opining.

Abrasion

It is a superficial injury where there is destruction of epidermis and superficial layer of dermis. It is produced by friction and/or pressure between the skin and some rough object/surface. These are simple injuries that bleed slightly and heal rapidly, usually without scar formation [*scars can form in deeper abrasions involving dermis*].

In the living, abrasions readily escape notice if the victim is examined in poor light or if the skin is wet. They become readily visible when the skin gets dried.

Different types of abrasions are *scratch, graze and pressure/imprint/pattern/impact abrasion* depending upon their manner of causation. Friction over skin with a pointed object will produce a scratch. Rubbing of a large uneven surface over the skin shall produce a graze while perpendicular impact over the skin shall result in pressure/imprint/pattern/impact abrasion (Figs 9.2A to D).

Contusion [Bruise]

In contusion, there is extravasation of blood into the skin, subcutaneous or deeper tissues due to rupture of blood vessels by blunt force trauma. Continuity of skin is not lost in this type of injury. Bruise is a term used when the extravasation is readily visible through skin externally (Figs 9.3A to C). For deeper extravasations, term contusion is used.

Table 9.1 Types of injuries

Causation	*Different injuries*
Mechanical injuries	Contusion, abrasion, lacerated wound, incised wound, stab wound, chop wound, firearm wound, fracture, dislocation
Thermal injuries	Hypothermia, frostbite, trench foot, immersion foot, heat cramps, heat stroke, heat exhaustion, burns, scalds
Chemical injuries	Corrosive acid, corrosive alkali, irritant juice
Miscellaneous	Injuries due to electrocution (Joule burn), lightening, X-rays, radioactive substances, microwave burns

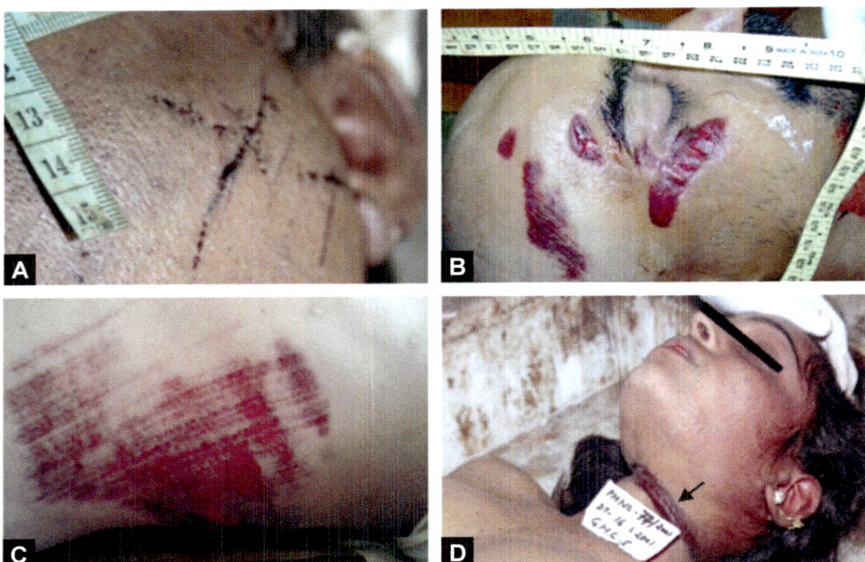

Figs 9.2A to D Types of abrasions: (A) Scratch abrasions; (B) Abrasions during impact (fall); (C) Graze abrasion; (D) Patterned abrasion (arrow)

Extravasation produced by an impact from patterned object usually lies in the subepidermal layer and may correspond with the pattern of the object producing it. Such bruises are called as *intradermal bruises*, for e.g., bruises produced by whip, cane, tyre or bicycle chain. Normally, the contusion produced by impact from hard, blunt object lies in the subcutaneous tissues and is called as *subcutaneous bruise*; it has blurred edges and is raised above the surface. If blood collection is large, it is termed as *hematoma*. Such a contusion appears immediately after the injury. If the extravasation occurs in deeper tissues, it is termed as *deep contusion*. External evidence of injury in such cases is usually a swelling which is readily appreciated when compared with the opposite side. Such a contusion may take hours or days to appear at the surface. This phenomenon is called as *delayed bruising*. Delayed bruising has medicolegal significance in that when injured persons are examined immediately after the assault, they may not show any contusion but when examined after a few hours or a day following the injury, the body shows contusion on the surface. Therefore, in case of any suspicion in injured persons about deeper extravasations, they may be called again after a day or two to look for any delayed contusion. A bruise can also occur at a place other than the site of impact due to traveling of the extravasated blood along the tissue planes under gravity—*an ectopic bruise*. Some common instances of such ectopic bruises are black eye seen in blow to forehead or fracture of roof of orbit, bruise behind the ear due to fall on vertex or fracture of posterior cranial fossa (Battle' sign), bruising above knee on outer aspect in fracture shaft femur, and bruising around ankle due to blow over calf muscles (Fig. 9.3A). Contusion occurs readily in lax tissues like eyelids, face and genitalia than taut tissues like palm and soles. Obese, alcoholics, women, children, old aged, persons with poor physique and those having bleeding tendencies get easily bruised from even minor trauma.

A blow with a rod or stick may produce two parallel linear hemorrhages with intervening skin remaining unchanged—*'railway line or tramline bruise'* (Fig. 9.3B). The width of normal area of the skin between the two lines of contusion usually corresponds to the thickness of the offending object. There is a misconception that a blow with rod or stick will always produce a railway track bruise but it is not always so.

Many a times, to substantiate a false charge of assault, artificial bruises are produced since true bruise can rarely be self-inflicted. To differentiate them, following points must be kept in mind (Table 9.2 and Fig. 9.3D).

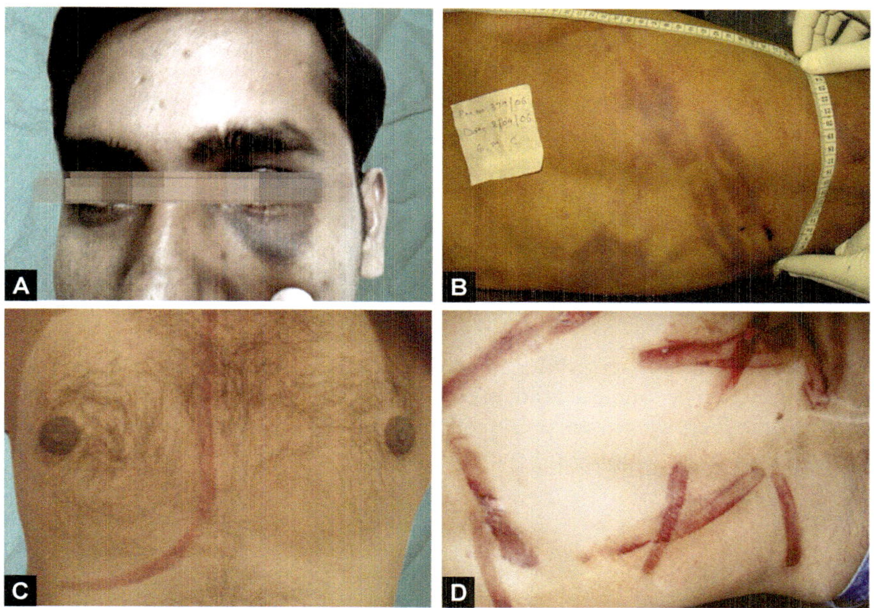

Figs 9.3A to D Various types of contusions. (A) Contusion around left eye; (B) Tramline contusion; (C) Contusion by hard, flexible instrument; (D) Artificial bruise (*Courtesy:* Dr KH Chavali, AIIMS, Raipur)

Table 9.2 Artificial and true bruise

Features	*Artificial bruise*	*True bruise*
Cause	Irritant juice, for e.g., marking nut, *Calotropis* or *Plumbago rosea*	Trauma
Site	Usually exposed accessible parts	Anywhere
Margins	Well-defined and regular, margins showing small vesicles	Ill-defined margins with no vesicles
Itching	Present	Absent
Other areas	Staining/vesication of the tips of fingers due to the act of applying the juice	No such change

Lacerated Wound [Tear/Rupture]

It is the tearing of skin, mucosa and underlying tissues as a result of application of *blunt* force.

These injuries have irregular, contused margins and deeper tissues are unevenly divided as a result of which strands of tissues are seen crossing the deeper parts of the wound (Fig. 9.4). On closer examination, hair bulbs and blood vessels are found crushed in the wound. These wounds bleed less as compared to incised wounds because the torn margins of blood vessels retract easily. These wounds are frequently contaminated with foreign matter; infections too are common as compared to incised/stab wounds. Upon healing, lacerated wound leaves permanent scar due to damage to part or whole of true skin. Unlike abrasion and contusion, which are two dimensional injuries, laceration is a three dimensional injury.

Different types of lacerations are: split laceration, stretch laceration, avulsion laceration, cut lacerations/chop wounds (Figs 9.5A to C).

- *Split lacerations* are produced at places where the overlying skin is tightly stretched over bone underneath, without much intervening tissue, like in scalp, eyebrows, cheeks, lower jaw, back of forearm and shin. The skin gets crushed between the hard object and underlying bone. It gets split and looks like an incised wound. On closer examination with magnifying lens, all the features of lacerated wound are found. Adjoining hairs can be shaved before examination.
- *Stretch lacerations* are produced when skin along with subcutaneous tissues are stretched beyond the point of elasticity of skin.
- *Avulsion lacerations* are produced because of grinding compression and stretching of skin commonly seen in accidents with industrial machinery.

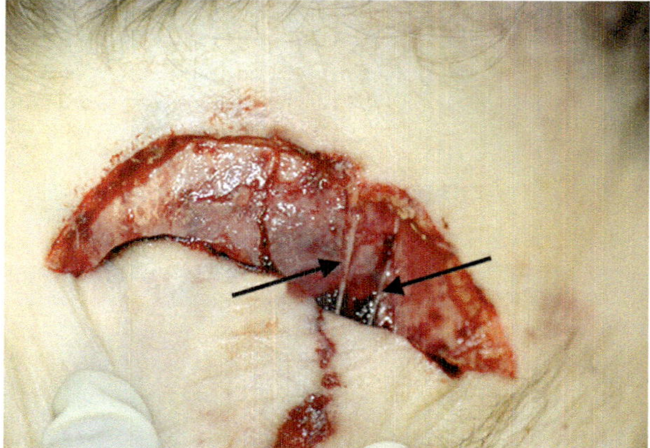

Fig. 9.4 Lacerated wound with 'tissue bridging' (arrows) (Image reprinted with permission from eMedicine.com, 2011. Available at: http://emedicine.medscape.com/article/1680082-overview and Prof. Joseph A Prahlow, Forensic Pathologist, Indiana University School of Medicine, South Bend, Indiana)

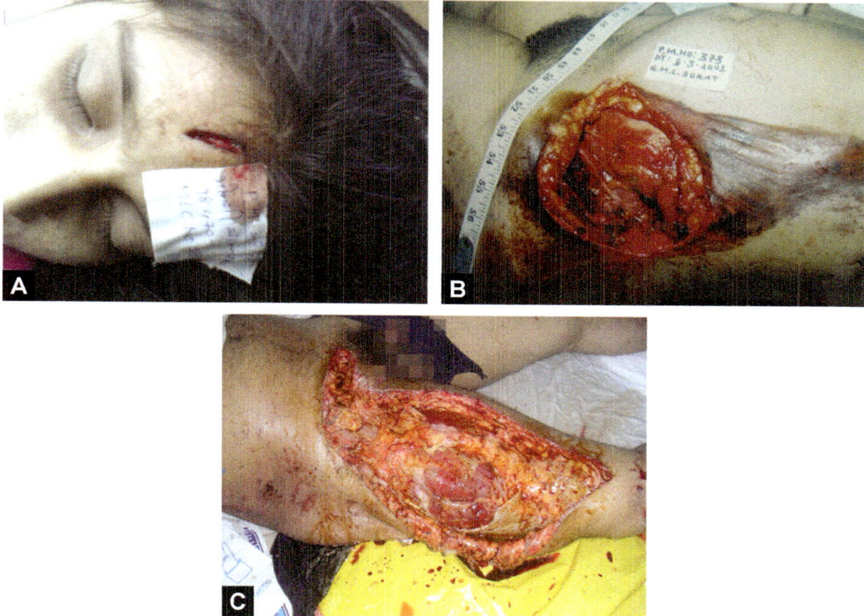

Figs 9.5A to C Types of laceration: (A) Split laceration; (B) Stretch laceration; (C) Avulsed laceration

- *Cut lacerations*/chop wound are produced by heavy weapon with a sharp cutting edge. Margins are not smooth and edges show abrasions and contusions. The abrasion or bruising is due to the weight of the offending weapon. In chop wounds, the underlying bone may also show an even cut. These wounds are usually inflicted by not so sharp, uneven, rusty edges of heavy weapon like axe or chopper.

With regards to laceration of internal organs, however severe a blunt impact may be, there may be no external evidence of injury or there may be minimal injury with massive internal injury; especially true for abdominal injuries.

Combinations of abrasion, contusion and laceration: It is very common to find a combination of abrasions, contusions and lacerations together or as integral parts of one another. A single object may result in abrasion with first blow, contusion with second blow and laceration with third blow or all three can occur with a single blow too. Many a times, it becomes difficult to differentiate an imprinted injury to be an abrasion or contusion.

Incised Wound [Cut/Slash/Slice]

Incised wound is an injury produced by sharp cutting weapon having clean cut margins. Length of an incised wound is more than its breadth or depth that differentiates it from a stab wound which is deeper than its length. Shape is usually elliptical or spindle shaped (Figs 9.6A and B).

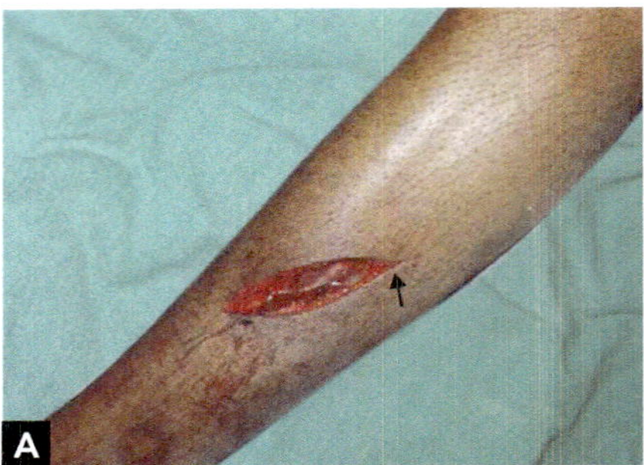

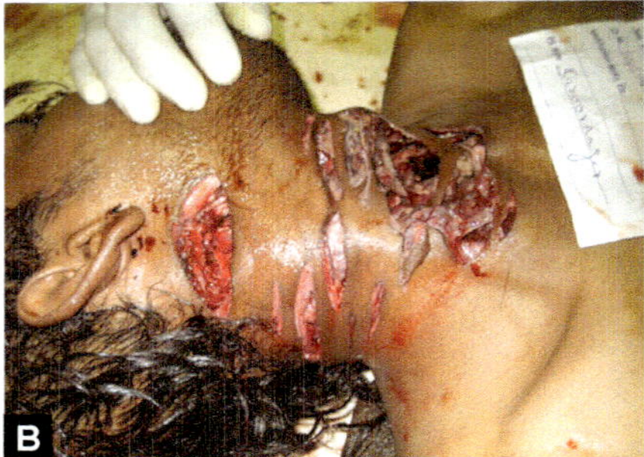

Figs 9.6A and B Incised wounds: (A) Incised wound with tailing (arrow); (B) Multiple incised wounds (*Courtesy:* Dr. P Harikrishna, Osmania Medical College, Hyderabad)

Margins of these wounds are clean cut without any bruising or abrasion of the edges and there is usually no loss of tissues. Bleeding is profuse, since cut vessels are unable to retract and close down. The underlying tissues too are evenly cut. Normally, the edges are straight but when inflicted over lax tissues like eyelids/ front of neck/scrotum, margins may be irregular and there may be multiple cuts with intervening normal tissue even by a single blow. These wounds are usually gaping (when placed across the pattern of connective tissue—Langer' lines). The length and width of the wound has no relation to the length, width, thickness or edge (single or double) of the offending weapon.

These are deeper at the beginning because more pressure is exerted at this point by the weapon—the head of the wound. Towards the end, the wound becomes increasingly shallow till finally the weapon rises above the surface—tailing of the wound. The wound shows maximum retraction of edges at its center, i.e. gaping (Fig. 9.6A).

Suicidal incised wounds, especially on throat and front of wrist are quite common. The suicider (person) makes repeated, horizontal, parallel, shallow, half-hearted, tentative cuts on the neck/wrist before he picks up the courage to make the final fatal cut. Since these preliminary, shallow cuts denote the initial hesitation or nervousness on the part of the suicider, they are called *hesitation cuts (exploratory cuts/tentative cuts/feeler strokes).* Hesitation cuts often involve the skin and are usually seen at the beginning of the incised wound.

In homicidal injuries, incised wounds are found on the palms, fingers, back of elbow or back of the trunk, sustained in an instinctive attempt to shield oneself from an attack with a sharp cutting weapon in self-defense which are called *defense wounds (protective cuts).* The natures of defense wounds vary with the kind of weapon used in assault. If a blunt weapon is used, defense wounds like contusions or lacerations are seen in same locations described above.

Sometimes, wounds are inflicted by the victim upon oneself to charge an enemy with assault or to make simple injury look grievous. These wounds are called *self-inflicted/fabricated wounds* and can be diagnosed by their being multiple, superficial, directed towards center of the body and only over accessible parts of the body.

Many a times in an assault, the sharp cutting weapon is used tangentially or at an angle to the body. As a result, there is flapping at one margin of the wound at the cost of the opposite margin. This is called *beveling*. Beveling gives clue regarding the position of the victim and assailant along with the direction of force applied.

Wounds produced by glass are usually lacerated but resemble incised and stab wounds. Margins of the wound almost always show tiny side cuts due to the irregularities of glass whereas if sharp pointed part of glass enters the skin, it gives a stab-like appearance. Particles of glass are usually found in the wound.

Chop Wound [refer Cut Laceration]

This is an injury produced by heavy, sharp-cutting weapon. The wound is similar to incised wound but the margins show abrasion/bruising. The abrasion or bruising is due to the weight of the offending weapon. The mode of infliction varies in chop wounds. The direction of force is perpendicular to the body whereas in incised wound, it is tangential. In chop wounds, the underlying bone may also show an even cut (Figs 9.7A and B).

Stab Wound

Stab wound is produced by a pointed weapon, usually sharp, sometimes blunt, having depth more than length or breadth. Such a wound entering a body cavity is called *penetrating wound,* and when it comes out of the body at the opposite end, it is termed *perforating wound.*

The margins are usually clean cut, may be ragged or contused if a blunt pointed weapon is used (for e.g., poker with blunt tip). While examining the surface wound of a stab, one should note down whether the margins are clean cut or not, and whether the angles are acute or comparatively blunt. This helps in identifying the offending weapon. A double-edged knife as well as a single-edged one with a pointed double-edged tip can both produce a stab wound with both ends acute, whereas a single-edged weapon generally produces a stab injury with one end acute and other comparatively blunt (Fig. 9.8). At times, a double-edged weapon thrusted upto the hilt can produce a surface wound with one sharp end and the other blunt (the sharp margin of the knife is usually blunt at the hilt).[6] Abrasion/contusion may be present around the wound due to impact of the hilt in such cases (Fig. 9.9). Depth needs to be measured in case of stab wounds. In a living person, before surgery, depth may be assessed clinically but under no instance the wound should be probed, since it may enlarge the track and also dislodge

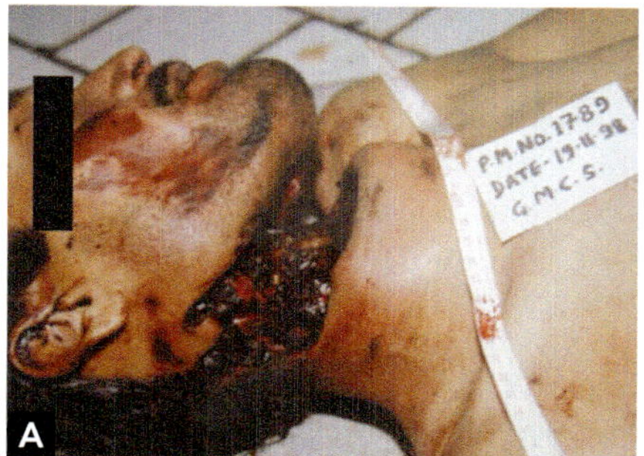

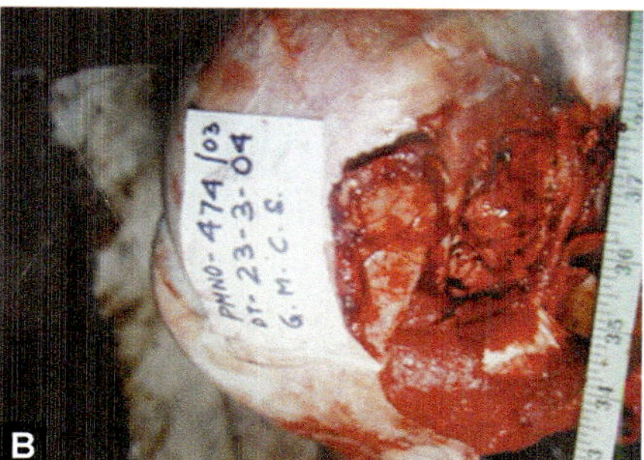

Figs 9.7A and B Chop wounds: (A) Over neck; (B) Over head

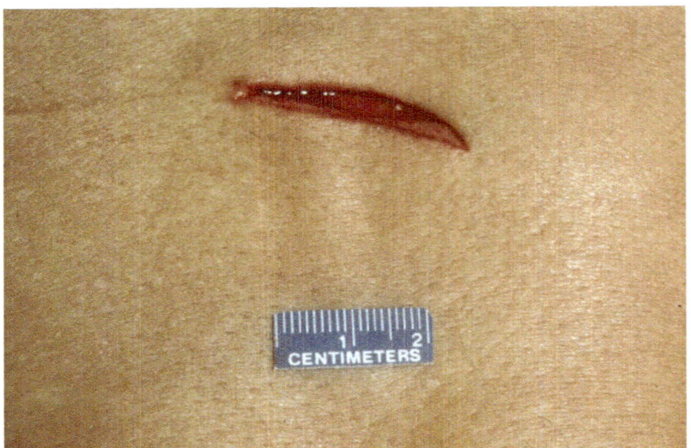

Fig. 9.8 Stab wound with single edged weapon
(Image reprinted with permission from eMedicine.com, 2011. Available at: http://emedicine.medscape.com/article/1680082-overview and Prof. Joseph A Prahlow, Forensic Pathologist, Indiana University School of Medicine South Bend, Indiana)

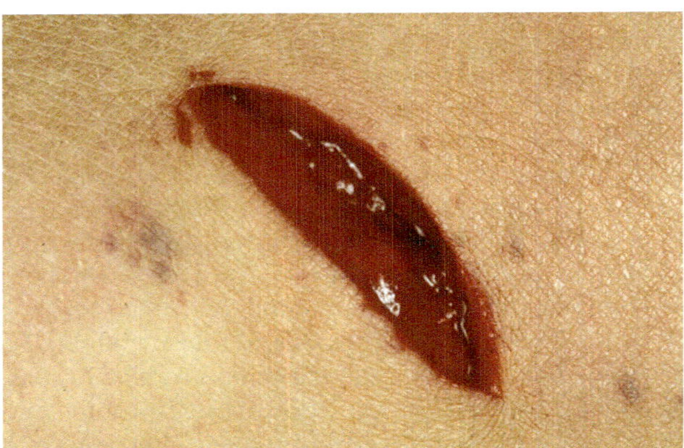

Fig. 9.9 Stab wound with hilt guard mark
(Image reprinted with permission from eMedicine.com, 2011. Available at: http://emedicine.medscape.com/article/1680082-overview and Prof. Joseph A Prahlow, Forensic Pathologist, Indiana University School of Medicine South Bend, Indiana)

a clot already formed and result in hemorrhage. If such probing is absolutely necessary, it should be carried out in an operation theater.

It should be remembered that length of the surface wound of a stab is due to the width of the blade of the weapon and width of the wound is due to the thickness of the blade. Because of elasticity of skin, width is always greater than the thickness of the weapon. As far as length of the wound is concerned, it is usually equal to or larger than the width of the blade of weapon at a given depth (distance from the tip of the weapon). Sometimes, the length of the stab wound is smaller than the width of the blade of weapon at a given depth. This is possible because of retraction of skin outwards at the wound margins. This makes the angles to come closer (studies have shown that the length of the wound can come closer by 0.5 cm following skin retraction). Therefore, it is advisable to approximate the margins of a gaping stab wound before recording the dimensions (Figs 9.10A and B).[6]

[*A tradition is being followed at places to write every injury as CLW. Various full forms have come forward like cut-lacerated wound, contaminated lacerated wound or contused lacerated wound. The fact is that most of the clinicians are not aware of different nomenclatures of mechanical injuries. Therefore, they write every injury as CLW. This creates a problem while one is asked to identify a weapon. It has been observed by the author that the RMP who has prepared the injury report invariably says 'yes' to any weapon shown during court evidence to have caused the injury. There is no terminology like CLW.*]

Fracture

A fracture is loss of continuity of a bone, especially that of the periosteum (Fig. 9.11). Usually, a fracture can be detected by palpation but this should never be done as there is a chance of displacement of the fractured ends. It is advisable to get an X-ray done for proper documentation and confirmation, and opinion kept reserved till such confirmation.

Firearm Wound

Firearms are essentially of two types, smooth bored weapons or rifled weapons. Shotguns are the most common types of smooth bored weapons. They may

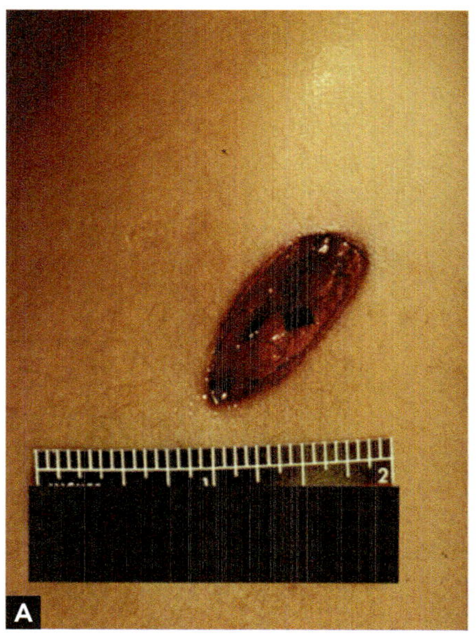

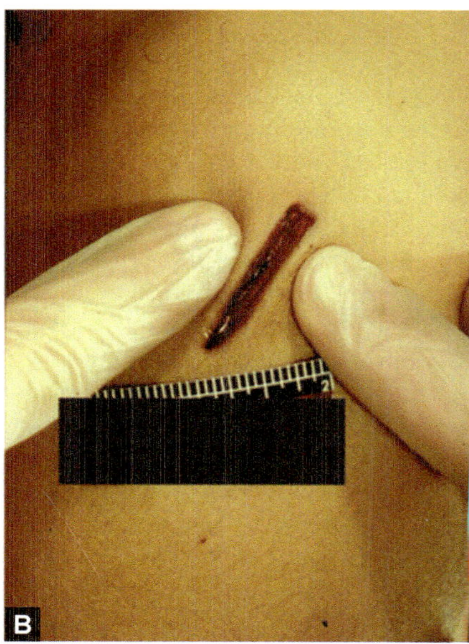

Figs 9.10A and B (A) Gaping wound; (B) After re-approximation of the wound edges (Image reprinted with permission from eMedicine.com, 2011. Available at: http://emedicine.medscape.com/article/1680082-overview and Prof. Joseph A Prahlow, Forensic Pathologist, Indiana University School of Medicine South Bend, Indiana)

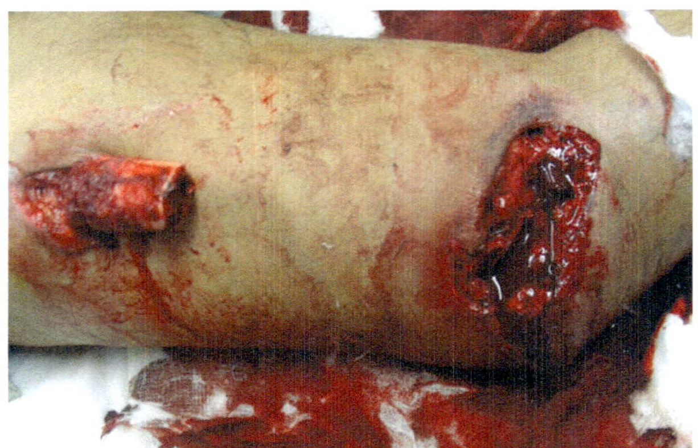

Fig. 9.11 Fracture shaft of femur

be either single barreled or double barreled. Their ammunition consists of a cardboard or plastic cartridge case with a brass base containing primer. Inside the main part of the cartridge are a layer of gun powder, one or more felt or card wads and a mass of pellets (lead shots of variable size).

Rifled weapons are characterized by rifling on the inner surface of the barrel which imparts gyroscopic steadiness to the bullet (the ammunition) and also leaves characteristic scratches (rifling marks unique to that weapon) over the surface of the bullet.[1] Two types of firearm wounds are seen—one produced by smooth bore weapon/shotgun (pellets and wads are discharged) and the other by rifled weapon (a bullet is discharged).

When a shotgun is discharged, the wad/s and the lead pellets emerge together *en masse*, gradually diverging in a cone shape as the distance from the weapon increases. In wounds from shotgun, depending upon the distance, there may be a single wound of entry or a central large hole with surrounding multiple entry wounds of individual pellets or only multiple pellet wounds. Along with the pellets and wads, flame, smoke and unburnt gunpowder too comes out of the firearm that leaves its mark around the entry wound. Thus, an entry wound of a shotgun shows (Fig. 9.12A):

1. A central inverted hole
2. Singeing of hairs
3. Deposit of smoke as blackening
4. Impregnation of unburnt gun powder particles as tattooing

Singeing of hairs, blackening and tattooing may not be present on the skin if the wound is through a clothed part. Effect of burning, blackening and tattooing are then present on the overlying cloth, depending upon the distance of fire.

In wounds from a rifled firearm, following features are observed from inside to outside (from the center of the wound to its periphery) (Fig. 9.12B):

i. Entry wound with inverted margins
ii. Grease/dirt collar
iii. Abrasion/contusion collar
iv. Singeing of hairs
v. Blackening due to smoke
vi. Tattooing due to unburnt gunpowder

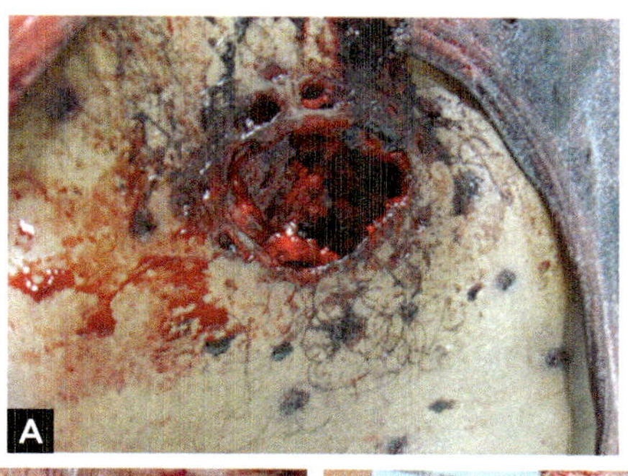

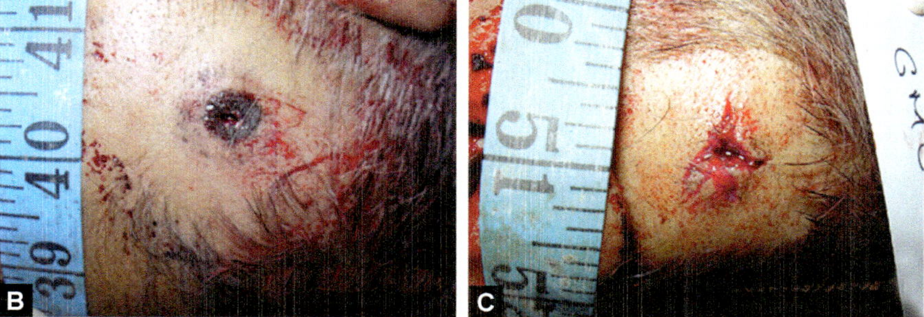

Figs 9.12A to C Firearm wounds: (A) Shotgun entry wound; (B) Rifled firearm entry wound; (C) Rifled firearm exit wound

Bleeding is usually less from entry wound as compared to exit wound. Exit wound shows the following features (Fig. 9.12C):

i. Larger than the size of entry wound
ii. Irregular in shape
iii. Margins are everted
iv. Bleeding is more as compared to entry wound
v. No abrasion collar/dirt collar, blackening, tattooing, singeing of hairs

Normally, abrasion collar is absent at the exit wound. But, if the skin at the exit wound is supported, the exit wound appears as a circular defect surrounded by a margin of abrasion resembling a wound of entrance—*shored exit wound*. In atypical cases, there can be multiple entry and exit wounds from a single shot; bullet passing through the sides of individual/in squatting position.

Care must be taken when cleaning bullet wounds to remove blood and debris, as smoke soiling of the wound margins or surrounding skin can easily be wiped away.[1] At surgery, the bullet must be handled with gloved hand or with soft rubber tipped forceps. It should not be allowed to come in direct contact with any hard surface, as it can alter the surface markings required to identify the crime weapon. The recovered bullet must be marked by scratching one's initials on its base with a sharp pointed instrument to facilitate its subsequent identification in the court but *never on the sides*. Bullet/pellets/wads which are to be further examined by ballistic expert, must be wrapped in cotton wool and preserved in empty match box or similar container, taking care that it does not touch the floor or walls of the container and then sealed properly.

Injuries by Bomb Explosion

Bomb explosions result in combination of injuries. These include injuries by:

1. Disruptive effects
2. Burns
3. Blast effects
4. Flying missiles
5. Falling masonry
6. Fumes

While describing them, all the features should be noted in the injuries. Multiple injuries are observed like burns, lacerations, incised wound or total disintegration of the body part (Fig. 9.13).

Hypothermia: This condition results from continued exposure to low temperatures where the body temperature is less than 35°C. The victim has cold skin, generalized muscular stiffness, depressed reflexes, low blood pressure and slow pulse rate.

Frostbite: It is tissue necrosis from vascular spasm or thrombosis due to exposure to cold. Exposed parts of the body are involved like tip of nose, ears, fingers and toes.

Trench foot: It is tissue necrosis of the foot due to sustained exposure to cold and moist conditions, usually seen in soldiers.

Immersion foot: It is tissue necrosis of the foot due to sustained exposure to cold water.

Heat cramps: They are painful spasms of voluntary muscles due to loss of salt and water from perspiration following strenuous work.

Heat exhaustion: It is collapse of a person without any elevated body temperature following exposure to hot and humid atmosphere.

Heat stroke: It is the impairment of heat regulating mechanism following failure of cutaneous circulation and sweating.

[All above injuries are uncommon; hence no detailed description has been included]

Flame Burns

These are the injuries produced by application of dry heat. The burns may be epidermal, dermo-epidermal or deep as per Wilson's classification. Singeing

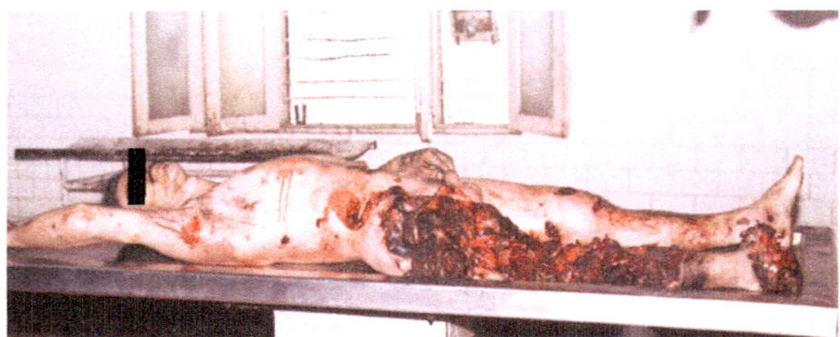

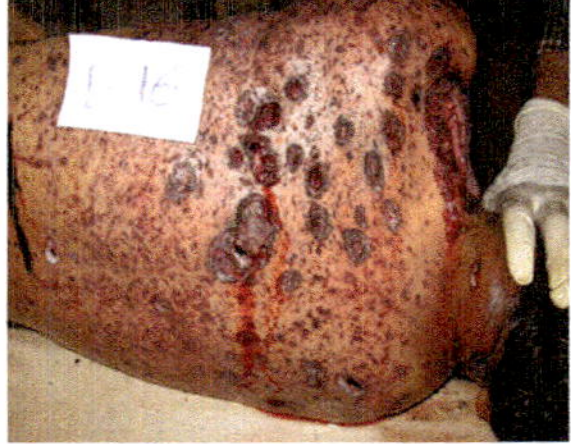

Fig. 9.13 Blast injuries (*Courtesy:* Dr P Harikrishna, Osmania Medical College, Hyderabad)

of hairs, blackening and vesication are present in these injuries (Fig. 9.14). The severity of burns depends on the percentage of body surface involved. It is believed that involvement of more than 1/3rd of body surface does not have good prognosis. Total area involved can be calculated on the basis of 'Rule of Nines'. As per this rule, following areas constitute 9% of body surface each (head including face, front of chest, back of chest, front of abdomen, back of abdomen, whole right upper limb, whole left upper limb, front of right lower limb, front of left lower limb, back of right lower limb, back of left lower limb); remaining 1% is for the perineum (Fig. 9.15). The above area distribution is to be used for adults. For different age groups, Lund and Browder chart is used for calculating body surface area involved (Fig. 9.15 and Table 9.3).[7]

Scalds: These are the injuries produced by application of moist heat from liquids at or near their boiling temperature. These burns show vesication and trickling. Burning of clothes, singeing of hairs, deposition of carbonaceous material and charring of tissues are absent in these injuries (Fig. 9.16).

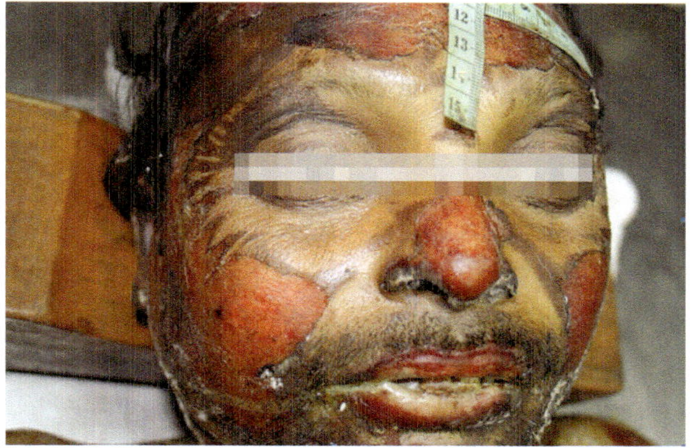

Fig. 9.14 Flame burns

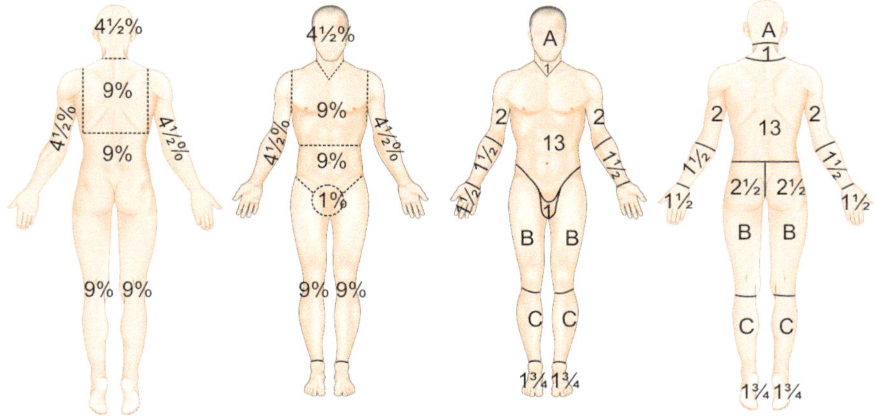

Rule of nines | Lund and Browder chart

Fig. 9.15 Calculation of surface area burnt

Table 9.3 Calculation of body surface area involved (Lund and Browder chart)

Area	*Age (years)*					
	0	1	5	10	15	*Adult*
A = ½ of head	9½	8½	6½	5½	4½	3½
B = ½ of one thigh	2¾	3¼	4	4½	4½	4¾
C = ½ of one leg	2½	2½	3¾	3	3¼	3½

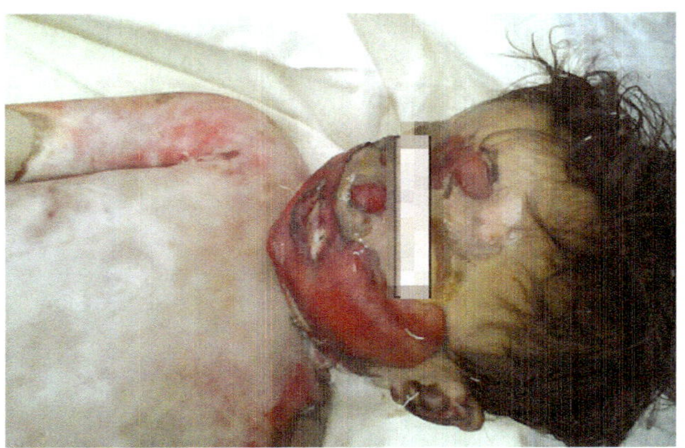

Fig. 9.16 Scalds

Burns produced by corrosives/irritants: These injuries are characterized by inflammation and discoloration of skin, ulcerated patches, discoloration of clothing and presence of chemical in the stains (Fig. 9.17). Alkalis give a soapy feel to touch. Singeing of hairs and vesication is absent in these type of burns.

Electric burns: The entry point of electricity is an ulcerated crater with everted and corrugated margins and necrosed tissue (Joule burn). The red line of demarcation seen in flame burns is usually absent. The exit wound is a lacerated wound with everted and irregular margins (Figs 9.18A to B).

Lightning burns: Burns appear as zigzag lines, often found over moist areas of skin. It may appear like branching of a tree due to rupture of subcutaneous vessels giving an arborescent pattern that fades with time (also called arborescent marks/Lichtenberg's flowers).

X-ray burns: Skin is red and inflamed (dermatitis), may vesicate, degeneration of finger nails, shedding of hairs and epidermis with formation of ulcers. On healing, radiating scars are formed with pigmentation of surrounding skin. There may be deeper sloughing, resulting in bluish discoloration of skin externally. These injuries have a tendency to turn malignant.

Microwave burns: Tissues with more water content are affected. Burns have a sandwich effect with involvement of skin and muscle sparing subcutaneous fat.

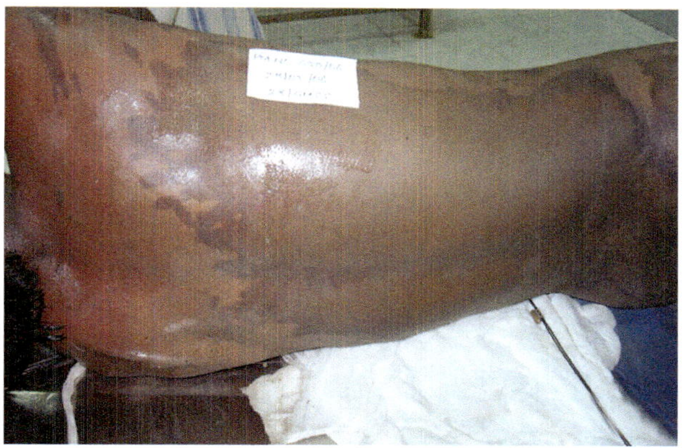

Fig. 9.17 Corrosive acid burns

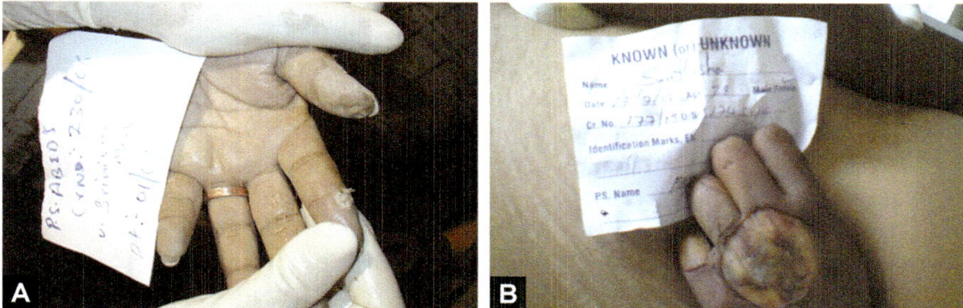

Figs 9.18A and B (A) Entry wound; (B) Exit wound of electrocution
(*Courtesy:* Dr P Harikrishna, Osmania Medical College, Hyderabad)

Column No. 3 [Site of Injury]

This column is to write down the site of injury over the body. It is imperative to note down the exact site of injury. First, the general location must be noted like on the right upper limb, or scalp. Then, the precise location should be determined using fixed anatomical landmarks. At least two parameters should be taken. The site should include the part of body involved (i.e. front of chest/back of abdomen/outer aspect of right or left arm) and distance from two fixed points over the body like the midline, nipple (in case of men), ear canal or umbilicus. In case the injury is over the limbs, it should be mentioned whether it is on front/back/inner aspect/outer aspect of upper third/middle third/lower third of arm/forearm/thigh/leg.

Column No. 4 [Size of Injury]

This column is to write down the size of injury determined with the aid of a measuring scale. Normally, any injury has three dimensions, length, width and depth but abrasion and contusion are to be described in two dimensions (as abrasion involves epidermis and part of dermis where depth cannot be measured while in contusion, as bleeding is subcutaneous, exact depth cannot be measured). One should also note the shape of the wound, using simple terms like circular, triangular, V-shaped, cresentric or oval and try to outline them on the appropriate body chart. Wounds have got depth, but often it is not possible to estimate this clinically or see the base.

Ideally, the size should be measured and no guess work should ever be done. This is easier said than practically possible, especially in living subjects.

Column No. 5 [Nature of Injury]

This column is to point out the nature of injury. Legally, injuries are of two types—*simple hurt* and *grievous hurt.*

Section 320 of the IPC enlists the following as grievous hurt:[8]

1. Emasculation.
2. Permanent privation of sight of either eye.
3. Permanent privation of hearing of either ear.
4. Privation of any member or joint.
5. Destruction or permanent impairing of the powers of any member or joint.
6. Permanent disfiguration of the head or face.
7. Fracture or dislocation of a bone or tooth.
8. Any hurt, which endangers life or which causes the sufferer to be during the space of 20 days in severe bodily pain or unable to follow his ordinary pursuits.

Dangerous hurt means any hurt that poses an imminent danger to the life of a person and is included in the definition of grievous injury. Hence, it should not be taken as a separate entity but as a subsection of grievous injury. There is a fine line of distinction between a bodily injury that is 'dangerous to life' and one which is 'likely to cause death'.

Although, grievous hurt has been discussed in detail in the next chapter, the author would like to highlight some of the contentious issues concerning Sec. 320 IPC along with case laws:

a. To make out the offence of voluntarily causing grievous hurt, there must be some specific hurt, voluntarily inflicted and coming within any of the eight kinds enumerated in this section. Where the injury was caused on the abdomen with a sharp edged weapon and the doctor stated that the injury was penetrating into the abdominal cavity touching the interior surface of the stomach, not involving any important structure or organ involving danger to life, it was held that the accused had caused simple hurt and not grievous hurt [*Jagdish Chand* vs. *State of HP, 1992 CrLJ 3076 (HP)*].[9]
b. In clause 2 and 3 of Sec. 320 IPC, the gravity of injury lies in permanent deprivation of use of organ of sight and hearing. To be counted as grievous, the loss may be partial or complete but it needs to be permanent. Permanent does not mean that the loss should be incurable [*for e.g., if an injury produces corneal opacity, there is loss of sight though it can be cured by corneoplasty. But as the resulting opacity is permanent it is considered grievous hurt, and its cure by surgery does not minimize the gravity of offence*].
c. Where a girl's cheeks were branded with red hot iron which left scars of a permanent character, it was held that the disfigurement contemplated by this section was caused [*Anta Dadoba, (1863) 1 BHC 101*]. Similarly, when the

accused went with a razor to the house of a dancing girl and cut the bridge of her nose with it, which according to doctor permanently disfigured her face, the case clearly fell within clause 6 of Sec. 320 IPC [*Gangaram, 1984 CrLJ 180 (Raj)*].

d. A partial cut of the skull vault has been held to be fracture within the meaning of this clause and hence punishable under Sec. 326 IPC [*Naib Singh* vs. *State of Punjab, AIR 1986 SC 2192: 1986 CrLJ 2061: (1986) 4 SCC 401*].[9] For application of this clause, it is not necessary that a bone should be cut through and through, or that the crack must extend from the outer surface to the inner surface, or that there should be displacement of any fragment of the bone. It has been held that a mere partial cut of the bone amounts to fracture and is, therefore, a grievous hurt within the meaning of clause 7 of Sec. 320 [*Narinder Singh* vs. *Sukhbir Singh, 1992 CrLJ 2616 (P&H)*][9].

e. Many a times, healing of wounds is deliberately prevented so as to prolong the hospital stay to 20 days or more in order to convert simple hurt into grievous hurt. Under these circumstances, opinion of the treating doctor is taken into consideration before coming to a conclusion.

The clause 8 speaks of two things: (1) any hurt which endangers life, and (2) any hurt which causes the sufferer to be during the space of 20 days (a) in severe bodily pain, or (b) unable to follow his ordinary pursuits.

The line between culpable homicide not amounting to murder and grievous hurt is a very thin line. In the former, the injuries must be such as are likely to cause death and in the latter, the injuries must be such as to endanger life [*Abdul Wahab, (1945) 47 Bom LR 998, FB*]. Any injury can be said to endanger life if it itself may put the life of the injured in danger [Ramla, (1963) 1 CrLJ 387].[9]

The mere fact that a man has been in hospital for 20 days is not sufficient; it must be proved that during that time he was unable to follow his ordinary pursuits [*Vasta Chela, (1894) 19 Bom 247; the accused in a quarrel inflicted an injury on the victim by the blade of a scissors, and there was no evidence that the victim was in severe bodily pain or was unable to follow his ordinary pursuits for 20 days, so clause 8 of Sec. 320 IPC was not attracted*]. On the other hand, where the accused caused hurt to a woman who remained in the hospital for 17 days only, out of which her life was danger for three days, it was held that he had caused grievous hurt [*Bassoo Rannah, (1864) 1WR (Cr) 9]*. Where the accused persons, after raping a girl of 11 years, thrust a stick into her private parts and she died of injuries thereby caused, it was held that while the accused could be convicted under this clause, in the absence of evidence that the injury was sufficient in the ordinary course of nature to cause death, they could not be convicted under Sec. 302 IPC [*Ghuraiyaa* vs. *State of MP, 1990 Cr LJ 1129*].[9]

Where the medical evidence showed that the injury on the forehead which caused death was by a *lathi* and not by an iron rod as deposed to by witnesses, and the internal injury could not be correlated with the external injury caused by the accused, it was held to be a fit case where the accused should be convicted only under Sec. 325 IPC [*Mohinder Singh, 1985 Cr LJ 1903: AIR 1986 SC 309*][9].

Where the accused acting on the sudden spur of the moment squeezed the testicles of the deceased, as a result of which he had a shock resulting in cardiac arrest and sudden death, the Supreme Court came to the conclusion that it was a case falling under clause 8 of this section, i.e. causing hurt that endangers life.

It was a case of grievous hurt punishable under Sec. 325 IPC and not that of a simple hurt punishable under Sec. 323 IPC [*State of Karnataka* vs. *Shivlingaiah, AIR 1988 SC 115: 1988 Cr LJ 394: 1988 SCC (Cr) 881*][9].

The arrack supplied was mixed with methyl alcohol resulting in many deaths. The court concluded that the person responsible for the mixing had knowledge that the consumption of such substance was likely to cause serious adverse effects. Some of the victims lost eyesight. The court said that the maximum sentence under the section was properly awarded [*EK Chandrasenan* vs. *State of Kerala, AIR 1995 SC 1066: (1995) 2 Cr LJ 1445*].[9]

The authors of the Code observed: 'We have found it very difficult to draw a line between those bodily hurts which are serious and those which are slight. To draw such a line with perfect accuracy is, indeed, absolutely impossible; but it is far better that such line should be drawn, though rudely, than that offences some of which approach in enormity to murder, while others are little more than frolics which a good-natured man would hardly resent, would be classed together [*Note M, p. 151*]'.[9]

A question every medical officer is asked in the court of law during his deposition is whether the injury/injuries caused to the victim is/are sufficient in ordinary course of nature to cause death or not. The medical officer should remember that these are those injuries which by virtue of their own effects can prove fatal and death is highly probable. The fact, that in exceptional cases, death may not occur or life might be saved by proper and timely treatment is immaterial.

It is the treating doctor or the autopsy surgeon that has to decide the nature of a particular injury depending upon its type, site and involvement. Also one must never forget that it is ultimately the Presiding Officer of the court, Judge/Magistrate that finally decides on whether an injury is simple or grievous. A medical practitioner's opinion is only to guide the court.[8]

Column No. 6 [Type of Weapon]

Depending upon the type of injury, the possible weapon/s that could have produced the injury is to be mentioned in this column. One need not have to name a particular weapon like sword or stick or knife. Common weapons of offence are grouped into:

1. Hard blunt objects, for e.g., sticks or stones.
2. Light weapons with a sharp cutting edge, for e.g., knife or razor.
3. Heavy weapons with a sharp cutting edge, for e.g., hatchet or axe.
4. Pointed weapons, for e.g., dagger or needle.
5. Firearms, for e.g., shotgun or rifle.

Column No. 7 [Age of Injury]

The column is to note down the age (time since infliction) of the injury mentioned. It can be approximately inferred as follows:

Age of abrasion[10]

Fresh	Red
12–24 hours	Dark red scab
1-2 days	Brownish red scab

3-5 days	Dark brown scab
5-7 days	Reddish hypopigmented area

Age of bruise[10]

Fresh	Red
12–24 hours	Dark red
1–3 days	Blue/bluish red
3–5 days	Brown (due to hemosiderin)
5–7 days	Green (due to biliverdin)
7–12 days	Yellow (due to bilirubin)

Age of lacerated, incised and stab wounds[10]

Unsutured	
Inflamed skin edges	Up to 24 hours
Appearance of infection	More than 36 hours
Sutured	
Inflamed edges	Up to 24 hours
Edges easily separated	1–3 days
Edges difficult to separate	3–7 days
Red, soft, tender scar	1–4 weeks
Pale, firm, nontender scar	More than 4 weeks

Age of burns[8]

Redness	Immediate
Vesication	1 hour
Drying of exudates from burnt area	12–24 hours
Dry brown crust	24–48 hours
Pus from infection	2–3 days [not before 36 hours]
Separation of slough	1 week
Separation of deep slough	2 weeks
Presence of red granulation area	> 2 weeks

Age of fracture[8]

Organisation of blood clot	48 hours
Development of osteoid matrix	3 days
Callus formation	10–14 days
Conversion of callus into hard bone	8–12 weeks
Complete bony union	No opinion

Dislocation of a joint: Age of the dislocation can be ascertained from the color changes of the associated bruise.[8]

Falling-off of a tooth	
Bleeding stops from socket	24–48 hours
Cavity gets filled up with granulation tissue	7–10 days
Alveolar process smoothens	14–21 days
New bone filling seen on X-ray	6 months–1 year

As per the observation of the Hon'ble Supreme Court, doctor's evidence on the point of time so far as duration of injuries is concerned, can never be absolute [Ram Swaroop and other vs. State of UP, AIR, 2000, SC 705].[5] The author himself has experienced that the data available is not absolute. Further research is the need of hour to come to an approximate conclusion with regards to timing of injuries.

Column No. 8 [Remarks]

This column is for any remarks to be made by the examining doctor. The condition of the injury at the time of examination may be mentioned. If any investigation is to be advised, it is mentioned here and the opinion kept reserved till arrival of the investigation report. Apart from investigations, if any expert opinion is sought, the same can be mentioned too.

The report should always be signed by the medical practitioner to authenticate it along with date, his/her full name, qualifications, designation and registration number, current employment and qualifications at appropriate place.

Recently, various courts in Delhi, Haryana and Punjab has directed the medical practitioners to prepare computerized medicolegal and postmortem report since their handwriting is not legible and lot of time is wasted in deciphering the said reports. The Hon'ble Punjab and Haryana High Court has ordered for web-based software for such reports where the concerned doctor can upload the reports. However, the basic tenets of the report remains the same. It is contemplated that in future the concerned Presiding Officer of the court where this case come up for hearing, the public prosecutor, and the defense counsel would be able to download the said report and thus save invaluable time. It has also initiated the process of 'video-conferencing' for recording of evidence.[11]

OPINIONS SOUGHT/REQUIRED IN CASE OF INJURIES

1. **What could be the relative position of the victim and assailant?**
   A very guarded opinion is to be given considering whether the victim was standing, sitting or lying down. Due consideration must also be given to the direction of the injury in the body. A perfect opinion is usually not possible.
2. **By what weapon/instrument, could these injuries be caused?**
   Depending upon the type of injuries, a generalized opinion has to be given whether the injuries could be produced by hard blunt impact, sharp cutting instrument, soft/hard flexible instrument, dry flame, heated liquid or corrosive substance.

   Most of the times, recovered weapon is being shown in the court for an opinion. The weapon should be closely examined and injuries corroborated. It may happen that few of the injuries may be possible while rest may not be possible with the shown weapon. When multiple weapons are shown, each injury should be again read thoroughly to find out which injuries are possible by a particular weapon.

3. **About what time could these injuries have been inflicted?**
   Opinion about timing of the injuries can be tendered based on the data available [already mentioned above]. One must be careful not to go by the history of the case, as it may be misleading many a times.
4. **Whether these injuries, singly or collectively were sufficient to produce death of the injured person?**
   Answer to this depends upon the type of injuries present over the body. There may be a single injury over vital part of the body along with other simple injuries, or there might be multiple injuries, but not involving any vital part of the body. There are many instances where a person dies after an assault with multiple contusions without any other fatal injury. The question is that whether a person can die as a result of such individually nonfatal contusions. The answer is *yes,* because even a small bruise can lock in around 10 ml of blood in the extravascular areas. This blood becomes unavailable for circulation. Therefore, a single bruise may not be sufficient to cause death but multiple bruises involving large areas are sufficient to produce death from hemorrhage.[10]

   Contrary to the above, even a minute single contusion or bleeding at certain specific locations can result in death. These are hemorrhage in brainstem, contusion of right atrium involving the SA node or bleeding into the respiratory tract producing laryngospasm.
5. **What was the degree of force involved in the stabbing incident?**
   Forensic experts are sometimes asked to estimate or quantify the degree of force required to create a wound. The answer to this question is considered significant in determining an alleged assailant's intent to cause harm. Quantifying the exact force used in a stabbing incident is considered to be a difficult area due to the large number of variables present, such as sharpness of the weapon, the area of the body and alignment with cleavage lines of the skin, the angle of attack and the relative movement of the person stabbing relative to the victim being stabbed. The radius of the blunt edge at the tip is important for controlling the penetration ability of a kitchen knife. There is a direct correlation between the cross-sectional area of a screwdriver head and the amount of force required for penetration. Screwdrivers with larger cross-sectional areas require a significantly greater force to penetrate (forces in the region of 100–120 N) but 'sharper' slotted screwdrivers penetrate with much lower forces (~30 N).
6. **In case of firearm injuries**
   a. *What kind of firearm has been used?*
      This can be inferred from the type wound present and the type of ammunition recovered from the body, if there was no exit. Recovery of a bullet indicates rifled firearm, while presence of pellets/wads indicated smooth bored firearm. The stains on the body/clothes of the victim also are helpful. Rifled weapons employ cartridges with smokeless powder which does not cause much blackening of the skin, because it burns up entirely, while the black powder of shotguns causes blackening of the skin. Therefore, if undue blackening is seen, it suggests that a shotgun has been discharged.[12]

b. *What could be the probable range/distance of fire?*
From firing with shotgun, contact wounds are produced by holding the distal end of firearm against the skin. This usually leaves a circular or oval entrance wound, depending upon whether the barrel was perpendicular or tangential to the skin surface. Margins are usually clean cut but may be bruised or abraded due to the so called 'recoil' impact of the distal end of barrel. Wound margins and the tissues within the base of the wound are usually blackened by smoke and there may be charring of the wound margins or singeing of hairs by flame. There may be severe disruption of the tissues inside and they may get discolored pink because of carbon monoxide.

At close range, with the weapon at 15 cm from the body, the entrance wound is still usually round or oval with fairly clean cut margins. Clothing or the skin may show burning from the flame and there may be blackening and tattooing. Blackening is usually seen up to 20–40 cm while tattooing usually is usually seen upto a distance of a meter or so. The wads travel a relatively short distance, rarely being found beyond 2 meters.[1]

Up to a meter, the pellets tend to travel as a compact mass and thus usually cause a single circular hole with ragged margins [rat hole like appearance]. With increasing range of fire, from about 1 to 3 meters, the pellets start to scatter and cause variable numbers of satellite pellet holes surrounding a large central hole. At long ranges, there is no main entrance wound, only 'peppering' of the skin from individual pellets.[1]

From firing with a rifled weapon, in contact wounds, the entrance hole may be bordered by the imprint of the distal end of the barrel. The margin may be charred and parchmented by flame, and the surrounding skin may be pink in color due to the effects of carbon monoxide. Blackening and tattooing is absent but the subcutaneous tissues within the depth of the wound are commonly soiled.

In close range wounds, singeing due to flame is rarely seen beyond 15 cm with blackening extending up to 30 cm. Tattooing is often present up to 60 cm. Typical features may not be present, if clothing is interposed between the distal end of the weapon and the skin surface.[1]

At larger distances, entry wound margins may be irregular and wound size is usually larger than the size of the bullet. It is inadvisable to express an opinion on the caliber of the bullet based on the size of the entrance wound, nor is it possible to state confidently from the appearance of the entry wound whether the bullet was fired from a particular type of rifled weapon (revolver, pistol, or rifle).[1]

c. *From what direction firearm has been discharged?*
The place from where a firearm has been discharged can be deduced from the direction of injury and the range. If the line joining the wounds of exit and entry or the wound of entry and the site where the bullet/pellets are lodged is projected forwards, it generally indicates the direction of fire. If the bullet enters the clothes perpendicularly, fibers of the cloth are more or less perfectly cut, while if it enters obliquely, the fibers of the cloth are frayed.

If bullet enters through the skin perpendicularly, entrance wound is roughly circular with uniform abrasion collar. The bullet hole is at the center of the area of blackening or tattooing, if present. If it enters obliquely, the shape is oval, the broad end of the wound indicating the point of initial contact of the bullet. The edge of the wound from where the missile has entered is beveled, and the other is overhanging. The abrasion collar is wider on the side from which it has entered. Also the position of the entrance wound is eccentric in relation to the blackening or tattooing, latter being more on the side from where the firing has taken place.[12]

7. **Can there be a fatal internal injury present without any external injury?**
   The answer is yes.
8. **Is it possible by the victim to carry out any volitional activity after receiving the injuries?**
   Unless it can be proved that a particular injury would be immediately incompatible with life, it is not possible to state that the injured could not have performed some activity.
9. **Would the victim have survived, had he been given immediate medical treatment?**
   The answer is difficult since it depends on the nature and extent of injuries as there is always an individual variation.

CONCLUSION

The present chapter gives a detailed overview on how to examine a case of injury, correct nomenclature to be used, how to interpret medicolegal issues and prepare a valid MLR. A badly prepared report is worse than no report being prepared at all. A correctly interpreted and neatly prepared MLR goes a long way in ensuring justice in the court of law.

REFERENCES

1. Crane J. Injury. Clinical forensic medicine. McLay WDS (ed). 3rd edn. New York: Cambridge university press; 2009. p. 99-111.
2. Manohar VR. Powers of superior officers of police. Ratanlal and Dhirajlal's The Code of Criminal Procedure. 20th edn. New Delhi: Lexis Nexis; 2012. p. 59-64.
3. Paramand Katara vs. Union of India and Others, (1989) 4 SCC 286.
4. Pattipati Venkaiah vs. State of AP (1985) AIR 1985 SC 1715, 1985 CrLJ 2012.
5. Karmakar RN. Forensic medicine and toxicology–oral, practical and MCQ. 3rd edn. Kolkata: Academic Publishers; 2011. p. 287-325.
6. Saukko P, Knight B. The pathology of wounds. Knight's forensic pathology. 3rd edn. London: Arnold; 2006. p. 136-73.
7. Vij K. Thermal deaths. Textbook of forensic medicine and toxicology–principles and practice. 5th edn. New Delhi: Elsevier; 2011. p. 159-72.
8. Mukherjee JB. Injuries. Forensic medicine and toxicology. 2nd edn. Kolkata: Allied Publishers; 1994. p. 258-474.
9. Manohar VR. Of hurt. Ratanlal and Dhirajlal's The Indian Penal Code. 33rd edn. New Delhi: Lexis Nexis; 2011. p. 665-96.
10. Mathiharan K, Patnaik AK. Injuries by mechanical force. Modi's Medical Jurisprudence and Toxicology. 23rd edn. New Delhi: Lexis Nexis; 2005. p. 685-730.
11. CRM No. 18934 of 2013 in MRC No. 8 of 2007, P and B High Court (State of Punjab vs. Mohinder Singh). Available from: http://yaruran26.rssing.com/browser.php?indx=14248871anditem=347.
12. Krishnan MKR. Wounds. Handbook of forensic medicine. 4th edn. Hyderabad: Kothari book depot; 1973. p. 130-219.

Medicolegal Aspects of Injuries

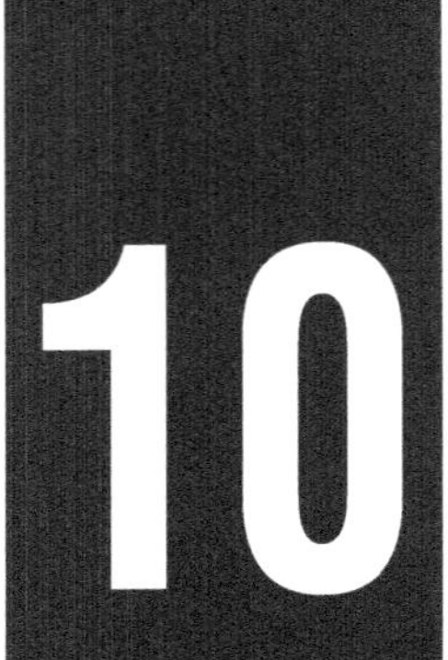

Anil Kohli

'The injuries we do and those we suffer are seldom weighed in the same scales.'
Aesop (Greek fabulist)

ABSTRACT

Trauma, a common presentation in the emergency department, is also a source of confusion to many doctors with regard to its medicolegal aspect. This is especially so in the case of grievous hurt. This article discusses the various Indian laws in relation to trauma. Problems faced by doctors are discussed and interpretation of the various laws in relation to trauma, especially with regard to the different clauses of grievous hurt has been attempted in light of various judgments by the courts of law that could be accessed. Suggestions have been given on how a doctor should approach a medicolegal case and opine on the matter.

Keywords: Grievous hurt, Sec. 320 IPC, trauma, law, opinion, nature of injury, dangerous injury, injuries endangering life.

INTRODUCTION

Trauma is a common presenting feature of patients in the emergency department. There exists an urgency to treat the patients, and at the same time the injuries have to be properly documented, so that they can be explained at a later stage to the legal authorities in the interest of justice. Expert opinion by a doctor in medicolegal cases is usually given in the following circumstances:

- After personally examining a case which has come to a doctor for the first time.
- On findings documented earlier in a case seen by some other doctor (the person is not examined).
- As member of board of doctors assigned a case or reviewing a case already seen.

Doctors are generally asked to opine on the nature and manner of injuries sustained by a victim. Sometimes, queries are not limited to these points only, and opinion on age of injury and type of injury can also be sought.

Injury Characteristics Documented in Medicolegal Cases

When examining a victim of injury, doctors should ensure that all the characteristics of the injury are taken into consideration and documented (Table 10.1).

Table 10.1 Characteristics of injuries to be documented

Opinion	*Injury characteristic*
Type of injury	Abrasion, bruise, laceration, stab, incise, gunshot
Age of injury	Color, scab formation, granulation tissue formation
Causation of injury (whether by blunt objects, sharp objects, heavy objects, firearm)	Wound margins/edges—clean cut, irregular, contused. Presence of abrasion collar (in firearm injury) Crush injuries Wound shape—spindle, wedge, irregular, stellate
Manner of infliction (whether suicidal, accidental, homicidal or self-inflicted)	Hesitation cuts, defense wounds Foreign bodies in and around wound, like grease, dirt, paint
Nature of injury	Simple, grievous or dangerous (endangering life)

Incomplete examination or documentation may cause problems later on for the doctor in the courts of law.

As already discussed in previous chapter, it is not necessary to give the exact age of the injury, as this is not possible most of the time. A similar opinion was also voiced by the Supreme Court of India in Ramswaroop vs. State of UP[1], where the Honorable Court said that 'It is well known that a doctor can never be absolutely certain on the point of the time so far as duration of injuries is concerned'.

Sometimes, it may not be possible to deduce the manner of infliction and the doctor should not hesitate in admitting this fact.

Difficulties in Interpreting Indian Laws

Sometimes, help of a medical expert is required for interpreting many sections of the Indian Penal Code (IPC) which involve trauma, and hence they should be well versed in these sections and their interpretations. The expert, many a time, faces difficulty in interpreting many terms outlined in these sections of the IPC.

One of the common problems faced by doctors is with regard to 'grievous hurt' or 'grievous injury' as it is mistakenly more commonly called. Which injury should be labeled grievous and which should be said to be simple? Another difficulty is with regard to dangerous injuries, injuries endangering life, injuries likely to cause death and injuries sufficient to cause death in ordinary course of nature. These are the terms mentioned in the Indian Penal Code (IPC) and form the basis for convicting persons under the IPC.

What exactly these terms denote is sometimes not clear to many doctors and so these terms have been explained along with the relevant legal pronouncements involving them. This would be of immense help to medical experts who have to opine on injuries in medicolegal cases in the context of whether the injuries are simple, grievous, endangering life, likely to cause death or sufficient to cause death in the ordinary course of nature.

DEFINITION

The dictionary meaning of injury is 'harm or damage that is done or sustained'.[2] Medical dictionaries define injury as 'wound or trauma, harm or hurt, damage inflicted on the body by an external force'.[3]

Trauma or *injury* refers to 'a body wound or shock produced by sudden physical injury, as from violence or accident'. In medicine, a *wound* is a type of injury in which skin is torn, cut or punctured (an *open* wound) or where blunt force trauma causes a contusion (a *closed* wound). In some countries, unlike India, *wound has been legally defined* as an injury that breaks the continuity of the skin. There must be a division of the whole skin and not merely a division of the cuticle or upper layer. A single drop of blood is sufficient to constitute wound but it must fall outside the body. The legal definition of injury in India is discussed below.

DISCUSSION

Sections of the IPC concerning injury/trauma are discussed below along with the decisions of courts of law relevant to these Sections.[4]

Sec. 44 IPC (Injury): The word 'injury' denotes any harm, whatever illegally, caused to any person in body, mind, reputation or property.

Sec. 299 IPC (Culpable homicide): Whoever causes death:

i. By doing an act with the intention of causing death, or
ii. With the intention of causing such bodily injury as is likely to cause death, or
iii. With the knowledge that he is likely by such an act to cause death.

Explanation 1: A person, who causes bodily injury to another who is laboring under a disorder, disease or bodily infirmity, and thereby accelerates the death of that other, shall be deemed to have caused his death.

Explanation 2: Where death is caused by bodily injury, the person who causes such bodily injury shall be deemed to have caused the death, although by resorting to proper remedies and skilful treatment the death might have been prevented.

Explanation 3: The causing of the death of child in the mother's womb is not homicide. But it may amount to culpable homicide to cause the death of a living child, if any part of that child has been brought forth, though the child may not have breathed or been completely born.

Sec. 300 IPC (Murder): Except in the cases hereinafter excepted, culpable homicide is murder,

- *Firstly:* If the act by which the death is caused is done with the intention of causing death, or
- *Secondly:* If it is done with the intention of causing such bodily injury as the offender knows to be likely to cause the death of the person to whom the harm is caused, or
- *Thirdly:* If it is done with the intention of causing bodily injury to any person, and the bodily injury intended to be inflicted is sufficient in the ordinary course of nature to cause death, or
- *Fourthly:* If the person committing the act knows that it is so imminently dangerous that it must, in all probability, cause death or such bodily injury as is likely to cause death, and commits such act without any excuse for incurring the risk of causing death or such injury as aforesaid.

In second clause, knowledge should be possessed by the offender that victim is in a particular state of health that internal harm caused to him is likely to be fatal, not with standing the fact that such harm would not in the ordinary way of nature be sufficient to cause death of a person in normal health. Intention to cause death is not a requirement of this subclause. Thus, *injuries likely to cause death* are those in which the offender causes injuries which are not fatal in the ordinary course of nature, but are fatal in the case of that particular person, by reason of knowledge of that person's physical infirmity, disease or subnormal state of health. There should be intention to injure and knowledge about the consequences of injury relating to that particular person. For example, causing death by a fist blow intentionally given, knowing that the victim is suffering from enlarged liver/spleen/diseased heart and such blow is likely to cause death of that particular person. It is not necessary that the offender intended to cause death. He is culpable, even if intention was limited to infliction of injury (Rajwant vs. State of Kerala[5]).

In third clause, intention has to be to inflict the injury. Whether intention was to kill the victim or not, is not material. As compared to 'knowledge', 'intention' requires something more than the mere foresight of the consequences, namely, the purposeful doing of a thing to achieve a particular end.

Injuries *sufficient to cause death in the ordinary course of nature* are those in which the sufficiency is the high probability of death. Examples are:

- Stab injuries on the abdomen or chest which are injuring an internal organ or large blood vessel
- Stab injuries or traumatic rupture of heart
- Blunt injuries causing rupture of spleen, liver or an internal organ
- Bleeding due to sharp or blunt injuries to large blood vessels anywhere in the body
- Severe injuries of brain like hemorrhages, contusions, edema, diffuse axonal injury
- Extensive burns, scalds or bruising
- Incised wounds of neck involving trachea or major blood vessels of neck
- Ligature marks of hanging and strangulation or marks of smothering
- Compound fractures of skull.

Clause Third of Sec. 300 IPC Distinguished from the Second Clause of Sec. 299 IPC

In Sec. 299 IPC, instead of words 'likely to cause death' (second clause) the words 'sufficient in the ordinary course of nature' have been used.

The difference between the second clause of Sec. 299 and clause 'thirdly' of Sec. 300 is one of degree of probability of death resulting from the intended bodily injury. To put it more broadly, it is the degree of probability of death which determines whether a culpable homicide is of the gravest, medium or lowest degree. The word 'likely' in second clause of Sec. 299 *conveys the sense of 'probable' as distinguished from a mere possibility*. The words 'bodily injury .... sufficient in the ordinary course of nature to cause death', in clause thirdly of Sec. 300, mean that death *will be the most probable result of the injury* having regard to the ordinary course of nature (State of Andhra Pradesh vs. Rayavarpu Punayya).[6] Therefore, injuries 'sufficient in the ordinary course of nature to cause death' pose a greater danger to the life of the victim than 'injuries likely to cause death'.

Exception 1: **When culpable homicide is not murder**—Culpable homicide is not murder if the offender, whilst deprived of the power of self-control by grave and sudden provocation, causes the death of the person who gave the provocation or causes the death of any other person by mistake or accident.

The above exception is subject to the following provisions:
- *Firstly:* That the provocation is not sought or voluntarily provoked by the offender as an excuse for killing or doing harm to any person.
- *Secondly:* That the provocation is not given by anything done in obedience to the law or by a public servant in the lawful exercise of the powers of such public servant.
- *Thirdly:* That the provocation is not given by anything done in the lawful exercise of the right of private defense.

Exception 2: Culpable homicide is not murder if the offender, in the exercise in good faith of the right of private defense of person or property, exceeds the power given to him by law and causes the death of the person against whom he is exercising such right of defense without premeditation and without any intention of doing more harm than is necessary for the purpose of such defense.

Exception 3: Culpable homicide is not murder if the offender, being a public servant or aiding a public servant acting for the advancement of public justice, exceeds the powers given to him by law, and causes death by doing an act which he, in good faith, believes to be lawful and necessary for the due discharge of his duty as such public servant and without ill-will towards the person whose death is caused.

Exception 4: Culpable homicide is not murder, if it is committed without premeditation in a sudden fight in the heat of passion upon a sudden quarrel and without the offender having taken undue advantage or acted in a cruel or unusual manner.

Explanation: It is immaterial in such cases which party offers the provocation or commits the first assault.

Exception 5: Culpable homicide is not murder when the person whose death is caused, being above the age of 18 years, suffers death or takes the risk of death with his own consent.

Sec. 319 IPC (Hurt): Whoever causes bodily pain, disease or infirmity to any person is said to cause hurt.

Infirmity is a bodily ailment or weakness or condition or disease producing weakness. It could even be due to the administration of poison or alcohol. It can be temporary mental impairment, hysteria or terror.

Disease is an abnormal condition affecting the body of an organism and affecting its normal function.

Sec. 320 IPC (Grievous hurt): The following kinds of hurt *only* are designated as 'grievous' (Table 10.2).

Simple hurt is not defined in law. However, an injury which is neither serious nor extensive but heals rapidly without leaving permanent deformity or disfiguration is simple hurt.

Table 10.2 Grievous hurt

Clause	*Kinds of hurt*
First	Emasculation
Second	Permanent privation of the sight of either eye
Third	Permanent privation of the hearing of either ear
Fourth	Privation of any member or joint
Fifth	Destruction or permanent impairing of the powers of any member or joint
Sixth	Permanent disfiguration of the head or face
Seventh	Fracture or dislocation of a bone or tooth
Eighth	Any hurt which endangers life or which causes the sufferer to be during the space of twenty days in severe bodily pain or unable to follow his ordinary pursuits

GRIEVOUS HURT

The eight clauses of grievous hurt are an exhaustive list of injuries which define grievous hurt for this section of the IPC. No hurt outside this list can be termed as grievous. Many times, there is confusion amongst doctors on the interpretation of some of these clauses. In some cases, judgments by the courts of law are available which have cleared the ambiguities in these cases. There will, however, be instances when the doctor may not be able to form a definite opinion about the nature of the injuries, and the doctor should then stick to the medical facts and leave the final decision to the courts of law.

'Grievous' means any serious injury and it is not necessary that it should be dangerous. All dangerous injuries are grievous but not all grievous injuries are dangerous. Grievous hurt has been legally defined and doctors have to give their opinion within the framework of the existing law. Sometimes, an injury may seem to be trivial to a doctor but if it falls under any of the categories mentioned in Sec. 320 IPC, the opinion has to be grievous. On the other hand, some injuries may seem grievous because they are on a vital part of the body, but are not actually grievous. On many occasions, it becomes difficult to opine whether a hurt is grievous or not. Hence, there is a need to illustrate and explain the clauses of Sec. 320 IPC, i.e. grievous hurt in detail.

Emasculation

Emasculation is depriving a male of masculine vigor or depriving him of his virility.[7] It covers both sterility and potency in a male. Impotency caused must be permanent (question as to whether treatable or untreatable is immaterial) for the injury to be called grievous.

Therefore, emasculation could be by removal of genitalia, i.e. penis or testicles (castration) or injury to spinal cord at the level of L2 to L4 vertebra resulting in impotency. Castration is any surgical or chemical action by which male loses functions of the testicles or a female loses function of the ovaries. In this section, only male castration comes under emasculation and not female castration. (Female castration can, however, be a grievous injury under clause 4 or clause 8).

If only one testis gets damaged or removed and the other testis with intact male organ is present, then it is not called emasculation as sterility or impotency have not been caused. However, it is still a grievous injury under clause 4, which is, privation of any member or joint.

Privation

Privation is an act, condition or result of deprivation or loss. It is a state of being deprived. Loss of hair/nails would not come under the category of privation of member.

Sight

Sight means visual perception. It is the power or function of seeing or range of vision. Three aspects of vision are visual acuity, field of vision and visual functioning. Visual functioning refers to the degree to which or the ability of a person to use vision for all daily activities.

A legal definition of blindness is given in 'The Persons with Disabilities (Equal Opportunities, Protection of Rights and Full Participation) Act, 1995.[8] This Act was enacted for job opportunities and disability estimation. Under this Act, blindness refers to a condition where a person suffers from any of the following conditions:

- Total absence of sight
- Visual acuity not exceeding 6/60 or 20/200 (Snellen) in the better eye with correcting lenses
- Limitation of the field of vision subtending to an angle of 20 degree or worse.

Some experts have suggested that those with diminution of vision after an injury (i.e. someone having visual acuity of 6/6 initially which gets reduced to say 6/9 after injury) would also be said to be suffering from loss of sight. But this interpretation can sometimes present with practical difficulties. A person could fake partial loss of vision after an injury by purposely reading one or two lines less (in Snellans chart) than what he/she could really read. Another example is of a person hiding the fact that he/she had reduced visual acuity long before the injury, in order to implicate the person responsible for the injury. But to consider only complete loss of vision would be unfair to those people who are able to appreciate only hand movements after injury. One way to get out of this dilemma would be to consider only those victims with vision restricted to finger counting or hand movements as a result of trauma to be those with loss of sight. Alternatively, the definition of low vision in the 'The Persons with Disabilities (Equal opportunities, Protection of Rights and Full Participation) Act, 1995' or the WHO definition of low vision could be used. 'Person with low vision' means a person with impairment of visual functioning even after treatment or standard refractive correction but who uses or is potentially capable of using vision for the planning or execution of a task with appropriate assistive device. However, low visual acuity is not quantified in the Act. World Health Organization (WHO) defines low vision as visual acuity less than 6/18 or visual field of less than 10 degrees.

Hearing

Unlike blindness, there is no definition of legal deafness but hearing impairment has been defined in the 'The Persons with Disabilities (Equal Opportunities, Protection of Rights and Full Participation) Act, 1995'.

'Hearing impairment' means loss of 60 decibels (Db) or more in the better ear in the conversational range of frequencies. Profound hearing impairment occurs with hearing loss between 61–70 Db. Total deafness is said to occur with loss > 91 Db.

The case cited in Box 10.1 illustrates the confusion caused by labelling slight hearing loss/loss of visual acuity as grievous.

Member

The term 'member' as used here, means an organ, limb or tissue, being a part of an individual and capable of performing a distinct function. As such, it includes the eyes, ears, nose, mouth, hands, feet, and in fact, all distinct parts of the human body designed to perform a distinct function.

Loss of a distinct part or organ of the body does not require proof that such loss amounts to an impairment of one's bodily health. Loss is enough.

Dislocation of Joint

A joint is a place where two or more bones or muscles join. Privation of joint implies loss of joint leading to the joint being unable to perform its normal function. In Sec. 7 of 320 IPC, it is clearly mentioned that dislocation of the joint

Box 10.1 Fallacies of labelling slight hearing loss as grievous

AIIMS docs get a clean chit[9]

Three senior doctors of AIIMS who were summoned by the trial court recently for allegedly fabricating the medical report of a woman in a dowry harassment case have come out unscathed with the court giving them a clean chit. Stating that it was a 'bonafide mistake' by doctors, Additional Session's Judge directed that no further proceedings be initiated against them. 'It is clear from medical records that some bonafide mistake or error might have been committed by doctors in interpreting legal provisions and doctors have been guided by their own medical literature in giving their opinion on injuries sustained by the woman,' the court said. 'In the circumstances, I am of the considered opinion that from the material on record, benefit of doubt may be extended to all three doctors and no further proceedings be initiated against them,' the court added. Later, holding a press conference, one of the doctors said. 'The case was referred to the Forensic department in December 2008 and after going through the medical reports of the patient, we found that the injuries were grievous in nature, therefore, we had written that in our report. The ENT report shows that there is mild conductive hearing loss caused to the patient. This could be due to physical injury or other medical reasons like infection etc, but in this case the woman did not have any other medical problem.' The three doctors had quoted medical literature to prove that injuries suffered by the patient were grievous in nature. 'Any physical damage which is partial can be termed grievous in nature. She was suffering from partial hearing loss. We were able to convince the Judge that we had purely gone by medical books, while terming the injury grievous in nature and had not fabricated records, but we could not convince him that it was actually grievous in nature.'

is a grievous injury. However, nothing is mentioned about the *dislocation of the implanted joint.*

In Australia, damage to artificial aids like broken dentures, damaged artificial limbs, or damaged prosthesis are included in classification of injuries that qualify for workers' compensation claim.[10]

In a case in Patiala, Punjab (2005),[11] doctors declared an injury leading to privation of implanted joint as grievous, as they felt that dislocation of joint cannot be declared as simple in nature.

Disfiguration

Disfiguration is change in configuration or personal appearance. Disfigure means to deface or mar the appearance or beauty of someone. The word 'disfigure' must be distinguished from the word 'disable'. To disfigure is to do an individual some external injury which detracts from his/her personal appearance, but does not weaken him/her, but to 'disable' is to do something creating a permanent disability and not a mere temporary injury. Disability is restriction or lack of ability (resulting from an impairment) to perform an activity in the manner or within the range considered normal.

Disfigurement may be caused by amputation of an individual's ear or nose, in which case there would be sufficient disfigurement without consequential disability so as to constitute grievous hurt under this clause. A nasty cut on the face leaving a permanent scar would be another instance of this species of injury. Branding also may leave a permanent scar causing disfigurement.

The Supreme Court of Alaska defined 'disfigurement' in a civil law context.[12] The court held that, for purposes of this statute, a 'disfigurement' is an injury that 'impairs or injures the beauty, symmetry or appearance of a person, or that which renders a person's appearance unsightly, misshapen or imperfect'.

Another court judgment held that 'If a reasonable person would see the injury as detracting from the plaintiff's appearance, the injury has caused disfigurement'. Other courts agree that, if a scar is observable from a normal social distance (for e.g. at arm's length distance) it constitutes a disfigurement. A United States court held that 'even a small but noticeable scar on a person's face ... is a disfigurement'. Disfigurement is severe, if a reasonable person would find that the injury mars the [victim's] physical appearance and causes a degree of unattractiveness sufficient to bring negative attention or embarrassment.

Reasonable healing period must be allowed before disfigurement may be assessed. Otherwise, a victim might claim to be disfigured based on his condition immediately after being injured, when a wound that will eventually heal completely still appears gruesome.

Therefore, opinion of disfigurement in cases involving healing of wound should ideally be given after complete healing, as then only can it be judged whether disfigurement is permanent or not. However, if the doctor feels that there may be an inordinate delay in healing of the wound, or on the request of the law enforcement authorities, the doctor, in the interest of justice, can give an interim opinion regarding the nature of the injury. The doctor can state that the wound on healing is likely or unlikely to leave a scar which is likely or unlikely to disfigure the person, and give the final opinion after complete healing of the wound.

Fracture of Bone

There has been a lot of controversy regarding what constitutes fracture of bone. The medical dictionary defines fracture as 'any break in continuity of a bone'. Various textbooks of Forensic Medicine have given guidelines in this regard. According to Modi's Textbook of Medical Jurisprudence and Toxicology,[13] the dimension in respect of the depth of the cut in the bone must be mentioned. JB Mukherji's Textbook on Forensic Medicine and Toxicology[14] states that fracture will be considered as grievous injury, if the cut in the bone or break in the continuity of the bone extends deep up to the medullary cavity.

A ruling of the **High Court of Rangoon** (1937)[15] was to the following effect. The primary meaning of the word 'fracture' is '*breaking*' though it is not necessary in case of fracture of the skull bone that it be divided into two separate parts because it may consist merely of a crack, but if it is a crack, it must be a crack which extends from the outer surface of the skull to the inner surface. The view taken in this case was that unless the crack extends to the inner surface which means the entire depth of the bone, it may not amount to a fracture.

In 1942, the **Patna High Court**[16] held that 'where the evidence is merely that a bone has been cut and there is nothing whatever to indicate the extent of the cut, whether deep or a mere scratch upon the surface, it is impossible to infer from that evidence alone that grievous hurt has been caused within the meaning of the definition in Sec. 320 IPC'.

In 1954, **Rajasthan High Court**[17] held that fracture means 'breaking' of a bone. Fissured fracture is one in which there is no displacement of the fragments, and this condition may be caused by direct or indirect violence usually resulting from a fall or a blow from a blunt object. These fissures may extend far and wide from the point struck may implicate one or both tables, and not infrequently run down into the base. A scratch or a cut which does not go across the bone cannot be said to be a fracture of a bone within the meaning of Sec. 320 IPC. Both outer and the inner tables of the skull bone may be considered to be bones by themselves and fracture of outer or the inner table by itself can be taken to be a fracture of a bone within the meaning of Sec. 320 IPC. A crack which does not involve both the tables of the skull bone may amount to a fracture of a bone. A fissured fracture of the outer table of the skull bone would, therefore, bring the case within the definition of a grievous hurt.

In a later case in 1956, **Rajasthan High Court**[18] held that when the dimensions of a cut of a bone are not known, it may be difficult to say whether it is a grievous hurt. The Judges said 'it seems that the point urged by the learned counsel for the petitioner that unless the crack extends to the inner side, the hurt cannot be said to be grievous within the meaning of Sec. 320 IPC does not appear to be justified. As explained by the learned public prosecutor, there can be a cut, though the division or split resulting from the cut need not be complete. If a cut resulted only in a scratch and did not go deep to any length into the bone, it cannot be deemed a fracture; otherwise, it should be deemed to be one'.

In the **Madras High Court** (1965)[19] it was discussed whether the cutting of a bone to a slight extent would be a grievous hurt within the meaning of Sec. 326 IPC. This court also held that it is not necessary that the cut has to extend to the inner surface of the bone to constitute a fracture.

The **Supreme Court of India** in 1970[20] finally ended this controversy and defined fracture with regard to Sec. 320 IPC. The Supreme Court in Hori Lal and Anr vs. State of UP stated that 'It did not agree with the assumption that if the evidence is merely that a bone has been cut and there is nothing whatever to indicate the extent of the cut, whether a deep one or a mere scratch on the surface of the bone, it will be difficult to infer that the injury is a grievous hurt within the meaning of Sec. 320 IPC. In our view, these assumptions are misleading. It is not necessary that a bone should be cut through or that the crack must extend from the outer to the inner surface or that there should be displacement of any fragment of the bone. If there is a break by cutting or splintering of the bone or there is a rupture or fissure, it would amount to a fracture within the meaning of clause 7 of Sec. 320 IPC. What we have to see is whether the cuts in the bones noticed are only superficial or do they affect a break in them.'

In view of this, it can be concluded that even if the extent of the cut is not mentioned, it will amount to grievous hurt if there has been a break in the bone. Thus, the Supreme Court in its judgment defined fracture within the meaning of Sec. 320 IPC.

In 1993, in the **Orissa High Court**,[21] a question arose as to whether without knowing the extent of cut to a bone could it be conclusively said that there has been a fracture to that bone. In the case under appeal, the extent of cut to the scapula-bone was not ascertainable but since the doctor deposed that he could see the nature of the injury to be grievous, it had to be taken that there was break in the bone by the cutting and as such, the injury was grievous within the meaning of clause 7 of Sec. 320 IPC.

Hurt which Endangers Life and Dangerous Injuries

Hurt which endangers life is any bodily injury of such a nature that, if left untreated, would *endanger life* whether or not medical treatment is or could have been available. The words 'any hurt which endangers life' mean that the life is only endangered and not taken away. It means placing a person in danger of death, i.e. death may be probable.

Dangerous injury has not been defined in the IPC. However, medical literature defines dangerous injuries as those which cause imminent danger to life by their direct or imminent effects, because of being extensive in nature, involving important structure of body or organs and also being likely to prove fatal in absence of surgical aid, for e.g. injury to internal organs or large blood vessels.

There is confusion amongst the medical profession and the legal fraternity with regards to the terms dangerous injuries and injuries which endanger life. However, the courts of law have taken up this issue and their judgments have cleared the air to a great extent. Doctors may wonder why they should get involved in such matters which are best left to the courts. A judgment of the Punjab and Haryana high court (Atma Singh vs. State of Punjab)[22] very aptly tell the reasons why doctors have to address these issues:

'When the doctor is required to carry out medicolegal examination of the injury suffered in a criminal assault, he is required to examine the injury from two standpoints: (1) for the purpose of opining the kind of weapon used to inflict the injury in question and, (2) to form an opinion regarding the degree of seriousness of the injury in order to enable to see as to what offence has the accused committed by inflicting the injury in question. The Indian Penal Code recognizes from standpoint of seriousness only four types of injuries:

1. Simple injuries.
2. Grievous injuries.
3. Injuries of the kind inflicted with intent to commit murder described in clause 'Firstly' and 'Secondly' of Sec. 300 IPC.
4. Injury sufficient to cause death in the ordinary course of nature envisaged by clause 'Thirdly' of Sec. 300 IPC.

There is no provision in the IPC which envisages or refers to an injury described as 'dangerous to life'. The medicolegal examination of an injured person is intended to enable the investigating agency and the court to find out the nature of the offence. Therefore, the doctor examining an injured person has to opine that the injury in question is one or the other of the type recognized in the IPC for the purposes of a given offence'.

Hence, a doctor has to opine an injury as:

- Simple
- Grievous
- Endangering life (clause 8 of grievous hurt)
- Likely to cause death
- Sufficient to cause death in the ordinary course of nature.

These are types mentioned in the IPC and form the basis for convicting persons under various sections of the IPC. Injuries likely to cause death and those sufficient to cause death have already been discussed. To get a proper understanding of injuries endangering life, it is important to first discuss the legal position outlined by the courts in this regard.

Judicial Opinion Regarding Injuries Dangerous to Life and Injuries Endangering Life

The Punjab and Haryana High Court in 1973 held that expression 'dangerous to life' is somewhat milder and subdued as compared to the expression 'endangered life' used in clause 8 of Sec. 320 IPC.[23] Therefore, an injury which is described by the doctor as 'dangerous to life' cannot be held to be one which endangered life. Justice SC Mittal, deciding Jagrup Singh's case expressed himself in the following words while interpreting clause 'Eighthly' of Sec. 320 of the IPC: 'Clause 8 refers to injuries which are not only dangerous but which endangers life—a much stronger expression. This term is designedly used to exclude cases of hurt, which, however, dangerous to life do not put life in a given case in danger. The question is one of degree and must be ascertained in each case to what extent the hurt bears proximate relation to the risk of life'.

Justice SS Dewan, in Harbans Singh vs. State of Punjab,[24] observed as did Justice SC Mittal, that the term 'dangerous to life' is milder than the expression 'endangers life'. He merely followed his earlier decision holding that an injury described as dangerous to life cannot be considered grievous.

Justice AS Bains (in Surjit Singh vs. State of Punjab), merely followed the decision in Jagrup Singh's case and held that an injury described as 'dangerous to life' would not satisfy the requirement of clause 8 of Sec. 320 IPC and would not be a grievous injury.[22]

Justice Arijit Pasayat and Justice BP Singh (Supreme Court of India) in Niranjan Singh vs. State of Madhya Pradesh said that 'the term endangering life is much stronger than the expression dangerous to life'.[25]

Justice Palekar, in Jai Narain Mishra vs. State of Bihar,[26] discussed a penetrating wound chest wall deep on the right side of the chest caused with a *bhala* and described by the doctor as 'dangerous to life' and a grievous injury. In the later part of the judgment (para 11), this injury was described as one 'endangering life'. The expression 'dangerous' is an adjective and the expression 'endanger' is verb. An injury which can put life in immediate danger of death would be an injury which can be termed as 'dangerous to life'. Therefore, when a doctor describes an injury as 'dangerous to life', he means an injury which endangers life in terms of clause 8 of Sec. 320 IPC, for, he describes the injury 'dangerous to life', only for the purpose of the said clause. Instead of using the expression that this was an injury which 'endangered life' the injury was described as 'dangerous to life', meaning the same thing both the times.

The Punjab and Haryana High Court in 1980[22] said "when a doctor describes an injury as 'dangerous to life' one has to see what had the doctor intended to convey thereby. Is one to hold that since injury has not been described by the doctor as one which *endangered life,* so the concerned injury cannot be held to be grievous on the ground that an injury described as 'dangerous to life' is not as serious an injury which 'endangers life'. It appears that the doctors who had been conducting the medicolegal examinations have been using the term 'dangerous to life' as synonymous with an injury which 'endangers life'. Even the courts at times have considered an injury described as dangerous to life as an injury envisaged in clause 'Eighthly' of Sec. 320 IPC". They were firmly of the view that wherever a doctor describes an injury as 'dangerous to life' and the nature of the injuries is such which could merit such a conclusion, then such an injury has to be treated as 'grievous hurt' of the description mentioned in first portion of clause 8 of Sec. 320 IPC.

Medically, it is very difficult to categorize injuries into injuries endangering life and dangerous injuries as the distinction is virtually nonexistent. The views of various courts of law on this issue have also been discussed above (Refer to Box 10.2 also). Taking the above viewpoints into account, it is recommended that the medical expert should desist from trying to differentiate between injuries endangering life and dangerous injuries. Hence, it would be advisable for doctors to consider injuries endangering life as dangerous injuries and vice versa. This is one clause of grievous hurt where the role of the doctor is important as he uses his medical knowledge to ultimately decide whether an injury is endangering life or not and does not have to rely on any legal guidelines in clause 8 of Sec. 320 IPC.

Ordinary Pursuit

'Ordinary pursuit' means day to day personal activities of an individual like attending nature's call, taking food or bath, or wearing clothes. Stay in hospital for twenty days does not amount to grievous hurt, until the doctor certifies that the patient was unable to follow his ordinary pursuits or was in severe bodily pain during this period (Bombay High Court, Abdul Sajid Abdul Sadiq vs. State of Maharashtra).[28] It is held by the courts that 'in the absence of any evidence to that effect, it will not be possible legally to draw such inference inasmuch, as an

Box 10.2 Injuries endangering life as opined by courts of law

Stabbing on any vital part, squeezing the testicles (State of Karnataka vs. Shivalingaiah),[27] thrusting *lathi* into rectum so that bleeding is caused, have all been held as hurts that endanger life and thus grievous hurts. In another case, the Supreme Court (Neelam Bahal Anr vs. State of Uttarakhand, Criminal Appeal 1012 of 2009), the doctor had mentioned two incised wounds on the victim, one on the left side of chest with unknown depth and another on the left shoulder which was bone deep. The doctor had also opined the general condition of the patient to be very bad with very weak pulse, and blood pressure (BP) could not be recorded. However, the doctor did not mention the nature of the injury. The court held that because of the fact that the victim remained in hospital for 15 days, and had unrecordable BP on admission, the injuries were grievous as life had been endangered.

injured person may be quite capable to follow his ordinary pursuits long before twenty days are over, and yet for the sake of permanent recovery or greater ease or comfort be willing to remain as a convalescent in a hospital'. It was pointed out that mere fact that the sufferer did not attend his duty for the statutory period or that he remained in hospital for that period is no indication of his inability to follow his ordinary pursuits.

SOME GRIEVOUS INJURIES INVOLVING DIFFERENT REGIONS OF THE BODY

Eye

Grievous injury involving the eye can be caused even when the vision remains normal. Permanent disfiguration of face occurs when injuries to the eyes leave residual defects after healing, like ptosis, entropion or squint. Privation of eye can occur due to dislocation of lens, breaking of zonules or stripping away of whole or part of eyelid.

Injuries dangerous to life or endangering life can occur, when injuries involving the eye lead to involvement of the cranium which may prove fatal immediately or from delayed complication like meningitis and endopthalmitis.[29]

Ear

An ear injury may involve the outer ear, ear canal or the eardrum. Hearing loss can occur due to injuries to the eardrum (perforation) or damage to the ear ossicles. Permanent disfiguration of face can occur when injuries lead to loss of pinna of the ear.

Injuries dangerous to life can occur when injuries involving the ear lead to infections of the middle ear with complications, like meningitis or brain abscess which could prove fatal.

Skin

A person with burn injuries to the face resulting in scarring or tattooing will have permanent disfiguration. Grievous hurt can occur when burn injuries involving the skin lead to the person being admitted to the hospital and unable to follow his/her ordinary pursuits or be in severe bodily pain for a period of at least 20 days.

Injuries dangerous to life can also occur due to potentially life-threatening burn injuries (because of the risk of hypovolemic shock). Three risk factors for death after burns have been identified: an age of more than 60 years, burn size of more than 40% of body surface area and inhalation injury. Mortality is a function of the number of risk factors present. When burn size of more than 40% of body surface area, age greater than 60 years and presence of inhalation injury are taken as risk factors, patient's mortality is 0.3% with no risk factors, 3% with one risk factor, 33% with two risk factors and approximately 90% with all three risk factors. This rule is applicable to all patients younger than 90.[30-32]

Potentially life-threatening burns can occur in persons either less than 10 years of age or greater than 50 years of age who have partial thickness burns involving more than 30% of the total body surface area (TBSA) and in those between 10 and 50 years of age with partial thickness burns involving more than 35% TBSA.[30-32]

The Baux Score is the sum of age and the percentage of TBSA burned. There is a strong association between this sum or score and case fatality for both men and women. A sum of age and burn size (Baux Score) of 110 was associated with death in approximately 50% of cases. Baux Score of 140 or more is non-survivable.[30-32]

For patients with an inhalation injury, a sum of age and burn size (Baux Score) of 100 was associated with death in approximately 50% of cases, compared with 110 for those without. Thus, a revised Baux Score, i.e. Age + Percent Burn + 17 has been suggested for those with inhalation injuries.[30-32]

Therefore, doctors should desist from using the yardstick of 40% of TBSA burnt to classify the burns as simple or grievous, since inhalational injuries and age of the person also play a significant part in assessing whether burns are endangering life. If the doctor who initially saw the patient in the emergency is not well versed in opining on the seriousness of the burns, it is better that the opinion on the nature of the burns is left to the specialist who will be treating the patient.

Brain

Concussion: Traumatic brain injury can lead to unconsciousness. It is by definition not a life- threatening injury. Simple isolated concussion has a good recovery.

Subdural hemorrhage: Poor prognostic indicators (leading to endangering of life) are:

- Pupillary inequality
- Decreased GCS score (less than 8 initially and post-resuscitation, less than 7 on admission)
- Postoperative elevated intracranial pressure
- Ischemic damage to brain
- Hypotension/hypoxia
- If bleed is larger than 3 cm (which then requires surgery)
- On CT scan, hypodensity of SDH (isodensity has good prognosis).

Subarachnoid hemorrhage: Prognosis depends on location and amount of bleeding.

Diffuse axonal injury

- *Grade I:* involves gray-white matter interfaces (most commonly: parasagittal regions of frontal lobes, periventricular temporal lobes)
- *Grade II:* Involves corpus callosum in addition to grade I locations
- *Grade III:* Involves brainstem in addition to grade I and II locations (most commonly: rostral midbrain, superior cerebellar peduncles, medial lemniscus and corticospinal tracts).

  Grade II and III diffuse axonal injuries endangers life.

WEAPONS

Webster's New World Law dictionary has defined weapon as an implement used or designed to be used to kill or injure a person.[33] A concealed weapon is a weapon that is carried by someone, but is not visible to the ordinary observer's eye. It has also defined dangerous and deadly weapons.

Dangerous weapon is an implement or device that is capable of causing serious bodily harm or death; not to be confused with a deadly weapon. A dangerous weapon may be deadly; a deadly weapon must be dangerous.

Deadly weapon is any firearm or other device (crossbow, longbow, bomb, grenade, and so on), substance (poison), or material (dagger, cutlass), that when used in the manner, it was intended to be used, will be likely to cause death.

The terms dangerous weapon and deadly weapon have been used in Indian law.

Dangerous Weapon

A dangerous weapon has been defined in the IPC.

Sec. 324 IPC: *Voluntarily causing hurt by dangerous weapons or means:* Whoever, except in the case provided for by Sec. 334 IPC, voluntarily causes hurt by means of any instrument for shooting, stabbing or cutting, or any instrument which, used as a weapon of offence, is likely to cause death, or by means of fire or any heated substance, or by means of any poison or any corrosive substance, or by means of any explosive substance, or by means of any substance which it is deleterious to the human body to inhale, to swallow or to receive into the blood, or by means of any animal, shall be punished with imprisonment of either description for a term which may extend to three years or with fine or with both. Hence, a dangerous weapon is any instrument for shooting, stabbing or cutting, or any instrument which, used as a weapon of offence, is likely to cause death. Thus, one can see that this definition is very subjective and its interpretation may vary from person-to-person. To highlight this point, the following case serves as an interesting illustration.

In Mathai vs. State of Kerala (2005) an appeal was filed in the Supreme Court regarding conviction of a person for causing offence punishable under Sec. 326 IPC (of voluntarily causing hurt by dangerous weapons or means).[34] In the appeal, it was to be decided whether the factual position indicates that any grievous hurt was caused and whether the weapon used was a dangerous weapon. The doctor who examined the injured noticed following injuries, namely, a lacerated wound over the left posterior partial region of the head and a fracture of the left upper second incisor tooth involving the pulp and the root. The injuries were caused by a stone. The inevitable conclusion was that a grievous hurt was caused. However, the court felt that it is not that in every case a stone would constitute a dangerous weapon. It would depend upon the facts of the case. The expression 'any instrument which used as a weapon of offence is likely to cause death' has to be gauged, taking note of the heading of the Section. What would constitute a 'dangerous weapon' would depend upon the facts of each case and no generalization can be made. The heading of the Section provides some insight into the factors to be considered. The essential ingredients to attract Sec. 326 IPC are: (1) voluntarily causing a hurt; (2) hurt caused must be a grievous hurt; and (3) the grievous hurt must have been caused by dangerous weapons or means. As was noted by the Supreme Court in State of UP vs. Indrajeet alias Sukhatha, there is no such thing as a regular or earmarked weapon for committing murder or for that matter a hurt.[35] It is not that in every case a stone would constitute a dangerous weapon. It would depend upon the facts of the case. The facts involved in a particular case, depending upon various factors like size, sharpness, would throw light on the question whether the weapon was a dangerous or deadly weapon or not. In the instant case, considering the size of the stone which was used, as revealed by material on record, it cannot be said that a dangerous weapon was used.

The expression 'an instrument which used as a weapon of offence is likely to cause death' should be construed with reference to the nature of the instrument and not the manner of its use (Supreme Court of India, Anwarul Haq vs. State of UP).[36]

The mere fact that it is a stone or that it is a granite stone is not sufficient in the absence of better evidence to conclude that the said weapon was a dangerous weapon under Sec. 324 IPC (Kerala High Court, Chandran vs. State of Kerala).[37]

Deadly Weapon

In some other more serious offences, the expression 'deadly weapon', has been used like for e.g., in Secs. 397 and 398 IPC. Deadly weapon, however, has not been defined in Indian law. The facts involved in a particular case, depending upon various factors like size, or sharpness of the weapon would throw light on the question whether it was a dangerous or deadly weapon or not.

A deadly weapon is usually defined as a firearm or any object designed, made or adapted for the purposes of inflicting death or serious physical injury, i.e. weapons which can kill.[38] This includes, not only weapons which are intended to do harm like a gun or knife, but also blunt instruments like clubs, baseball bats, monkey wrenches, an automobile or any object which actually causes death.

INFORMING POLICE ABOUT CASES OF TRAUMA

There is some confusion amongst doctors on whether they should inform the police when they are treating an injured person, if the person does not consent for intimation of his injuries to the police. What action can be taken against the doctors if they fail to do so? In this regard, some relevant sections of the Indian law are discussed below.

Sec. 39 CrPC (Public to give information of certain offences)
This section has twelve sub-sections, out of which sub-section 5 relates to offences affecting life. The relevant section is reproduced below.

- Every person, aware of the commission of or of the intention of any other person to commit any offence punishable under any of the following sections of the Indian Penal Code (45 of 1860), namely:

----

v. Secs. 302, 303 and 304 (i.e. to say, offences affecting life).

When offences affecting life occur, i.e. injuries which can kill a person are present, the doctor has to inform the police as this is a requirement of Sec. 39 CrPC.

Sec. 176 IPC (Omission to give notice or information to public servant by person legally bound to give it)
Whoever, *being legally bound to give* any notice, or to furnish information on any subject to any public servant as such, intentionally omits to give such notice or to furnish such information in the manner and at the time required by law, shall be punished with simple imprisonment for a term which may extend to one month, or with fine which may extend to ₹ 500, or with both; or, if the notice or information required to be given respects the commission of an offence or is required for the purpose of preventing the commission of an offence or in order to the apprehension of an offender, with simple imprisonment for a term which may extend to six months or with fine which may extend to ₹ 1000, or with both.

Sec. 201 IPC (Causing disappearance of evidence of offence, or giving false information to screen offender)
Whoever, knowing or having reason to believe that an offence has been committed, causes any evidence of the commission of that offence to disappear with the intention of screening the offender from legal punishment or with that intention gives any information respecting the offence which he knows or believes to be false,

a. If a capital offence—and if the offence which he knows or believes to have been committed is punishable with death, shall be punished with imprisonment of either description for a term which may extend to seven years, and shall also be liable to fine.
b. If punishable with imprisonment for life—and if the offence is punishable with imprisonment for life, or with imprisonment which may extend to ten years, shall be punished with imprisonment of either description for a term which may extend to three years, and shall also be liable to fine.
c. If punishable with less than ten years' imprisonment—and if the offence is punishable with imprisonment for any term not extending to ten years, shall be punished with imprisonment of the description provided for the offence, for a term which may extend to one-fourth part of the longest term of the imprisonment provided for the offence or with fine or with both.

Sec. 202 IPC (Intentional omission to give information of offence by person bound to inform)
Whoever, knowing or having reason to believe that an offence has been committed, intentionally omits to give any information respecting that offence

which he is legally bound to give, shall be punished with imprisonment of either description for a term which may extend to six months or with fine or with both.

Comments

Assuming that the prosecution has not positively proved that the death was homicidal, yet from the medical evidence, it is clear that it was not a natural death, and consequently, the death should at least be noted as one of suicide. Even in the cause of suicide, an offence of abetment punishable under Sec. 306 is inherent. Therefore, even in the case of suicide, there is an obligation on the person who knows or has reason to believe that such a suicidal death has occurred, to give information (Bhagwan Swarup vs. State of Rajasthan, 1991).[39]

The words 'which he is legally bound to give' play a major role in interpreting these sections. Section 43 IPC states that the word 'illegal' is applicable to everything which is an offence or which is prohibited by law or which furnishes ground for civil action; and a person is said to be 'legally bound to do' whatever it is illegal for him to omit. Persons legally bound to furnish information are, for e.g. the police, village headman, village accountant, owner or occupier of land and head of family. The public are under legal obligation to inform for certain offences specified under Sec. 39 CrPC. Experts feel that Secs. 176 and 202 IPC do not put any legal binding on the doctors to inform. Legally, the doctor is not duty bound to inform the matter to the police, unless the patient or her relatives express their desire to do so or if the police seeks information about a particular case. However, we are duty bound to keep complete detail records of such cases including all the investigation reports, the samples taken, if any, and the clinical records. In case, at a future date, if any authority (either police or judiciary) asks for these documents, then we are duty bound to handover the copies of these documents to the concerned authority and support the criminal investigation process. *However, many hospitals argue that they are duty bound to notify the police of all medicolegal cases, even though there is no legal provision explicitly stating which cases must be recorded as medicolegal cases.*[40]

Some experts feel that doctors are still responsible under Sec. 202 IPC to inform the police. They have voiced a fear that, if doctors do not inform the police, then Sec. 201 IPC may be used by the police against the doctors, as it may be said that they have caused disappearance of evidence. But, by keeping detailed records of the cases, where the police have not been informed, including all the investigation reports, preservation of samples, if any, and the clinical records, the concern of this section of experts can be addressed.

It is evident that the above sections of IPC regarding intimation to the police are interpreted by different legal luminaries, doctors and judiciary in different ways. Varied opinions have been expressed in this regard, and every individual case will have to be treated on its merits as no blanket rule can be followed. What the doctor should do in such cases still needs discussion and debate, and the opinions expressed above should not be interpreted as a statement of fact.

Recently, an amendment to Criminal Procedure Code has brought some clarity to this issue (Box 10.3). It has now been specified that for certain offences, the police have to be informed of the incident. Therefore, for injuries falling under Sec. 326A IPC, the police have to be informed. However, does Sec. 357C IPC apply

Box 10.3 Intimation to police of certain offences

In April 2013, an amendment to Sec. 357 of the CrPC titled Sec. 357C was introduced which states that 'all hospitals public or private whether run by the central government, the state government, local bodies or any other person should immediately provide the first aid or medical treatment free of cost to the victims of any offence covered under Secs. 326A, 376, 376A, 376B, 376C, 376D and 376E of the IPC, and should immediately inform the police of such incident'. Denial of treatment of rape victims is punishable under Sec. 166B IPC with imprisonment for a term which may extend to one year or with fine or with both. *In this section, it has been stated that the hospitals are to inform the police of incidents/ offences falling under these sections of the IPC.*

One of these sections involves trauma and has been introduced in the IPC in 2013. This is Sec. 326A IPC and it states—'Whoever causes permanent or partial damage or deformity to, or burns or maims or disfigures or disables any part or parts of the body of a person or causes grievous hurt by throwing acid on or by administering acid to that person or by using any other means with the intention of causing or with the knowledge that he is likely to cause such injury or hurt, shall be punished with imprisonment of either description for a term which shall not be less than ten years but which may extend to imprisonment for life and with fine'.

only to hospitals or also to doctors treating patients in their own clinics? This point will need further clarification.

CONCLUSION

India is a common law country. Common law refers to law and the corresponding legal system developed through decisions of courts, rather than through legislative statutes. When there is no authoritative statement of the law, Judges have the authority and duty to make law by creating precedent. The body of precedent is called 'common law' and it binds future decisions. Issues, on which no law exists or clarity is lacking, court judgments are taken as precedent for future judgments.

Grievous hurt is a legal definition and not a medical one. The doctor should not be expected to keep abreast of all the legal judgments which have been delivered in this regard. Therefore, when the doctor is not sure whether to label an injury as simple or grievous, it is best that he refrains from giving such opinion and just sticks to the presentation of medical facts so that the courts can give a final opinion. Similarly, when opining on whether an injury endangers life or not, if the doctor feels that the case will require opinion of the field/speciality in which the injury falls, it is best left to the expert of that field (specialist) to give an opinion in this regard.

Burn injuries is an example in which some doctors apply 40% TBSA burns as yardstick for all people for classifying injuries endangering life and thus grievous hurt. This is erroneous, as an expert would know that the age of the patient, body surface area involved and presence of inhalational injury are factors affecting the severity of the burn injuries, and thus, the prognosis in such cases (in many cases, burns of less than 40% TBSA may be grievous). They all have to be taken into account for assessing what burns are endangering life and what are not.

For injuries to the skull leading to brain hamatoma, diffuse axonal injury, brainstem injury, concussion or brain edema, the opinion of neurosurgeon should be taken regarding the nature of injuries. Similar would be the case for other injuries involving different specialities of medicine. Hence, an ophthalmologist, orthopedician or surgeon, as the case maybe, would be proper persons to give such opinions.

It is also not necessary that opinion regarding nature of injury be given when patient is initially examined. In some conditions, the patient may need to be followed up so that some manifestations of injury appearing after a period of time can be ascertained. An example is retinal detachment appearing some time after injury.

As grievous injury is a legal definition and not a medical one, the law in India regarding grievous injury needs further clarity to remove the confusion which sometimes arises. Doctors can then opine based on the legal requirements of the law. Whenever the doctor is not sure about the nature of the injury, he/she should stick to the medical facts of the injuries and leave it to the honorable courts to form a final opinion.

REFERENCES

1. Ram Swaroop & Ors. vs. State of U.P., AIR 2000 SC 715, 2000 (1) ALD Cri 457.
2. Thefreedictionary.com [homepage on the internet]. [cited 2012 July 14]. Available from: http://www.thefreedictionary.com/injury.
3. Medical-dictionary.the freedictionary.com [homepage on the internet]. [cited 2012 July 14]. Available from: http://medical-dictionary.thefreedictionary.com/Wounds+and+injuries.
4. Indian Penal Code, 1860.
5. Rajwant vs. State of Kerala. AIR 1966 SC 1874.
6. Rayavarpu Punayya vs. State of Andhra Pradesh. AIR 1977 SC 45.
7. Thefreedictionary.com [homepage on the internet]. [cited 2012 July 14]. Available from:
http://www.thefreedictionary.com/emasculate
8. Wbhealth.gov.in [homepage on the internet]. Kolkata: Department of Health and Family Welfare, Government of West Bengal. [cited 2012 July 14]. Available from: http://www.wbhealth.gov.in/mental/Acts_Rules/Person_Disabilities.pdf.
9. AIIMS docs get a clean chit. The Times of India. 2009 Jan 7. [cited 2012 July 14]. Available from: http://articles.timesofindia.indiatimes.com/2009-01-07/delhi/28014595_1_medical -report-clean-chit-doctors#ixzz1FDtafNhj.
10. Safeworkaustralia.gov.au [homepage on the internet]. Canberra: Safework Australia. [cited 2012 July 14]. Available from: http://www.safeworkaustralia.gov.au/sites/SWA/about/Publications/Documents/208/TypeOfOccur-renceClassificationSystem_3rdEdition_2004_PDF.pdf.
11. Gorea RK, Garg A, Aggarwal AD. Traumatic dislocation of implanted joint. *Medicolegal Update* 2005; 5: 53.
12. Allen Charlie Akaran vs. State of Alaska. [cited 2012 July 14]. Available from: http://www.lexisone.com/lx1/caselaw/freecaselaw?action= OCLGetCaseDetail&format=FULL&sourceID=beehde&searchTerm=eHdL.eEca.aadj.edUQ&searchFlag=y&l1loc=FCLOW.
13. Mathiharan K, Patnaik AK (eds). Modi's textbook of medical jurisprudence and toxicology. 23rd edn. New Delhi: Lexis Nexis Butterworths; 2005. p. 745.
14. Karmakar RN (ed). JB Mukherji's Forensic Medicine and Toxicology. 3rd edn. Kolkata: Academic publishers; 2007. p. 321.
15. Po Yi Maung vs. Ma E Tin, AIR 1937 Rang 253.
16. Mutukdhari Singh vs. Emperor, AIR 1942 Pat 376.
17. Kalya and Ors. vs. The State, 1955 CriLJ 579.
18. Parma vs. The State, AIR 1956 Raj 39, 1956 CriLJ 270.

19. Mokkasamy vs. Unknown, Madras High Court, 1965 CriLJ 48.
20. Hori Lal and Anr vs. State of UP, AIR 1969, 1970 SCR (2) 237.
21. Subash Chandra Panda and Ors. vs. State, 1994 CriLJ 1429.
22. Atma Singh vs. State of Punjab, Punjab-Haryana High Court, 1980 CriLJ 1226.
23. Jagrup Singh's vs. State of Punjab, 1973 Chand LR (Cri) 253 (Punj).
24. Harbans Singh vs. The State of Punjab, Crl. Appeal No, 1007 of 1975 (1979).
25. Judis.nic.in [homepage on the internet]. New Delhi: Supreme Court of India [cited 2012 July 14]. Available from: http://judis.nic.in/supremecourt/imgs1.aspx?filename=29149.
26. Jai Narain Mishra vs. State of Bihar, AIR 1972 SC 1764, 1973 (0) BLJR 241, 1972 Cri LJ 469.
27. Shivalingaiah vs. State of Karnataka, (1988) Cr LJ 394: AIR 1988 SC (115).
28. Abdul Sajid Abdul Sadiq vs. State of Maharashtra. Bombay High Court, 2003 (4) MhLj 306.
29. Sharma D, Mathur PN, Saini OP. Ocular injury and its medicolegal implications. *J Indian Acad Forensic Med* 2008; 30: 227-30.
30. American Burn Association. National Burn Repository 2009. Version 5.0. [cited 2012 July 14]. Available from: www.ameriburn.org/2009NBRAnnual Report.pdf.
31. Ryan CM, Schoenfeld DA, Thorpe WP, Sheridan RL, Cassem EH, Tompkins RG. Objective estimates of the probability of death from burn injuries. *N Engl J Med* 1998; 338: 362-66.
32. Osler T, Glance LG, Hosmer DW. Simplified estimates of the probability of death after burn injuries: extending and updating the Baux score. *J Trauma* 2010; 68: 690-97.
33. Yourdictionary.com [homepage on the internet]. Webster's new world *law dictionary* [cited 2012 July 14]. Available from: http://www.yourdictionary.com/weapon.
34. Indiakanoon.org [homepage on the internet] [cited 2012 July 14]. Available from: http://indiankanoon.org/doc/1043893/.
35. Indiakanoon.org [homepage on the internet] [cited 2012 July 14]. Available from: http://indiankanoon.org/doc/724729/.
36. Indiakanoon.org [homepage on the internet] [cited 2012 July 14]. Available from: http://indiankanoon.org/doc/1522453/.
37. Indiakanoon.org [homepage on the internet] [cited 2012 July 14]. Available from: http://indiankanoon.org/doc/1486547/.
38. Uslegal.com [homepage on the internet] [cited 2013 October 31]. United States: US Legal, Inc. Available from: http://definitions.uslegal.com/d/deadly-weapon/.
39. Bhagwan Swarup vs. State of Rajasthan, (1991) Cr LJ 3123 (3133) (SC).
40. Jagadeesh N. Legal changes towards justice for sexual assault victims. *Ind J Med Ethics* 2010; 7: 108-12.

An Approach to a Case of Poisoning

Sandeep Puri

*'All things are poison and nothing is without poison.
It is the dose only that makes a thing not a poison.'*
Paracelsus (Swiss German physician and alchemist)

ABSTRACT

Poisoning is a significant public health problem worldwide. Acute poisoning (fatal and non-fatal poisonings) is one of the most common reasons for visiting emergency department. Knowledge of the epidemiology of poisoning is important to the emergency physicians so that it is helpful in planning rational use of resources for the management, prevention and research of poisoning. It is also essential that they have rapid access to toxicological information and diagnostic facilities.

Acute pesticide poisoning from suicidal, occupational, accidental and intentional exposure is a major problem in the developing world. Self-poisoning is the most common method in women and the second most common method in men attempting suicide. In developed countries, poisoning exposure has mostly been associated with medicines, alcohol and household chemicals.

A case of suspected poisoning may present with variable features including abdominal pain, vomiting, tremors, altered mental status, seizures, cardiac dysrhythmias and respiratory depression. These may be the only clues to diagnosis when the cause of toxicity is unknown at the time of initial assessment and management. Many conditions may mimic these signs and symptoms of poisoning, including seizures, alcohol intoxication, stroke and insulin reaction. Sometimes, symptoms of poisoning can take time to develop. One should suspect poisoning if someone suddenly becomes sick for no apparent reason.

Detailed history of poison (what, how much, how, when, why and what else) should be taken. The approach should be in methodological manner with characterizing toxidromes and managing accordingly. Vitals need to be monitored with basic ABCs, decontamination, antidote, supportive care and elimination. Factors generally associated with unfavorable prognosis are unstable vital signs (including decreased consciousness, shock, respiratory distress, abnormal heart rate and abnormal body temperature), history of major disease and old age.

Samples should be taken, packaged and sealed appropriately and sent to the forensic science laboratory with suitable storage through this process. The nature and amount of sample is a critical determinant of methods to choose for proper toxicological analysis. Reports provided by the toxicologist may be introduced as evidence in a court of law. The treating physician is sometimes asked to interpret and substantiate their findings and any associated opinions. This chapter discusses the various issues related to poisoning since it is necessary that the medical practitioner be thoroughly knowledgeable and familiar with legal issues surrounding a poisoning case and be professionally comfortable in a court room environment.

Keywords: Toxicology, common poisons, manner of poisoning, diagnosis of poison, interpretation of toxicology results, analysis of poison.

INTRODUCTION

Poisoning and overdoses are common forms of deliberate self-harm worldwide. Although, suicidal intent is often far lower than for self-immolation and hanging, the mortality rate is high due to toxicity of the poisons used and poor medical care. Patients generally present with varying degree of signs and symptoms in emergency and it can be challenging for the medical officer.[1] The final outcome in a poisoning case depends on type of poison consumed, lethality, amount consumed and medical care available.

In most patients, the point of first contact is with the emergency department at the primary health care or the hospital, and the initial toxicology is done at the hospital laboratory. The hospital laboratories are generally not equipped to perform full forensic toxicology screens, hence, many potential poisonings are misdiagnosed. Unfortunately, in many cases the samples for toxicological testing from the initial hospital admission are either of insufficient quantity, are destroyed or are never collected by police personnel, so, follow-up testing is never there. The actual analysis is performed in a forensic science laboratory in few cases only.

Results of toxicology testing may assist the courts in establishing the truth, either by providing evidence of presence of poison/drug or by absence of it. Allegations of drugging prior to rape or robbery may be refuted or confirmed. The rape victim may have been given drugs by the assailant to reduce consciousness and memory. An opinion as to whether the individual was telling the truth or lying can be of value to the police/court. There is a good chance of checking the truth of statements provided that a blood or urine sample is taken within about 12 hours of the incident. Nowadays, testing methods are sensitive to nanogram amounts of drugs and hence it may be detected in blood. Sometimes, drug use is often suspected, but can only be confirmed by testing.[2,3]

This chapter discusses the common poisons encountered, signs and symptoms, diagnostic tests and medicolegal issues that may arise in subsequent court proceedings (Box 11.1).[2-5]

DEFINITIONS

Some of the definitions which a medical practitioner should be familiar with:[1-2,5-7]

- **Poison:** It is a substance (solid, liquid or gaseous) which if introduced in the living body or brought into contact with any part thereof will produce ill health or death by its constitutional or local effects or both. It can be any substance, including medications, that is harmful to our body if too much is taken, inhaled, injected or absorbed through the skin. Thus, almost anything is a poison.

Box 11.1 Questions a medical practitioner may need to answer

- Whether poisoning is the cause of his/her condition?
- What is the identity of the poison or the offending substance?
- How was it administered? (the route and mode of entry)
- When the poison/drug was administered?
- What are its effects?
- Was it ingested acutely or cumulatively?
- If multiple substances are detected, do they possess additive or synergistic toxic activity?
- Was it a dangerous or lethal amount?
- Was ingestion accidental or intentional?
- Whether there is unlawful poisoning by a third party?
- Whether the presence of the toxin/drug may affect a person's behaviors or ability to make rational/ reasoned judgment?
- Whether performance-enhancing drugs were used by the individual?
- Whether the individual used drugs in the workplace? Is this person taking an illegal substance?
- Whether parents consumed drugs in alleged history of abuse of children (in some countries)?

In law, the real difference between a medicine and a poison is the intent with which it is given. If the substance is given with the intention to save life, it is a medicine, but if it is given with intention to cause bodily harm, it is a poison. The law does not make any difference between murder by means of poisons or by any other means.

- **Toxicology:** It is the branch of science that deals with properties, actions, toxicity, detection, estimation, treatment and fatal dose in relation to the poisonous substances.
- **Toxidrome:** A toxidrome or toxic syndrome is a constellation of clinical examination findings that assists in the diagnosis and treatment of the patient who presents with an exposure to an unknown agent.
- **Clinical toxicology:** It is primarily concerned with the identification of poisons and drugs as an aid to the diagnosis and treatment of acute and chronic poisoning. It is done by examining and evaluating the signs and symptoms of the patient and analyzing the specimens collected. As a result, the proper course of treatment is taken.
- **Forensic toxicology:** It is the application of knowledge of poisons and drugs to the elucidation of questions that occur in judicial proceedings. It involves not only the analysis, identification and quantifying of a poison or drug in biological specimens (fluids and tissues), but also the ability to interpret the results of analysis. It must be correlated with the circumstances of the case to determine what role, if any, the detected substances played.

  The difference between the clinical toxicologist and the forensic toxicologist is the judicial element.
- **Hospital toxicology:** It is concerned with individuals admitted to hospital with suspected poisoning, and its prime aim is to assist in the treatment of the patient.
- **Postmortem toxicology:** It investigates the role of poisons and drugs in causing or contributing to the individual's death.

- **Acute poisoning:** It is caused by an excessive single dose or doses of a poison, taken over a short interval of time.
  An acute pesticide poisoning is any illness or health effect resulting from suspected or confirmed exposure to a pesticide within 48 hours. Warfarins, superwarfarins and coumarins are an exception as the onset of symptoms or laboratory findings may be delayed by > 48 hours.
- **Chronic poisoning:** It is caused by smaller doses over a period of time, resulting in gradual worsening, for e.g., poisoning with arsenic, phosphorus, lead and opium.
- **Subacute poisoning:** It shows features of both acute and chronic poisoning.
- **Fulminant poisoning:** It is caused by massive dose of poison where death occurs rapidly, sometimes without preceding symptoms.

Legal provisions

- Sec. 284 IPC states that whoever causes hurt/injury with rash or negligent conduct with respect to poisonous substance shall be punished with imprisonment up to 6 months with/without fine (up to ₹ 1000).
- Sec. 328 IPC deals with administering of any poison, stupefying or intoxicating agent with the intent to cause hurt and facilitate the commission of an offence. Punishment is imprisonment up to 10 years and fine.

HISTORY

For many centuries, poisoning has been a popular method of homicide. The reasons are that almost any natural substance in the right dose can be poisonous, and many poisons mimic common medical conditions, leading doctors to believe that the victim died of natural causes. Till 1700s, it was very difficult to prove poisoning by scientific evidence. Autopsies were rarely performed and chemical tests were not in vogue. Hence, convictions associated with homicidal poisoning were based only on circumstantial evidence like discoloration of the dead body, poisons found at victim's neighborhood or animal testing, or by confession or by torture, rather than the identification of the actual poison within the victim. In 1781, Joseph Plenic suggested that the detection and identification of poison in the organs of the deceased was the only precise indication of poisoning.[5,8-10]

The first person to suggest a chemical method for the detection of poisons was Dr Hermann Boerhaave. His method was relatively crude, consisting of placing substances suspected of containing poison on red-hot coals, then testing for odors. In 1751, the first homicide trial to feature toxicological testimony from medical experts was in England. In this trial, four doctors testified that the victim's 'preserved quality' of the organs at autopsy were suggestive of arsenic poisoning. During that time, arsenic was the most common poison of choice and was known as the 'poison of poisons' and 'inheritance powder', since many relatives used it to eliminate aging patriarch.[8,9]

The origin of modern analytical forensic toxicology is often attributed to a Spanish-born French toxicologist and chemist Mathieu Orfila (also known as the 'Father of Toxicology') who wrote '*Traité des poisons*' or Treatise of General Toxicology in 1814. In it, he summed up all known poisons at that time and suggested classifications. It was his analysis of autopsy materials to identify poisons and the subsequent accounting of such, represented the first systematic approach to the identification of poisons. Orfila in 1840 was also involved in court room toxicological testimony in the trial of Marie Lafarge in France for poisoning her husband to death with arsenic. In 1836, English chemist James Marsh discovered an accurate way to detect arsenic in the body. In 1842, Hugo Reinsch developed the test that 'plates' arsenic onto copper wire, turning it black. This was followed by Max Gutzheit's semiquantitative test in 1879, again involving precipitation of arsenic. This latter test remained a hallmark in arsenic testing for almost 100 years, and all substances of toxicological interest were analyzed via precipitation or plating techniques. Then, instrumental techniques became the norm which offered substantial improvements in selectivity and sensitivity. Today, the field is dominated by instrumental methods, especially mass spectrometric techniques, for e.g., GC-MS (gas chromatography-mass spectrometry), LC-MS (liquid chromatography-mass spectrometry), related tandem mass spectrometric techniques (GC-MS/MS; LC-MS/MS) and ICP-MS.[8-10]

EPIDEMIOLOGY[11-15]

According to World Health Organization, in 2002, an estimated 350,000 people died worldwide from unintentional poisoning.

In 2009, 31,758 (76%) of the 41,592 poisoning deaths in the United States (US) were unintentional (second only to motor vehicle crashes as a cause of unintentional injury for all ages), and 3,349 (8%) were of undetermined intent. In 2010, unintentional poisoning caused about 831,295 emergency department visits, and poison control centers reported receiving calls about 2.4 million human poison exposure cases.

In the United Kingdom, poisoning accounts for an estimated 10–20% of admissions and 5–10% of the workload of emergency department. Episodes of self-poisoning are on the rise, with the rates being the highest in Europe.

The most commonly encountered poisons in emergency set-up are pesticides, pharmaceuticals, drugs of abuse and ethanol (alcohol).[4] Medicines and house hold products are also common and important causes of morbidity. There is also a possibility of poisoning with a wide range of other compounds including volatile substances, rodenticides or insecticides, metals and anions and natural toxins. Type of poison consumed varies in different regions depending on availability of pesticides or drugs, cost and addiction.

Pesticides

Pesticide self-poisoning is the single largest cause of acute poisoning deaths worldwide (most widespread in rural areas of developing countries). It accounts for 30% of suicides globally, although official data from India underestimates the incidence of suicides. Pesticides are commonly taken in acts of self-poisoning in India, China, Bangladesh, Malaysia, Pakistan, Nepal, Sri Lanka and South Korea. The proportion of all suicides using pesticides varies from 4% in the European Region to over 50% in the Western Pacific Region. This proportion is not concordant with the volume of pesticides sold in each region; it is in the pattern of pesticide use and the toxicity of the products, not the quantity used that influences the likelihood they will be used in acts of self-harm.

Most common cause of lethal pesticides self-poisoning worldwide are WHO toxicity class I and II organophosphorus (OP) insecticides. Unintentional oral or dermal exposure to WHO Class I OP pesticides can cause severe poisoning but the doses are usually lesser than with intentional poisoning, resulting in fewer deaths. WHO Class II OPs are generally less toxic in unintentional poisoning and less likely to cause severe poisoning. Class II OPs are highly toxic in intentional overdose. Other classes of pesticide that are common causes of significant and/or fatal poisoning include carbamate (less toxic than OP pesticides) and organochlorine insecticides, the fumigant aluminum phosphide (mortality rate of 59–70%) and the herbicide paraquat. Less common causes of significant poisoning include the herbicides chlorphenoxy acetic acid derivatives and propanil, some pyrethroid insecticides, avermectins and amitraz.

Thallium containing rodenticides (banned in the US) are still used in some tropical countries and accidental poisonings are common. Self-poisoning cases with propanil, an aromatic anilide herbicide have been reported from Sri Lanka. Pyrethrins self-poisoning have been reported from India and Sri Lanka.

Medicines

Medicines are used throughout the developed and developing world's cities for self-harm. In general, they cause few deaths compared to pesticides. Chloroquine is an exception to this rule.

Central nervous system (CNS) acting drugs are most commonly used for self-harm throughout the developing world cities. In most case studies, barbiturates were most commonly found, followed by benzodiazepines, antidepressants and antiepileptics. Of the analgesic drugs, paracetamol (acetaminophen) is a common poison in some regions of the developing and developed world. Salicylates have been reported as common causes of childhood poisoning.

Chloroquine has been used for self-poisoning in parts of Africa, Asia and Pacific. Quinine is used for self-harm in Europe. Dapsone was reported as common cause of accidental poisoning in children in India, with few cases of deliberate self-poisoning.

Herbal or Traditional Medicines

Traditional medicines are mostly of plant origin but may incorporate mineral or animal products. Traditional medicines are a common cause of accidental poisoning but a rare cause of intentional self-poisoning.

Households Products

Household products including kerosene oil (most common), dettol, bleach and strong acids, such as sulphuric acid are commonly reported. Some cases involving hair dye (paraphenylenediamine), traditional hair remover containing arsenic sulphide and calcium oxide, or barium sulphide and potassium permanganate have been reported.

Corrosives

Corrosives are used widely in industry and the home. Self-poisoning with hydrochloric and sulphuric acid is a major problem in Taiwan, Morocco and India.

Industrial Chemicals

Copper sulphate has been used for self-harm in South Asia. Other chemicals that have been used for self-poisoning include potassium cyanide, turpentine, chromic acid and ethylene bromide in India.

Plants

Poisonous plants, such as yellow oleander, thorn apple (*Datura stramonium*), oduvan (*Cleistanthus collinus*) and superb lily (*Gloriosa superba*) are used for homicide, suicide and inducing abortion.

Drugs

The most commonly abused drugs are methamphetamine, amphetamine, cocaine, marijuana, opiate narcotics (morphine, codeine and heroin), phencyclidine (PCP), lysergic acid diethylamide (LSD) and methylenedioxymethamphetamine (MDMA, 'ecstasy').[3,16]

APPROACH TO A SUSPECTED CASE OF POISONING

The initial approach to the poisoned patient is basically similar in every case, irrespective of the toxin, just like the initial approach to the trauma patient management, irrespective of the mechanism of injury. It starts with initial evaluation and stabilization followed by a thorough evaluation to identify the agent(s) involved and assessment of the severity of exposure. The possibility of concomitant trauma or illness must be recognized and addressed before initiation of decontamination.

The sections that follow give an overview of some of the most common classes of poisons or drugs that may be encountered in the emergency with a flow chart of the general approach to the poisoned patient.

Clinical Presentation

The emergency medical officer needs to be familiar with signs of poisoning because patients may present with symptoms which he/she may attribute to some organic disorder or disease, although the patient has been exposed to poisons.[4] The clinical presentation of occult ingestion varies, depending upon the type and amount of ingested poison or drug, and can range from asymptomatic to critically ill. One should suspect poisoning if there is an acute onset of multiorgan system dysfunction, abdominal pain, vomiting, altered mental status (alteration of sensorium and orientation), respiratory depression, cardiac dysrhythmias, unexplained metabolic acidosis, seizures or there are unusual symptoms, and a definite diagnosis of a specific disease cannot be made.[17] In literature, there are well documented instances of failure by clinicians to suspect poisoning when it was otherwise.

History

History in suspected case of poisoning is of paramount importance not only for medically managing the patient but also from legal point of view. In some cases, there may be useful history regarding ingestion or exposure to particular substances present in the home, workplace or local environment which can help. This often yields clues as to what the cause of toxicity might be, and therefore, suggest which tests should be performed as a priority.

History should be quick and focused (Box 11.2).[2,4-6,18,19] An attempt must be made to obtain as much information about the patient as possible. As far as possible, history should be taken from the patient, close relative or eye witness. The history should include not only the clinical picture but also any previous medical history, details of drugs or other substances to which the patient may have had access, and in cases of accidental poisoning, substances to which the patient may have been exposed. Reliability of history should be assessed and facts corroborated.

Physical Examination

If the patient is unstable, detailed physical examination may not be possible. Once the patient is stable, a comprehensive physical examination can reveal signs of specific poison.

Identification of Poison from Clinical Features

Specific clinical manifestations, examination of the vital parameters like body temperature, pulse rate, blood pressure and respiratory rate, and systemic examination can provide clues to the nature of poison consumed and help in the differential diagnosis (Tables 11.1 and 11.2).[6,7]

Neurological examination is extremely important in a suspected poisoned patient, particularly if patient has presented with altered mental status. Seizures are a common presentation of variety of drug and toxin overdoses. Table 11.3 illustrates the abnormal neurological features due to certain poisons.[20]

Box 11.2 Details of history

- Type or nature of toxin(s)
- Time and place of exposure
- How much taken (quantity)? (tablet, bottles or syringes found near the body should be submitted)
- Route of administration (i.e. ingestion, intravenous, inhalation, dermal)
- What are the dominant symptoms? What systemic features are present?
- Why has the exposure occurred (accidental, suicidal, euphoria, iatrogenic)
- Date and time when last seen in normal health
- Date and time of illness and where found (at work , in bed, outdoors)
- Time and details of last meal
- Any relationship between food or medicine taken and the toxic manifestations
- History of all drugs taken, for e.g. vitamins, herbal medications, over-the-counter drugs
- Occupation history of patient (detail of end-product of factory or firm)
- Any recent foreign travel?
- Whether patient was given treatment in some other hospital? Details.
- History of psychiatric illness or previous suicide attempts
- Whether there is a family history regarding psychiatric illness?
- Any other information that could be useful such as pregnancy, comments made by the patient, witnesses or suspect, details of suspect

Table 11.1 Clinical features associated with poisoning

Vitals	Poisoning suspected
Hyperthermia	Cocaine, lysergic acid diethylamide (LSD), methylene dioxymethamphetamine (MDMA), nicotine, antihistamines, salicylates, sympathomimetics, anticholinergics, antidepressants or antipsychotics
Hypothermia	Carbon monoxide, opioids, oral hypoglycemics, insulin, alcohol or sedative-hypnotics
Bradycardia	Opiates, physostigmine, anticholinesterase drugs, ethanol or digoxin
Tachycardia	Anticholinergics, antihistaminics, antipsychotics or sympathomimetics
Hypertension	Cocaine, anticholinergics, amphetamine, nicotine, sympathomimetics or caffeine
Hypotension	Rodenticides, heroin, opiates, sedative-hypnotics, antidepressants or antihypertensives
Rapid respiration	Paraquat or nerve agents
Slow respiration	Sedative-hypnotics, alcohol, opioids, barbiturates or salicylates (hypoventilation)
Miosis	Opiates, organophosphates, sedative-hypnotics, cholinergics, pilocarpine or phenothiazines
Mydriasis	Atropine (datura), amphetamines, cocaine, sympathomimetics or anticholinergics
Lacrimation, nystagmus	Alcohol or phenytoin

Table 11.2 Systemic examination and poison suspected

System	Poisoning suspected
Nose	Nasal septum complications (cocaine)
Kidneys	Rhabdomyolysis (ethanol, quinine, heroin, colchicine or chlorophenoxy acids)
Chest	Radiography (metals)
Abdomen	Diarrhea (organophosphates) Obstruction (opiates, sympatholytics such as atropine) Radiography (lead, thallium, condoms packed with illicit drugs)

Differential Diagnosis of Coma

It may be difficult to suspect a case as poisoning simply on the basis of clinical examination when circumstantial evidence is lacking, since coma induced by poisons and drugs is not readily differentiated from that caused by disease conditions. Some conditions that mimic the signs and symptoms of poisoning includes hypoglycemic coma, cerebrovascular accident, brain damage, meningitis, exhaustion (after seizures), withdrawal symptoms, allergic reactions (shock) and viral infections. In these situations, toxicological analyses is

Table 11.3 Neurological features and possible poisoning/overdoses

Appearance	*Poisoning suspected*
Restlessness, agitation or seizures	Amphetamines, cocaine, lysergic acid diethylamide (LSD), overdose or withdrawal of opiates or ethanol, organophosphates, oral hypoglycemics, tricyclic antidepressants, insulin, salicylates, sympathomimetics, anticholinergics or lithium
Drowsiness, coma	Ethanol, heroin, lead, insulin, carbon monoxide, organic solvents, cyanide, antidepressants, anticonvulsants, antipsychotics, lithium or heavy metals
Disturbances in: motor functions	Alcohol or benzodiazepines
speech	Alcohol or drugs of abuse
movement disorders	Cocaine, amphetamines, hallucinogens, butyrophenones or ethylene glycol

useful either to confirm poisoning as the cause of coma or to rule it out in favor of an organic disorder that requires alternative investigations.[6]

Other Indicative Features

Some poisons have characteristic odors that may be detected on the patient's body, clothes, breath and samples of vomit which may help to identify the nature of poisoning. Characteristic odor produced by certain commonly used poison is given in Table 11.4.[6,7,21] Changes in skin can also be useful indicator to reveal the type of poisoning (Table 11.5).[6] However, these clues should be interpreted with caution and are not a substitute for proper toxicological evaluation.

Some poisons may produce a collection of symptoms (toxidromes) that can assist in making diagnosis and also useful for anticipating other symptoms that may occur. Table 11.6 enumerates the symptoms seen in such toxic syndromes which need to be carefully elucidated in any suspected case of poisoning.[1,17,20]

Some features of other commonly encountered poisons or drugs:[17,22]

1. **Aluminum phosphide**: The symptoms produced usually involve the cardiovascular and respiratory systems. Symptoms include irritability, restlessness, drowsiness, tremors, parasthesia, vertigo, diplopia, ataxia, cough, dyspnea, retrosternal pain, abdominal pain and vomiting. Patient may have hypotension, tachycardia, oliguria, anuria, cyanosis, pulmonary edema, tachypnea and seizures. *No specific antidote* is available. Treatment is symptomatic.
2. **Rodenticide poisoning**: Many poisons can be used as rodenticides.
   i. Anticoagulants like warfarin present with various hemorrhagic manifestations, prolonged prothrombin, partial thromboplastin and thrombin time with normal fibrinogen, fibrin degradation products and platelets.
   ii. ANTU (α-Naphthylthiourea): Poisoning produces local gastric irritation, vomiting, hypersalivation, pulmonary edema, ataxia, tachycardia and subnormal temperature.

Table 11.4 Odors associated with poisoned patients

Odors	*Potential agents or situation suspected*
Garlic	Arsenic, malathion, parathion, yellow phosphorus, aluminum phosphide or zinc phosphide (phosphine)
Kerosene-like/petrol	Organophosphorus or other pesticide formulation
Nail polish remover/ acetone	Propanol, toluene, aromatic hydrocarbon sniffing or metabolic acidosis
Fruity	Ethanol (except vodka), cleaners or esters
Ammonia	Ammonia
Bitter almonds, silver polish	Cyanide
Phenolic	Disinfectants, cresols or phenols
Formaldehyde	Formaldehyde or methanol
Foul	Bromides or lithium
Hemp, burnt rope	Marijuana
Mothballs	Camphor or naphthalene
Smoke	Nicotine or carbon monoxide
Organic solvents, sweet	Diethyl ether, chloroform or dichloromethane
Peanuts	Rodenticide
Rotten eggs	Disulfiram, hydrogen sulfide or hepatic failure
Turpentine	Turpentine, wax, solvent of parathion or polish

Table 11.5 Skin changes and poisoning

Skin signs	*Poisoning suspected*
Dry	Anticholinergics, antihistamines, tricyclic antidepressants or parasympatholytics
Perspiration	Organophosphates, acetylsalicylic acid, cocaine or parasympathomimetics
Gooseflesh	Strychnine, lysergic acid diethylamide (LSD) or opiates withdrawal
Needle marks	Parenteral injections: drugs of abuse or insulin
Color	• Red: Anticholinergics, boric acid or carbon monoxide • Blue: Nitrates, nitrites, aniline dyes or ergotamine • Yellow (jaundice): Liver damage (alcohol, borate, nitrites, mushrooms, metals, paracetamol, phosphorus or solvents) • Black, necrosis: Sulfuric acid or burning
Blisters, rash or bullae	Paraquat or barbiturates

Table 11.6 Toxidromes

Toxidrome	*Clinical features*	*Common poisons*	*Treatment*
Sympathomimetic (Stimulant)	Hypertension, tachycardia, pyrexia, pupillary dilatation, diaphoresis and occasionally altered mental status	Cocaine or amphetamines	Benzodiazepines
Cholinergic (Organophosphate and carbamates)	Bradycardia, respiratory depression and pinpoint pupils SLUGE [salivation, lacrimation, urination, defecation, gastrointestinal (GI) distress and emesis] CNS: seizures and coma Muscle: fasciculations and paralysis Decreased oxygen saturations on pulse oximetry	DDT, parathion, malathion or diazinon	Atropine Pralidoxime (for organophosphate insecticides)
Anticholinergic (Antimuscarinic syndrome)	Tachycardia, hyperthermia (mild to severe), agitation, delirium, seizures, mydriasis, dry and flushed skin, urinary retention and decreased intestinal motility	Datura, atropine, scopolamine or antihistamines	Physostigmine
Opiate	Respiratory depression and oxygen desaturations, miosis (except meperidine), decreased GI motility, bradycardia, hypothermia and coma	Morphine, codeine, oxycodone, diacetyl morphine, fentanyl, meperidine, methadone or imidazolines	Naloxone
Sedative hypnotic* (Benzodiazepines)	Sedation or coma, normal vital signs, diplopia, ataxia, impaired motor function, slurred speech, anterograde amnesia, anxiety, hallucinations and delirium	Alprazolam, flunitrazepam, oxazepam or temazepam	Flumazenil

*Benzodiazepine ingestion generally does not develop respiratory compromise (common misconception) but in intravenously administered and severe cases, the patient may present with coma, respiratory depression, hypoxemia, hypotension, bradycardia, cardiac arrest and death.

iii. Bromethalin is a neurotoxin; it causes cerebral edema and posterior paralysis.
iv. Barium containing rodenticide cause headache, weakness, nausea, abdominal pain or shortness of breath.
v. Thallium ingestion may cause acute gastrointestinal distress, anorexia, myalgias, painful neuropathy and hair loss.
vi. Strychnine ingestion may cause anxiety, muscle twitching or facial grimacing.
vii. Zinc phosphide poisoning may cause pulmonary edema.
viii. Arsenic ingestion causes nausea, vomiting, bloody diarrhea and garlic taste in mouth.

3. **Corrosives**: Symptoms of corrosive ingestion depend on type of corrosive, amount and morphologic form of the agent. It causes perforation and necrosis of gastrointestinal tract in acute stages, and later on leads to esophageal stricture, antral stenosis and may even cause esophageal carcinoma. Endoscopy should be done to assess the degree of damage.
4. **Phenol** (carbolic marasmus): It has a corrosive action on mucosa and skin. Symptoms include burning pain and white necrotic lesions in the mouth, esophagus and stomach, vomiting and bloody diarrhea. After skin exposure, there occurs pain, numbness and blanching. Systemic features include headache, dizziness, salivation, hypotension, ventricular arrhythmia, respiratory distress, cyanosis, pallor, seizures, coma, hemolytic anemia and pulmonary edema. Treatment includes activated charcoal/gastric lavage.
5. **Paracetamol poisoning**: It presents initially with nonspecific symptoms (first 24 hours) like vague abdominal pain, nausea, vomiting, pallor and sweating which progress to develop features of acute liver failure later on (3–5 days). Symptoms include hypoglycemia, acidosis, encephalopathy, cerebral edema, sepsis and coagulopathy. Acute kidney failure can also occur. Specific treatment is with N-acetylcysteine.
6. **Salicylate poisoning**: Common symptoms include nausea, vomiting, tinnitus, hyperventilation, hyperactivity, fever, confusion and seizures. In severe cases, rhabdomyolysis, acute renal failure and respiratory failure can occur. Salicylate poisoning is suspected in elderly patients taking aspirin with unexplained altered mental status, tachypnea and fever and unexplained metabolic acidosis. Treatment includes activated charcoal, alkaline diuresis with potassium chloride and hemodialysis in severe cases.
7. **Solvent abuse**: Symptoms include lethargy, confusion, dizziness, headache, restlessness, incoordination, derealization and depersonalization. Common examples are acetone, chlorinated hydrocarbons, naphthalene and trichloroethane.

Biochemical Tests

Biochemical tests that determine the physiological status of the patient are more important in terms of the immediate management of the patient and some of the abnormalities found can also be diagnostic of the type of agent involved (Table 11.7).[6] These, together with the clinical manifestations and history, provide the basis for the order in which the toxicological tests are carried out. The results of biochemical tests are usually available before any toxicological tests have been completed.

Table 11.7 Biochemical and hematological abnormalities in poisoning

Abnormalities	*Indication*
Acid-base disturbances	
Metabolic acidosis	Methanol, ethylene glycol, salicylates, ethanol, cyanide, amphetamines, MDMA or iron
Metabolic alkalosis	Alkali ingestion or chronic use of diuretics or laxatives
Respiratory acidosis	Opiates, barbiturates or tricyclic antidepressants
Respiratory alkalosis	Salicylates (aspirin) or amphetamines
Increased anion gap	Ethylene glycol
Increased osmolar gap	Alcohols or glycols
Electrolyte disturbances	
Hypocalcemia	Ethylene glycol or oxalates
Hyperkalemia	Potassium salts
Hypokalemia	Insulin, oral antidiabetic drugs or chloroquine
Hypernatremia	Sodium chloride or sodium bicarbonate
Hyponatremia	MDMA
Glucose	
Hypoglycemia	Insulin, oral antidiabetic drugs, ethanol (children) or paracetamol (with liver failure)
Liver enzymes	
Raised transaminases	Paracetamol, amphetamines, MDMA, iron, *Amanita phalloides* or strychnine
Hematological	
Anemia, raised zinc protoporphyrin, basophilic stippling	Lead
Carboxyhemoglobin	Carbon monoxide
Methemoglobinemia	Chlorates or nitrites
Raised prothrombin time	Paracetamol or coumarin anticoagulants

However, when the patient's condition is serious and the diagnosis is not clear, toxicological tests may be crucial and the analytical results must be furnished quickly (usually within 1–2 hours of the patient's arrival) if they are to have any bearing on diagnosis and treatment. Ideally, the toxic substance can be both identified and quantified within this time frame. When this is not possible, a qualitative result still has considerable value if the symptoms are consistent with the identified toxin.[6]

Emergency Department Assays

In emergency, following assays should be available:[10,17]

- **Finger stick:** This test should be done in the patient with altered metal status (blood glucose level).

- **Chemistry:** A basic metabolic profile should be done on any patient with suspected poisoning. The importance of this analysis include bicarbonate (low bicarbonate indicates metabolic acidosis) and creatinine levels.
- **Testing for organophosphorus (OP):** If pesticide poisoning is suspected, a test for cholinesterase inhibitors should be carried out as this may help to identify the presence of OP and/or carbamate compounds. Diagnosis is made by serum and RBC cholinesterase levels which decrease by 50%. Some carbamate herbicides and fungicides, such as the dithiocarbamates do not inhibit cholinesterases to any significant degree and are relatively nontoxic in humans.
- **Blood gas:** In most cases of poisoning, pH is of significance, hence, venous blood gases rather than arterial blood gases (ABG) should be done. However, if adequate oxygenation is a concern (for e.g., cyanide, carbon monoxide poisoning and methemoglobinemia) then an ABG should be sent.
- **Serum drug screen:** In general, screening includes acetaminophen, salicylate, tricyclic antidepressant (unreliable as it cross-reacts with many therapeutic agents) and ethanol concentrations.
- **Urine drug screen:** Many of the assays produce false-positive or false-negative results. It may cause confusion to the medical practitioner who may attribute a patient's condition to intoxication rather than a medical emergency.

Electrocardiograph: The ECG is important tool for toxicological evaluation, and certain poisoning and overdoses produce characteristic ECG changes that may help in diagnosis.

Imaging: In general, there is a limited role of diagnostic imaging in toxicology, except it may reveal radiodense material in the stomach or gut in the following ingestions: chloral hydrate, heavy metals, iron, phenothiazines and presence of 'rosettes' or elongated packets in the GI tract of body packers.

Management

The general approach and initial management of the patient who is suspected to have ingested or inhaled an unknown poison is outlined in Flow chart 11.1.[1,5,17-20,22] (For specific issues relating to management of common poisoning and drug overdoses, the reader may refer to any standard textbook of toxicology).

DUTIES OF A MEDICAL PRACTITIONER IN SUSPECTED POISONING

In the emergency room, medical practitioners come across many cases of poisoning. They should be aware of the correct medicolegal procedures and ethical principles that ought to be followed when managing such patients. Due to medicolegal complexities, large number of poisoning cases are either referred to other hospitals citing nonavailability of facilities or not reported to police due to the fear of investigative and legal proceedings. Whenever a medical practitioner comes across a case of suspected poisoning, he should perform the following duties:[7,23-25]

- In case of emergency, every effort should be made to save the life of the patient
- Maintain confidentiality
- Send the police information/intimation

Flow chart 11.1 Management of a case of poisoning

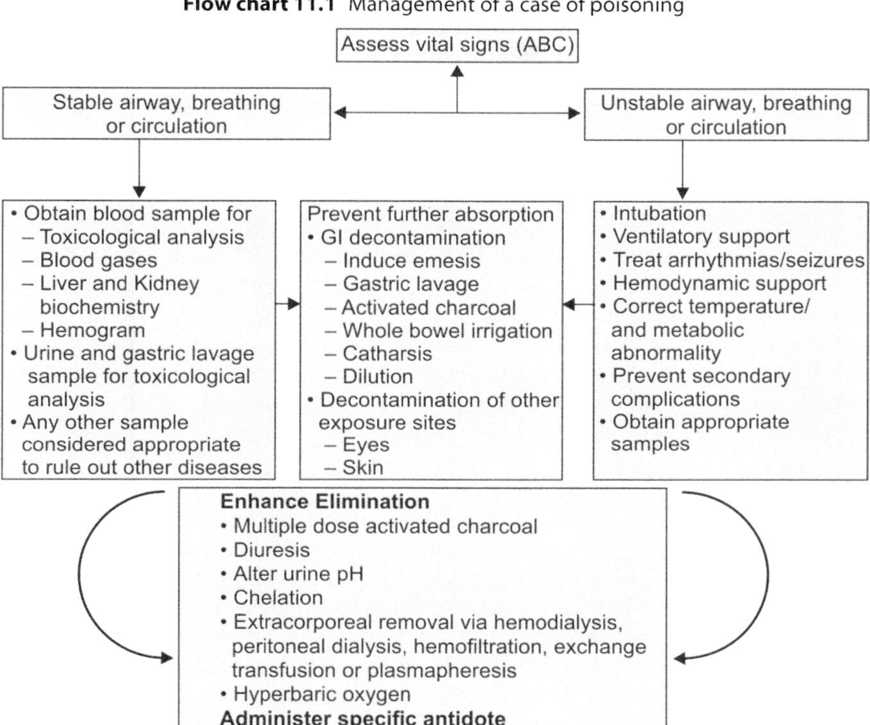

- Prepare a medicolegal report
- Collect and preserve all necessary samples
- Forward samples for analysis
- In case of imminent death, arrange for recording the dying declaration
- Maintain proper records.

Treatment

The first and foremost duty of a medical practitioner is to save the life of the patient. A doctor working in a government hospital cannot refuse treatment of a patient of poisoning. A private practitioner has the right to choose a patient and hence, can refuse to treat a case of poisoning. But, he/she should not refuse cases requiring emergency treatment.[26] However, in such cases, the doctor-patient relationship is not established, as the patient was only given life saving treatment. Once he is stable, then he is in a position to give consent for further treatment and/or medicolegal examination. Therefore, it is unethical for any doctor to refuse treatment in case of emergency, like poisoning.

A medical practitioner must remember that he is protected against any harm done in good faith to a patient in an emergency as per Sec. 92 IPC. In case of suspected poisoning or in cases of absence of any obvious signs and symptoms of poisoning, observation of the patient for at least 24 hours is a good practice and can help avoid suits of negligence being filed against them.

Preparing a Medicolegal Report

Medicolegal report (MLR) is prepared immediately after the examination is done. MLR should be prepared in suspected poisoning cases brought dead in the emergency. In all other cases, consent should be sought prior to the preparation of medicolegal report.

Procedure of Police Information

In all medicolegal cases, doctor must inform the nearest police station in writing along with receipt of acknowledgement of information or may inform telephonically and note down the diary number (DD or the Daily Docket number). According to the Hon'ble Supreme Court, information regarding name, age, sex of the patient and the exact place of occurrence of the incident should be sent to the police station and treatment of the patient should be started.

Dying Declaration

If the patient is conscious but seriously ill and on the verge of death, a dying declaration relating to the circumstances and cause of his impending death should be recorded. Ideally a Magistrate should be called, but if death appears imminent or there is a delay in arrival of Magistrate, then doctor should record the dying declaration [Sec. 32 (1) IEA]. It is preferable to record it in the language of the patient and in his own words. Even in the presence of Magistrate, a doctor's presence is essential to testify that patient is in full possession of his senses, and there is no abnormality of judgment or incoherent thinking.

Death of a Patient with Suspected Poisoning

The following are the do's and don'ts in case of a suspected poisoning patient is brought dead or dies in the emergency or any other department of the hospital:

i. Police should be informed immediately and death certificate should not be issued—even if the patient was admitted and the treating doctor is certain of the type of poison and how the death was caused. He/she may record in the bed head ticket the cause of death, for e.g., 'In my opinion, the death was due to acute phenobarbitone poisoning'.
ii. The body is send to the hospital mortuary for preservation, till the legal formalities are completed and the police releases the body to the lawful heirs.
iii. The dead body should never be released to the relatives; it should only be handed over to the police.
iv. A medicolegal postmortem examination is requested to confirm the cause of death.
v. Any residual antemortem specimens should be obtained as a matter of urgency from the hospital pathology laboratory (not only biochemical, pathology and hematology, but also immunology, transfusion medicine and virology departments may be a source of such specimens) and submitted for toxicological analysis.

Medical Records

In every case of suspected poisoning, the doctor must keep and maintain detailed and meticulous records of the case. He/she should be aware of the possibility that medical records may be perused by the legal counsel in a court of law. Therefore, the history, all relevant clinical findings and observations must be legibly recorded. If the history was obtained from a relative or a bystander, that fact should be mentioned and the name of the person must be recorded.

CONFIDENTIALITY AND REPORTING

It is essential to maintain strict confidentiality as in other clinical cases. All information regarding the patient that a doctor comes across during the course of his treatment has to be kept secret. The reasons revealed by the patient for suicidal or homicidal poisoning should be clearly recorded in the hospital case sheet or medicolegal report, but should not be discussed with relatives or friends of the patient without his/her prior permission.[7]

Sometimes, the patient may state that he has consumed the poison in a suicidal attempt and request the medical practitioner not to inform police. Almost all patients attempt suicide due to sudden impulse and many, for trivial reasons. They regret their suicidal act with the exception of patients with severe organic psychiatric disturbances. Steps should be taken to protect patients from further suicidal attempts (poisoning or otherwise).

Under these circumstances, there is a dilemma between professional secrecy at one hand and privileged communication/breach of confidentiality on the other. Initially, out of compassion, the treating doctor may not inform the police so as to protect the patient's and his/her family from further trauma of humiliation and harassment. But, he has to safeguard himself against legal complications that may arise later on.[23-25]

If the medical practitioner is working in a government hospital, he/she is bound by the service guidelines to inform the legal authorities of all the cases of poisoning regardless of their manner, whether suicidal, accidental or homicidal.[7]

A private medical practitioner is not legally bound to inform the police of all the cases of poisoning. He only has a legal obligation to inform in homicidal cases of poisoning as per Sec. 39 CrPC. He is not bound to inform the legal authorities if he is sure the case is suicidal or accidental in nature. Under Sec. 39 CrPC, Sec. 309 IPC (attempt to commit suicide) and sections relating to accidents are not included for the sections which require the public to give information. However, following needs to be pondered upon when deciding not to inform the police officials or Magistrate:

- If an investigating officer inquires about a case of poisoning, regardless of its nature, the medical practitioner is expected to report all details to him failing which he can be penalized. Under Sec. 175 CrPC, one is bound to supply such information if he is summoned by the investigating police officer or Magistrate. Noncompliance or concealing any such fact is punishable under Sec. 202 IPC (imprisonment of either description up to 6 months or fine or both).
- Section 43 IPC describes the word 'illegal' and 'legally bound to do'. The word 'illegal' is applicable to everything which is an offence or which is prohibited

by law, or which furnishes ground for a civil action, and a person is said to be 'legally bound to do' whatever it is illegal in him to omit. Thus, it is the duty of the medical practitioner not to do anything illegal or hide illegal acts. Attempted suicide is a criminal offence and attempted suicidal poisonings should be informed to the police. However, he/she is not liable for giving notice, if the case has already been reported to the police by the village headman/village watchman or any other officer required under the law to give such information under Sec. 40 CrPC.

- The medical practitioner does not know the circumstances of the poisoning. He/she may not be in a sound position to label the case for one or the other category. His only source of information is what is told by the patient himself or by the relatives. The patient may retract his statement later or it may be tutored, induced, fraudulent or unreliable, and additional evidence may come forward pointing towards criminality. The Supreme Court has held that even the dying declaration may not be reliable. Furthermore, in the current state of affairs, the public is quite knowledgeable about the law of the land, the relatives/attendants may hide some facts or there may be an element of bias in the history given. This may be for their own benefits or for insurance claims/pension benefits. Therefore, the patient's or relative's statement about self-poisoning cannot be a ground for not reporting to police. For example, in case of a married lady, the husband or in-laws may give the history of suicide at the time of admission, later on the parents of the patient may allege that it is a case of homicide and she was forcefully given the poison. In some cases, it may emerge later that even though the patient knowingly took the poison himself, he/she was instigated or compelled or forced to do so by other person(s) or circumstances created by them. In such cases, the person(s) might be liable for abetment to suicide which is a criminal offence. The medical practitioner can be charged with suppression of evidence or failure to inform the police of a possible criminal act or collusion in a criminal act and may be dragged into the group of parties for murder by not informing the police. Noncompliance or concealing any such information or failure to inform the police in a case of homicidal poisoning makes the doctor liable for prosecution under Sec. 176 IPC (punishment is simple imprisonment of 1 month or fine of ₹ 500/- or both). Giving false information on such matters is punishable under Sec. 177 IPC (punishment is of simple imprisonment for 6 months or fine of ₹ 1000 or both).
- If police information is not sent at the time of admission, and death ensue from poisoning, then dying declaration may not be recorded as information was not provided to the police officials.
- The State Medical Council is likely to hold this act of not informing the legal authorities as professional misconduct.
- Suicidal poisoning are unnatural acts and it is in the interest of the society to investigate and prevent such unnatural acts.

Hence, it is desirable to report all cases of poisoning to police. In spite of all these, if using his/her own discretion, the medical practitioner decides not to inform the police, he/she should take all steps necessary for a regular MLR and maintain the records and preserve the samples including clothings accordingly, in a documented manner. This will help him/her, if there is a police inquiry later on.

Moreover, it is not for the medical practitioner to decide whether the poisoning was suicidal, homicidal or accidental. It is not his/her role to determine who administered the poison, whether he himself or somebody else. That is typically the role of the police or the courts.

If the circumstances are not clear, especially when the patient is unconscious, or if the poisoning is suspected as homicidal, he/she should consult a senior colleague. Patients should be protected from further homicidal attempts, if necessary, through the help of the police.

In case of accidental poisoning, for e.g., a case of poisoning arising out of a public eating place or contamination of public drinking water, where further exposure to other people is anticipated, he must inform the public health authorities concerned due to his duty towards the State. Accidental poisoning, especially in children, usually has no medicolegal implications, unless there is gross neglect by some individual (child abuse) or institution.

CIRCUMSTANCES OF POISONING[2,6,7]

Once a patient with a history of poisoning or suspected of poisoning is admitted, the circumstances of poisoning should be determined. Poisonings are either intentional or unintentional. If the person taking or giving a substance did not mean to cause harm, then it is an unintentional poisoning. Unintentional poisoning includes the use of chemicals or drugs for nonmedical purposes in excessive amounts, such as an 'overdose'. Nonmedical use includes misuse or abuse of a drug prescribed.

Intentional Overdose/Attempted Suicide/Parasuicide Attempts

Self-poisoning is the most common method in women and the second most common method in men attempting suicide. Risk factors include mental health problems, substance abuse especially alcohol, social and economic stresses, domestic violence and nonavailability of protective factors like family and social support.

Self-poisoning often occur immediately after an acute relationship crisis—conflicts within the family or breakdown of romantic relationships (especially in females). Self-harm, in particular self-poisoning, is used for many reasons—to gain attention, express distress or get revenge—not just for ending life. Sometimes, someone may instigate to commit suicide (abetment to suicide)—breach of trust, false promise of marriage, shame and deception. Many deaths from self-poisoning occur in people who do not intend to die; they die because the poisons ingested are very toxic, there is a delay in getting medical facilities and patients are difficult to treat.

Mental disorders, particularly psychological disease are an important risk factor for self-harm and deliberate poisoning. Affective disorders (MDD, obsessive disorder, anxiety disorder and antisocial personality disorder) and family histories of affective disorders are associated with attempted suicide.

Accidental

Accidental poisoning usually takes place in the domestic environment with young children and the elderly particularly at risk.

Poisonings are common among young children ('at risk' group 1–4 years) as they explore their environment and put new objects into their mouth. Accidental poisoning usually occurs when the child is unsupervised. There is an increased incidence in poisoning following recent disruption in households, such as a new baby or moving house or where there is maternal depression. Children may gain access to pharmaceutical products, cleaning agents (bleach, disinfectants), pesticides, alcoholic drinks and cosmetics.

The confused elderly may misjudge their intake of medications or poisoned by inappropriate handling of toxic household products. Both are susceptible to acute or chronic poisoning with carbon monoxide emitted by burning '*angithi*' (stove) or faulty domestic heating appliances.

The workplace is another environment in which accidental poisoning occurs.

Homicidal

Homicidal poisoning is relatively rare and an infrequently established crime. Several difficulties come with the detection of homicidal poisonings. Presenting symptoms and signs are often misdiagnosed as natural disease.

The lethal agent of choice has changed over the years. In earlier years, traditional poisons such as arsenic, cyanide and parathion were frequently used. Such poisonings are nowadays rare, and instead, narcotics are more commonly detected in victims of this crime. In one study, the agents of choice in both Sweden and North America were hypnotics and sedatives, analgesics, antipsychotics and carbon monoxide.[27]

Malicious

There may be allegation of malicious administration of drugs or poisons by a third party. Individuals who are administered substances without their knowledge to facilitate robbery or sexual abuse may also be admitted to hospital. Victims of so-called date-rape may be administered drugs such as γ-hydroxy butyrate (GHB), flunitrazepam, barbiturates or alcohol to induce confusion and amnesia, and facilitate sexual abuse.[3,6]

Deliberate poisoning in children by parents, guardians or siblings has been reported. In non-accidental poisoning in children, mothers are the most frequent perpetrators. They do so to attract sympathy and attention at the expense of the child's illness (Munchausen's syndrome by proxy). Symptoms are induced via the administration of drugs. A history of poisoning is usually lacking at the time of presentation. Most poisoning episodes in childhood and adolescence are of low lethality and little or no treatment is required.[6]

Drug Abuse

Alcohol and solvent abuse are the most common forms of drug abuse in children (United Kingdom). In 2009, 28,754 (91%) of all unintentional poisoning deaths were caused by drugs in the US. The drugs most commonly involved were the prescription painkillers—methadone, hydrocodone and oxycodone, followed by cocaine and heroin. Among those treated in the emergency for nonfatal poisonings involving nonmedical use of prescription or over-the-counter drugs, opioid pain medications and benzodiazepines were involved most frequently.

Iatrogenic

Iatrogenic intoxications occur through inappropriate medical treatment in which a patient or relative sue the medical practitioner for neglect. In children, the most common offender is diphenoxylate with atropine (Lomotil). This combination is toxic to some children at therapeutic doses. The most frequently fatal drug is digoxin. Some cases of toxicity following overdoses of medications or wrong injections and vaccination have also been reported.

Occupation

Most of the farmers are unfamiliar with pesticide safety practices, such as compliance with instruction on the label, proper spraying techniques, proper use of protective equipment and safe pesticide disposal. Consequently, farmers are at high-risk of being harmed by pesticide exposure.

COLLECTION, PRESERVATION AND FORWARDING OF SAMPLES

Samples can be divided into:[3-6,21]

i. Blood and related fluids (for e.g., 'whole blood', blood cells, CSF, plasma, serum and cord blood).
ii. Body fluids other than blood (for e.g., gastric aspirate, saliva, vaginal fluid, amniotic fluid, breast milk, semen and peritoneal fluid).
iii. Excretory fluids/residues (for e.g., urine, sweat and bile) and exhaled air.
iv. Other clinical samples (for e.g. stomach wash, hair, nail clippings, nasal swabs and vomit).

Usually, toxicological procedures require the collection of blood, urine, stomach contents and 'scene residues'—material found at the scene of incident, like tablets, empty containers or aerosol canisters (Table 11.8). However, other specimens such as hair, sweat, saliva and exhaled air have also been used to determine poisoning and/or drug use.

1. **Blood:** It is the most useful specimen collected, since poison or drug present in the medium can best be correlated to the physiological effect, and assesses the likelihood of recent exposure to poisons or drug use. In a suspected case, 10 ml blood is taken from an adult (proportionally smaller volumes from young child) as soon as possible, after admission to hospital. A heparinized or EDTA whole blood sample will give either whole blood or plasma as appropriate. Additionally, 2 ml of blood should be collected in a fluoride/oxalate tube, if ethanol is suspected. This prevents the production of bacterial ethanol which can yield a false positive result. If possible, it is recommended to preserve 10 ml of clotted blood (unpreserved blood sample).

Table 11.8 Sample preservation and its requirements

Sample	*Quantity*	*Preservative*	*Advantage*	*Disadvantage*
Whole blood	10 ml	Lithium heparin or EDTA tube, fluoride/oxalate if alcohol is suspected	Detect parent compound, interpretation of quantitative data	Limited volume, low concentrations of basic drugs
Urine	20–50 ml	No preservative, sodium fluoride is added if alcohol is suspected	Large volume, high concentration of many poisons	Not always available, quantitative data not useful
Gastric contents	25–50 ml	No preservative	Large amount of poison, if ingested	Not useful in case of inhalation or injection
Scene residues	As appropriate	No preservative	Large amount of poison	May not have taken the poison
Saliva	As available	No preservative	Noninvasive, qualitative information	Small volume, low concentration, quantitative analysis not possible
Hair/nail clippings	About 100–200 head hair	No preservative	Readily available	Gives an idea of exposure data for days/weeks/months
Exhaled air	As required	No preservative	Noninvasive, large volume available	Analyte must be volatile

The tubes/vials used for clinical use contain only about 0.1% (w/v) fluoride, whereas about 2% (w/v) fluoride (40 mg sodium fluoride per 2 ml blood) is needed to inhibit microbial action in such specimens. Addition of fluoride also helps to protect other labile drugs such as clonazepam, cocaine and nitrazepam from degradation. The use of disinfectant swabs containing alcohols, and heparin anticoagulant solutions that contain phenolic preservatives should be avoided.

2. **Urine:** This, along with blood, is the most frequently collected specimen. Urine is useful, since it is often available in large quantity and may contain higher concentrations of poisons or drugs or metabolites than blood—ideal for qualitative screening. The presence of metabolites may sometimes assist identification of a poison, if chromatographic techniques are used. A 50 ml specimen is collected in a sterile container from an adult and sealed. No preservative should be added. The sample should be obtained as soon as poisoning is suspected, ideally before any drug therapy has been initiated. Strong smelling poisons such as camphor, ethchlorvynol and methylsalicylate can sometimes be recognized in urine because they are excreted, in part, unchanged.

3. **Stomach contents:** This includes vomit, gastric aspirate or stomach washout. Stomach washout (gastric lavage) is obtained soon after admission, since large amounts of poison may be present while metabolites are usually absent. It is important to preserve the first sample of any lavage fluid because later samples may be very dilute. About 50 ml without preservative should be taken for analysis. However, all stomach contents should be retained and the volume noted. Stomach contents are especially useful, if poison(s) which are not easy to measure in blood, such as cyanide have been taken orally.
4. **Exhaled air:** Measurement of concentrations of volatile substances in exhaled (expired) air by infrared or other devices is essential in roadside testing for ethanol, and valuable in assessing exposure to poisons such as carbon monoxide.
5. **Saliva:** It is best collected by absorption onto an absorbent material or a device which stimulates production of saliva. It should be collected at least 30 minutes after a meal, consumption of beverage or drug, and the oral cavity is free from food material.[3] For qualitative work, such as testing for drugs of abuse, oral fluid is normally collected. Oral fluid collection for forensic purposes has the advantage that sampling can be carried out while the donor is under observation, hence it is more difficult to adulterate or substitute the specimen. Collection of saliva or oral fluid require cooperative individuals, and collection is noninvasive and reflects current drug or alcohol usage. Saliva concentrations are much higher than blood for some drugs, for e.g. amphetamines, whereas it is lower in cases of barbiturates and benzodiazepines.[3]
6. **Sweat:** Sweat can be collected by using suitable absorbent devices such as sweat patches or forehead wipes. Drugs detected in sweat include alcohol, amphetamines, cocaine, benzodiazepines, barbiturates, opioids and phencyclidine.[3]
7. **Hair and nail clippings:** Many metal ions, drugs and their metabolites are sequestered in hair and nail as they are formed, and are not metabolized further. These samples may be useful if chronic exposure is suspected, for e.g. in cases of drug abuse (particularly opiates and methadone) where establishing recent drug use is very important, and for poisons that may have been eliminated from other commonly sampled fluids and tissues before sample collection. The target analytes in hair are mostly the parent drugs. Cocaine, δ-tetrahydrocannabinol (THC), heroin and 6-acetylmorphine for heroin, and benzodiazepines are found in higher concentration than their metabolites. Acidic drugs tend to have lower concentrations than basic drugs.[3] However, the information is qualitative in nature.

   If a single exposure to a poison is suspected, as in drug-facilitated sexual assault (DFSA), but the suspected agent is not detected in blood or urine, waiting for 1–2 months for head hair to grow and then performing segmental analysis may reveal the presence of the drug.

In general, biological specimens should be stored at 4°C before transport to the laboratory. Exceptions to this include hair and nail, which are stable at room temperature, and filter-paper adsorbed dried blood which is a convenient way of storing and transporting blood samples for specified analyses, if refrigerated transport and storage is not feasible.

In medicolegal cases, sample integrity is of prime concern as evidence may have to be produced in court. Precautions to ensure sample integrity include:[21]

i. Proper sample labeling,
ii. Use of tamper-proof containers, and
iii. Proper accompanying documentation (chain-of-custody documents).

All relevant specimens should be collected and properly labeled with the patient's name, admission or CR number, nature of sample, collection site, preservative used, date and time of collection. They should be sealed with a tamper-proof device under the doctor's supervision. They are handed over to the investigating officer after obtaining proper receipt, along with the medicolegal report and a proper requisition letter detailing the tests to be conducted on such samples. Failure to manage this stage correctly can ruin subsequent analysis. If the samples have been collected on the request of the police, the fact is to be mentioned in the report and no requisition is necessary.

It is the duty of a medical practitioner to collect and preserve all evidences suggestive of or confirmatory to poisoning. Failure to do so is punishable under Sec. 201 IPC [punishment is imprisonment of either description up to 7 years depending upon the nature of offence (trying to shield the accused)]. In this case, the onus of proving a nondeliberate omission to collect and preserve the samples would lie on the medical practitioner.[7]

General Methodology in Toxicological Examination

The main steps in any toxicological examination are usually the following:[2]

a. *Detection* of any drugs or poisons in the samples submitted by means of screening procedures.
b. *Identification* conclusively of any drugs, metabolites or poisons present by means of specific physicochemical tests.
c. *Quantification* of those drugs, metabolites or poisons present.
d. *Interpretation* of the analytical findings in (b) and (c) in the context of the case, the information given and the questions asked by the investigating officer.

CONFIRMATORY DIAGNOSIS

The methods and instrumentation used in a clinical toxicology laboratory are similar to those used in forensic toxicology laboratories. The circumstances surrounding the case will usually determine the types of toxicological tests that are required. There are different screens specific for the type of substance to be assayed. A given laboratory will follow an algorithm to handle the analysis.

Ideally, the toxicological laboratory should have the capability to identify and quantify pesticides, pharmaceutical agents, illicit drugs, gases, solvents, toxic metals and a host of other industrial and environmental poisons in biological fluids. Practically, few laboratories can offer such a comprehensive menu, and resources are concentrated on testing 'common drugs and poisons'.[2]

If the poison for which the toxicologist has to test is not specified by name, the request to 'test for poisons' is a major problem. A broad range of substances with very different chemical nature may need to be tested for. In some instances, the toxicologist may be provided with history of the case giving an indication that a poisonous substance may be present which is not likely to be picked up in the usual 'routine' tests mostly applied to the samples. This enables the toxicologist to apply additional analyses for the types of poisons suspected to be present. This has its own limitation too, because the amount of sample may be little, methods of analysis may not be available in the laboratory where particular poisons are not commonly encountered, and time and cost factor. However, applying these additional tests may confirm or rule out recent ingestion or exposure. Hence, in all suspected cases of poisoning, it is important to obtain as much information as possible and submit it to the toxicologist. It will assist the toxicologist to use the most directly useful methods of analysis and to interpret the results in context of the case.[2,4]

The following documents should be enclosed along with the samples:[2,21]

i. Complete case history of the patient (even though in many incidents of suspicious poisoning there may be no obvious indication of poisoning from case history).
ii. Past medical history including current or recent prescription medications.
iii. Signs and symptoms on admission that might suggest poisoning.
iv. Details of emergency hospital treatment and medication given.
v. Laboratory investigations (including biochemical tests and toxicological investigations).
vi. Circumstances of poisoning and details of poison or drug suspected.
vii. Copy of medicolegal report.

In many instances, belongings found alongside a victim of poisoning or the location and circumstances may give guidance about possible substances present. For example, in cases of accidental or intentional poisonings with pesticide or drugs, labeled containers or tablets strips may be found close by which may help in identification of the compound.[4]

The detailed discussion of techniques for detection of poisons and drugs are beyond the scope of this chapter. Only a brief mention of some techniques utilized by forensic science laboratory is given below.

Toxicological Screening

Toxicological screening methods can be divided into limited, specific or extensive ('general unknown') screening. In forensic toxicology, unless specific information is available indicating that a particular poison or drug should be targeted for analysis (for e.g. relatives brought a labeled pesticide product found alongside the patient), a broader screening procedure should be employed to identify the active components.[3,5] The Volatile Screen is frequently used for the detection of ethanol. A Drugs of Abuse Screen is commonly used for amphetamines, cocaine, marijuana, and so on. When the cause is unclear, a General Drug Screen is employed. Acidic/Neutral Screen is primarily used to detect barbiturates, muscle relaxants, and so on. Basic Drug Screens are more specific for the detection of drugs such as cocaine and antidepressants. Pesticides are considered as a separate category from drugs, although they fall in the category of 'organic nonvolatile' substances isolated by solvent extraction.[2,5]

The nonspecific initial tests in a series are valuable for determining the presence or absence of a particular class of compounds. Colorimetric tests to detect the presence of phenothiazines would give initial information about a drug class present. This would be followed by more specific tests to identify the actual compound, as well as provide quantitative data. Another example of a type of initial test would be an immunoassay that determines the presence of barbiturates. Confirmatory tests are mandatory to identify the particular drug within the class detected.[5]

Fast Limited Screening

Immunoassays: Commonly available immunoassays, such as fluorescence polarization immunoassay (FPIA), enzyme multiplied immunoassay technique (EMIT), radioimmunoassay (RIA) and enzyme linked immunoabsorbent assay (ELISA) give quick qualitative results and in some cases, a semiquantitative result in plasma for a variety of substances or groups of compounds. Their limitations in terms of specificity and sensitivity must always be considered when interpreting results.[3,5,6]

Toxicological Screening by Chromatography

Thin-layer chromatography (TLC): TLC is usually applied to urine sample or, if this is not available, to stomach contents that have been purified prior to extraction.

Organophosphorus (OP) compounds

Initial screening procedures help identify individual pesticides but are not geared to quantifying the levels that are present. Some color tests are very useful preliminary indicators of the class of compound and can confirm the constituents of a proprietary formulation.[4,5]

Phosphorus test can be used to detect OP compounds; although with limited sensitivity of the test, it is not able to detect OP compounds in blood, and the sodium dithionite test is used for diquat and paraquat. The furfuraldehyde test is used for carbamates in the same matrices.

Visualization reagents are available which produce a variety of colors to facilitate differentiation. A large number of pesticides react with more than one reagent. For example, silver nitrate in solution or rhodamine in ethanol followed by an overspray of sodium hydroxide in ethanol can be used to visualize OP compounds, carbamates, chlorinated hydrocarbons, chlorinated phenoxy acids, pyrethroids, substituted ureas and triazines. Some reagents are considerably more specific and can be used to confirm a particular pesticide class. OP compounds can be visualized using 4-(4-nitrobenzyl) pyridine and tetraethylenepentamine.[4,5]

While color tests are useful to indicate preliminary classes, they are generally restricted to stomach contents and nonbiological materials and will only detect a rather restricted range of pesticides. Thin layer chromatography (TLC), gas chromatography (GC) and liquid chromatography can be used to screen for a far wider range of substances. The method of choice, regarded as the reference method for identification and confirmation of the presence of pesticide in different materials, is GC-MS (Gas chromatography-mass spectrometry). High-performance liquid chromatography (HPLC) and combined liquid chromatography mass spectrometry (LC-MS) are also used as confirmation methods.[4,5]

Phosphides

Hydrogen phosphide (commonly known as phosphine) is usually generated by the action of water on metallic phosphides (aluminum, magnesium or zinc). The ammonium molybdate test is used for phosphorus and phosphides in stomach contents and nonbiological materials. The commercially available detector tubes for the test may be used as qualitative and quantitative procedures for stomach contents and nonbiological materials. Phosphine can also be determined in biological samples by using GC and NPD (nitrogen-phosphorous) detection.[4]

INTERPRETATION OF TOXICOLOGICAL RESULTS

Forensic toxicology is not an exact science. The techniques used to detect and quantitate poisons and drugs are often accurate, but the exact meaning of those findings is subject to the experience and interpretation of the experienced medical practitioner. In practice, interpretation is complex as well as vital.

The foremost question asked by the legal counsel is whether the individual was exposed to poison or drug? The answer is given based on the outcome of a thorough toxicological analysis that is capable of detecting significant concentrations of any substance that could logically be present.

The highest concentrations of a poison or drug are found at the site of administration. Stomach contents may contain large amounts of unabsorbed poison or drug in case of oral ingestion.[5]

If a poison or drug or drug metabolites is conclusively identified in a properly collected sample, then the person who provided the sample must have taken it. The presumption of toxicity must be further evaluated, taking other physical and circumstantial evidence into consideration. The prehospital events, medical and social history must be correlated with toxicological data. Therefore, interpretation should include the subject's blood concentrations of all drugs capable of causing impairment, as well as evidence that the subject was impaired. The medical practitioner familiar with the effects of poison or drug may be able only to offer an opinion that the observed symptoms are consistent or not consistent with the effects of the detected drugs. However, to conclude that since the drug was present, regardless of concentration, the subject must have been impaired without having evidence of symptoms of intoxication is speculation or assumption, not objective interpretation.[2]

Questions may be raised as to whether the exposure was intentional or unknowing. The medical practitioner should give unbiased interpretation, and must give consideration to alternative explanations for apparently incriminating findings. He/she should be aware of circumstances that can produce positive tests in a person who has not abused the drug (Box 11.3).[1,16] Sometimes, definitive testing may be required if someone challenges a positive urine test results, since presence of drug or metabolites in urine is useless for demonstrating impairment.

A negative result must be interpreted from an understanding of the sensitivity of the analytical method. It implies that the analyte targeted by the test was not present, or if present, was at a concentration below the detection limit. If methods of sufficient sensitivity are used, negative findings mean that either nothing was ingested or something outside the scope of analysis was involved. There is no universal method of analysis for all substances, particularly where the requirement is to be able to detect, identify and quantify the substance, typically at low concentrations and in complex matrices such as organ, tissues and blood. Most of the numerous screening procedures reported in literature are too limited to permit a confident negative report, and there is always the possibility of an unexpected substance being involved in any particular case.

The other questions that may be asked are:[5]

- What was the route of administration?
- What dose was administered?
- Is the concentration enough to have caused injury or death, or altered the victim's behavior enough to cause injury or death?

Box 11.3 Positive/negative urine drug screen and its possible/alternate explanations and implications

- **Amphetamines:** Amphetamines cross-reacts with over-the-counter cold medications or diet products. Diet supplement phenylpropanolamine may have traces of amphetamine. Several pharmaceuticals (for e.g. nasal inhalers) contain or are metabolized to methamphetamine (l-deoxyephedrine).
- **Opioids:** Consuming pastries with poppy seeds may contain traces of morphine and codeine (testing for the alkaloid thebaine derived from poppy seeds may help to distinguish food from drug). Moreover, this screen frequently misses the presence of the synthetic opioids, such as fentanyl and meperidine.
- **Cocaine:** Drinking coca tea. This test is very reliable for the identification of recent use (detects the metabolite benzoylecgonine), but in no way confirms intoxication.
- **Cannabinoids:** Using hemp seed oil or hemp seed confections. Like cocaine, detection of the tetrahydrocannabinolic acid metabolite is a reliable indicator of use; however, its presence does not have any bearing upon the diagnosis of intoxication.
- **Benzodiazepines:** Detection of benzodiazepines most commonly depends upon the detection of oxazepam; commonly used benzodiazepines (such as lorazepam) are often missed by this screening.
- **Phencyclidine (PCP):** Screening assays may cross-react with dextromethorphan, ketamine and diphenhydramine to produce a false-positive result.

The route may be interpreted from the site where the highest concentration of a poison was found. A large quantity of unabsorbed poison or drug in the gastrointestinal (GI) tract (lavage sample) indicates oral ingestion. Higher concentrations of toxicant or drug in the lungs compared to other tissues may indicate inhalation, while compounds located in tissue surrounding an injection site indicates an intramuscular or intravenous injection. Detection of drug combustion breakdown products within fluids or tissues reveals that smoking was the route of drug administration (for e.g. cocaine and its pyrolysis product anhydroecgonine methylester). The concentration may be interpreted from quantitative analysis and fatal dose compared with reference levels.

Limits on Interpretation

The information available from a toxicological analysis depends to some extent on the sample. Blood samples provide more information about drugs which might currently be affecting the individual, whereas urine samples are better at revealing what drugs the individual has been exposed to in the past several days. Following should be taken into consideration before giving the final opinion:[16]

- The emergency room specimens sometimes yield the only reliable evidence of the individual's state of intoxication at the time of admission. For example, drugs administered by physicians, including morphine, haloperidol, lignocaine (lidocaine), atropine and others will not usually be found in admission specimens, whereas drugs taken prior to hospitalization will. Hence, the nature of the sample can also impact on the interpretation of results.
- Drugs may no longer be detectable, if victims of drug-facilitated sexual assault tend to contact the medical services several days after the incident.

- Most toxicological investigations are restricted to a few analytical tests for a range of 'common drugs and poisons', unless the medical examiner has made a request to examine for (additional) specific chemicals. He/she should make the courts aware of this fact, as assumption is often made by legal counsel (and other parties) that the toxicological investigations were exhaustive, and all drugs and poisons were included in the testing processes.
- The 'routine' screens for alcohol and other drugs, particularly drugs of abuse should be asked for, because the finding of alcohol and/or other drugs may be pertinent to the case. For example, if a factory worker is involved in workplace accident and if high levels of alcohol is found in the blood or urine, then it may put a different complexion on an investigation of the incident.
- For many drugs, the amount of drug seen in the blood in one person when the substance is taken as prescribed may be the same as the level in another who suffers severe toxicity or even death. For example, methamphetamine is taken for the treatment of obesity, blood level of 200 ng/ml was seen in therapeutic use, as well as reported fatal overdoses. Cocaine has been found toxic over a large range with deaths occurring at concentrations ranging from 0.01 to 78 mg/l.[28] The concentration of drug and its active metabolites(s) in blood is important, but other factors must also be considered. Individual variability and tolerance can affect the degree of impairment at any given blood drug concentration. Hence, considerations must include the chronicity of drug use, age of the person, health of the person (presence of heart, liver or kidney disease), use of multiple substances and genetic factors that may lead to a reduced metabolism.
- Commercially available pesticides preparations usually contain an active substance mixed with filler (solids) or dissolved in an organic solvent (liquids). Although, certain pesticides are unlikely to cause acute toxicity, the vehicle in which they are formulated (toluene, xylenes, butan-1-ol, cyclohexanone, farbasol and solvent naphtha) may itself be toxic and, in some cases, can be the main causative agent for the symptoms observed. This needs to be taken into consideration in clinical forensic toxicology both in terms of the analytical methods applied to samples and the interpretation of results.

The medical practitioner should be able to put forward his/her opinion to counter the arguments offered by the defense counsel of the suspect who tested positive for a drug. The defense may range from passive exposure, to subject's unknowing consumption of a food or beverage containing the drug, to transfer through semen from a drug-abusing partner to handling contaminated money (cocaine-positive drug test). The possible motivation for someone to administer the drug should be considered, as well as the opportunity to do so without detection. Moreover, the amount of cocaine in semen is insufficient to produce a positive urine test. Passive exposure to marijuana smoke does not yield urinary concentrations of δ–tetrahydrocannabinol (THC) metabolites above 40 ng ml/l.

CONCLUSION

As can be seen from above discussion, toxicology is a complex science, and poisoning is a significant cause of morbidity and mortality in developing as well as in developed countries. In majority of the cases, the poison or drug can be identified from a careful history, detailed physical examination and commonly available laboratory tests.

The circumstances surrounding poisoning are quite different and may not be apparent as from those surrounding the industrial/vehicular accidents. Moreover, as doctor is not an investigating officer and can never be sure about the manner of poisoning (suicide, accident or homicide), it is advisable to report each and every case of suspected poisoning. This will be in the best interest of the medical practitioner by which he/she can avoid complications arising at some later stage.

Interpretation is sometimes difficult. In expert opinions about poisonings, each case must be approached diligently and must look at all possibilities, examine each piece of evidence with objectivity and process the findings into a logical and consistent explanation. There may be unavailability of data on concentrations of poisons in various biological materials, occurring normally and in poisoning cases. Furthermore, the nature of the substance, mode of action and metabolism in the human body may itself cause problems. The true meaning of these results should be taken in context with all of the other information obtained including the clinical findings and factual evidence, and should be interpreted only by a competent, trained forensic medical practitioner. It can be a tedious and laborious job, but the search for the truth is never easy and is always fulfilling.

REFERENCES

1. Halcomb SE, Brenner S, Mullins ME. Medical emergencies. In: Foster C, Nevillie F, Mistry NF, Parvin F. Peddi PF, Sharma S (eds). The Washington manual of medical therapeutics. 33rd edn. London: Wolters Kluwer and Lippincot William and Wilkins; 2010. p. 917-97.
2. Moffat AC, Osselton MD, Widdop B, Jickells S, Negrusz A. Introduction to forensic toxicology. Jickells S, Negrusz A (eds). Clarke's analytical forensic toxicology. Cambridge: Pharmaceutical press; 2008. p. 1-12.
3. Drummer OH. Toxicology/methods of analysis - antemortem. Siegel J, Knupfer G, Saukko P (Eds). Encyclopedia of forensic sciences. 1st edn. Philadelphia: Academic press; 2000. p. 1397-1403.
4. Flanagan RJ, Kala M, Braithwaite R, de Wolff FA. Other substances encountered in clinical and forensic toxicology. In: Jickells S, Negrusz A (eds). Clarke's analytical forensic toxicology. Cambridge: Pharmaceutical press; 2008. p. 79-129.
5. Branch S. Forensic and clinical toxicology. In: Hodgson E (ed). A textbook of modern toxicology. 3rd edn. New York: Wiley Interscience; 2004. p. 399-409.
6. Uges DRA, Hallworth M, Moore C, Negrusz A. Clinical toxicology, therapeutic drug monitoring, in utero exposure to drugs of abuse. In: Jickells S, Negrusz A (eds). Clarke's analytical forensic toxicology. Cambridge: Pharmaceutical press; 2008. p. 219-60.
7. Biswas G. General toxicology. Review of forensic medicine and toxicology. 2nd edn. New Delhi: Jaypee brothers; 2012. p. 411-26.
8. Ramsland K. Forensic toxicology. Available from: http://www.trutv.com/library/crime/criminal_mind/forensics/toxicology/2.html.
9. A history of toxicology. Available from: http://toxicologyproject.weebly.com/history.html.
10. Wennig R. Forensic toxicology. Available from: http://www.eolss.net/sample-chapters/c09/E6-12-23-00.pdf.
11. Eddleston M. Patterns and problems of deliberate self-poisoning in developing nations. *Q J Med* 2000; 93: 715-31.

12. Eddleston M, Dawson AH. Triage and clinical management of patients with acute pesticide self-poisoning presenting to small rural hospitals. *Clin Toxicol* 2012; 50: 455-57.
13. Gunnell D, Eddleston M, Phillips MR, Konradsen F. The global distribution of fatal pesticide self-poisoning: Systematic review. *BMC Public Health* 2007; 7: 357-71.
14. Senarathna L, Buckley NA, Jayamanna SF, Kelly PJ, Dibley MJ, Dawson AH. Validity of referral hospitals for the toxicovigilance of acute poisoning in Sri Lanka. World Health Organization. Available from: http://www.who.int/bulletin/volumes/90/6/11-092114/en/.
15. Poisoning factsheet-home and recreational safety. Injury center. Available from: http://www.cdc.gov/homeandrecreationalsafety/poisoning/poisoning-factsheet.htm.
16. Hearn WL. Toxicology/Interpretation of Results. Siegel J, Knupfer G, Saukko P (eds). Encyclopedia of forensic sciences. 1st edn. Philadelphia: Academic press; 2000. p. 1391-97.
17. Olson KR. Poisoning. In: McPhee SJ, Papadakis MA, Rabow MW (eds). Current medical diagnosis and treatment. New York: McGraw Hill and Lange; 2012. p. 1518-47.
18. Erickson TB, Thompson TM, Lu JJ. The approach to the patient with an unknown overdose. *Emerg Med Clin N Am* 2007; 25: 249-81.
19. Erickson TB, Aks S, Gussow L. Diagnosis and management of the overdosed patient: a rational approach to the toxic patient. *EM Practice*; 2001. p. 1-25.
20. Leikin JB. Approach to toxicology. In: Leikin JB, Paloucek FP (eds). Poisoning and toxicology handbook. 4th edn. New York: Informa healthcare; 2008. p. 35-53.
21. Flanagan J, Taylor A, Watson ID, Whelpton R. Sample collection, transport and storage. Fundamentals of analytical toxicology. Wiltshire: John Wiley and Sons; 2007. p. 21-48.
22. Kumar R, Singh B, Singh N, Singh J. Review of management of common poisoning in India. *Medicolegal Update* 2005; 5(2) [Internet]. Available at: http://www.indmedica.com/journals.php?journalid&issueid&articleid=861&action=article.
23. Pillay VV. Procedure of examination in medicolegal cases. Medicolegal pocket book for casualty medical officers. Mangalore: Sharada Press; 1997. p. 9-10.
24. Harish D, Chavali KK. The medicolegal case-should we be afraid of it? Anil Aggarwal's internet journal of forensic medicine and toxicology 2007; 8(1) [Internet]. Available from:
http://www.anilaggrawal.com/ij/vol_008_no_001/others/pg/pg001.html.
25. Medicolegal issues: Guidelines to medical officers. Available at: http://indianarmy.nic.in/writereaddata/Documents/medico_legal.pdf.
26. Parmananda Katara Vs Union of India. AIR 1986 SC 2039.
27. Finnberg A, Junuzovic M, Dragovic L, Ortiz-Reyes R, Hamel M, Davis J, Eriksson A. Homicide by poisoning. *Am J Forensic Med Pathol* 2013; 34: 38-42.
28. Molina DK, Hargrove VM. Fatal cocaine interactions: a review of cocaine-related deaths in Bexar County, Texas. *Am J Forensic Med Pathol* 2011; 32: 71-77.

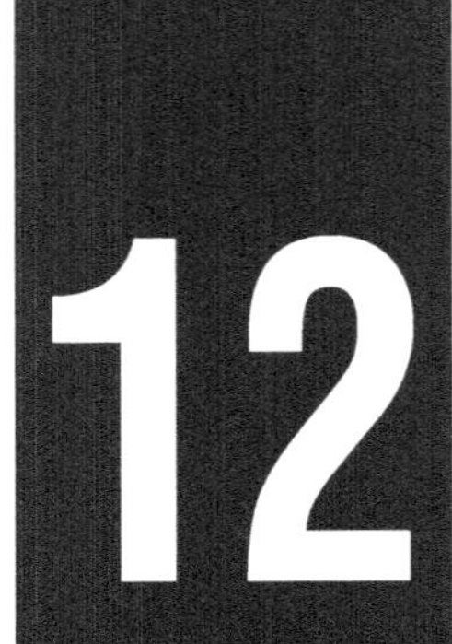

An Approach to a Case of Alcohol Intoxication

Sandeep Puri

'In vivo veritas: In wine [there is the] truth.'
Latin phrase

ABSTRACT

Alcohol intoxication has been identified as an important risk factor in injury occurrence, particularly road traffic accidents and violent crimes. Alcohol misuse is a common presentation to the Emergency Department (ED). The criteria of ICD-10 and DSM IV for alcohol misuse are not straightforward. The emergency medical practitioners are expected to be aware of this and clinically assess for presence of alcohol intoxication in injured persons brought to the ED. In case of medicolegal cases of injury, they are also required to collect and send blood samples to the forensic science laboratory. In India, the maximal permitted ethanol concentration for driving is 30 mg/100 ml of blood; drivers exceeding this limit may be imprisoned and/or fined. However, ethanol concentrations are not predictive of intoxication as it is a clinical diagnosis. Sometime, serious medical conditions may coexist in the intoxicated patients. These conditions are frequently missed when the patient is thought to be drunk.

It is implicit that those who have alcohol in the body must have drunk it, although the defense may attribute this to the prescribed medication that the person is taking. Hence, a thorough understanding of the metabolism, effects, consent associated sampling, examination and medicolegal issues is essential for any medical practitioner in the ED. The interpretation of results from the extrapolation of blood alcohol concentrations (BACs) and influence and interferences caused by some medications has been discussed.

Keywords: Intoxication, ICD Y90, ICD Y91, clinical examination, tests for incoordination, interpretation of blood alcohol concentration, medicolegal aspects of intoxication.

INTRODUCTION

Alcohol (ethanol, C_2H_5OH) is a commonly consumed beverage and most frequently detected drug by toxicology laboratories. It has health and social consequences via intoxication (drunkenness), dependence (habitual, compulsive and long-term drinking), and other biochemical effects. Alcohol is significant in clinical forensic medicine because of its association with violent crimes, traffic violations and assessments regarding fitness for detention.[1,2]

Ethanol is a colorless, odorless, flammable liquid with a warm burning taste produced by the fermentation of fruits and grains by yeast. Raw materials commonly used for starting this process include corn, molasses, fruit juices, grain, rye and barley. Fermented beverage has a maximum alcohol content of 14–15% by volume (percent v/v) as the yeast dies. The final product is either artificially sweetened or fortified with additional alcohol and mixed with congeners. Congeners are organic compounds added to beverage to impart the characteristic flavor and unique odor which is usually perceived by the doctor (or any other observer) in the breath of the individual (since ethanol is odorless). There are numerous alcoholic beverages depending on the locality, custom, traditions, social and political settings (Table 12.1). In hard liquors like whiskey, brandy, scotch, gin, vodka and rum, the alcoholic contents range from 35 to 50% which is brought about by distillation (superheating a mixture of alcohol and water with capture and cooling of the steam thus formed, to increase the percent alcohol concentration by volume).[1-4]

A beverage that contains at least 0.5% alcohol is considered an alcoholic drink. The concentration written on the labels of most bottles is volume of alcohol per volume of drink (v/v). In European Union, the alcohol content of drinks is referred to by percentage alcohol by volume (percent v/v). This is equivalent to the number of milliliters of pure alcohol per 100 ml of the drink. 'Proof' is the quantity of alcohol in beverages in the United States. The term proof equals twice the percentage of alcohol by volume. So, the common 80 proof whisky sold in the US contains 40% alcohol by volume. In India, the spirit (whisky, rum or brandy) is usually 42.8% by volume and 75 proof.[1,4]

The emergency medical officers are expected to clinically assess for the presence of alcohol in suspected cases of alcoholism brought to the emergency, and are also required to collect and send blood samples to the forensic science laboratory. They may have to appear in the court of law and appraise the judiciary regarding the patient from time to time (Box 12.1).[5,6] However, the level of training among these practitioners regarding clinical assessment of alcohol and other drugs of abuse, and preservation of samples are not very satisfactory. The most commonly used method of assessing for presence and extent of alcohol intoxication remains crude—sniffing for smell of alcohol in breath and checking slurring of speech.[5] Emergency room protocols for identifying a drunk driver or victim are also not standardized across countries and states, and BAC testing may not be available as a standard tool for screening in some emergency rooms, particularly in developing countries like ours. Therefore, the identification of a drunken driver or accident victim may still rely on a thorough clinical examination to determine alcohol intoxication, which without continuous training can lead to misleading results.[6] Moreover, they are usually not acquainted with

Table 12.1 Approximate percentage of alcohol by volume in beverages

Beverage	*Alcohol by volume*
Spirits (whisky, brandy, rum, gin, vodka)	35–50%
Port (fortified with brandy), sherry	17–21%
Wine	10–15%
Champagne	10–13%
Beers, stout, cider	4–8%

Box 12.1 Questions that may be asked in the court of law

What are the various symptoms which can be associated with alcohol intoxication?
How do you diagnose a case of drunkenness?
Is this quantity sufficient to cause symptoms in this person?
What is your opinion regarding alcohol consumption?
Was this patient suffering from any addictions, psychiatric disease or any other medical condition?
Is there any other disease which can mimic these symptoms?
How can you say that person was under the influence of alcohol?
Whether the suspect was driving under the influence of drugs and/or alcohol?
What are various tests available?
What is the accuracy and specificity of the tests used?
Is this person habituated of taking alcohol?
Can anything else produce false positive tests?
Can this test be false negative?

International Classification of Diseases (ICD-10) codes for alcohol intoxication. Hence, a thorough understanding of the metabolism (absorption, distribution and elimination), various signs and symptoms, examination, medicolegal reporting and opinion writing and medicolegal aspects of alcoholism including the provisions of Motor Vehicle Act in a suspected case of drunkenness is essential for any doctor working in the emergency department.

DEFINITIONS

Some definitions which a medical practitioner should be familiar with:[2,4,7-9]

- **Intoxication** is a condition that follows the administration of a psychoactive substance and results in disturbances in the level of consciousness, cognition, perception, judgment, affect or behavior, or other psychophysiological functions and responses (WHO).
- **Alcohol intoxication** is a physiological state which occurs after ingestion of large amount of alcohol in a short period of time.
- **Drunkenness** (inebriation) is an altered state of an individual affecting cognitive and motor activities that results from an elevated level of ethanol in the blood.

  'Drunkenness' is one aspect of 'intoxication' and with regard to alcohol describes a physiological state, whereas 'drunkenness' also involves social and behavioral component.
- **Binge drinking** ('heavy episodic drinking') is a pattern of drinking alcohol that brings blood alcohol concentration level to ≥ 0.08 g% and this corresponds to consumption of 5 or more drinks in a male or 4 or more drinks in a female (7+ alcohol units per session for women / 10+ units for men in United Kingdom) in about 2 hours.
- **Hangover (veisalgia)** is the experience of various unpleasant physiological effects following heavy consumption of alcoholic beverages.

- **Hazardous drinking** is defined as when a person drinks over the recommended weekly limit of alcohol (21 units for men and 14 units for women).
- **Harmful drinking** is defined as when a person drinks over the recommended weekly amount of alcohol and experiences health problems that are directly related to alcohol.
- **Alcohol withdrawal syndrome** is a cluster of symptoms observed in 6-48 hours in persons who stop drinking alcohol, following continuous and heavy consumption.
- **Alcohol dependence (alcoholism)** is a condition characterized by harmful consequences of repeated and compulsive alcohol use, and may sometimes be associated with physiological dependence, i.e. tolerance or symptoms of withdrawal.
- **Alcohol abuse** is defined as repetitive problems with alcohol use in any one of these four life areas—social, interpersonal, legal and occupational—or repeated use in hazardous situations, such as driving while intoxicated.
- **Proof of spirit** indicates a mixture containing 57.1% by volume or 49.28% by weight of absolute alcohol.
- **Standard drinks or units of alcohol** are a measure of specified amount of pure ethanol in alcoholic beverages expressed in grams used as a guideline in some countries.
- **Human performance toxicology** deals with the effects of alcohol and other intoxicating substances on a subject's ability to drive a motor vehicle or engage in other potentially hazardous activities.

Explanations

ICD-10 has defined harmful use as harm experienced after alcohol consumption in the absence of dependence. The 'Y' codes have been developed for alcohol intoxication. The Y90 classifies alcohol consumption by blood alcohol level and the Y91 code classifies alcohol consumption according to clinical assessment of intoxication (Tables 12.2 and 12.3).[5]

Table 12.2 ICD Y90 codes

Code	*Blood alcohol level*
Y90.0	< 20 mg/100 ml
Y90.1	20–39 mg/100 ml
Y90.2	40–59 mg/100 ml
Y90.3	60–79 mg/100 ml
Y90.4	80–99 mg/100 ml
Y90.5	100–119 mg/100 ml
Y90.6	120–199 mg/100 ml
Y90.7	200–239 mg/100 ml
Y90.8	≥ 240 mg/100 ml
Y90.9	Presence of alcohol, level not specified

Table 12.3 ICD Y91 codes

Code	Category	Signs and symptoms
Y91.0	Mild alcohol intoxication	Smell of alcohol in breath, slight behavioral disturbance in functions and responses or slight difficulty in coordination
Y91.1	Moderate alcohol intoxication	Smell of alcohol in breath, moderate behavioural disturbance in functions and responses or moderate difficulty in coordination
Y91.2	Severe alcohol intoxication	Severe disturbance in functions and responses, severe difficulty in co-ordination or impaired ability to cooperate
Y91.3	Very severe alcohol intoxication	Very severe disturbance in functions and responses, very severe difficulty in coordination or loss of ability to cooperate
Y91.9	Alcohol involvement, not otherwise specified (NOS)	Alcohol use by and large is heavily stigmatized in the public eye

Unit of Alcohol

One unit of alcohol is defined as 10 ml (8 g of pure alcohol) in UK, 10 g (12.7 ml) in Australia and 14 g in US. A standard drink is 30 ml of spirits; 330 ml can of beer or 100 ml glass of wine. Thus, in terms of the alcohol it contains, a standard drink or unit will be the same—regardless of whether it contains beer, distilled spirits, wine, or a mix of any of these beverages.[3-5]

To calculate standard drinks, the following formula is used: Volume of container (litres) × % alcohol by volume (ml/100 ml) × 0.789 = Number of standard drinks.

Hangover

It is a set of symptoms including thirst, headache, nausea, diarrhea, fatigue and the 'shakes' typically occurring after the intoxicating effect of the alcohol begins to wear off. It may be associated with decreased occupational, cognitive or visual-spatial skill performance. While a hangover can be experienced at any time, it is generally experienced in the morning after a night of heavy drinking. 'Dark' drinks with more congeners, such as brandy, wine (especially red) and whiskey are associated with more severe effects, while with 'clear' drinks such as gin and vodka the effects are less.[4,10]

In addition to the physical symptoms, a hangover may also induce psychological symptoms including heightened feelings of depression and anxiety, and an independent risk factor for cardiac death.

Alcohol Dependence

Alcohol is both physically and psychologically addictive, and some individuals become dependent on it. It has a moderate to high abuse potential with up to 10% of users becoming dependent and developing into alcoholics. Dependent means that a person feels that they are unable to function without alcohol and the consumption of alcohol becomes an important, or sometimes the most important factor in their life. This not only interferes with physical and mental health but affects the family and social responsibilities. An alcoholic will continue to drink despite serious health, family or legal problems. Alcohol dependence is defined under fourth edition of the *Diagnostic and Statistical Manual of Mental Disorders* (DSM-IV) as repeated alcohol-related difficulties in at least three of seven areas of functioning particularly tolerance and withdrawal that occur over a 12-month period.[2] Those seven areas include:

i. Tolerance which is defined by increased amounts of alcohol to achieve same degree of intoxication.
ii. Withdrawal symptoms.
iii. Alcohol is imbibed in greater amounts or over longer time periods than intended.
iv. Persistent desire and/or unsuccessful efforts to reduce or stop alcohol use but these are not successful.
v. Great deal of time is spent in obtaining alcohol or recovering from the negative consequences of alcohol use, for e.g., hangover.
vi. Important social, occupational or recreational activities are diminished or given up completely because of alcohol dependence.
vii. Continued use, despite knowledge of alcohol-related harm (physical or psychological) which are either caused by or intensified by drinking alcohol.

Alcohol Abuse

Alcohol abuse is defined as a pattern of drinking that result in one or more of the following situations within a 12-month period:[7,10,11]

- Failure to fulfill major work, school or home responsibilities.
- Drinking in situations that are physically dangerous, such as driving a car or operating machinery.
- Having recurring alcohol-related legal problems, such as being arrested for driving under the influence of alcohol or for physically hurting someone while drunk.
- Continued drinking despite having ongoing relationship problems that are caused or worsened by the drinking.

The main features differentiating alcohol dependence from alcohol abuse are evidence of tolerance, the presence of withdrawal symptoms and the use of alcohol to relieve or avoid withdrawal. In alcohol abuse, there is no significant psychological or physiological dependence on alcohol.

Alcohol Withdrawal

In chronic alcoholics, there is dependence and tolerance of the central nervous system to the effects of alcohol. Depending on their level of dependence, a person can experience withdrawal symptoms if they suddenly stop drinking alcohol. Withdrawal symptoms can be both physical and psychological. It may present as a mild picture of uncomplicated alcohol withdrawal or as the more severe delirium tremens of alcohol withdrawal (DSM-IV criteria).[2,12]

Signs and Symptoms

The earliest sign of alcohol withdrawal seen 5–10 hours after stopping of alcohol is tremors of the hands ('shakes' or 'jitters'). This accompanied by insomnia, nightmares, anxiety and GI symptoms, and autonomic hyperactivity (sweating, hypertension, tachycardia, tachypnea, fever) and grand mal (generalized) seizures in the next 24–48 hours. *Delirium tremens* is a state of intense acute withdrawal seen in less than 5% cases, and characterized by delirium (mental confusion, agitation and fluctuating levels of consciousness), tremors and autonomic over-activity (for e.g., marked increase in pulse, blood pressure and respiration).[2,12]

Many alcoholics may develop symptoms of withdrawal when in custody which can have serious consequences. The doctor should assess the degree of dependence, and then initiate treatment to prevent the potentially fatal complications of delirium tremens and convulsions.

EPIDEMIOLOGY

In various epidemiological studies conducted over the last many years, it has been found that alcohol contributes to traumatic outcomes that kill or disable at a relatively young age. This results in the loss of many years of life, disability or death. Worldwide, alcohol causes 1.8 million deaths (3.2% of total) and 58.3 million (4% of total) of Disability-Adjusted Life Years (DALYs). In 2009, the Delhi drunken driving report prepared by the Campaign against Drunken Driving found out that the capital loses 1,500 people every year in accidents caused by drunk drivers. The report added that the highest mortality in such accidents was among those below the age of five years and in the 21–34 year age group. Around 17% of government hospital beds are occupied by road accident victims in drunken driving cases.[12] Another study indicated that 26% of attempted suicides and 15% of road traffic injuries were linked to alcohol. Another constant finding in most of the studies was that men are the primary consumers of alcoholic beverages with a reported 49.6% in one village in Punjab.[5]

The US Preventive Services Task Force (USPSTF) has updated its guidelines for screening and behavioral counseling interventions in primary care to reduce alcohol misuse. With approximately 30% of the US population engaging in risky drinking behaviors, the USPSTF recommends that clinicians screen all adult patients 18 years of age or older for alcohol misuse, as well as provide patients engaged in risky or hazardous drinking with brief behavioral counseling interventions to reduce alcohol misuse.[9]

METABOLISM

It is a fact that an individual who exhibits the signs and symptoms of intoxication and tests positive for alcohol must have ingested it, although it can be absorbed through lungs after breathing alcohol/air mixtures for several hours (blood alcohol concentration of up to 50 mg/100 ml has been reported). Once ingested, it is absorbed into the body through passive diffusion that occurs through the mucosa of the gastrointestinal tract (GIT); the rate of absorption being maximum in the duodenum as its mucosa is thinner and blood supply is more abundant than the stomach.

As soon as alcohol enters the blood stream, elimination begins. About 5–10% of the total alcohol absorbed is excreted unchanged in the breath, urine and sweat.

The concentration of alcohol in the breath and urine mirrors the concentration of alcohol in the blood. This allows the estimation of BAC from its levels in the urine and breath. The overall elimination (90-95% alcohol is metabolized in the liver by *alcohol dehydrogenase*) is fairly constant as the enzyme becomes saturated at low alcohol concentration and soon reaches it maximum working capacity. Rates of elimination of alcohol can vary from person to person with the range from 15–25 mg/100 ml per hour (average rate is 17–18 mg/100 ml/h), with chronic alcoholics having well-developed liver enzyme systems often achieving a higher level of elimination. A person's blood alcohol concentration (BAC) level is represented by the amount of ethanol in a given amount of blood. It is measured as milligrams of ethanol per deciliter of blood (mg/dl). The rate of absorption is much faster than the rate of elimination, giving rise to the characteristic blood alcohol curve (Fig. 12.1). Peak BAC level usually occurs in 30–60 min (range 20 min to 3 hours) after ingestion, but the time to peak levels are influenced by many factors. One standard drink will raise the BAC by about 17 mg/dl.[1-4,13]

FACTORS DETERMINING ALCOHOL ABSORPTION

The shape of the BAC is influenced by large number of variables, many of which are either not quantifiable or discoverable in a specific case. The major determinants of the timing and peak of the BAC include body size, gender, amount and type of beverage ingested, duration of drinking, and the presence and type of food (Table 12.4). These are important in calculating the peak BAC or extrapolating from a given level.[2-4,14]

Body water content: Alcohol is more soluble in water than in fat. This means that tissues rich in water, for e.g., muscle, take up more alcohol than do tissues rich in fat. Hence, the peak levels depend on both weight and gender of the individual.

- *Body weight and build:* Following absorption, an individual with larger total body water will dilute more alcohol than an individual with a smaller volume of body water. Hence, if same quantity of alcohol is consumed by different sized individual, a lower peak will be reached in the large sized individual. Similarly, a leaner person with a greater muscle mass provides a larger volume for alcohol to be distributed as compared to a person who weighs the same but has a higher percentage of body fat. Hence, if there are two individuals of equal weight, then the person with low body fat will be affected less than the person with a higher level of body fat.

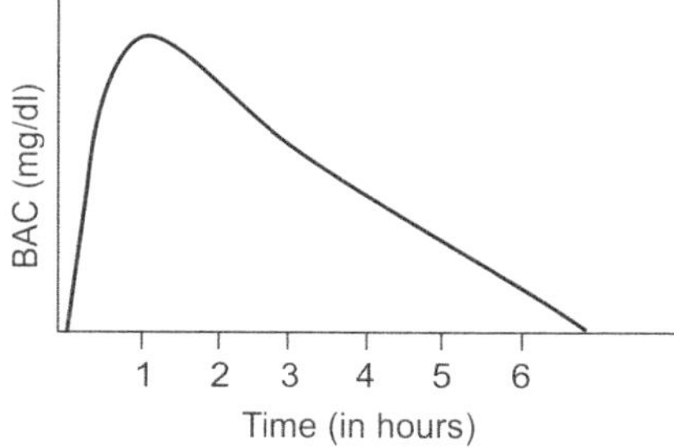

Fig. 12.1 Blood alcohol curve

Table 12.4 Factors affecting rate of absorption of alcohol

Factors enhancing absorption	*Factors decreasing absorption*
Femaleness	Maleness
Empty stomach	Full stomach
Drugs: Cholinergic agents, parasympathomimetic agents, aspirin, erythromycin, metoclopramide or H_2-receptor antagonists	Drugs: Anticholinergic agents, sympathomimetic agents, nicotine or caffeine, chlorpromazine, tricyclic antidepressants, antidiarrheal agents, amphetamines or opiates
Gastric resection, gastric ulcers or gastritis	Malignant gastric neoplasm or pyloric stenosis
Carbonated drinks	Fatty foods

- *Gender:* Females usually have a smaller body mass and a higher proportion of body fat than their counterparts. They exhibit higher peak alcohol levels than the males of same weight after consuming the same amount of alcohol.

Time of gastric emptying: A delay of the emptying of the stomach into the small intestine will delay absorption of alcohol, whereas anything which hastens stomach emptying will increase the absorption.

- *Type of drink:* Beverages with concentration of 10-20% of alcohol is maximally absorbed. Alcoholic drinks of lesser strength are absorbed slowly because of a lower concentration gradient (as alcohol is absorbed by passive diffusion). Besides, intake of large volumes may also delay gastric emptying and cause further slowing of absorption. Drinks with higher alcohol content irritate the stomach and pyloric sphincter causing increased secretion of mucus and delayed gastric emptying, thus slowing absorption.
- *Duration of drinking:* If alcohol is ingested slowly over a prolonged period, it will be eliminated at the same time, giving rise to a much lower peak alcohol concentration and a flatter BAC curve.
- *Presence of food:* The presence of food in the stomach reduces the rate of gastric emptying, dilutes the alcohol that enters the stomach, and limits the contact between the alcohol and the gastric mucosa. Hence, blood peak values will be lower and there will be a slower rise of the BAC on a full stomach, as compared to an empty stomach (Fig. 12.2). Absorption of alcohol is faster when the stomach is empty; the empty stomach, allows rapid passage of the alcohol into the small intestine. Moreover, the rate of alcohol absorption depends not only on the presence of food, but also on the type of food present. Fatty foods such as milk, cream and butter coat the gastric mucosa and delay the stomach-emptying time, the reduced BAC is due to combination of delayed and reduced absorption of alcohol.

Physiological factors and genetic variation: Factors, such as stomach wall permeability, blood supply to the alimentary tract and the rate of gastric emptying vary from person to person and from time to time in the same person. All of these affect the shape of the blood alcohol curve.

Other factors: Some other individual parameters, such as gastric surgery (may lead to a more rapid absorption), medication use and mode of taking the drinks

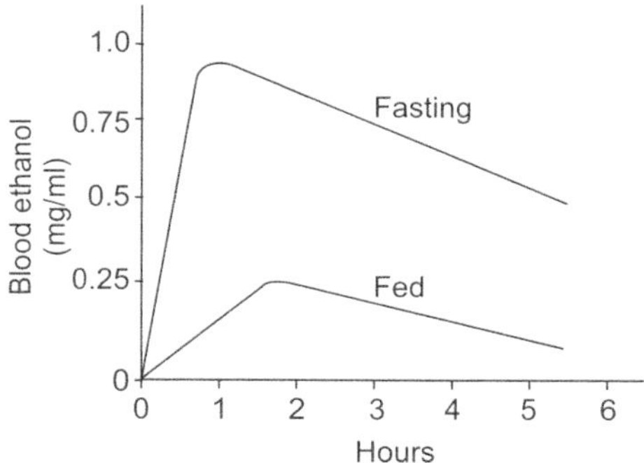

Fig. 12.2 Blood alcohol curve in relation to presence of food

(carbonated drinks hasten absorption as the bubbles greatly increase the surface area carrying alcohol) are important factors in assessing blood alcohol levels and peak alcohol levels.[13]

In short circuit operations like Billroth I and II, gastro-jejunostomies and Roux en-Y gastric bypass (for weight loss) with the absence of a functional pylorus, alcohol will move directly into the small intestine. Diffusion is fast and effective. The BAC of these subjects will reach peak levels much earlier than expected. In these cases, the result of back calculation using the Widmark formula will not be a true reflection of the intoxication level during the incident.

ACTION

Alcohol is a psychoactive substance and the predominant pharmacodynamic action is as a central nervous system (CNS) depressant. As a CNS depressant, it acts as a sedative, hypnotic and an anesthetic. In small doses, it interferes with cortical function but in larger doses alcohol may depress medullary processes that regulate homeostatic control of autonomic body functions (controlling respiration and circulation). The apparent stimulatory effects of alcohol occur because it acts first on the higher centers of the brain (neocortex) that govern inhibition, control judgment and morals. It impairs reaction time and affects an individual's ability to execute a range of motor tasks.[1,2,4]

The physical effects are dependent predominantly on the amount consumed. In contrast, the subjective intellectual and emotional effects are strongly influenced by the 'set' and 'setting.' The 'set' is individual's underlying personality traits, i.e. mood and attitudes of the individual at the time of consumption which may become unmasked. The 'setting' refers to the external circumstances in which the consumption occurs.[1,2]

SIGNS AND SYMPTOMS OF INTOXICATION

Clinical signs for alcohol intoxication can be useful for screening in areas where the use of breath analyzers or quick blood analysis for alcohol intoxication is not routine or available. This would increase the power for brief intervention and referral to treatment in emergency rooms. Signs and symptoms of alcohol intoxication vary with amount of consumption, type of drink and duration over which it is taken. As mentioned earlier, different alcoholic beverages contain different levels of alcohol.

Following are the effects of acute alcohol intoxication:[1-4]

I. **Neuropsychiatric effects**
   a. It causes impaired judgment, incoordination, memory disorders, impulsive and aggressive behavior, stupor and coma, thus increasing the risk of accidents and injury.
   b. Some psychiatric syndromes temporarily show up during heavy drinking including an alcohol-induced mood disorder (sadness), alcohol-induced anxiety disorder and alcohol-induced psychotic disorder characterized by auditory hallucinations and paranoid delusions.
   c. Temporary anterograde amnesia is an episode of blackout in which the person forgets all or part of what occurred during a drinking session.
   d. It causes snoring and exacerbates sleep apnea.
   e. It reduces deep sleep and leads to disturbing dreams.
   f. Hangover syndrome.

II. **Gastrointestinal system:** Patient may present with pain abdomen, vomiting and hematemesis due to following effects:
   a. Esophagitis, gastritis, pylorospasm and Mallory-Weiss lesion which is a longitudinal tear in the mucosa at the gastroesophageal junction.
   b. Acute pancreatitis.

III. **Cardiac and respiratory system:** Patient may have symptoms like palpitations, dyspnea, edema and cough due to cardiovascular involvement in the form of:
   a. Atrial or ventricular arrhythmias without any underlying heart disease which is known as *holiday heart syndrome.*
   b. Increased risk for coronary artery disease and cardiomyopathy due to chronic heavy drinking. These patients present with unexplained arrhythmias or heart failure.
   c. Respiratory depression due to CNS depressant effect.
   d. Vomiting in a comatose patient leading to aspiration pneumonia.
   e. Diuresis which can occur independent of the amount of alcohol taken.

IV. **Musculoskeletal system**
   a. Acute alcohol ingestion can cause acute alcoholic myopathy which can cause rhabdomyolysis with myoglobinuria, acute tubular necrosis and acute renal failure.
   b. Orthopedic injuries, like fractures or dislocation can occur under the influence of acute alcohol intoxication which can produce pain and loss of mobility.

The physiologic effects of alcohol are more pronounced when the blood level is rising as compared to levels attained at peak or plateau, or when the level is falling. This is known as the *Mellanby effect* and is believed to result from an acute tolerance to alcohol that develops during intoxication. Signs of intoxication at different BAC levels in absence of tolerance are given in Table 12.5. In summary, the progressive effects which become more pronounced with steadily increasing BAC, consist of intellectual deterioration, followed by impairment of motor coordination, loss of consciousness, respiratory depression, circulatory collapse and death.

Table 12.5 Signs of intoxication at different BAC levels

BAC levels (mg/100 ml)	*Degree of Impairment*
20–40	Impairment of fine motor control, reaction time, mood state and judgment.
50–140	Low to moderate impairment in cognitive function and gross motor skills.
150–190	Impaired movement and speech, serious mental and physical impairment, euphoria, irritability and aggressiveness.
200–290	Nausea, vomiting, visual impairment and changes in mental state.
300–390	Generally induces partial amnesia ('blackout'), hypotension and hypothermia.
≥ 400	Alcohol poisoning, coma and risk of death regardless of tolerance or whether individual is alcohol-dependent.

Death from Alcohol Poisoning

A BAC in the range of 350–450 mg/100 ml is generally taken as minimal lethal level, although survival at much higher concentrations is well documented in literature. Alcohol intoxication may result in death owing to respiratory or circulatory failure, or as a result of aspiration of stomach contents in the absence of a gag reflex. Death associated with BAC < 350 mg/100 ml suggests other underlying complicating factors. Usually, there is an interaction between alcohol and some other drug that has also been ingested. In some, low levels of BAC may trigger a lethal cardiac dysrhythmia in a susceptible person, or the presence of a pre-existing disease or gastrointestinal surgeries may hasten death. Hence, caution must be maintained in interpretation in light of the great variation of human response to alcohol ingestion.[2,4]

Management of Acute Alcohol Intoxication

Brief outline is given in Flow chart 12.1.[4] (For details refer to any standard textbook of toxicology).

EXAMINATION OF SUSPECTED CASE OF DRUNKENNESS

Conditions under which these cases are brought for examination

These cases are brought by police for medical examination in the following circumstances:[6,15,16]

a. Person was found in a drunken condition and was unable to take care of himself or behaving in a disorderly manner in a public place.
b. Person may be involved in some crime like rape, assault or homicide, as a victim or assailant.
c. In cases of road traffic accidents, medical examination of victim or driver may be required for determining alcohol consumption and/or drug intoxication.

Flow chart 12.1 Management of an intoxicated patient

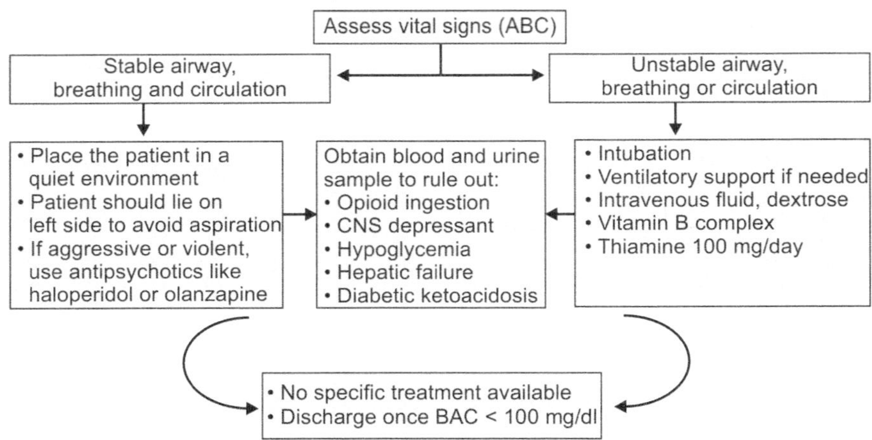

The medical practitioner needs to carry out an examination in the above mentioned cases to ascertain whether:

i. There is a condition present that might be due to alcohol and/or drug
ii. There is a condition that may mimic intoxication
iii. The person's ability to drive is impaired
iv. The person is fit for detention.

The police will then require a specimen for analysis, provided the doctor has advised them that there is a condition present that might be due to alcohol and/ or drug.

Consent

Informed consent is established before the examination and the person is explained that the information *will not be* treated confidentially. The examining doctor may explain the individual in a manner as suggested in Box 12.2.[15,16]

In case a person fails to give consent, he may be medically examined without his consent [even if reasonable force is required for doing it (Sec. 53 CrPC)], if following criteria are fulfilled:[4,16]

i. The person is an accused and has been arrested on charge of committing an offence punishable under law.
ii. There are reasonable grounds for believing that an examination of his person will afford evidence as to the commission of the offence.
iii. The requisition for medicolegal examination is from an officer of the rank of a sub-inspector of police or above acting in good faith in his aid and under his direction.

For example, in a road traffic accident case, the police may bring a person suspected of drunk driving for medical examination, but he refuses the same. The correct procedure for the doctor would be *not* to conduct the examination

Box 12.2 Informed consent

i. I have been asked to examine you to ascertain whether in my opinion, you have a condition which might be due to alcohol or drugs. You should be aware that any conversation with me might not be treated confidentially.
ii. This examination would culminate in the preparation of a medicolegal injury report.
iii. All relevant investigations needed for medicolegal purpose would be done.
iv. The findings of the report may go against you if they do not tally with the history given.

Signature of the person Signature of the doctor

forcefully. However, if the police arrest that person and bring him for MLR under Sec. 53 CrPC, then reasonable force can be applied.

History

History in a case of suspected alcohol intoxication is very important, both for medical management and medicolegal report writing. Specific history should be noted as given in Table 12.6. History should be corroborated from close relatives, friends or contacts. However, obtaining accurate and reliable information about a person's drinking habits can be extremely difficult, because the average person tends to underestimate or deliberately lie about the amount of alcohol consumed. Information about the time of drinking and type of liquor may be correct. The longer the time between an injury and admission to an emergency room, the less likely a person is to report previous drinking, even with a positive BAC.[17]

Take a full medical history including details of any current medical problems, and details of recent events, particularly about any road traffic accident that led to the event. Past or present medical history (with specific reference to diabetes, epilepsy, hypertension, asthma, and visual and hearing problems), past surgical and psychiatric history is noted. Details of medicines taken (prescribed, over the counter and illicit) in the past or present, and any previous attempts of self harm should be recorded. Social history and relevant educational history to assess

Table 12.6 Specific history regarding alcohol and/or drug intake

Amount consumed
Type of drink
Duration of intake
Symptoms at the time of presentation
Time of first and last drink and food (am/pm)
Period of regular use
Quantity used per day
Frequency of use
Any drug used
Experience of withdrawal

learning disability should be noted. Effort should be made to rule out methanol poisoning, as it is a common adulterant in indigenous alcoholic drinks.[4]

Previous brain injuries will have an effect on coordination, walking abilities, intelligence, nystagmus, memory, and/or behavior. A post epileptic stupor is one of the conditions which is often confused with intoxication.

Any previous injury in the upper or lower limbs will affect his performance of the tests. Lower limb injuries are important because the examiner will later on determine the gait and ability to turn around. A person with paralysis or other neurological defects will not be able to perform coordination tests.

Examination

Detailed general and systemic examination is done to exclude any metabolic conditions, diseases and injuries. The following are noted:[4,13,18,19]

i. General demeanor/appearance of patient and state of clothes for any soiling.
ii. Any *injuries* present. Injuries could have been sustained in a motor vehicle accident or as a result of resistance to arrest. Careful documentation of these injuries needs to be done. Compare the characteristics of the wounds with the allegations made by the subject. Wound identification is important, as well as the time element attached to it.
iii. *Gait* is observed for any unsteadiness, staggering, bumping into people or furniture. The best way is to watch him approaching the examination facility, or to ask the person to go to the weighing machine, and while doing so, watch the gait. The person must be unaware that he is subjected to a gait test. While he is walking, watch for orthopedic defects that may cause this abnormality. Gait on turning (normal, unsteady, stumbling) is also noted. A little bit of postural hypotension should not be interpreted as an unsteadiness or gait abnormality. Avoid asking the person to rise from a chair and then walk in a certain direction.
iv. *Orientation and memory:* Ask him about incidents which have occurred few hours prior to examination to check his memory (clear, vague or confused) and mental alertness. Ask him about the date, time and place where he is at present (good, moderate, bad or indefinite).
v. *Behavior:* Whether noisy, jovial, boastful, rude, emotional, talkative, excited, nervous or uncontrollable. If the subject is cooperative, state it.
vi. Note his *face*, whether normal, flushed or pale. Alcohol is known for its vaso-dilatatory effect and redness of the face is indicative of this effect.
vii. Record whether the patient can understand, and whether his *speech* is normal, thick and slurred, stuttering or confused. Speech is also observed for incoherence, unintelligible, aggressive, offensive or over precise.
viii. Examine the *tongue*, whether dry, moist and clean or furred. Dry tongue is seen in thirst, and waning phase of BAC. Moist tongue may be indicative of having taken any drink including water.
ix. *Signs of vomiting and salivation:* As soon as the alcohol concentration inside the intestines reaches a concentration of about 20%, an ileus will follow. An ileus is responsible for vomiting. If there is vomiting, it usually is an indication of over indulgence. Nausea is responsible for abnormal

salivation. Salivation and drooling may also be the result of suppression of swallowing reflex. It is, therefore, only found in the severely intoxicated.

x. *Smell of alcohol:* Strong, moderate, faint or none. This aspect of the observation is very much debatable. The smell is dependent on the capabilities of the examiner, and smell acuity differs from person to person. The smell of the breath may confirm that alcohol has been taken and the type of drink, but is no guide whatsoever to the amount. For instance, certain liquors like vodka have a lesser odor than that of beer.

xi. *Ears:* Examine the ears for any discharge and any chronic disease. Any middle ear condition may have an impact on the balance and the maintaining thereof in the subject (vertigo, ataxia) or inability to hear questions or commands.

xii. The person is asked to copy a few lines from a book or newspaper and *handwriting* should be assessed. Note the time taken, ability to write in line and any repetition or omission of words. The individual can be asked to sign his name and compared with his driving license. Drawing simple patterns, such as triangle and diamond may be preferable, if the person is illiterate.

xiii. *Examine for drug abuse:* Look for needle marks, shivering, yawning, rhinorrhea, gooseflesh and lacrimation.

xiv. *Eyes:* Examine the eyes, noting the state of the conjunctiva (normal or congested), pupillary size (normal, equal, unequal, mydriasis or miosis), response to light, visual fields and acuity (reading the time on a clock across a room), and the presence of nystagmus (coarse, fine, continuous or absent). Note should be made of use of spectacles or contact lens and any other abnormal eye findings. In drunkenness, drooping and swollen eyelids, congestion of conjunctiva and horizontal nystagmus may be seen and convergence test is negative (difficulty in convergence).

Conjunctiva: Alcohol is known for its vaso-dilation and hence suffusion. Other conditions and diseases can irritate the conjunctival vessels as well like pyrexia, allergic conjunctivitis, Beçhet syndrome, sleepless night, swimming pool chlorine or pH imbalance.

Response to light: The person is asked to look at an object in the room while a light is shone into the eye. This will eliminate the possibility of pupil size change as a result of accommodation. The reaction may be normal, delayed (intoxication), or non-reacting (severe intoxication).

Nystagmus: The head is held in the neutral position. The subject is asked to follow with the eyes of an object held about 30–40 cm in front of him/her. The object is moved from side to side to a maximum angle of about 45° (Fig. 12.3). If the object is moved to a more acute angle, they muscles of eye movement will be stressed and nystagmus can be elicited in a sober person.

xv. *Tests to determine incoordination:* Co-ordination is defined as the smooth recruitment, interaction and cooperation of separate muscles or groups in order to accomplish a definite motor act. Watch the patient unbutton his shirt, dressing, undressing or handling objects like picking up a pen. Carry out a series of standardized field impairment tests (FITs) to check muscle coordination. These consist of Romberg test (marked, moderate, weak or

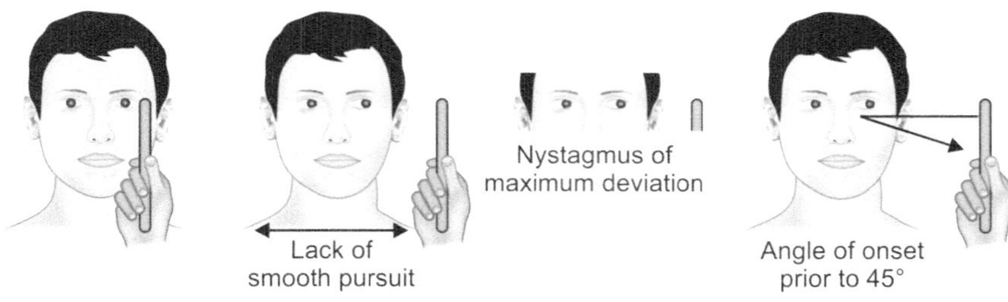

Fig. 12.3 Horizontal gaze nystagmus test

absent), Walk and Turn test, One Leg Stand test and a Finger Nose test (Box 12.3).

xvi. *Knee reflexes* are elicited to check whether normal, exaggerated or depressed. Reflexes are equally depressed in intoxication. Sometimes, the subject may exaggerate to impress the examiner but they are usually not equal in magnitude. In sober subjects, hyper reflexes are encountered with upper motor neuron abnormalities and hyporeflexivity with lower motor neuron pathology. Reflexes can have a pendular quality in cerebellar ataxia (hypotonia). It is important to elicit other reflexes during the examination (abdominal, ankle) in order to eliminate or confirm neuropathology.

xvii. Examine the *cardiovascular system* noting pulse, blood pressure, temperature and heart sounds.

xviii. *Respiratory* (hurried, slow, shallow, deep, stertorous, sighing or gasping, any added sounds) and *gastrointestinal system* (soft, tender, bowel sounds, enlarged liver or spleen, ascites) examination are done both to exclude other diagnosis and to find out complications related to acute or chronic alcohol consumption.

Some specific effects of alcohol intoxication are discussed below:[2,19]

i. *Slurred speech:* Speech production is a complex motor activity. Slurring or stuttering is due to incoordination of the tongue muscle that results in improper formation of words. It is a sensitive index of alcohol intoxication, since it requires a high degree of coordination. Changes in speech are produced at BAC > 100 mg/dl (moderate to strong intoxication), although the effects of lower BAC have been variable. Normal speech defects may be seen in chronic stuttering and defects of the tongue and mouth. The test may consist of asking the person to read a passage, but it will become obvious during normal conversation.

ii. *Nystagmus:* The effect of alcohol on the CNS can be observed in the eyes, since they are connected with the CNS. Alcohol can cause nystagmus through two mechanisms. By acting on the vestibular system, it can cause positional alcohol nystagmus (PAN), detected when the patient is lying supine with the head turned to either the left or right. Horizontal gaze nystagmus (HGN) results from the inhibition of the smooth pursuit system and the impaired

Box 12.3 Standardized field impairment test

- **Romberg test:** The person is asked to stand up straight with feet together and arms down by the sides. When told to start, he should tilt his head back slightly and close his eyes (*this is demonstrated by the examiner but he/she should not close his/her eyes*). Tell him to keep the head tilted backwards with eyes closed for about 30 secs, and then bring his head forward. Assessment is based on ability to stand still during instructions, whether he sways excessively or unable to complete the test (positive sign). Comment on his internal body clock (whether he is able to judge 30 secs). The essential feature is that the patient is unsteadier than with open eyes. With severe intoxication, a positive Romberg is seen even with open eyes or in the sitting position (Fig. 12.4).

  Romberg is often regarded as a test for coordination of the lower limbs. It is, however, a test for loss of position sense (proprioception and semi-circular canals in the middle ear) or sensory ataxia in the legs and not a test for cerebellar ataxia.
- **Walk and turn test:** Identify a real or imaginary line. The examiner puts his left foot on the line, then his right foot on the line in front of the left touching heel to toe (*demonstrate*). The person is asked to do the same and put his arms down by the sides and keep them there throughout the entire test (Fig. 12.5).

  When told to start, the person should take nine heels to toe steps along the line. On each step, the heel of the foot must be placed against the toe of the other foot (*demonstrate*). When the ninth step has been taken, he then leaves the front foot on the line and turns around using a series of small steps with the other foot. After turning, he then takes another nine heel to toe steps along the line. Tell him to watch his feet at all times and count each step loud and not to stop until the test is completed. The person is assessed as whether he is able to stand during instructions, start too soon or late, stops walking, incorrect turn, misses heel to toe, steps off line, raises arms and incorrect step count.
- **One leg stand test:** The person is asked to stand with his feet together and arms by the sides. When told to start, he should raise his foot 6–8 inches off the ground, keeping his leg straight and toes pointing forward, with the foot parallel to the ground (*demonstrate*). Arms are by the sides and he should keep looking at his elevated foot while counting out loud in the following manner, 'one…two…three…four…' and so on until the examiner tells him to stop. The person is assessed as to whether he sways, hops, puts his foot down or raises arms (Fig. 12.6).
- **Finger nose test:** The person is asked to stand with his feet together. The arms extended with both hands out in front or on sides, palms side up and closed with the index finger of both hands extended (*demonstrate*). When told to start he should tilt his head back slightly (*demonstrate*) and close his eyes. When the examiner instructs he should move that hand to touch the tip of his nose with the tip of that finger and lower his hand once done (*demonstrate*). The examiner calls out the hands in the following order: left, right, left, right…The person is assessed whether he sways his body, use incorrect hand, and any other comments (Fig. 12.7).
- **Mirror test:** Ask the subject to perform the same hand movements as you do. Spread the fingers of one hand, touch each individual fingertip with the contralateral index finger or thumb. Reverse the hands and repeat the movement. The doctor does the same and the subject has to interpret the 'mirror image'.
- Flex the elbow to a right angle and ask the subject to pronate and supinate continuously and rapidly (good test for dysdiadochokinesia or cerebellar ataxia). When it is abnormal, the movements will be slow, awkward and incomplete, and the rhythm is irregular.

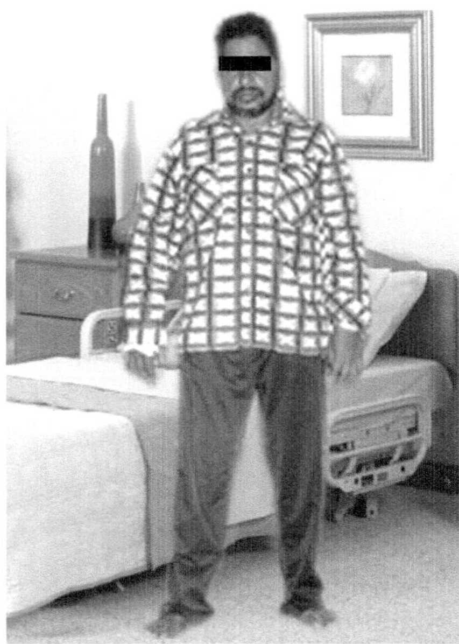

Fig. 12.4 Romberg test: Patient is unable to stand still and sways to either side

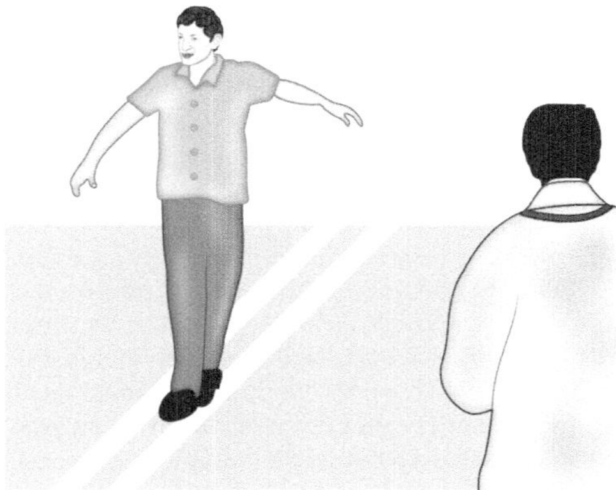

Fig. 12.5 Walk and turn test

ability to maintain eccentric gaze brought about by alcohol's effect on ocular movements via neural mechanisms.

- *PAN:* Initially, PAN I nystagmus is seen in the direction towards which the head is turned (30 minutes after alcohol ingestion), but after 5–6 hours, the PAN II nystagmus is seen in the opposite direction to which the head is turned.
- *HGN:* They are jerky movements of the eyeball when the gaze is directed to one side (Fig. 12.3). The fast phase of HGN is in the direction of gaze

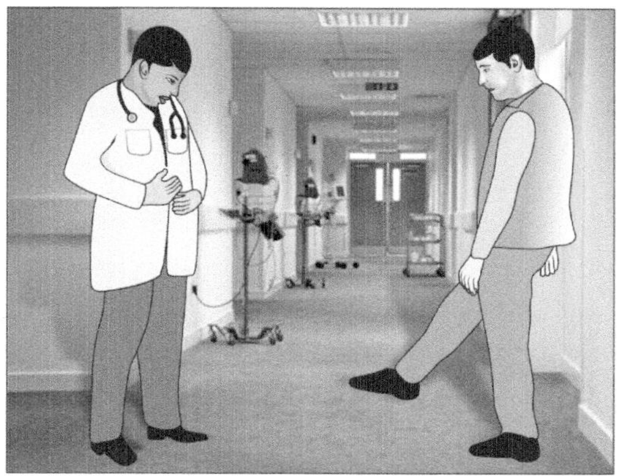

Fig. 12.6 Stand on one leg test

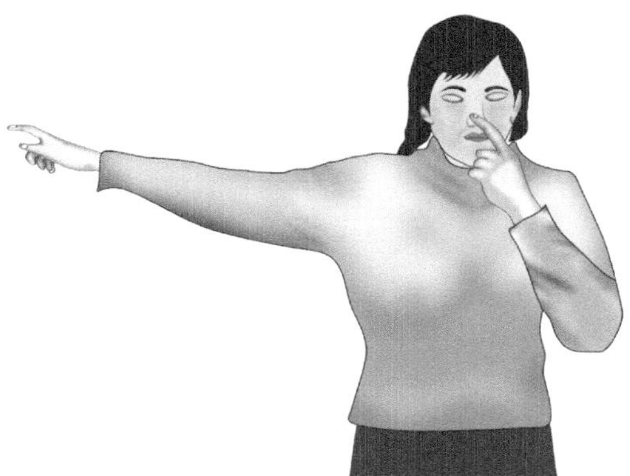

Fig. 12.7 Finger nose test

and it becomes intensified at a more eccentric gaze position. An angle of onset of 40° or less from the midline is a sensitive indicator of a BAC > 100 mg/dl (it is noticeable even at 80 mg/dl). HGN may be noted in several pathological conditions, including ingestion of sedative and tranquilizing drugs, hence its presence should not be taken as proof of alcohol intoxication (Table 12.7).

iii. *Pupillary changes:* In the early stages of alcoholic intoxication, the pupils dilate, then becoming pinpoint as the level of intoxication advances, particularly when the state of coma is reached. Alcohol may slow the pupillary response to light, such an effect being one of the more reliable eye signs of intoxication, although it is difficult to detect clinically.

iv. *Cardiovascular effects:* Moderate doses of alcohol cause a slight increase in pulse rate and blood pressure. However, with higher intake, there is depression of cardiovascular functions.

v. *Metabolic effects:* Emergency medical officers should be aware that hypoglycemia may accompany alcohol intoxication because of inhibition of

Table 12.7 Nystagmus seen in other conditions

Opto-kinetic	Errors in refraction and macular lesions
Weak ocular muscles	Injury to cranial nerves III, IV and VI
Cerebellar injuries	Vestibular lesions
Brainstem lesions	High cervical cord lesions

gluconeogenesis. It develops within 6–36 hours of heavy drinking, typically seen in an undernourished individual or one who has not eaten for the previous 24 hours. The usual features of hypoglycemia, such as flushing, sweating and tachycardia are often absent, and the person may present in coma.

DIAGNOSIS OF INTOXICATION

Ethanol concentrations are not predictive of intoxication, despite the legal limit of 30 mg/dl for driving. Intoxication is a clinical diagnosis. The terms *alcohol intoxication* and *drunkenness* are often used interchangeably. The diagnostic features of alcoholic intoxication developed by the American Psychiatric Association include a requirement that there must have been recent ingestion of alcohol. The diagnostic criteria for alcohol intoxication as per DSM-IV and ICD-10 are given in Boxes 12.4 and 12.5.[2,3]

Pathological States Simulating Alcohol Intoxication

The importance of a comprehensive examination cannot be overemphasized since many other medical or drug-related (non-alcohol) conditions may simulate acute alcohol intoxication (Box 12.6).[2,4] The DSM-IV criteria require that these conditions must be excluded before the diagnosis of alcohol intoxication is made. This is particularly important when assessing an intoxicated individual in police custody, because failure to exclude any pathological conditions may lead to death in police custody. Detailed history and physical examination should be done to exclude these conditions.

Box 12.4 Diagnostic criteria for alcohol intoxication (as per DSM-IV)

- Recent ingestion of alcohol
- Clinically significant maladaptive behavioral or psychological changes (for e.g., inappropriate sexual or aggressive behavior, mood lability, impaired judgment, impaired social or occupational functioning) that developed during or shortly after alcohol ingestion.
- One (or more) of the following signs, developing during or shortly after alcohol use:

Slurred speech	Unsteady gait
Incoordination	Impairment in attention or memory
Nystagmus	Stupor or coma

- The symptoms are not due to a general medical condition and are not better accounted for by another mental disorder.

Box 12.5 Diagnostic criteria for alcohol intoxication (as per ICD-10)

The 'Y' codes of ICD consisted of a checklist of signs of intoxication the patient displays as well as the severity of these signs. These included:

Smell of alcohol on breath	Conjunctival injection and/or flushed face
Impairment of speech (for e.g., slurring)	Impairment of motor coordination
Impairment of attention and/or judgment	Elated (euphoria) or depressed mood
Disturbances in behavioral responses	Disturbances in emotional responses
Impaired ability to cooperate	Horizontal gaze nystagmus

The medical officers are expected to rate the presence of each item on a 4 point severity scale.

Based on these signs, the medical officers are expected to make a judgment whether the patient is in the state of:

- Very severe alcohol intoxication (very severe disturbance in functions and responses, very severe difficulty in coordination or loss of ability to cooperate)
- Severe alcohol intoxication (severe disturbance in functions and responses, severe difficulty in coordination or impaired ability to cooperate)
- Moderate alcohol intoxication (smell of alcohol on breath, moderate behavioral disturbance in functions and responses or moderate difficulty in coordination)
- Mild alcohol intoxication (smell of alcohol on breath, slight behavioral disturbance in functions and responses or slight difficulty in coordination)
- Alcohol involvement, not otherwise specified
- Not intoxicated at all

Box 12.6 Conditions that can mimic acute alcohol intoxication

- Craniocerebral trauma and cerebrovascular accidents (stroke).
- Metabolic disorders (for e.g., diabetic ketoacidosis, hypoglycemia, hyperglycemia, uremia or hyperthyroidism).
- Neurological conditions associated with dysarthria, ataxia, tremor, drowsiness (for e.g., multiple sclerosis, intracranial tumors, Parkinson's disease, epilepsy or acute vertigo).
- Effects of drugs, either prescribed or illicit (for e.g., insulin, cocaine, anticonvulsants, narcotics, antihistamines, sedatives, analgesics, tranquilizers, hypnotics or rarely antibiotics, such as streptomycin or sulfonamides).
- Psychiatric disorders (for e.g., hypomania or general paresis).
- Febrile illnesses.
- Carbon monoxide poisoning.

One frequently explored defense is that the accused was taking prescribed medication. The combination of alcohol and many of these drugs usually creates either an accumulative or a synergistic effect that promotes higher levels of CNS depression and hence increased impairment. If medication per se has a suppressive effect on the CNS, alcohol will enhance the effect. But, relatively few drugs interact with alcohol pharmacokinetically leading to significantly altered BAC. Before a court hearing, it is recommended that the doctor do research and at least find out what the direct effects and the half-life of the medication in question is.

Sometimes, the defense is made that the subject took a bottle of cough medication. Most cough mixtures contain 10% or less of alcohol. If a person with an average body mass of 70 kg took 500 ml of cough mixture, the total alcohol consumed will be about 50 ml. If these are substituted in the Widmark formula, then C = 0.08 g/dl. Two tablespoons will have a volume of about 50 ml and the alcohol content will be 5 ml (3.95 g). The difference created will be in the order of 0.008 which will have almost no effect on the BAC. It has to be taken in 'bottle quantities' to make a difference.[19]

LAB EVALUATION

a. **Blood analysis for alcohol levels:** Blood alcohol content, blood alcohol concentration (BAC), blood ethanol concentration, or blood alcohol level is most commonly used as a measure of alcohol intoxication for legal or medical purposes. Although, the degree of impairment may vary among individuals with the same blood alcohol content, it can be measured objectively, and is therefore legally useful and difficult to contest in the court. Most countries prohibit operation of motor vehicles and heavy machinery above prescribed levels of blood alcohol content. Operation of boats and aircraft are also regulated.[8,20-22]

   Advantages[1]
   - More reliable than breath test.
   - If the time since alcohol ingestion is known and single specimen was obtained, then one can extrapolate the result and estimate peak alcohol level because absorption and elimination of alcohol follow a relatively constant curve.

   Disadvantages[22]
   - Needs time for reporting, and levels may drop by the time patient reaches hospital.
   - Person might not give consent for sampling.
   - Levels might not have reached to peak level if he is tested soon after ingestion of alcohol.
   - They may be falsely high if skin cleanser used contains alcohol, or laboratory instruments and containers have been contaminated with foreign substances or have been left exposed to air, and in diabetics.
   - Delay in processing may also give incorrect value.

b. **Urine analysis:** It should be done in a patient who resents blood sampling or if medical reasons are there for failure to take a sample. When urine is analyzed for alcohol, the assumption is that there are 1.3 parts of alcohol in the urine for every 1 part in the blood, even though the actual ratio can vary greatly.[1,20]

   Disadvantage
   - Levels may not be as accurate as direct blood alcohol estimation.
   - Urine concentration does not follow a constant pattern, so extrapolation cannot be done.

- Result may be affected by the amount of urine present in bladder before the consumption of alcohol.

c. **Breath analysis:** Measurement of alcohol in an exhaled sample of breath is another indirect method of estimating blood alcohol levels. On an average, the ratio of blood alcohol content to breath alcohol content (the *partition ratio*) is 2100 to 1. In other words, there are 2100 parts of alcohol in the blood for every part in the breath. However, the actual ratio in any given individual can vary from 1300:1 to 3100:1, or even more widely. This ratio varies not only from person to person, but within one person from moment to moment.[20-22]

   Advantage: Law enforcement personnel can administer this test quickly at the scene where alcohol intoxication is suspected. When a breathalyzer or similar instrument is used, the instrument automatically converts the breath alcohol level to BAC (Fig. 12.8).[1]

   Disadvantage: Caution has to be taken in interpreting blood alcohol levels by breath analyzer because:[21]

   - Breath analyzer can detect certain substances similar to alcohol like acetone in diabetics, and in dieters certain bread products, environmental substances like paint removers, gasoline and lacquers.
   - They are very sensitive to environmental and person's temperature and can produce false high and false low readings.
   - Physical activity and hyperventilation can lower BAC levels.
   - Low hematocrit can produce falsely high BAC.
   - Improper usage and improper calibration of breathalyzer can produce false readings.

Hospital and Laboratory Testing

Alcohol dehydrogenase test

Hospital and clinical laboratories commonly employ the enzymatic *alcohol dehydrogenase test* to determine BAC. This quantitative test is based on the

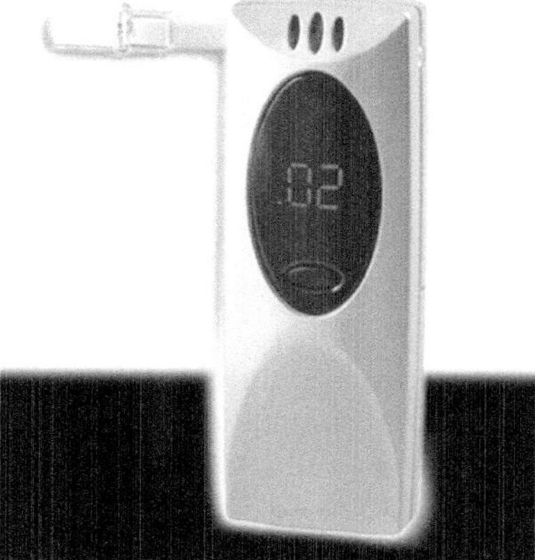

Fig. 12.8 Breath analyzer

oxidation of ethanol to acetaldehyde by alcohol dehydrogenase (ADH) in the presence of coenzyme nicotinamide adenine dinucleotide (NAD) and is applicable to serum and plasma. The NAD is reduced as a byproduct of the oxidation reaction of alcohol. The resultant reduction product is measured by a spectrophotometer. This is a quick, easy and automated method. Several commercial ADH kits are available and the test can be performed on routine clinical chemistry analyzers. However, it lacks the specificity because the presence of other alcohols such as isopropanol and other higher alcohols may interfere chemically and yield an inconclusive, false-positive or spurious result. Methanol and acetone do not react and therefore a gas chromatographic method for alcohols is much preferred.[13,20]

Tests like γ-glutamyl transferase (γ-GT), carbohydrate-deficient transferring (%CDT) and mean corpuscular erythrocyte volume (MCV) are biomarkers for chronic alcohol abuse which can help to distinguish habitual from non-habitual drinkers.[21]

In toxicology laboratory, there are several techniques to determine BAC, but the most common and one of the most reliable is Gas Chromatography/ Flame-ionization detectors (GC-FID). GC provides a quantitative analysis of volatile and semi-volatile organic compounds found in a variety of matrices (gases, liquids and solids) in foods, medical specimens, plastics, environmental samples and occupational monitoring samples. FID is useful for determining the concentration of specific compounds. It is said that GC is the 'gold standard' for specific identification and quantification of BAC. Headspace chromatography is completely specific for ethanol.[1,13,20]

In contrast to the practices of clinical laboratories, which analyze either serum or plasma from living subjects for BAC, samples used in most toxicology laboratories is whole blood preserved in sodium fluoride. Under most physiological conditions, serum or plasma contains about 10–12% more water than the same volume of whole blood, so the levels of alcohol are correspondingly slightly higher in these samples (alcohol has an affinity for water). The average ethanol ratio of whole blood to serum or plasma is approximately 1:1.16, with a reported range of 1.12–1.17. The following ratios can be used for conversion of these blood components to whole blood: serum = 1.12–1.17; plasma = 1.10–1.35. Using either serum or whole blood produces essentially equivalent results for clinical and forensic purposes, as long as the final report of analytical results clearly specifies the analyte (serum, plasma, whole blood).[1]

MEDICOLEGAL REPORT WRITING

Medicolegal reports (MLR) are to be prepared immediately after the examination is done. Care should be taken, since the certificate of drunkenness from a medical practitioner is produced as evidence in the court of law.

The opinion at the time of the examination is given as 'the person is strongly/ moderately/slightly/not under the influence of alcohol/a drug having narcotic effect.' This conclusion is based on the total clinical picture found during the examination and interview, and not on a single symptom or sign.

Final opinion in a suspected case of drunkenness is given as:[4]

i. Person has not consumed alcohol: No smell of alcohol in breath and no physical findings of alcoholism. Negative chemical analysis.
ii. Person has consumed alcohol but is not under its influence: Negative clinical findings but positive chemical analysis report.
iii. Person has consumed alcohol and is under its influence: Positive smell of alcohol in breath and positive findings of intoxication. Blood, urine or breath analysis reveals alcohol concentration above statutory level.

MEDICOLEGAL ASPECTS OF ALCOHOLISM

Drunkenness is a behavior found across cultures and geographic borders, particularly in young individuals and represents a considerable public health issue. It can be asserted as a defense in civil and criminal actions in which the state of mind of the defendant is an essential element to be established in order to obtain legal relief. Social outcomes of binge drinking include an increased risk for road traffic accidents, injuries, violence due to psychopharmacologic effect and loss of productivity or absenteeism from work. Risk factors for these outcomes include genetic or temperamental traits, antisocial personality disorder, parental modeling of heavy drinking and aggression, and poor relations with parents.[5,9]

Alcohol and Driving

Even at low doses, there is clear evidence that alcohol impairs driving performance. More recent research showed a significant increase in crash risk at BAC levels of 40 mg/dl. Studies have also found that at 100 mg/dl to 150 mg/dl, accident risk is twenty five times more than at 10 mg/dl. To minimize the potential harm that can result from impaired driving, government has formulated various legal instruments for the conduct of road traffic in India, viz. the Motor Vehicles Act, 1988 (MVA 1988), Central Motor Vehicle Rules, 1989 (CMV 1989), State Motor Vehicles Rules and the Rules of Road Regulations, 1989. They also prescribe penalties which has set maximum legally permissible BAC levels for drivers at 30 mg/dl (in Kerala, a policy of zero tolerance is followed). This is much lower than the BAC limits allowed in most states in the US, Canada, much of Europe and the UK (in the range of 80 mg/dl).[4,5]

Box 12.7 describes the important sections related to alcohol intoxication. Sec. 202 MVA empowers the police to arrest a person without warrant who commits offences like drunken driving, dangerous driving, taking vehicle without authority or a person committing an offence and refusing to give his name and address. Sec. 203 MVA empowers police to submit a person driving motor vehicle in a public place to breath test and arrest without warrant, if test is positive. Under Sec. 204 MVA, the person has to undergo medical examination and blood or urine analysis within 2 hours, otherwise he has to be released from the custody.[23] In a recent judgment, the Bombay high court held drunk driving cases as non-cognizable offences.[24]

Recently, a Delhi Motor Accident Claim Tribunal (MACT) has suggested that an accident victim should also undergo medical check-up to verify if he was driving

Box 12.7 Relevant sections of Motor Vehicles Act, 1988 (MVA)

Sec. 184: Driving dangerously: Any person who drives a motor vehicle at a speed or in a manner which is dangerous to the public, is to be punished with imprisonment up to 6 months or with fine of ₹ 1000 (first offence), and for subsequent offence imprisonment is up to 2 years and/or with fine up to ₹ 2000, if committed within 3 years.

Sec. 185: Driving by a drunken person or by a person under the influence of drugs
If a person, while driving or attempting to drive a motor vehicle has in his blood alcohol of > 30 mg/dl (the clause of 30 mg/dl was added by an amendment in 1994) or is under the influence of a drug to such an extent that he is incapable of exercising proper control over the vehicle, then he is punished with an imprisonment of 6 months and/or fine of ₹ 2000 (first offence). If the second offence is committed within 3 years, the punishment is 2 years and/or fine of ₹ 3000.

- 'Drugs' are specified by the Central Government by notification in the Official Gazette, which are deemed to render a person incapable of exercising proper control over a motor vehicle.
- The government is planning to amend the Motor Vehicles Act, 1988. The proposed amendment seeks to penalize the driver according to the amount of alcohol in his blood. Present penalty would be for BAC of up to 60 mg/dl, from 60–150 mg/dl penalty would be imprisonment for a term up to 6 months and/or fine up to ₹ 5,000, and BAC exceeding 150 mg/dl, imprisonment for a term up to 1 year and/or fine up to ₹ 10,000.

Sec. 197: Taking vehicle without authority (without having either the consent of the owner or other lawful authority) should be punished with imprisonment up to 3 months and/or with fine up to ₹ 500. If a person, unlawfully by force or threat of force or by any other form of intimidation, seizes or exercises control of a motor vehicle, then he should be punished with imprisonment up to 3 months, and/or fine up to ₹ 500.

Sec. 202: Power to arrest without warrant: A police officer may arrest without warrant any person who in his presence commits an offence punishable under Sec. 184 or Sec. 197, provided that the person arrested in connection with an offence punishable under Sec. 185 is subjected to a medical examination referred to in Secs. 203 and 204 by a medical practitioner within 2 hours of his arrest, failing which he should be released from custody.

Sec. 203. Breath tests

i. A police officer may require any person driving or attempting to drive a motor vehicle in a public place to provide one or more specimens of breath for breath test there or nearby (done as soon as reasonably practicable after the commission of such offence), if the police officer has reasonable cause to suspect him of having committed an offence punishable under Sec. 185.
ii. If a motor vehicle is involved in an accident in a public place, and a police officer has reasonable cause to suspect that the person who was driving at the time of the accident, had alcohol in his blood or that he was driving under the influence of a drug (referred to in Sec. 185) he may require the person to provide a specimen of his breath for a breath test:
    a. In the case of a person who is admitted as an indoor patient at the hospital,
    b. In the case of any other person, either at or near the place where the requirement is made, or, if the police officer thinks fit, at a police station specified by the police officer.

    The indoor patient is *not required* to provide such a specimen if the medical practitioner in immediate charge is not first notified, or objects on the ground that it would be prejudicial to the proper care or treatment of the patient.

Contd...

Contd...

iii. The police officer may arrest that person without warrant, except while that person is at a hospital as an indoor patient, if a breath test carried out by him indicates the presence of alcohol in the person's blood beyond the legal permissible limit.
iv. If a person refuses or fails to provide a specimen of breath for a breath test, and the police officer has reasonable cause to suspect him of having alcohol in his blood, the officer may arrest him without warrant except while he is at a hospital as an indoor patient.
v. A person arrested under this section, while at a police station will be given an opportunity to provide a specimen of breath for a breath test.
vi. The results of a breath test are admissible as evidence.

- 'Breath test', means a test for the purpose of obtaining an indication of the presence of alcohol in a person's blood carried out on one or more specimens of breath provided by that person, by means of a device of a type approved by the Central Government for the purpose of such a test.

Sec. 204. Laboratory test

i. A person arrested under Sec. 203 is to be produced before a medical practitioner for a specimen of his blood for testing:
   a. If breath test indicates the presence of alcohol in the blood, or
   b. If the person has refused, omitted or failed a breath test.

   If the arrested person is a female and the medical practitioner happens to be male, then the specimen should be taken only in the presence of a female attendant.
ii. If the person admitted an indoor patient may be required by the police to provide a specimen of his blood for a laboratory test:
   - If breath test indicates the presence of alcohol in the blood, or
   - If the person, whether at the hospital or elsewhere, has refused, omitted or failed a breath test and there is reasonable cause to suspect him of having alcohol in his blood.
iii. The indoor patient is not required to provide such a specimen if the medical practitioner in immediate charge is not first notified, or objects on the ground that it would be prejudicial to the proper care or treatment of the patient.
iv. The results of a laboratory test are admissible as evidence.

- 'Laboratory test' means the analysis of a specimen of blood made at an established or recognized Central Government or a State Government laboratory.

Sec. 205: Presumption of unfitness to drive: In any charge of an offence punishable under Sec. 185 if it is proved that the accused, when requested by a police officer had refused, omitted or failed to consent to providing a specimen of his breath for a breath test or a specimen of his blood for a laboratory test, his refusal (unless reasonable cause is there) is presumed to be circumstance supporting any evidence given on behalf of the prosecution, or rebutting any evidence given on behalf of the defense, with respect to the condition at that time.

the vehicle in an inebriated state. Tests relating to blood alcohol content will help to ascertain whether the victim himself is guilty of contributory negligence. If the doctor while examining the victim suspects alcohol, then he should provide the investigating officer with the person's blood sample to ascertain the level of alcohol.[25]

Alcohol and Insurance

As per the Motor Vehicles Act, 1988 it is mandatory for every owner of a vehicle plying on public roads, to take an insurance policy to cover the amount which the owner becomes legally liable to pay as damages to third parties as a result of accidental death, bodily injury or damage to property. A certificate of insurance must be carried in the vehicle as a proof of such insurance. An important exclusion under all the policies is when driving with invalid driving license or under the influence of alcohol. Similarly, alcohol related injuries are a notable exclusion in claiming accident insurance. The victim of accident or any disease related to alcoholism, if found guilty of contributory negligence, and insurance company may not be liable to pay to him.[5,9]

Consequently, people are most anxious to avoid any mention of alcohol use in contiguity to accidents or injuries in medical records of such events. It is not uncommon for money to change hands in order to falsify the record.[5]

Alcohol and Crime

Sec. 85 IPC states that 'Nothing is an offence which is done by a person who at the time of doing it, is, by reason of intoxication, incapable of knowing the nature of the act, or that he is doing what is either wrong or contrary to law, provided that the thing which intoxicated him was administered to him without his knowledge or against his will'.[4]

Sec. 86 IPC states that 'In cases where an act done is not an offence, unless done with a particular knowledge or intent, a person who does the act in a state of intoxication shall be liable to be dealt with as if he had the same knowledge as he would have had if he had not been intoxicated, unless the thing which intoxicated him was administered to him without his knowledge or against his will'.[4]

As per these sections, it is clear that even if the person was so drunk that he was not capable of knowing whether the act he was committing was right or wrong, he is still punishable, unless the alcohol was given to him without his knowledge or against his will.[4,5]

Alcohol and Medical Practice

It is unacceptable to consume intoxicating substances while dealing with the patients. Under *Sec. 304A IPC*, if the patient dies while under treatment from a doctor who was intoxicated, guilty doctor can be imprisoned and State Medical Council may cancel the registration. In less serious cases, damages can be claimed by the patient.[4]

DEFENSES FOR NON-SUBMITTING OF SAMPLES

Numerous technical defenses for failure to provide a sample of breath, blood or urine are coming forward over the years. It is important for the medical practitioners to be aware of the most common ones. Under Sec. 205 of MVA, unless reasonable excuse is there, refusal to submit a sample of breath, blood or urine is presumed to be circumstance supporting any evidence given on behalf of the prosecution.

Failure to Provide Sample of Breath

Medically acceptable reasons include mouth, lip or facial injury, tracheotomy, chest wall injury and some neurological problems. Many cases have been challenged on the basis that the person has respiratory problems. It is often not possible for subjects with lung diseases (particularly COPD) to complete the required number of attempts because of the long periods needed for exhalation and recovery.[3]

A medical practitioner may be asked to examine a detained person to assess if a reasonable excuse exists. If there is doubt, the person may be given the benefit of doubt and recommend a blood/urine option.

Failure to Provide Sample of Blood

Medical reasons for failing to provide a blood sample include poor venous access, failure of the staff to take the sample and needle phobia. It is for the doctor to decide from where the sample should be taken, and it is generally accepted that up to three attempts are likely to be considered reasonable. A minimum of 2 ml of blood is required for analysis (1 ml is required by laboratory). If sufficient blood is not obtained at the first attempt, blood from initial attempt should not be mixed with blood from next. It is preferable that the blood is taken from one continuous sample. If the laboratory technician is unable to obtain an adequate sample after three attempts, then the procedure is abandoned. The police officer is informed that a medical reason for failing to provide a sample exists and he should then go for a urine sample.[3]

Needle phobia is sometimes complained of by the arrested person. In such cases, a detailed history is taken with specific attention to immunizations, body piercing, dental procedures, tattoos and current or past psychiatric history. It is also noted when the problem started and whether it is due to fear of needles or blood products. If the practitioner is unsure that needle phobia exists, it is best to act with caution and recommend a urine sample. The best way to get a successful prosecution is to obtain any sample for analysis.[3]

Failure to Provide Sample of Urine

Sometimes, the arrested person may fail to provide a urine sample. It is required that the police officer/examiner should be of the same gender as the arrested person. It is important for the practitioner to be aware of some of the reasons for failure:[3]

- Drugs acting on the bladder, for e.g., tolterodine, methadone
- Neurological problems affecting the bladder
- Embarrassment *(avoidant paruresis):* In order to pass urine, the urinary sphincter must relax for urine to flow from the bladder down the urethra. When other people are around, anxiety about urinating overstimulates the person's nervous system and the sphincter fails to relax. Failure to urinate heightens the person's anxiety, particularly if the bladder is already full. This is known as shy bladder, bashful bladder or bladder shyness. This condition affects men and women of all races.

RETROGRADE EXTRAPOLATION

The medical practitioner may be requested to determine whether the BAC of a person corresponds to the reported quantity of alcohol ingested or to the estimate of the quantity of alcohol consumed based on a measured blood level at a given time in circumstances where there is a delay between collection of the specimens and the actual occurrence (retrograde extrapolation). This extrapolation may be relevant in estimating BAC when driving and/or corroborating or contradicting the results of a later chemical test.

Retrograde extrapolation is the mathematical method by which a person's BAC at the time of driving is estimated by projecting backwards from a later chemical test. This involves estimating the absorption and elimination of alcohol in the intervening period between driving and testing. The minimal essential information necessary to make such estimations includes the individual's body weight, percent of alcohol in the drink, the number of alcoholic beverages consumed, the length of the drinking period and a given individual's excretion rate. Various formulas have been evolved to answer such questions. Of all the formulas, the Widmark equation, conceived by the Swedish physiologist Erik Widmark is most useful to provide retrograde and anterograde calculations for BAC estimations at a time different from the time of sample collection. The optimal specimen is one collected after a blood alcohol maximum is reached and the elimination phase begins. If the specimen is collected on the absorption side of metabolism curve, then total body distribution has not been achieved so that analysis of that sample will not properly reflect the BAC. A rough case example is cited to explain retrograde extrapolation (Box 12.8).[1,13,20]

Since it is often difficult to quantify the variables in the mathematical formulas, extrapolation remains controversial. In most of the states in US, laws have been enacted to facilitate this speculative task: the BAC at the time of driving is legally presumed to be the same as when later tested (as remote as 4 hours after the event) and extrapolation is unnecessary. There are usually time limits put on this presumption, and the defendant is permitted to offer evidence to rebut this presumption.

Box 12.8 Case example

Mr R was arrested at the scene of a road traffic accident which was 1 hour from the nearest hospital. The police officer responding to the call suspected that he was intoxicated, so he arrested Mr R and presented him to the doctor for examination. Blood was drawn for blood alcohol estimation. The accident occurred at 3:00 AM, the officer arrived at 3:30 AM, the ambulance arrived at 3:40 AM, and the individual arrived at the hospital at 4:45 AM. The individual was stabilized and blood was drawn for the alcohol estimation at 5:00 AM. The BAC of 5:00 AM sample was 20 mg/dl. The doctor was asked to estimate the BAC at 3:00 AM. Based on the established principles of alcohol metabolism (average human eliminates alcohol at a rate of about 17 mg/dl every hour), the BAC was near 54 mg/dl and, thus, the individual was probably driving with a BAC above the legal limit. However, the medical practitioner need to consider the following parameters that may affect that interpretation such as:

- Is this an average individual?
- Does he/she absorb and eliminate alcohol at the average rate?
- Was there any food in the stomach?

CONCLUSION

Alcohol is a major cause of morbidity and mortality in India. Clinical examination alone can identify 80% of intoxication of alcohol which involves recording the history and physical examination. The accuracy of the assessment depends on the reliability of the person and his relations and friends, and on the skill of the examiner. However, thorough assessment is a time-consuming and dexterous procedure. Difficulty is faced in making a clinical diagnosis in border line cases where the presentation is not obvious. The circumstantial evidence about the conduct of the person concerned is of vital importance. An incomplete clinical examination may lead to serious error. The smell of alcohol in the breath is a subjective index of alcohol taken or its presence in the body. If the time lag between ingestion of alcohol and time of examination is increased there are chances of excretion of alcohol, thus giving negative clinical findings. The duration elapsed between the alleged offence and the examination should be clearly stated in the report. The medical officer should make his clinical diagnosis uninfluenced by any knowledge of the results of the breath or chemical tests.

The medicolegal aspects of acute alcohol intoxication mainly concern driving while under the effect of alcohol and the regulation thereof. Sometimes, drivers involved in road traffic accidents are also frequently under the influence of two or more drugs. It is advisable to conduct a broad screen to include most of the common drugs suggested by the circumstances. Testing soon after the incident may assist in establishing the sobriety or otherwise of these drivers at the time of the accident. Determination of the level of blood alcohol remains the only approximate indicator, given the variable number of factors that may intervene. Hence, interpreting BAC is the most difficult aspect on the part of the doctor as the rate of absorption of alcohol is susceptible to both intraindividual and interindividual variation.

REFERENCES

1. Hunsaker DM, Hunasker JC. Postmortem alcohol interpretation. Medicolegal considerations affecting living and deceased persons. In: Tsokos M (ed). Forensic pathology reviews. Vol. 1. New Jersey: Humana Press; 2004. p. 307-40.
2. Stark MM, Norfolk G. Substance misuse. In: Stark MM (ed). Clinical forensic medicine: a physician's guide. 2nd edn. New York: Humana press; 2005. p. 285-326.
3. Wall IF. Alcohol, drugs and driving. In: McLay WDS (ed). Clinical forensic medicine. 3rd edn. New York: Cambridge university press; 2009. p. 89-98.
4. Biswas G. Inebriants: Alcohol. In: Review of forensic medicine and toxicology. 2nd edn. New Delhi: Jaypee brothers; 2012. p. 479-92.
5. Benegal V, Gururaj G, Murthy P, Taly AB, Kiran S, Chandrashekar R, Chandrashekar H. Report for the WHO injury and alcohol: emergency department study. Bangalore, 2002. http://www.nimhans.kar.nic.in/Deaddiction/lit/Alcohol and Injuries_WHO Collab.pdf.
6. Harish D, Chavali KK. The medicolegal case - should we be afraid of it? In: Anil Aggarwal's Internet Journal of Forensic Medicine and Toxicology [Internet]. 2007;8(1). Available from: http://www.anilaggrawal.com/ij/vol_008_no_001/others/pg/pg001.html.
7. Alcoholic beverage [Internet]. Available from: http://en.wikipedia.org/wiki/Alcoholic_beverage.

8. Binge drinking [Internet]. Available from: http://en.wikipedia.org/wiki/Binge_drinking.
9. Thompson W, Lande RG, Kalapatapu RK. Alcoholism [Internet]. Available at: http://emedicine.medscape.com/article/ 285913-overview.
10. Wiese JG, Shlipak MG, Browner WS. The alcohol hangover. *Ann Intern Med* 2000; 132: 897-902.
11. Schuckit MA. Drug and alcohol abuse: A clinical guide to diagnosis and treatment. 6th edn. New York: Springer; 2006.
12. Drunk at wheel? You could drive straight to jail. Indo Asian News Service. India Wed. 2011 Mar 2.
13. Logan BK, Gullberg RG, Negrusz A, Jickells S. Alcohol, drugs and driving. In: Jickells S, Negrusz A (eds). Clarke's analytical forensic toxicology. 1st edn. London: Pharmaceutical press; 2008. p. 299-322.
14. Langford NJ, Ferner RE. The medicolegal significance of pharmacokinetic interactions with ethanol. *Med Sci Law* 2013; 53: 1-5.
15. Millo T, Jaiswal AK, Behera C, Bhardwaj DN, Murthy OP. The medicolegal aspects of alcohol intoxication in India—a review: Indianjournals.com.
16. British Medical Association. Taking blood specimens from incapacitated drivers. Guidance for doctors from the British Medical Association and the Faculty of Forensic and Legal Medicine; 2007.
17. Pechansky F, Diemen LV, Soibelman M, Boni RD, Bumaguin DB, Fürst MC. Clinical signs of alcohol intoxication as markers of refusal to provide blood alcohol readings in emergency rooms: an exploratory study. *Clinics* (Sao Paulo). 2010; 65: 1391-92.
18. Faculty of Forensic and Legal Medicine. Section 4 RTA assessment. England and Wales: The FFLM [Internet]; 2012. Available from: http://fflm.ac.uk/upload/documents/1353340106.pdf.
19. Alcohol and the clinical examination. Available from: http://www.arrivealive.co.za/document/alcoholclinical.pdf.
20. Mozayani A. Toxicology in the crime laboratory. In: Mozayani A and Noziglia C (eds). The forensic laboratory handbook: procedures and practice. 1st edn. New Jersey: Humana press Inc.; 2006. p. 249-64.
21. Vanrell JP, Campos MLB. False-positive results in the alcoholmeter tests for exhaled air. In: Anil Aggrawal's internet journal of forensic medicine and toxicology [Internet]. 2003; 4(2). Available from: http://www.geradts.com/anil/ij/vol_004_no_002/papers/paper005.html.
22. Brautbar N. Principles and pitfalls in alcohol toxicity. Intoxication defense. http://www.environmentaldiseases.com/article-alcohol-toxicity.html.
23. The Motor Vehicles Act, 1988. Available from: http://www.tn.gov.in/sta/Mvact1988.pdf.
24. Thomas S. HC says drunk driving cases are non-cognizable offences. TNN [Internet]. 2013 Nov 29.
25. Government clears amendment to Motor Vehicle Act. Mar 1, 2012. Available from: http://articles.economictimes.indiatimes.com/2012-03-01/news/31113518_1_jail-term-fines-traffic-offences.

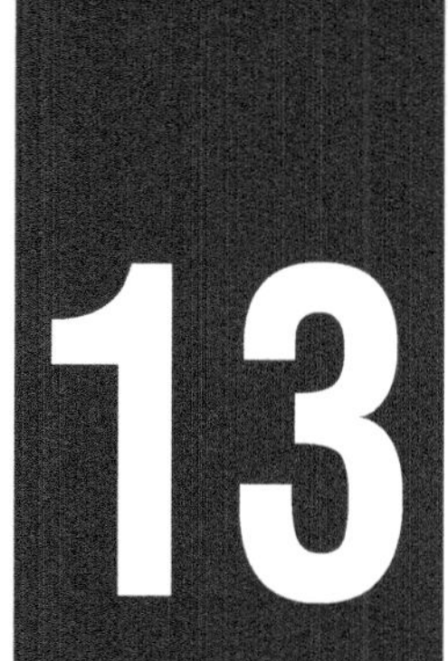

An Approach to a Case of Head and Neck Injury

Sarvpreet Singh Grewal, Punit Gupta

'Our profession, after all, deals partly with guess work; we do not deal in absolutes.'
Paul B Beeson (American professor of medicine)

ABSTRACT

Head and spine injury is a leading cause of morbidity, mortality and socioeconomic burden especially in developing countries like India. Common causes include road traffic accidents, assaults and fall from heights. Medicolegal issues are an important with regard to all the above situations and there are complex issues regarding the nature of injuries and their medicolegal aspects. This chapter discusses the mechanism, examination procedures, complications and medicolegal aspects of head and spine injuries.

Key words: Head injuries, spine injuries, concussion, DAI, EDH, SDH, SAH, cerebral edema, medicolegal aspects, grievous injury, dangerous injury.

INTRODUCTION

A head injury is any trauma that injures the scalp, skull or brain. It includes injuries to the face, mandible and special senses of smell, vision and hearing. The injury may range from an insignificant strike on the head to a serious brain injury. Sometimes, they are referred to as brain injury or traumatic brain injury depending on the extent of head trauma. Common causes of head injury are road traffic accidents (RTAs), assaults, home and occupational accidents and fall from height. It is one of the major causes of morbidity and mortality in all age groups and is rapidly becoming a socioeconomic problem and psychological burden, especially in the younger and reproductive age group. Currently, there is no effective treatment to reverse the effects of the primary brain injury sustained and the treatment is aimed at minimizing the secondary brain injury that can occur due to the effects of ischemia, hypoxia and raised intracranial pressure.[1]

In RTAs and fall from height, death is often caused by head and neck injuries. The head is targeted in assaults, since it contains the most vital organ of the body. An injury to the head can be easily fatal, especially in blunt force trauma and in firearm injuries.

From a medicolegal point of view, the consequences of head and neck injury falls in two categories: personal injury and medical negligence. The nature, mechanism and prognosis of injury need to be determined for cases in assault,

RTAs, and compensation claims. It is also essential to determine whether death occurred due to head injury or its complications, or due to some pre-existing pathology. Medical negligence may apply, if incorrect treatment has been administered or if appropriate treatment has not been undertaken. Therefore, a sound knowledge and understanding of head and neck trauma is essential to deal with the medicolegal issues raised by such injuries in court proceedings.[2] Opinion on medical negligence following the treatment of head injury will not be discussed in this chapter.

DEFINITIONS

The reader must be familiar with the following definitions:[3-6]

- **Closed head injury (nonpenetrating):** Damage to the brain without any fracture of the skull and/or penetration of duramater; most often results from blunt trauma like in automobile accidents (high velocity), or falls and assault (low velocity).
- **Open head injury (penetrating):** Disruption of cranial vault with opening through skin and cranial bones to expose damaged brain; most often associated missile wounds, stab/chop wounds, and motor vehicle or occupational accidents.
- **Missile injury**: Injury produced by moving object striking cranium; most often refers to bullet injury.
- **Primary brain injury** is the injury caused at the time of impact (for e.g. contusion, laceration).
- **Secondary brain injury** is brain damage arising from events developing subsequent to primary injury.
- **Acceleration/deceleration injury**: Damage produced by movement of brain within confines of cranial vault (tearing during violent movement or from impact of striking interior of skull or dural folds).

ANATOMY

An emergency medical practitioner should be well versed with the anatomy of the head and neck, since the unique nature of injuries to this area partly depends on its anatomy. A cross- section through the scalp and brain showing the various layers is shown in Figure 13.1.[7]

EPIDEMIOLOGY

Globally, head injuries contribute to about 10% of total deaths and 15% of disability-adjusted life-years (DALYs). According to WHO, RTAs are sixth leading cause of death in India with a greater share of hospitalizations, deaths, disabilities and socioeconomic losses in young and middle-age populations. In the United States, an average of 1.4 million traumatic brain injuries (TBIs) occur each year, including 1.1 million emergency department visits, 235,000 hospitalizations and 50,000 deaths.[2]

RTAs are the most common cause of TBI followed by falls and assaults. Alcohol involvement is seen in about 15–20% cases of TBI. In 2005, road traffic injuries resulted in the death of an estimated 110,000 and loss of about 3% of the

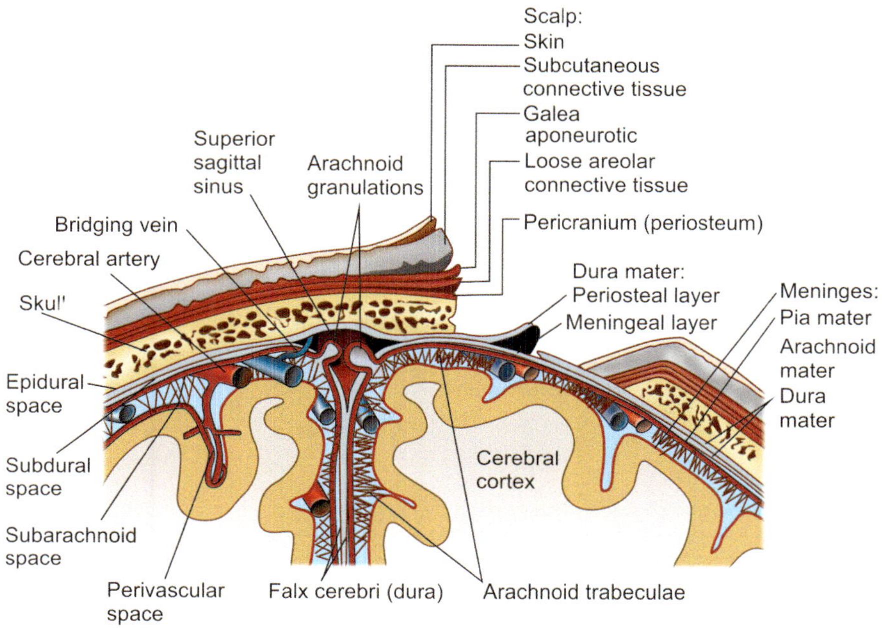

Fig. 13.1 Cross-section of scalp and brain

gross domestic product (GDP) in India. This continues to be rising, with nearly 10–30% of hospital registrations are due to RTA. A majority of victims of RTA are men in the age group of 15–44 years and belong to the poorer sections of society. Falls are a commoner cause of TBI in women, children and elderly. Moreover, a vast majority of those killed and injured are usually pedestrians, motorcyclists and pillions riders and bicyclists.[8,9]

CLASSIFICATION

Head injuries are commonly classified by a combination of cause, mechanism and consequences, both structural and functional (Table 13.1).[10,11] Classification by cause is chiefly of interest in epidemiological context. Mechanistically, a basic division is between blunt and penetrating injury, with gunshot and other missile wounds a major cause of the latter in some countries. A similar distinction is between closed and open head injury (Box 13.1). An open injury carries a much greater risk of intracranial infection and can be due to a direct penetrating injury or may occur in association with a blunt injury. A skull fracture per se is important only in indicating the risk of infection or of intracranial hemorrhage.

The Glasgow Coma Scale (GCS) is most often used to stratify severity of head injury. A post-resuscitation GCS score of 8 or less at the time of admission to hospital is now widely accepted as indicator of *severe head injury*. A *moderate head injury* is defined as an initial coma score of between 9 and 12, and *mild head injury* has been equated to a score between 13 and 15. The prognosis of the patient is directly related to the GCS at arrival. Other classifications based on the Revised Trauma Score and period of amnesia are less often used.[11]

Table 13.1 Structural injuries

Skull fractures	*Focal brain injuries*	*Diffuse*
Linear	Contusions/lacerations	Concussion
Comminuted	• Coup	Diffuse axonal injury
Depressed	• Contrecoup	Ischemic injury
Basilar	• Intermediate	Vascular injury
	Hemorrhages	Brain edema
	• Extradural hemorrhage	
	• Subdural hemorrhage	
	• Subarachnoid hemorrhage	
	• Intracerebral hemorrhage	
	• Intraventricular hemorrhage	

Box 13.1 Simple and compound head injury

Simple: There is no communication to outside. Hence, there is no CSF leak or brain matter coming out from wound. There is also no CSF rhinorrhea/otorrhea.
Compound: It can be:
i. Open: Brain is exposed to outside through scalp wound or skull fracture.
ii. Closed: When there is CSF rhinorrhea/otorrhea and X-ray skull or computed tomography (CT) scan head shows intracranial air.

MECHANISM OF SKULL FRACTURES[12-14]

Studies on experimental models have suggested the following mechanisms:

A moderately rapidly moving blunt object with small striking surface like a hammer, brick or a baseball bat may cause an area of depression, and most of the expended energy is absorbed in producing this depression. When the area under the point of impact is 'inbended', the immediate periphery is 'outbended'. When this force exceeds the limit of elasticity, fracture of bone occurs. In the inbended area, the bone is concave and compressed. As result of 'tearing apart forces' acting on the inner table, multiple radial fractures occur. Immediately away from the impact on the outer table, the bone is convex and stretched and a circular fracture is seen. Combination of these two mechanisms ultimately produces a *depressed communited fracture* which is circular in the case of a hammer blow.

A slowly moving object causing a localized blow may produce a depression at the site of impact but failied to cause a depressed communited fracture (as in the case of hammer blow) as not enough energy is expended. However, the energy of the blow may cause the skull to 'out bend' away from the site of intact. This is called 'struck hoop' analogy. These 'outbended' areas may produce *linear fractures* due to 'tearing apart forces' acting on the outer table which may extend towards the point of impact. If the energy is more, there may be more than one linear fracture produced as a result of outbending away from the site of impact.

A high kinetic energy blunt surface (for e.g. deceleration fall on a flat surface) would result in extensive communition with radial fracture lines extending from center of impact and circular fracture lines at varying distances around the area of impact (*stellate fracture*). At the point of impact, the inbending fails and a comminuted fracture occur due to tensile stresses of the inner table with several (3–6) linear fractures, which would extend outward from the center of impact. Simultaneously, linear fracture occur in the periphery due to outbending, which may extend towards the point of impact and merge with the linear fractures of the inner table. If the energy is adequate, there is a failure of the bone from inbending immediately around the point of impact at the junction between inbending and 'not-yet-inbended' bone causing a circular or curvilinear fracture lines at various distances from the point of impact. These semicircular fractures are initiated on the external surface of the skull.

It was found that impacts on certain areas of the skull produce fractures in specific areas of the skull, for e.g., impact on upper temporal or parieto-temporal areas cause fissured fractures running obliquely downwards across the temporal area. If impact is severe, there will be another fissured fracture which would run to the other side across the vertex.

When there is heavy impact on the top or side of the skull, a linear or fissured fracture would run down to the middle cranial fossa, crosses the middle cranial fossa along the petrous temporal bone or greater wings of the sphenoid to enter the pituitary fossa. Then it crosses the pituitary fossa to enter into the contralateral middle cranial fossa, sometimes dividing the base of the skull into two—'*hinged fracture*'. According to the rule, these fracture do not initiate at the point of impact instead they originate away and extend toward the point of impact.

When the impact is on the frontal area, a linear fracture would exend downward to the orbital margin, turn inwards and extends into the anterior cranial fossa. When the impact is on the occipital area, a linear fracture would typically extend vertically downward just to the side of the midline to the posterior cranial fossa and reaches the foramen magnum.

It should be noted that when there are two successive impacts on the head, the linear fractures caused by the second impact will terminate at those from the first impact when they meet, which is called '**Puppe's rule**'. By this rule, one would be able to identify the first impact from the second.

BIOMECHANICS OF BRAIN INJURY[14-16]

Head injury can be broadly classified into two types based on mechanical loading (Flow chart 13.1):

i. *Static:* Time period > 200 milliseconds (ms).
ii. *Dynamic:* Time period < 50 ms.

Brain injury is usually a brief event; the damage occurs in less than 200 ms and often in less than even 20 ms. Dynamic loading is usually the result of an impact, such as the head being struck a blow by a moving object or the head itself striking a relatively stationary surface. Injuries to the facial skeleton sometimes result in sufficient force being transmitted to damage the brain. Brain damage occasionally occurs without any head contact, as in impulsive loading, when the head is injured along with an acceleration-deceleration injury of the spine. In extremely rare circumstances, the head is slowly squeezed or crushed, and in such static loading, the majority of the force is dissipated in skull fracturing.

Flow chart 13.1 Pathological changes depending on mechanism of injury

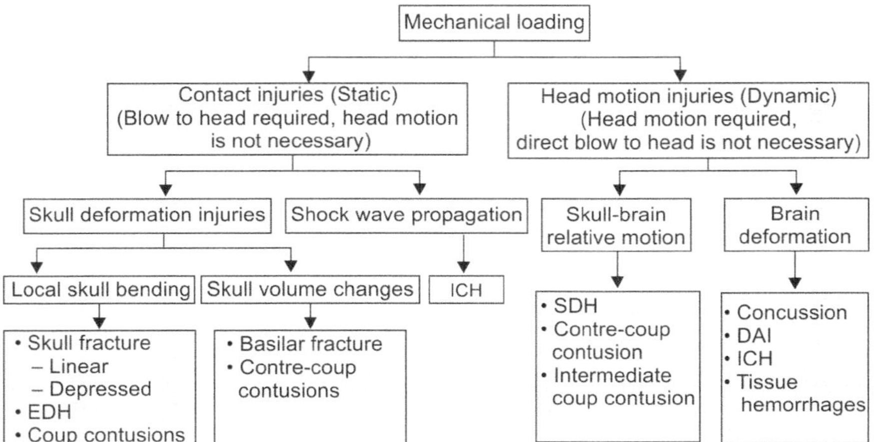

The biomechanics of traumatic brain injury involve both linear as well rotational forces. Linear forces result from straight acceleration-deceleration and can be associated with a coup injury (at the site of contact) and contrecoup injury (distant, usually opposite to the site of contact). While most high-speed head injuries involve linear component, rotational forces also act. It is these rotational forces that lead to twisting and shearing injuries in the brain parenchyma, particularly in the white matter fiber tracts (resulting in diffuse axonal injury). Rotational forces of lower magnitude are also present in milder forms of TBI, such as sports-related concussion.

Biomechanical forces in the pediatric population are different from those in the adults. Some of these differences result from the relatively large head size, reduced muscular strength and increased flexibility in the neck which may allow larger forces to be transmitted to the brain. Additionally, there is less CSF space around the younger brain, and the prominent bony ridges of the anterior and middle cranial fossa are less developed. These factors may contribute to the lower occurrence of focal lesions in pediatric population. The developing skull is thinner as compared to an adult skull, and therefore, more vulnerable to diffuse deformation. The open fontanels and the flexibility of the sutures may help dampen the force of injury, as compared to the adults. They also help to accommodate slower growing space-occupying lesions.

Inertial Injuries

Inertial injuries are commonly called 'acceleration' or 'deceleration' injuries which biomechanically can be considered as the same phenomenon. The brain is damaged by one or both mechanisms: through strains produced within the brain tissue itself, and through differential movements between the brain and the skull. Three types of acceleration are recognized. The most common and most serious is *angular acceleration* in which rotation is usually centered in the low cervical region. Angular acceleration alone is capable of producing almost every known traumatic brain lesion, except for a skull fracture or an epidural hematoma. *Translational acceleration* (for e.g., anterior to posterior) does not produce diffuse brain damage but may cause a variety of focal surface lesions. *Rotational acceleration* in the horizontal plane is a very damaging mechanism, producing both high surface forces and intracerebral damage, but it usually occurs in association with angular acceleration.

Strain within the brain tissue is best understood as the amount of deformation that it undergoes when a mechanical force is applied. Tensile strain refers to elongation of neural tissues and is the most important mechanism in head injury. Compression and shear strains also occur. The brain is virtually incompressible and has a low tolerance to tensile and shear strains. Slow application of strain is better tolerated by the brain than rapid strain which leads to the brain becoming brittle and breaking. The effect of acceleration on the brain depends on its duration and degree, and also on the brain's biophysical properties. With gradually longer durations of acceleration, the strains propagate deeply within the brain and it is these that are pre-eminent in causing concussion, diffuse axonal injury and prolonged traumatic coma. Shorter duration of acceleration shifts the focus of injury to the surface of the brain. Extremely short-lived acceleration, unless of an extremely severe degree, is damped by the brain's properties and does not produce injury.

Differential movements between the brain and the skull occur in acceleration-deceleration injury, because the inertia of the brain causes it to lag momentarily behind the movement of the skull. This may lead to rupture of subdural bridging veins and cause an acute subdural hematoma. Movement of the brain may also lead to tensile strains in regions of low pressure in the surface of the hemispheres. This is considered to be the mechanism that results in contusions distant to the site of impact.

Contact Injuries

Contact injuries occur both at the site and remote from the point of impact on the head and result in skull fractures and contusions. The length and direction of a skull fracture depends on the amount of contact energy absorbed by the skull and its thickness at the impact site. Fracture lines that run toward the base of the skull are guided between the solid buttresses of the sphenoid ridge and petrous temporal bone. A fracture at the base of the skull can also result from a blow to the face with transfer of the force through the maxilla or mandible.

The inward deformation of skull may lead to the brain being injured directly beneath the impact (compressive strain) and produce a contusion. However, a contusion can also result when the area of indentation rapidly snaps back into place and produces high negative pressure and tensile strain.

PATHOPHYSIOLOGY

The Monro Kellie doctrine states that the sum total of three components inside rigid skull remains constant (Brain + Blood + CSF). Therefore, if any one of primary component increases (cerebral edema or tumor), or if another process (intracranial space occupying lesion) occupies space, one of the component must be displaced or else intracranial pressure (ICP) will increase. Raised ICP in head injured patient is caused by cerebral edema, hyperemia, traumatically induced masses, hydrocephalus, hypoventilation and post-traumatic seizure. If ICP increases, it may cause various forms of brain herniation—uncal, transtentorial, central transtentorial, cerebellotonsillar. Transtentorial (tonsillar) herniation compresses the brainstem causing respiratory and cardiac failure and finally death.[17,18]

Biochemical Abnormalities

It has been seen that there is significant increase of glucose utilization within the first 30 minutes post-injury, after which glucose uptake diminishes and then remains low for about 5–10 days. Clinical studies in humans using Positron Emission Tomography (PET) have demonstrated comparable results. Although, it is difficult to capture the acute period of cerebral hyperglycolysis in a critically ill TBI patient, globally decreased glucose metabolism has been demonstrated, persisting chronically for weeks to months post-injury in patients. The initial hyperglycolysis described above results from disruption of ionic gradients across the neuronal cell membrane, activating energy-dependent ionic pumps; there is also an increasing evidence for impairment of oxidative metabolism following brain trauma.[19]

Acute injury to the brain also causes a rapid release of glutamate, the predominant excitatory neurotransmitter in the central nervous system. The indiscriminate release occurs as a result of extensive triggering of action potentials, synaptic neurotransmitter release and membrane disruption. This massive release of glutamate is a major source of potassium efflux into the extracellular space. The rise in the extracellular concentration of potassium also results from nonspecific breakdown of the plasma membrane, especially in areas of the brain damaged by a localized contusion or intracerebral hemorrhages. Glutamate also induces opening of ligand gated channels that are permeable to calcium. A number of studies have shown an increase in intracellular calcium concentration following various experimental traumatic brain injury models. Magnesium is one of the electrolytes that play a significant role in maintaining ionic balance within the injured cell. Several studies in experimental models of traumatic brain injury have shown a marked decrease in brain intracellular free and total magnesium concentration that lasts up to four days post-injury.[19]

FOCAL INJURY

Scalp Injuries

The easiest way to detect scalp injuries is by palpation, but shaving off the hair is necessary for proper documentation and photography.

1. **Scalp abrasion** is caused by a lateral rubbing action by a blow, a fall on a rough surface or by being dragged in a vehicular accident. They are simple injuries, bleed slightly, heal rapidly and scar is not formed. Large abrasions can cause severe pain and bleeding. Abrasions are modified by the presence of hair. Even if present, the medical officer may miss it, unless the scalp is shaven. Sometimes, impact/imprint abrasion may reproduce the pattern of the object causing it (patterned abrasions).[5,20]

2. **Contusion (bruise):** Presence of scalp contusion is indicative of blunt contact injury. The shape and size of the instrument (weapon or object) are usually not reproduced on the scalp due to blurring of the margins and presence of the hair which acts as a cushion. In superficial fascia, they appear as localized swelling due to the dense fibrofatty tissues, but contusions deep into the galea aponeurotica are diffuse due to gravity and loose aponeurotic tissues. Hence, bruises on the skull can gravitate around the eyes causing 'black eyes' or periorbital hematoma (Fig. 13.2). The soft fluctuant centers of scalp hematomas can masquerade as *depressed skull fractures.*[5,20,21]
3. **Laceration:** Lacerations are tears or splits of the skin caused by a blunt object, wherein localized portions of tissue are displaced by the impact of blunt force, which sets up traction forces and results in tearing of the tissues (Fig. 13.3). Scalp lacerations are *split lacerations*. Splitting occurs by crushing of the skin between the skull and some hard object, and they resemble incised wounds (incised looking lacerations) (Figs 13.4A and B). Careful examination in the depths of the wound will reveal the following features that may distinguish it from an incised wound:
   - Bruised/abraded margins
   - Presence of tissue bridges (fascia, nerves, blood vessels and hair bulbs) in the wound depth
   - Uncut head hair crossing the wound.

   Scalp lacerations are sometimes troublesome because of bleeding, especially from the superficial temporal artery (blood vessels in the fibrous

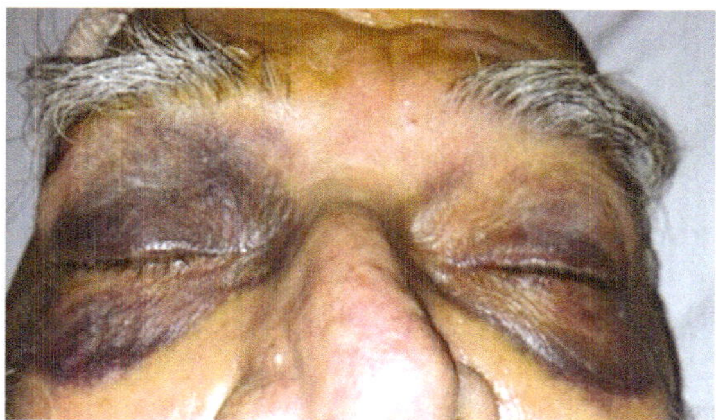

Fig. 13.2 Black eyes (Racoon eyes)

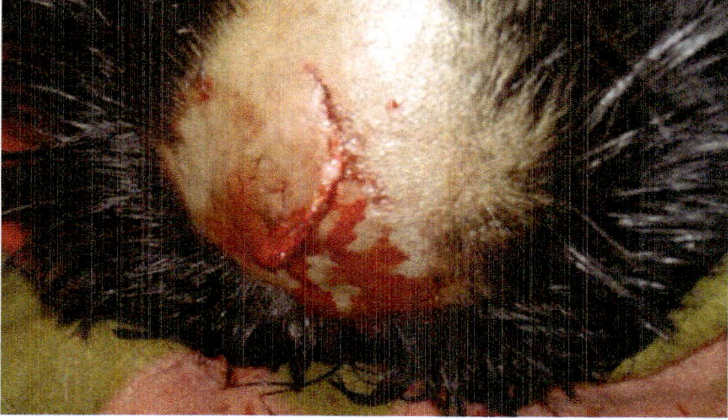

Fig. 13.3 Lacerated wound of scalp

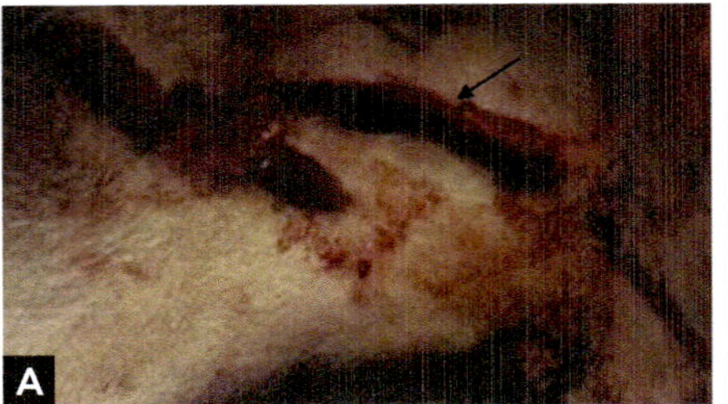

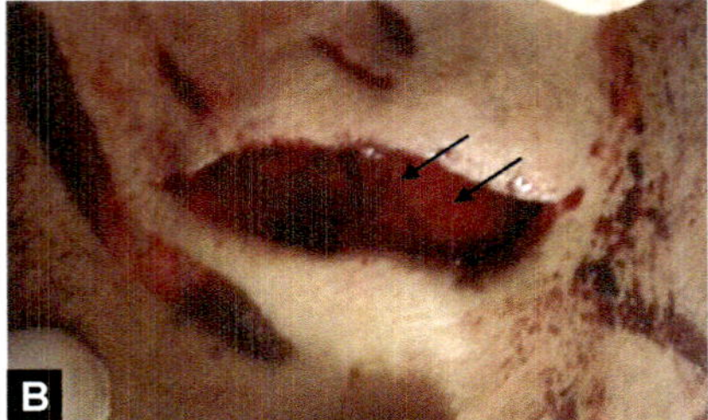

Figs 13.4A and B (A) Incised looking lacerated wound (arrow); (B) Tissue bridging (arrows)

layer, superficial to galea aponeurotica being held open once cut). They bleed profusely and may cause death if large enough and not treated early. Unlike bruises, scalp lacerations may reproduce the size and shape of the instrument, for e.g., a hammer blow onto the scalp may produce either a circular or semi-circular laceration depending on whether the full or part of the face of the hammer struck the scalp. All lacerations to the scalp should be explored and palpated to exclude a depressed fracture.

Avulsion: An avulsion is a laceration produced by sufficient force (shearing force) delivered at an acute angle to detach (tear off) a portion of a traumatized scalp from its attachments along the path of least resistance which is the loose areolar tissue layer. Scalp avulsion requires a strong tearing or shearing force. If the force is extensive enough, the avulsion will progress to the boundaries of galea at the supraorbital ridges and the zygomatic, mastoid and occipital nuchal line. Scalp avulsion may be lead to life threatening blood loss injury.[5,20-22]

4. **Incised wounds:** They have clean cut margins; hair bulbs are cleanly cut.[5]

   Infection is rare because of the rich blood supply. However, if an injury extending through the galea gets infected, it may spread through the emissary veins to involve the sagittal, lateral and cavernous sinuses causing septic complications, like meningitis and brain abscess.[5]

FACIAL INJURIES

Any injury to the head may also cause facial injuries. However, they are rarely fatal by themselves, unless the victim has asphyxiated from the blood entering into the air passages. The face has many prominences with complex contours such as chin, nose, cheekbones, eyebrows, ears and lips. They may be the first ones to receive the blows directed at the face producing characteristic injuries.[23]

Eyebrows are injured during falls and blows producing abrasions, lacerations and fractures of the frontal bone and orbital margin. Although the cartilaginous part of the nose escapes from being damaged, nasal bone is frequently fractured causing excessive and serious bleeding into the nasal passages, if the victim is unconscious. Direct impacts on the face can cause fractures of the mandible and maxilla. This also can cause dangerous bleeding into the air passages. Severe impacts like kicking and RTAs may totally detach the maxilla from the face. Injuries to the mouth and lips are very common in physical assaults including child abuse and wife battering. Punching or kicking on the mouth injures the lips when compressed between the inflicting object and teeth.[23]

SKULL FRACTURES

Skull fractures may occur without any brain injury. Most common are linear, communited, depressed and basilar fractures (Fig. 13.5).[5,12,14,24]

1. **Linear (fissure) fractures** are linear cracks passing over the vertex or across the skull base without any displacement of the fragments, and either involves the whole thickness of the bone or the inner or outer table alone. It appears as a fine linear hypodensity on radiograph or CT scan (Fig. 13.6). It is also called 'motorcyclist's fracture' as it is commonly seen in accidents involving motorcycles. 'Hinge fracture' is a linear fracture. Sometimes, a linear fracture may reach the skull sutures and opens up the suture line causing 'diastasis fracture'. This is often seen in the sagittal suture but rarely in closed metopic suture (in between the frontal bones).
2. **Depressed skull fracture:** When a portion of fractured bone is driven inwards, it is known as depressed fracture. It is also called *'fracture a la signature'* (**signature fracture**), as the shape often points towards the shape of the offending weapon. They are caused by blows with a heavy weapon having

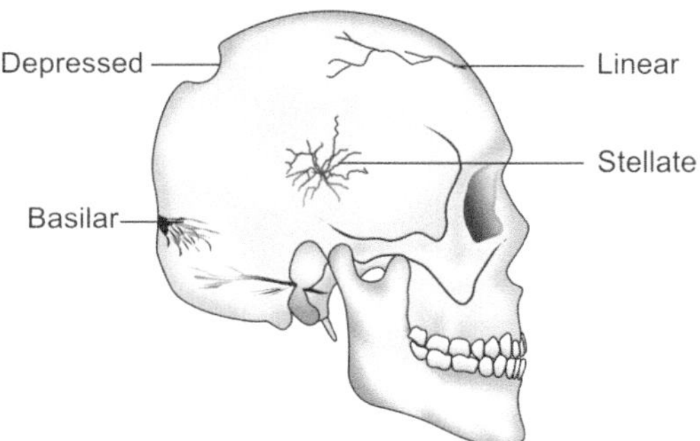

Fig. 13.5 Fractures of skull

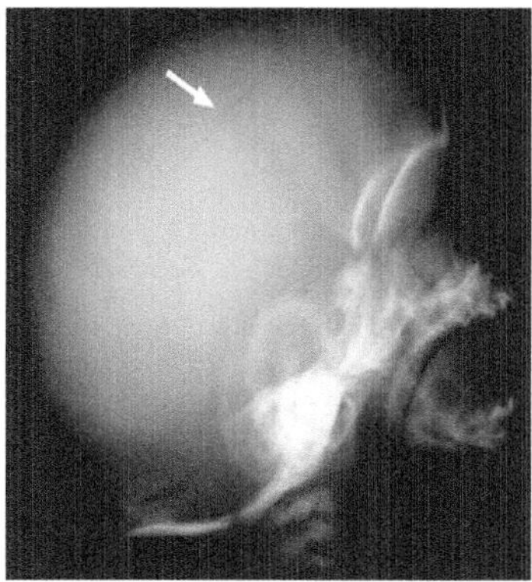

Fig. 13.6 Plain X-ray showing a linear fracture (arrow)

small striking surface, such as hammer, axe, brick, baseball bat or chopper. The part of the skull which is first struck shows maximum depression and are usually seen in the left frontal region (Fig. 13.7). There is no evidence that elevating a depressed skull fracture will reduce the subsequent development of post-traumatic seizures which are probably more related to the initial brain injury. Such fractures require immediate neurosurgical consultation. The decision to observe or operate immediately is made by the neurosurgeon. Fragments depressed more than 3–5 mm below the inner table are more likely to penetrate the dura and injure the cortex. CT is the best radiological study to identify a depressed skull fracture and underlying brain injury.

3. **Comminuted fracture (spider-web/mosaic fracture):** Two or more intersecting lines of fracture divide the bone into three or more fragments. Skull bone gets broken into multiple pieces by fracture lines which are haphazardly or concentrically arranged, or stellate if they radiate from the site of impact (Fig. 13.8). It is caused by vehicular accidents, fall from height on a hard surface or by blows with weapons having large striking surface, such as

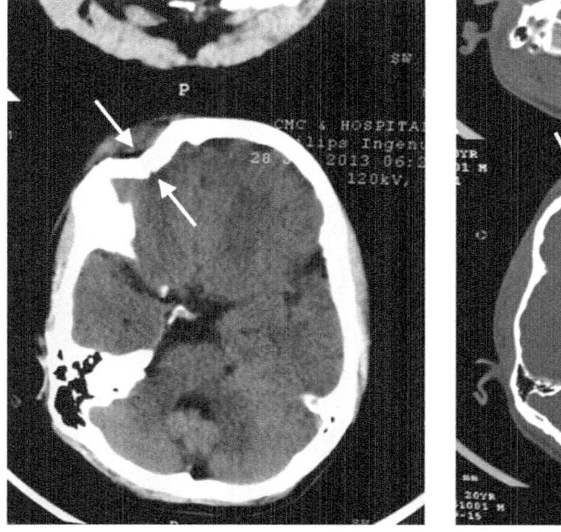

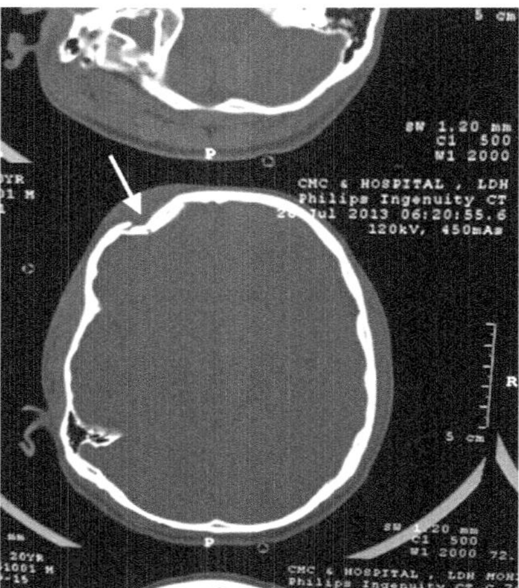

Fig. 13.7 Depressed fracture of skull (arrows)

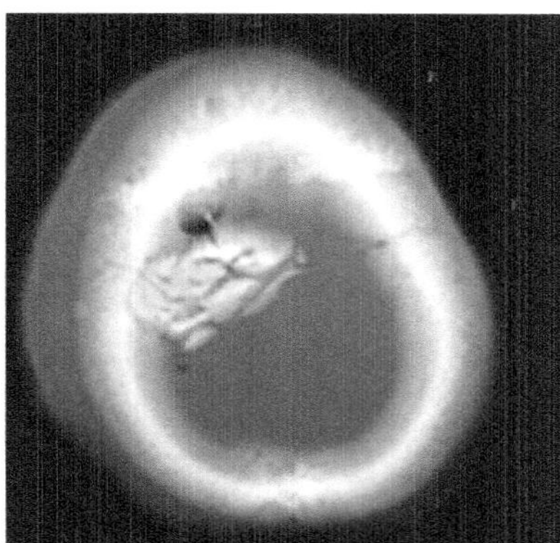

Fig. 13.8 CT scan bone window showing a comminuted fracture

heavy iron bar, or from a bullet. Comminuted fractures may be a complication of fissure fracture and the fragments of bone if displaced inward, form a depressed skull fracture.

4. **Basilar fracture:** The base of the skull is weak and hence, any diffuse impact to the vertex of the skull will produce basilar fracture. Most basal skull fractures are extensions of fractures through the cranial vault. CT scan is often poor for directly demonstrating basal skull fracture. Plain skull X-rays and clinical criteria (Box 13.2) are usually more sensitive. Sensitivity of CT diagnosis can be increased by the use of bone windows together with thin cuts (5 mm) and coronal images. Basilar fracture appears as linear lucencies through the skull base.

   Indirect radiographic findings (on CT or plain films) that suggest basilar fracture include: pneumocephalus (diagnostic of basal skull fracture in the absence of an open fracture of the cranial vault), air fluid level within or opacification of air sinus with fluid (suggestive). Other related findings include: fractures of the cribriform plate or orbital roof.

   In children, fractures are common in frontal and parietal bones. One third is closed, and these tend to occur in younger children as a result of the thinner, more deformable skull. Open fractures tend to occur with motor vechicle accidents, closed fractures follow accidents at home. Dural lacerations are

Box 13.2 Clinical signs of basilar fracture (Fig. 13.2 and Figs 13.9A to C)

1. CSF rhinorrhea and CSF otorrhea.
2. Subconjuctival hemorrhages.
3. Hemotympanum or laceration of external auditory canal.
4. Postauricular ecchymoses (Battle's sign).
5. Periorbital ecchymoses (Raccoon's eyes) in the absence of direct orbital trauma, especially if bilateral.
6. Cranial nerve injury:
   - CN VB and/or CNVIII: usually associated with temporal bone fracture
   - Olfactory nerve (CNI) injury: often occurs with anterior fossa basilar fracture and results in anosmia, this fracture may extend to the optic canal and cause injury to the optic nerve (CNII)
   - CN III through VI: can occur with fractures through the *clivus*.

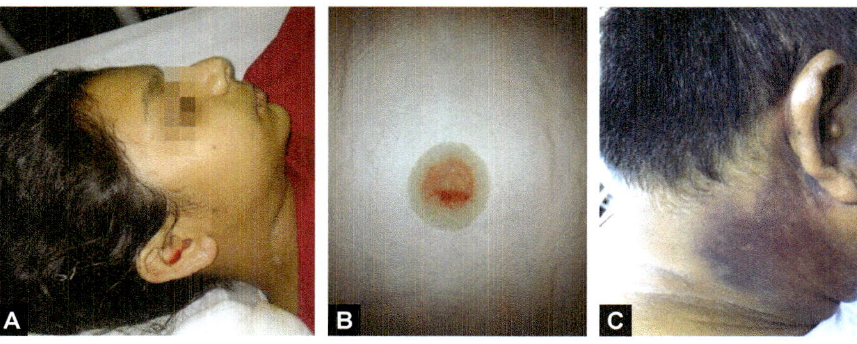

Figs 13.9A to C (A and B) CSF otorrhea with 'Halo sign'; (C) Battle sign

more common in compound fra ctures. Non-accidental trauma should be suspected in children below 2 years of age with depressed skull fractures, and they are more likely to develop epilepsy.

CRANIOFACIAL FRACTURES

Frontal sinus fractures: Frontal sinus fractures account for 5–15% of facial fractures. All frontal laceration should be explored digitally before repair. Digital palpation is sensitive to identifying frontal fractures, although false positives from lacerations extending through the periosteum can occur. A head CT should be obtained, if a frontal sinus fracture is suspected, to evaluate for posterior wall injury, brain injury and open fracture.

In the presence of a frontal sinus fracture, intracranial air (pneumocephalus) on CT even without a clinically evident CSF leak must be presumed to be due to dural laceration (although it could also be due to a basal skull fracture). Anesthesia of the forehead may occur due to supratrochlear and/or supraorbital nerve involvement. The risks of posterior wall fractures are not immediate, but may be delayed (some even by months or years) and include: brain abscess, CSF leak with risk of meningitis.

Fractures involving only the anterior table of the frontal sinus can be treated conservatively with referral to ENT or plastic surgery in 1–2 days. Fractures involving the posterior table require urgent neurosurgical consultation.

BRAIN INJURIES

Traumatic Brain Injury (TBI): It is defined as traumatically induced structural injury and/or physiological disruption of brain function as a result of an external force that is indicated by new onset of at least one of the following clinical signs, immediately following the event:

- Any period of loss of or a decreased level of consciousness
- Any loss of memory of events immediately before or after the injury
- Any alteration of mental state at the time of injury [confusion, disorientation or slowed thinking also known as alteration of consciousness (AOC)]
- Neurological deficits (weakness, loss of balance, change of vision, praxis, paresis/paraplegia, sensory loss or aphasia) that may not be transient
- Intracranial lesion.

It is important to consider TBI in the context of the skull and other structures above the neck, as well as to identify those 'isolated head injuries' and those with 'multisystem polytrauma' where other injuries may contribute to secondary brain injuries. The severity of TBI is usually classified by GCS. It should be clear that skull fracture itself is not TBI.

Brain Contusions

Brain contusions consist of heterogeneous areas of hemorrhage, brain necrosis and infarction. It is the most common lesion seen after head injury. An incidence on CT head of 30–40% is observed in head injury patients. They are caused by linear or more often laminar stresses (shear stresses). When it retains its shape, bruised and swollen, it is called 'contusion'. When the disruption is greater to produce macroscopic tearing, it is called 'laceration'. They are cone shape with base on the surface. They are usually multiple and are commonly associated with other intracranial hemorrhagic lesions.[25]

These may be of coup type, often associated with an overlying fracture (fracture contusion). Coup contusions are underlying the side of impact, whereas a contrecoup contusions lies far from side of impact, at frontal and temporal poles. Contusions of the medial cerebral hemisphere or corpus callosum may occur as a result of acceleration of brain against the falx cerebri. Small hemorrhagic lesions are also found in deep white and grey matter as a result of shearing that occurs with rapid acceleration and deceleration of the brain.[25,26]

Signs and symptoms vary according to the size and site of contusion and associated lesions, mass effect and edema. Contusion in speech area or in the motor cortex can cause permanent deficit. Large contusions or multiple contusions involving both frontal and temporal lobes (tetrapolar injury) can lead to raised ICP, brain shift and coma. In the period following injury, contused area becomes necrotic and heterogeneously hemorrhagic. Although, hemorrhage is eventually reabsorbed, the total mass may increase as a result of edema around the contused brain, leading to rise in ICP, decreased level of consciousness and appearance or exacerbation of the focal neurological deficits. Temporal contusions are notorious, as they are near the brainstem. Diagnosis is by CT scan and has a typical salt-pepper appearance (Fig. 13.10).[25,26]

INTRACRANIAL HEMORRHAGE

1. Extradural Hemorrhage (EDH)[27,28]

EDH refers to collection of blood between the skull and dura. Incidence of EDH is 1–3% of head trauma admissions. Ratio of male: female is 4:1. It usually occurs in young adults and is rare before age of 2 years or after 60 years (perhaps because the dura is more adherent to the inner table in these groups). The most common

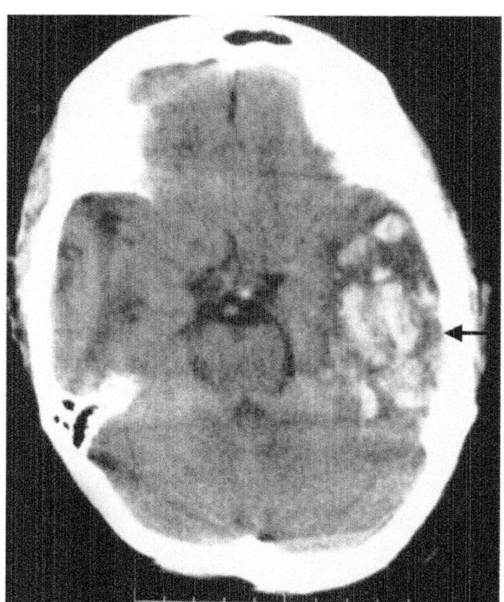

Fig. 13.10 CT head showing a left temporal contusion (arrow)

site is the temporoparietal region followed by frontal. A temporoparietal posterior fossa EDH occurs in 5–10% cases. Skull is usually fractured and meningeal vessels are torn (85–95% adults). Impact causes skull fracture due to inbending which strips the dura mater from the inner table. It disrupts the middle meningeal artery as it exits its bony groove at the pterion, causing arterial bleeding that dissects the dura from the inner table. Bleeding occurs where dura has been separated from the inner skull table, and the dura is further stripped by the hematoma. Another possibility is that dissection of the dura from the inner table may occur first, and then bleeding occurs into the space thus created. EDH is never considered to be a 'contrecoup' injury.

Source of bleeding: In 85% of cases, EDH is arterial in nature and the middle meningeal artery is the most common source of middle fossa EDHs. Remainder of cases are due to bleeding from middle meningeal vein or dural sinus. Association of hematoma and skull fracture is less common in young children because of skull elasticity.

Clinical presentation: The minimum collection of blood may vary from 35–100 ml before clinical signs appear. The classical presentation is seen in only 10–27% of cases. A brief post-traumatic loss of consciousness (LOC) followed by a lucid interval for several hours, then obtundation, contralateral hemiparesis, ipsilateral pupillary dilatation are seen in classical presentation. If untreated, it can go on to produce decerebrate rigidity, hypertension, respiratory distress and death. Deterioration usually occurs over few hours, but may take days and rarely, weeks (longer intervals may be associated with venous bleeding).

The lucid interval may be of variable duration, from as little as half an hour to more than a day, depending on how quick or slow the bleed is. However, the average interval is thought to be 4 hours. It should be noted that in some cases, this lucid interval is absent, as concussion merges with unconscousness caused by raised ICP.

Other presentations may be loss of consciousness at the time of impact. In a conscious patient, headache, vomiting, seizure (may be unilateral), hemiplegia, hyperreflexia and unilateral Babinski sign may be seen. Bradycardia is usually a late finding. In children, EDH should be suspected, if there is a 10% drop in hematocrit after admission. The diagnosis is confirmed on a plain CT, where it classically appears as a hyperdense biconvex space occupying lesion (Fig. 13.11). Fully conscious patients with less than 25 ml of blood and no midline shift in CT with mild head injury (GCS 14/15) can be kept under observation and conservative management. However, those with more than 25 ml of blood or midline shift and low GCS should be operated upon to remove the blood.

2. Subdural Hemorrhage[29]

Subdural hemorrhage (SDH) is a collection of fresh blood between the dura and pia arachnoid. It is seen in 5–22% of patients of severe head injury. Male to female ratio is 3:1 to 4:1. Falls, assaults and RTAs are the causative factors. It is commoner in older age group.

The magnitude of impact damage is usually much higher than EDH in acute subdural hematoma (ASDH) which generally makes this lesion a cause for higher mortality; there is often an associated underlying brain injury. Symptoms may

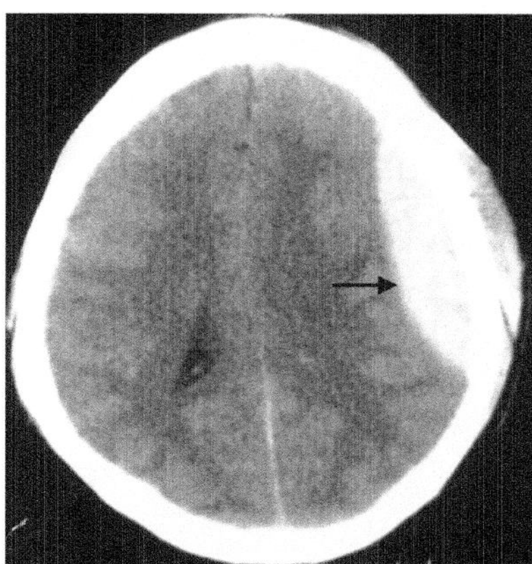

Fig. 13.11 CT head showing EDH of left parietal region (arrow)

be due to compression of the underlying brain with midline shift, in addition to parenchymal brain injury and possibly cerebral edema. The lesion is often seen alone in a close head injury with no skull fractures and scalp injuries. Unlike EDH which is confined to one place by the dura and the skull, SDH can move. The common mechanisms of traumatic ASDH:

a. Accumulation around parenchymal laceration (usually frontal or temporal lobe). There is usually severe underlying primary brain injury. Often no lucid interval. Focal signs usually occur later and are less prominent than with EDH.
b. Surface or bridging vessel torn from cerebral acceleration-deceleration during violent head motion. With this aetiology, primary brain damage may be less severe, a lucid interval may occur with later rapid deterioration.

Clinical signs: Similar to EDH, there can be a latent period or 'lucid interval' after the initial concussion and the position of SDH should never be interpreted as 'contrecoup'. When there is 'lucid interval', it should be longer than the average 4 hours for the more rapid arterial bleeding of EDH. In fact, this does not have a upper limit as ASDH can merge with the chronic variety. As with EDH, the minimal amount of blood before the clinical symptoms appear is thought to be between 35–100 ml.

The diagnosis is confirmed on a plain CT where it appears classically as crescentic hyperintense mass seen adjacent to inner table (Fig. 13.12). Edema is often present. The hemorrhage is usually over convexity, but may also be interhemispheric, along tentorium or in the posterior fossa. Membrane formation begins by about 4 days after injury (Table 13.2).

3. Subarachnoid Hemorrhage[30]

Trauma is the most common cause of subarachnoid hemorrhage (SAH). Traumatic SAH is usually a result of various forces that produce stress sufficient to damage superficial vascular structures running in the subarachnoid space. It may also arise when blood follows the path of CSF, as occurs in cases of intraventricular bleeding due to traumatic tears of the tela choroidea resulting from acceleration-deceleration injuries.

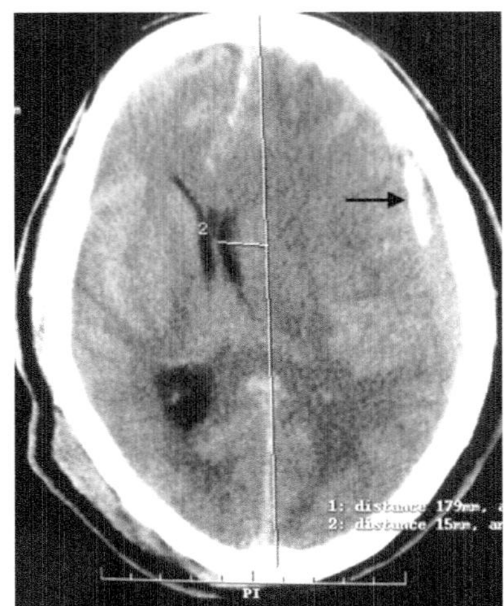

Fig. 13.12 CT head showing left SDH (arrow)

Table 13.2 ASDH density changes on CT with time

Time frame	*Density on CT*
1–3 days	Hyperdense
4 days to 2–3 weeks	Isodense
More than 3 weeks and less than 3–4 months	Hypodense (approaching density of CSF)
After about 1–2 months	May become lenticular shaped (similar to epidural hematoma) with density more than CSF but less than fresh blood

Post-traumatic SAH is associated with about 40% mortality. Furthermore, studies have found that traumatic SAH may predispose to cerebral vasospasm and diminished cerebral blood flow, therefore, increasing morbidity and mortality as a result of secondary ischemic damage. On a plain CT, SAH follows the contours of sulci and gyri. The overall sensitivity of CT is best within the first 12 hours (Fig. 13.13).

The blood in the subarachnoid space tend to mix with CSF. Therefore, unlike other hemorrhage, less likely to clot. Like SDH, it can gravitate down to lower position. Unlike SDH, the amount of blood present in most SAHs, from whatever cause, often seems insufficient to constitute a space-occupying lesion. It is able to diffuse more widely over the brain and displace CSF into the spinal theca. The total volume may be considerable, causing raised ICP, though some of this may be contributed by progressive cerebral edema. As blood in the subarachnoid space is irritant, even in small quantities, it seems possible that such sudden irrigation of the medulla may cause sudden collapse and death due to cardiorespiratory failure. There is an extensive vascular spasm that may have an effect on vital centers in the brainstem.

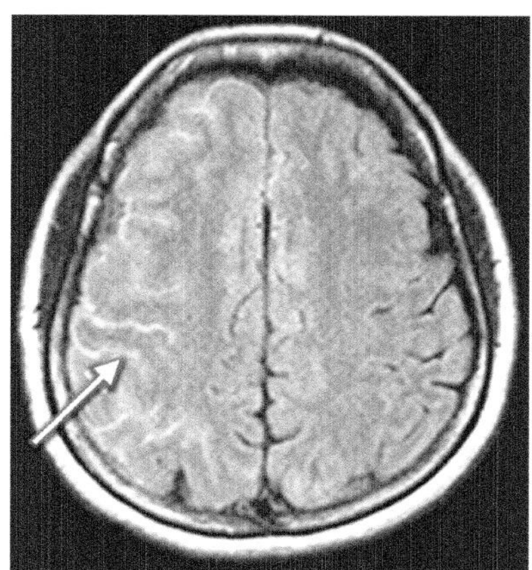

Fig. 13.13 CT head showing right SAH (arrow)

Traumatic Basilar Subarachnoid Hemorrhage

A blow from a fist, foot or any blunt object to the side neck/or head in the region between the angle of the jaw and ear may give rise to fatal SAH. This is due to tear or dissection of the basilovertebral artery which allows the blood to track along the upper part of the vessel and enter cranial cavity causing basilar SAH. In some cases, fracture of the transverse process of the first cervical vertebra may occur, hence, it is also called '*CV-One syndrome*'.

Mechanism: The mechanical force initiated by the blow to the side of the neck may cause tilting and rotation of the neck that could damage the vertebral artery in the vertebral canal, in addition to producing skin and soft tissue injuries on the side of the neck at the site of the blow. However, in some cases there may not be any external sign at all. However, some forensic pathologist believe that the vertebral artery damage is just a concomitant finding and the SAH is due to the damage to the intracranial vessels and not due to the vertebral artery damage. They are parallel findings and not cause and effect events.

4. Intracerebral Hemorrhage[31-33]

Intracerebral hemorrhages (ICH) are present in about 15% of fatal head injuries. They may be single or multiple and often complicate both penetrating intracranial wounds and closed head injuries. In patients with blunt trauma, ICH results from inertial loading of the head which produces shearing and tensile stresses within the brain tissue. This causes direct rupture of small vessels within the parenchyma at the moment of impact. ICH most frequently occurs in the white matter of the frontal and temporal regions (80–90% of cases). They are commonly associated with contusions, subdural hematomas and diffuse axonal injury because of common biomechanical mechanisms of injury. The complex of cerebral contusion and hematoma with concomitant hemorrhage into the subdural space is termed as '*burst lobe*'. The difference between a contusion and an intracerebral hematoma is one of degree, with hematomas having a greater blood content (at least two thirds of the volume of the lesion) and appearing more homogeneous.

Deep intracerebral hematomas occur in the basal ganglia, corpus callosum, centrum ovale and brainstem. In patients with these 'tissue-tear' hemorrhages, the associated contusions are more severe and the incidence of diffuse axonal injury is higher. In contrast to lobar hematomas, deep intracerebral hemorrhages are thought to arise from the shear strains arising from acceleration-deceleration forces.

Since the advent of CT, this has become a well-recognized entity, affecting 0.6–7.4% of all patients with head injury and having a reported mortality rate as high as 35–40% (Fig. 13.14). The time interval for the development of delayed intracerebral hematomas has continued to be a topic of debate, ranging from 6 hours to 30 days. Although these lesions may develop in areas of previously demonstrated contusion, they frequently occur in the presence of a completely normal initial CT. Patients with this diagnosis typically meet the following criteria: a definite history of trauma, an asymptomatic interval, an apoplectic event and the absence of vascular disease.

Various researchers have discussed possible mechanisms for the pathogenesis of delayed hematomas following trauma, such as increased vessel fragility, increased intramural pressure, increased capillary wall permeability, fibrinolysis and rupture of a post-traumatic aneurysm. Cranial trauma may increase the fragility of vessels by softening the brain around the wall of an artery, causing eventual rupture of the blood vessel, necrosis and hemorrhage. Intramural pressure may be increased by post-traumatic arterial hypertension. The loss of vascular autoregulation that often occurs after brain injury may increase capillary wall permeability, resulting in accumulation of toxic metabolites, tissue ischemia, perivascular edema and hemorrhage. Also, fibrinolysis and disseminated intravascular coagulation (DIC) has been found to be responsible for the development of up to 90% of reported delayed ICHs.

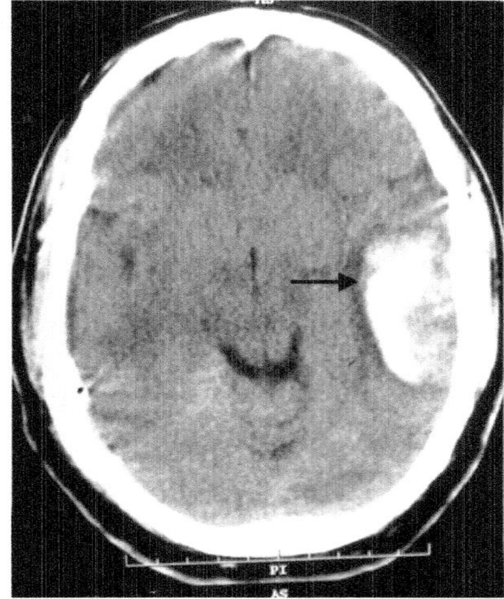

Fig. 13.14 Plain CT head showing ICH (arrow)

5. Intraventricular Hemorrhage

Intraventricular hemorrhage (IVH) was previously considered fatal. With the increasing availability of CT, post-traumatic IVH is readily diagnosed and has been found in 1.5–10% of all head-injured patients. Despite advances in diagnosis and treatment, this injury still carries a poor prognosis, particularly if there are associated brain lesions. In various reports, 60–80% of patients were either dead or in vegetative state following traumatic IVH. This poor outcome reflects the severity of the traumatic force and the general brain damage that is often associated with IVH. Isolated intraventricular blood in itself is not necessarily a poor prognostic sign. Acute hydrocephalus is uncommon, since the severe degree of cerebral edema and the presence of associated intracranial lesions are usually the cause of the increased intracranial pressure that occurs in nearly half of these patients.[34-37]

Pathogenic mechanisms that have been proposed for the cause of post-traumatic IVH include rupture of subependymal veins due to deformation by a negative pressure following sudden dilatation of the ventricular wall at the time of the impact, shearing injury resulting in laceration of the ventricular wall and perforating vessels, concomitant brainstem injury with blood extension into the ventricle, and spontaneous rupture of an unsuspected subependymal vascular malformation.[34-37]

OTHER TYPES OF FOCAL INJURY IN BRAIN

- *Cranial nerve avulsion:* Olfactory bulb injury resulting in anosmia is common after head injury, but other avulsions including the optic, facial and auditory nerves also occur.
- *Brainstem avulsion:* Severe hyperextension of the neck may result in brainstem avulsion, usually at the pontomedullary junction, and less commonly at the craniocervical junction. It results in immediate death, unless incomplete.
- *Focal vascular injury:* Carotid cavernous fistula resulting in pulsating exophthalmos and carotid or vertebral artery dissections may also occur with head injuries.
- *Pituitary infarction:* This may result from traumatic transection of the pituitary stalk or severe elevation of ICP.

DIFFUSE INJURY

Concussion[38-40]

Concussion is a clinical diagnosis, not a pathological entity. Cerebral concussions have been traditionally defined as a transient loss of consciousness without neuroanatomical evidence of parenchymal injury. When sustained in industrial accidents, motor vehicle collisions and assaults, cerebral concussions can have forensic and medicolegal implications, and treating doctors must decide when is it safe for the injured patients to return to work or resume driving.

Cerebral concussions also assume a significant role in sports. In contact sports and sports associated with high-speed and high-body inertia, the potential to injure the central nervous system (CNS) and spine is higher. Medical personnel assigned to the sports arena must determine, if athletes have been injured severely enough to preclude their continued participation in the event. Team doctors or coaches also must determine how soon injured athletes can participate in upcoming events. After a cerebral concussion, an athlete's risk for a second injury increases, and second-impact syndromes can have devastating outcomes. Repeated injuries can be cumulative and produce delayed neurophysiological and neuropsychological deficits.

Three grades of cerebral concussion are accepted for the evaluation and treatment of injured persons (Table 13.3). Athletes with Grade 1 concussions should be removed from competition. They should be examined immediately and at 5-minutes intervals for the development of mental status abnormalities or post-concussive symptoms both at rest and during exertion. Athletes may return to the arena, if mental status abnormalities clear within 15 minutes. A second Grade 1 concussion during the same competition, however, precludes athletes from further competition during the same day. They may return to competition only, if they remain asymptomatic at rest and during exercise for one week.

Athletes with Grade 2 concussions should be removed from competition for the remainder of the day. They should be examined onsite frequently for signs of increasing ICP and re-examined the next day. They should return to competition only after a doctor who has performed a full neurological examination has cleared the athlete. This medical clearance should be obtained after the athletes have been asymptomatic at rest and during exertion for one full week. Before returning to competition, neuroimaging studies are recommended for all athletes whose headache or symptoms of post-concussive syndrome persist longer than one week. Any abnormality on CT or MRI terminates the season for the athletes. If athletes sustain a second Grade 2 concussion during the same season, they should not be allowed to compete, until they have been asymptomatic at rest and during exertion for at least two weeks.

Athletes with Grade 3 concussions should be transferred from the field to the nearest emergency room by ambulance where a thorough evaluation should be performed. Athletes who are discharged home from the emergency department should be observed closely by a responsible adult for at least 24 hours or until all symptoms have resolved. Athletes with a Grade 3 concussion who lost consciousness for seconds only should be withheld from competition, until they have been asymptomatic at rest and during exertion for at least one week. Athletes who lose consciousness for minutes should return to competition only after they have been asymptomatic at rest and during exertion for at least two weeks. Athletes who sustain a second Grade 3 concussion during the same season should not return to competition, until they have been asymptomatic a minimum of one full month.

Table 13.3 Concussion grade

Grade I	*Grade II*	*Grade III*
Transient confusion No loss of consciousness Symptom resolve in less than 15 minutes	Transient confusion No loss of consciousness Symptom resolve in more than 15 minutes	Any loss of consciousness

Diffuse Axonal Injury[41-43]

Strich described diffuse brain lesions in patients with severe and prolonged post-traumatic dementia. She referred to the type of damage as diffuse degeneration of the white matter. Since then, a variety of synonyms have been applied to this condition, initiated by diffuse damage of nerve fibers at the time of injury. The term 'diffuse axonal injury' (DAI) has now gained wide acceptance as appropriately reflecting the underlying phenomenon.

The neuropathlogical findings in severe head injuries support the view that in most instances, immediate unconsciousness and coma are due to severe DAI resulting from the impact producing shearing forces in the white matter. The criteria for the diagnosis of DAI are histological and can be seen only microscopically with the use of suitable staining techniques. The earliest sign was shown by silver stains which demonstrated the appearance of axonal retraction bulbs or swellings throughout the white matter of the cerebral hemispheres, cerebellum and brainstem, after a patient had survived for at least 12 hours. In patients who have survived some weeks, standard histology shows large numbers of clusters of microglia throughout the white matter. Longer survival, particularly in vegetative state, results in long tract degeneration of the Wallerian type throughout the hemispheres, brainstem and spinal cord.

The clear correlation between severe axonal injury, and profound and persisting coma has raised the questions of the relationship between lesser degrees of injury and brief unconsciousness. Damage in the major hippocampal projection pathways like the fornices may underlie some of the persisting memory disturbances seen after concussive head injury.

Radiological investigations in life are now supporting the observations previously made at autopsy. Magnetic resonance imaging (MRI) has demonstrated a clear correlation between the occurrence of lesions in the subcortical white matter and loss of consciousness after injury. Lesions in the deep white matter were associated with more profound and more persisting impairment of consciousness. In contrast, brainstem lesions were uncommon in that study; some patients were in deep persisting coma, but no such lesions were detected. Atrophy of the fornix has also been observed.

The various clinical, pathological, radiological and neurophysical observations give rise to the hypothesis that the instantaneous loss of consciousness in a head injury represents a state of transient, but sometimes profound inhibition of arousal mechanisms within the hypothalamic and diencephalic brain system. There may be failure of facilitatory arousal systems or there may be active inhibition. DAI may be graded on MRI as given in Table 13.4.

The level of function before injury is a strong predictor of the potential for recovery of neurological function. Recently, the concept of 'individual vulnerability' has been advanced, which takes into consideration host factors including preinjury conditions (for e.g., medical diseases, psychiatric disorders, substance abuse, previous injury, learning disability), sociodemographic factors (for e.g., age, gender, economic status), and pending litigation or other compensation issues. All these preinjury factors may influence post-traumatic morbidity and mortality. The prognosis is better in grade I as compared to Grade II and Grade III. Patients who have no apparent lesion on conventional imaging and still do not regain consciousness will be shown to have DAI on MRI in many cases.

Table 13.4 Diffuse axonal injury grading

Severity	*Pathological findings*
Grade I	Involves grey-white matter interfaces, most commonly parasagittal regions of frontal lobes, periventricular temporal lobes and less commonly the parietal and occipital lobes, internal and external capsules and cerebellum
Grade II	Involves corpus callosum in addition to grade I locations. Most commonly involves the posterior body and splenium but does advance anteriorly with increasing severity of injury, and most frequently unilateral
Grade III	Involves brainstem in addition to grade I and II locations and most commonly seen in rostral midbrain, superior cerebellar peduncles, medial lemnisci and corticospinal tracts

Cerebral Edema

Although a number of factors contribute to the high mortality and morbidity associated with TBI, the development of cerebral edema with brain swelling remains the most significant predictor of outcome. Brain swelling can only occur with addition of water from the vasculature (vasogenic edema), since cytotoxic edema is essentially a compartment shift of water from the extracellular to intracellular compartment. As such, attenuating blood brain barrier permeability has increasingly become a promising approach to managing brain edema and associated swelling. Edema is harmful because it causes cell swelling; swelling that alters cellular metabolite concentration and therefore, cellular physiology, biochemistry and function. When the swelling involves not only the cells themselves but also the tissue parenchyma, there is a rapid increase in ICP which results in compression of blood vessels, reduced tissue blood flow and reduced oxygenation. This eventually shifts tissue down pressure gradients (herniation) that may crush vital brain centers such as those involved in respiration and cardiac function.[44,45]

Diffuse brain edema is a well defined entity. The CT picture is of absent third ventricle and basal cisterns, loss of sulci and differentiation of grey and white matter (Fig. 13.15). Although, this condition has been associated with children, it has also been seen in adults. Secondary deterioration (decline in consciousness, the development of new focal neurological signs or an increase in ICP) occurs in many cases and is common in adults than children. Features that may significantly associate with deterioration are the presence of prolonged coma (> 1 hour) after the injury, CT signs of DAI or SAH, or a recorded episode of hypotension.[44,45]

Diffuse vascular injury consisting of multiple small hemorrhages throughout the brain is virtually restricted to patients who die within 24 hours.

MISSILE HEAD INJURY

Impact of the head by an external object may result in a depressed skull fracture or penetration into the cranial cavity and focal brain damage. Damage to the brain is by direct intrusion, either by the foreign object such as a penetrating weapon, bullet or other missile, or fragments of skull in a compound fracture where the skull is disrupted. In these open wounds, the mechanism of the damage to the brain is evident.[46,47]

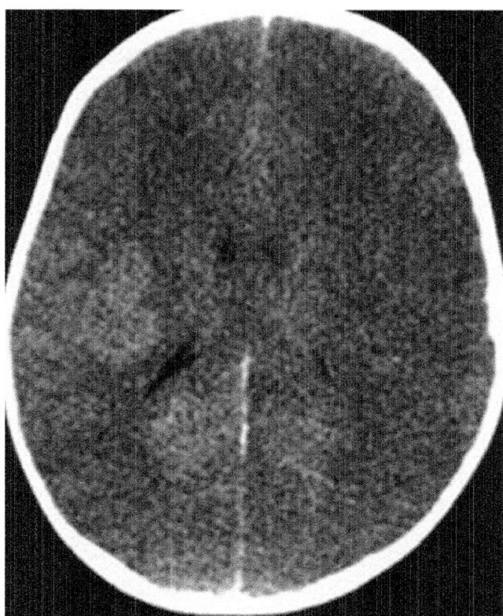

Fig. 13.15 CT scan showing cerebral edema

Penetrating injuries are common with gunshot wounds, but may also occur with stab wounds with knife or ice pick, particularly in the orbital and squamous temporal bones. Low velocity penetrating injuries may cause damage by direct injury to blood vessels, nerves and brain tissue and the complications caused by persisting hemorrhage and infection. High-velocity bullets (for e.g., rifles) often exit the skull (perforating injury) and may result in extensive brain damage from the massive shock wave.[46-48]

CLINICAL ASSESSMENT[49-50]

The main concern of the emergency medical officer for patients who have sustained a head injury is to accurately assess the important brain injuries and decide on the subsequent need for imaging and treatment of the injury. Attention should also be directed to co-existing injuries (for e.g., cervical spine injury) and to other concerns the medical officer may have (for e.g., nonaccidental injury, nontraumatic etiology such as seizure). The cervical spine should be immobilized in suspected cases. Early imaging is recommended which will reduce the time for detection of life-threatening complications and is associated with better outcomes. It is better not to wait for admission and observation for neurological deterioration. Hemodynamically unstable patients need evaluation of their head, chest, abdomen and pelvis. There should be no unnecessary investigations, and noncranial injuries leading to hemorrhage and hypotension should be dealt in priority.

History

Once stabilized, the clinical history should be obtained from the patient (if conscious), witnesses and paramedical staff. The history should include details of the mechanism of the injury—assault, ejection from vehicle, hit by motor vehicle or fall from height. It is important to gather information about mechanism as this can predict outcome. Pedestrians and cyclists fare worse than vehicle occupants, penetrating injuries fare worse than blunt and an ejection from a vehicle carries a higher risk of TBI.

Condition of the patient at the accident scene, age (elderly patients are prone to subdural hematomas), past medical history, medications, allergies, history of bleeding diathesis or anticoagulation therapy, smoking, alcohol or drug use and social circumstances should also be noted.

Symptoms depend upon the severity of the injury. Many patients with minor head injury may not have any symptoms when they reach the emergency department. In conscious patients, headache (most common complaint after mild head injury) due to somatic pain from a scalp injury is common. However, the headache seen due to raised ICP is aggravated by coughing, straining or bending, and is associated with nausea, vomiting and impaired consciousness. Post-traumatic amnesia, confusion, repetitive speech and disorientation are very common, even after relatively minor head trauma.

Focal neurological deficits affecting any part of the brain and cranial nerves can occur. Anosmia due to disruption of the olfactory pathways is one of the most common focal symptoms. History of seizures, CSF rhinorrhoea and otorrhea should be noted.

Examination

A comprehensive neurological examination is essential to detect subtle neurological abnormalities such as unequal pupils, cranial nerve deficit or peripheral limb weakness/abnormalities. The patient should be clinically evaluated so as to identify those at risk of traumatic intracranial pathology and, especially, those that require neurosurgical intervention. The neck should always be assessed for injury to the cervical spine.

The protocol that is usually followed is a case of head injury is given in Box 13.3.

Assessment of Consciousness

As mentioned earlier, GCS is the most universal scale for assessing the level of conscious as it is simple, quick, repeatable and has low inter-observer variation (Table 13.5). No other scale is more superior, and its use is recommended by the Brain Trauma Foundation and most other guidelines.

Repeated and regular assessment of the GCS is of importance in monitoring the condition of the patient. The GCS should be monitored at presentation as a baseline reading, and every 15–30 minutes thereafter. A GCS of 15 represents

Box 13.3 Examination protocol of head injured patient

i. Assessment of the level of consciousness and pupillary reactions
ii. Examination of the cranium
iii. Examination of cranial nerve function
iv. Examination of peripheral nerve function
v. Examination of the cervical spine

Table 13.5 Glasgow outcome scale and score

Feature	*Scale response*	*Score notation*
Eye opening	Spontaneous	4
	To verbal stimuli	3
	To painful stimuli	2
	No eye opening	1
Verbal response	Oriented	5
	Confused (conversation)	4
	Inappropriate words	3
	Incomprehensible sounds	2
	No verbal response	1
Motor response	Obeys commands	6
	Localizing pain	5
	Normal flexion to pain	4
	Abnormal flexion to pain	3
	Extension to pain	2
	No motor response	1

spontaneous eye opening, orientated (who is he, where is he, why is he and where he is) and obeying commands; E4,V5,M6. The focus should be not to miss brain injury, especially among those presenting with a GCS of 9–13. This group of moderate brain injury patients includes cases that may 'talk and die'. Intoxication and iatrogenic administration of sedating drugs can affect the level of consciousness, but they should not be assumed to be the sole cause of impaired consciousness without confirmatory imaging.

In clinical practice, documentation of the motor score causes most difficulty. If the patient is unarousable, a central painful stimulus is applied. Supraorbital pressure is most commonly used. Localization to pain is noted, if the patient raises the hand above the clavicle in response to central pain or tries to remove the stimulus in response to a sternal rub. Flexion is characterized by flexion at the elbow with the forearm in a supinated position and the wrist held in a neutral or flexed position. Abnormal flexion is observed when flexion occurs at the elbow but the forearm is pronated with a flexed wrist posture. Extension occurs when the elbow extends and the arm rotates into a pronated position. Again, the wrist is usually flexed.

If the patient is intubated or has a tracheostomy, the verbal response should be marked 'T'. This enables the eye opening and motor parameters to be used to assess the level of consciousness. Sometimes, severe periorbital swelling precludes accurate eye-opening responses. High spinal cord injury makes motor assessment difficult. However, the itemized GCS continues to provide useful information in such situations. When recording the GCS, the scores of individual components should be noted rather than just the total, as patients with the same total GCS but with different component scores may have differing outcomes. The motor component is regarded as predictive as the global GCS score.

Several studies have looked at the prognostic power of post-resuscitation GCS and shown a steep decline in mortality as GCS increases from 3 to 8 and then a shallow decline from GCS 9–15. A drop in GCS is also significant, predicting the need for surgical evacuation of a subdural hematoma.

Pupillary Reflexes

Pupil size and reactivity can be affected through a number of mechanisms after head injury: eye and optic nerve trauma, third nerve injury, brainstem dysfunction and drug administration. Hence, examination of the pupillary reflexes provides critical information about the integrity of the optic and oculomotor pathways.

In a normal person, shining a light into one eye causes direct contraction of the ipsilateral pupil and consensual contraction of the contralateral pupil. Light-sensitive afferent fibers travel via the optic nerve into both optic tracts synapsing in the pretectal nuclei of the midbrain. These projects bilaterally to the Edinger-Westphal nuclei which supply parasympathetic fibers to the oculomotor nerves. The oculomotor nerves emerge from the midbrain and travel anteriorly in the interpeduncular cistern and then along the ipsilateral free edge of the tentorium cerebelli before entering the cavernous sinus and orbit via the superior orbital fissure. The parasympathetic fibers cause contraction of the sphincter pupillae.

In patients with an expanding mass lesion, herniation of the medial temporal lobe (uncus) causes compression of the ipsilateral oculomotor nerve. The fibers to the ipsilateral sphincter pupillae cease to function, causing unopposed dilatation of the pupil which fails to contract on direct or consensual testing.

Unreactive pupils are associated with hypotension, reduced consciousness level and closed basal cisterns on CT brain scan. Bilateral unreactive pupils occur in 20–30% of severe TBI patients and predict a 70–90% chance of poor outcome. Asymmetrical pupils predict the presence of an operable mass lesion in about 30% of cases.

Pulsatile proptosis associated with orbital pain, ophthalmoplegia, reduced vision, chemosis and a bruit over the globe are the classical signs of a traumatic cavernous carotid fistula (CCF). Fundoscopy may reveal ocular injuries such as subretinal or vitreal hemorrhages.

External Examination

The scalp should be thoroughly inspected and palpated for signs of injury including abrasions, contusions, lacerations and any underlying bone fracture. These are commonly found in cases of assault with direct impact injuries. The damaged skin should be assessed for viability and the presence of foreign bodies within the wound.

Sometimes, depressed skull fractures can be palpated. Signs of skull base fractures should be looked for. The features associated with basilar fractures include subconjuctival hemorrhages, periorbital and postauricular ecchymoses (Battle's sign), CSF rhinorrhea and CSF otorrhea (Box 13.2).

The ears should be examined with an otoscope to detect any CSF otorrhea or hemotympanum—a dark red/blue appearance suggests blood behind the tympanic membrane. CSF rhinorrhea—blood mixed with CSF from the nose which does not clot and forms tracks on blotting paper.

The face should be examined for asymmetry, localized tenderness and fractures. Log-rolling is done for a careful examination of the posterior aspect of the head and whole spine (Figs 13.16A and B).

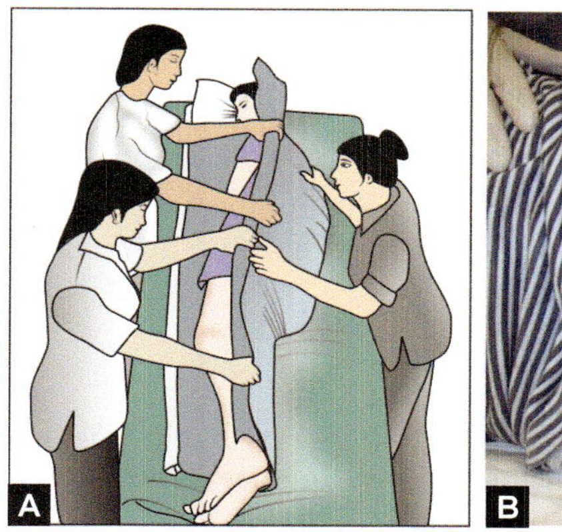

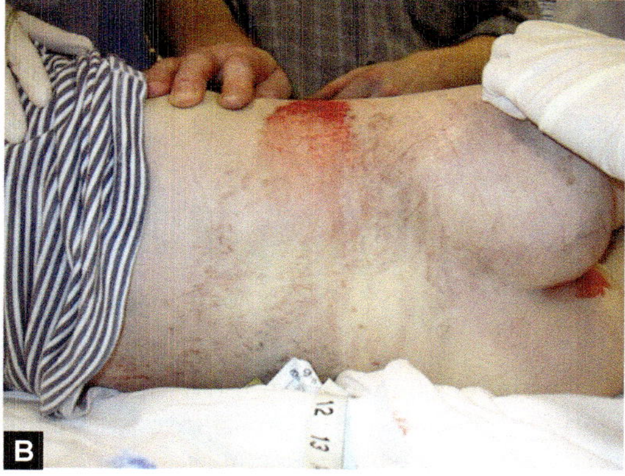

Figs 13.16A and B Log-rolling for examination of back

Cranial Nerves

The cranial nerves should be examined systematically in conscious and co-operative patients. In unconscious patients, the brainstem reflexes (pupillary, corneal and gag) and gaze palsies should be noted. Oculocephalic and vestibulo-ocular reflexes are not normally tested, unless ascertaining the presence of any brainstem dysfunction when undertaking brainstem tests.

i. Anosmia may occur due to tearing of the olfactory nerves at the cribriform plate. Patients with anosmia often report a change in the quality of taste sensation. Formal testing for sense of smell is done using test bottles of clove oil and peppermint solution.
ii. Visual acuity, visual fields and pupillary reflexes and tested. Diplopia may be reported with impaired eye movements. A complete oculomotor (CN III) nerve palsy results in a ptosis, ipsilateral pupillary dilatation unreactive to light directly or consensually and the eye in the 'down and out' position.
iii. Trochlear (CN IV) and abducent (CN VI) nerve palsies result in vertical and lateral gaze diplopia respectively. Superior orbital fissure fractures can result in CN III, IV, VI and the ophthalmic division of the trigeminal (CN V) nerve being injured.
iv. The trigeminal nerve is examined by testing sensation over the face and anterior scalp, and the strength of the muscles of mastication. Branches can be injured distally by facial fractures or more proximal nerve injury can occur at the petroclinoid ridge near Meckel's cave.
v. The facial nerve (CN VII) supplies the muscles of facial expression and can be disrupted by fractures of the petrous temporal bone causing a complete lower motor neuron type of facial palsy. The corneal reflex, elicited by lightly touching the lateral aspect of each cornea and inspecting for bilateral blinking, tests the integrity of the trigeminal and facial nerve pathways.
vi. Hearing loss should be characterized as either sensorineural or conductive; both commonly occur after head trauma.
vii. The gag reflex is tested by touching the soft palate or pharynx with a stick or tongue depressor and observing elevation of the uvula. The afferent limb of

the reflex tests the integrity of the glossopharyngeal (CN IX) nerve, whilst the vagus (CN X) causes contraction of the palatal musculature. Changes in the quality of voice are related to vagal injuries causing altered phonation.

viii. The spinal accessory nerve (CN IX) supplies the sternocleidomastoid and trapezius muscles.

ix. The hypoglossal nerve (CN XII) is rarely injured but does course through the anterior condylar canal and may be disrupted in fractures of the foramen magnum.

Peripheral Nervous System

A thorough examination of the peripheral nervous system may not be possible with a depressed level of consciousness and limb injuries. Injuries of the brachial plexus, rarely the lumbosacral plexus and the peripheral nerves can complicate the interpretation of abnormal findings.

Observation of movement is important in assessing spinal cord function and corticospinal tract injury. Any asymmetry is documented. Unilateral motor signs (for e.g., hemiplegia) may occur with an intracranial mass lesion which need further investigation.

Investigations

The primary investigation of choice is CT since, it is more sensitive than X-ray at detecting clinically important brain injuries. Plain X-rays of the skull should not be used to diagnose significant brain injury, except in cases of skeletal survey in children presenting with suspected nonaccidental injury. MRI is more sensitive than CT in detecting subtle brain lesions such as DAI and some small hemorrhages.

A urine toxicology screen and BAC should be done in suspected cases, as the combination of alcohol and head injury is a frequent presentation in the emergency department.

Management

The initial management includes the maintenance of the airway, breathing and circulation according to the principles of the Advanced Trauma Life Support (ATLS) care system as this also prevents secondary cerebral injuries. The level of consciousness, and pupil size and reaction should be determined when managing patients with TBI. A full assessment of the injuries determines the priorities of the treatment—whether the patient requires only observation and supportive care or urgent laparotomy or craniotomy.

Management of mild head injury is determined by the result of CT scan and the condition of the patient. Mild head injury patients who do not require neurological care are observed for at least 24 hours to ensure that no neurological deterioration takes place. The majority of the patients improves over a period of 24 hours and can be discharged subsequently. Written instructions should be given to the responsible guardian to monitor the patient for the next 24 hours. Patients should be advised about post-concussive symptoms lasting for weeks to months.

SPECIAL CONDITIONS/SITUATIONS

Coma, Brain Death and Persistent Vegetative State

Coma[51] is deep, sustained pathologic unconsciousness that results from dysfunction of the ascending reticular activating system in either the brainstem or both cerebral hemispheres. The eyes remain closed and the patient cannot be aroused. To be clearly distinguished from syncope, concussion or other states of transient unconsciousness, coma must persist for at least an hour.

Brain death[52,53] is the permanent absence of all brain functions, including those of the brainstem. Brain-dead patients are irreversibly comatose and apneic, and have lost all brainstem reflexes and cranial nerve functions. The American Academy of Neurology practice parameter on determining brain death outlines the process in detail. Key features include the following:

i. Unresponsiveness, absent brainstem reflexes (for e.g., pupillary, caloric, corneal, pharyngeal), and absence of effective respiratory movements in the presence of adequate oxygenation and arterial pCO_2 of 60 mm Hg.
ii. Clinical or neuroradiologic evidence of an etiology adequate to explain the clinical findings.
iii. Adequate observation period to guarantee irreversibility.
iv. Exclusion of reversible factors that can confound assessment, such as drug intoxication or body core temperature less than 90°F.
v. Use of serial examination or confirmatory tests (for e.g., EEG, blood flow studies) to assist in diagnosis, in situations of clinical uncertainty, but these are not routinely required for diagnosis.

The most common technical error is failure to perform an adequate apnea test with documentation of apnea at pCO_2 of at least 60 mm Hg. Complicating factors such as severe facial trauma, toxic levels of sedatives, tricyclic agents or neuromuscular blockers, or pre-existing pulmonary disease with high CO_2 retention may create confusion requiring additional studies or neurologic opinions. Judgment and experience are required to distinguish between spinal and cerebral motor responses or effective and ineffective movements on apnea testing.

The concept of brain death is important from the point of view of organ donation. However, it is a sensitive matter and it should be discussed with the relatives with great care. Families may reject the diagnosis of brain death for religious or other reasons. Hospital staff should not insist on suspending life support over vigorous family objection. Malpractice issues may be relevant, if the relatives believe that monetary gain is there for the hospital from the organ donation. Behavior that gives the appearance of absolute disrespect for the family or the dying patient could result in criminal penalties.

Locked-in syndrome[54,55] refers to a state in which consciousness and cognition are retained, but movement and communication are impossible because of severe paralysis of the voluntary motor system. This condition may result from abnormalities in the descending corticospinal and corticobulbar pathways at or below the pons. In such cases, breathing is possible. The locked-in syndrome can also be associated with diseases of the peripheral motor nerves or paralysis produced by the administration of neuromuscular blocking agents. Patients with this syndrome can usually establish limited communication through eye-movement signals. Diagnosis of the locked-in syndrome is established by clinical examination. Brain imaging may show isolated ventral pontine infarction, and nerve-conduction studies may demonstrate severe peripheral neuropathy. Positron-emission tomographic (PET) scans have shown higher metabolic levels in the brains of patients in the locked-in state rather than in patients in a persistent vegetative state.

Vegetative state is a clinical condition of complete unawareness of the self and the environment, accompanied by sleep-wake cycles with either complete or partial preservation of hypothalamic and brainstem autonomic functions. The clinical course and outcome of a persistent vegetative state depend on its cause. Three categories of disorder can cause such a state: acute traumatic and non-traumatic brain injuries, degenerative and metabolic brain disorders, and severe congenital malformations.

Persistent vegetative state[56,57] may be defined as a vegetative state present one month after acute traumatic or nontraumatic brain injury or lasting for at least one month in patients with degenerative or metabolic disorders or developmental malformations of the nervous system.

Recovery of consciousness from a post-traumatic persistent vegetative state is unlikely after 12 months in adults and children. Recovery from a nontraumatic persistent vegetative state after three months is exceedingly rare in both adults and children. For most such patients, life expectancy ranges from 2–5 years; survival beyond 10 years is unusual. The vegetative state can be diagnosed according to the following criteria:

i. No evidence of awareness of self or environment and an inability to interact with others.
ii. No evidence of sustained, reproducible, purposeful or voluntary behavioral responses to visual, auditory, tactile or noxious stimuli.
iii. No evidence of language comprehension or expression.
iv. Intermittent wakefulness manifested by the presence of sleep-wake cycles.
v. Sufficiently preserved hypothalamic and brainstem autonomic functions to permit survival with medical and nursing care.
vi. Bowel and bladder incontinence.
vii. Variably preserved cranial nerve reflexes (pupillary, oculocephalic, corneal, vestibulo-ocular and gag) and spinal reflexes.

POST-TRAUMATIC SYNDROME (POST-CONCUSSIVE SYNDROME)[58-60]

The post-traumatic syndrome refers to a group of symptoms that usually occur after a mild head injury. The existence of the syndrome is doubtful, but the patient complaints are usually consistent and doctors believe its existence. The symptoms include headache, dizziness, anxiety, impaired cognition and memory deficit. Neurological examination is normal. Rutherford and associates studied head injury patients at 6 weeks and 1 year after injury, and found that several factors are associated with a higher incidence of symptoms: female sex, headaches or abnormal CNS signs at 24 hours, and fall from a height.

Psychological testing is needed to assess whether a patient has experienced memory alterations, personality changes, task-oriented difficulties and similar dysfunction. This testing is especially needed in patients who demonstrate no objective manifestations on their physical examination, imaging studies or other testing.

Clinical Evaluation

Evaluation of a head injury patient with symptoms of post-traumatic syndrome should begin with a detailed history of the events surrounding the mechanism of injury. Family members should be interviewed to assess subtle changes in a patient's personality or behavior that may have occurred. Evaluation of pre-existing conditions, such as alcohol or drug dependency, psychiatric illness, or endocrinological disorders should be undertaken. The issue of ongoing or future litigation should be discussed to assess the potential for personal compensation in the situation.

A thorough neurological evaluation should be performed by a neurosurgeon, if possible. Even subtle abnormalities should be corroborated with objective testing. Motor and sensory examinations should assess weakness, tone and abnormal movements, as well as changes in the perception of external stimuli. Findings such as give-way weakness (*cogwheel weakness*) or glove and stocking hypoesthesia may be indicative of malingering or hysteria. Cerebellar function should be assessed by observation of gait and coordination. The neck and sub-occipital area should be examined for muscle spasm which may be responsible for the complaint of headache. Serial examinations should be undertaken at intervals to assess the consistency of findings and many symptoms may dissipate with time.

Radiological evaluation should be undertaken and include a review of the studies obtained during the initial hospital stay, with careful attention to abnormalities that may have been overlooked initially. Follow-up CT may show lesions such as chronic SDH, cortical atrophy (particularly in the frontal lobes) or hydrocephalus. MRI expands the diagnostic possibilities by demonstrating edema, resolving contusions, effusions or evidence of DAI. Other modalities such as PET, single photon emission CT and regional blood flow analysis may hold promise for the future, but have no current application in diagnosis or prognostication in post-traumatic syndrome. Electroencephalography (EEG) may be indicated, particularly in patients who have had seizure activity at some point in their clinical course.

The term 'neurobehavioral sequelae' is used to refer to the cognitive and behavioral effects of brain injury, including impairments of problem solving, memory, attention, language, perception and behavior that adversely affect global outcome and contribute to chronic disability seizures and focal neurological deficits (for e.g., hemiparesis). Assessment of neurobehavioral functioning is essential for clarifying the basis of chronic disability after severe closed head injury and to plan for post acute clinical management of the sequelae.

POST-TRAUMATIC AMNESIA[61,62]

Post-traumatic amnesia is the most common early neurobehavioral sequelae of closed head injury. Post-traumatic amnesia which continues after recovery of consciousness, may be *anterograde amnesia* (i.e., impaired episodic memory for events that occur within a specific spatiotemporal context) which is reflected by difficulty in recalling events in the hospital environment (for e.g., visitors, or names of medical staff) and recent events in the news or in the patient's life.

Retrograde memory loss can initially impair recall of events for months or years before the injury, a gap that tends to recede during the first few days of recovery. Traditional methods of assessing retrograde amnesia involve asking the patient to describe and date the last event in memory before the injury to estimate the duration of the gap. Information in the public domain (for e.g., titles of television shows) or autobiographical memory questionnaires may be used to assess retrograde memory loss.

Temporal disorientation during post-traumatic amnesia is characterized in most patients by displacement of the patient's time estimates into the past. The sequence of recovery of orientation is person, place and time in about 70% of patients, whereas the order varies in the other one third of head-injured patients. Although recovery of orientation to person, place and time is typically associated with resolution of post-traumatic amnesia, there are cases of persistent difficulty in episodic memory after return of full orientation. Serial administration of a brief bedside test, such as the Galveston Orientation and Amnesia Test can depict an early cognitive recovery curve that is related to long-term neurobehavioral outcome.

It has been found that about one half of survivors of severe closed head injury exhibit residual anterograde memory deficit as reflected by impaired learning and retention of new information. Episodic memory for events with a specific spatiotemporal context (for e.g., telephone calls from a specific person at a specific time) is the most intensively studied form of memory in head-injured patients. Tests involving verbal memory for word lists or short passages and recall of geometric designs have been used extensively in outcome studies. It has been postulated that a nonreactive pupil in a comatose patient reflects structural neurological deterioration, whereas a low GCS score is compatible with reversible cerebral dysfunction in patients with normal pupillary reactivity. In view of the vulnerability of the hippocampus to decreased cerebral perfusion, it is thought that high intracranial pressure would result in a chronic memory disorder. However, the results failed to provide support for a relationship between high intracranial pressure and residual memory deficit, while confirming the effects of a low GCS and pupillary abnormality.

There are few studies pertaining to the recovery of memory following closed head injury. In a study, the findings at 12 months were essentially unchanged from the 6-month memory test data. It was concluded that improvement in memory after severe closed head injury occurs primarily during the first 6 months on measures of verbal learning and memory and on visual recognition memory, whereas further gains are negligible, at least within the first year after injury. Memory generally recovers to the normal range within 1–3 months after mild closed head injury.

POST-TRAUMATIC EPILEPSY[63,64]

Seizures may occur soon after a head injury and have different characteristics than those that have a late onset. Seizures that occur within the first 7 days after injury are referred as *early post-traumatic seizures* and those that manifest afterwards as *late post-traumatic seizures.* Immediate seizures which happen within hours of injury are sometimes considered separately from other early seizures. The terms 'post-traumatic seizures' and 'post-traumatic epilepsy' are often used interchangeably, even though neurologists would generally require that at least two unprovoked seizures occur before a condition can be described as epilepsy.

Early Seizures

In unselected patients with head injury, the incidence of early post-traumatic seizures is about 2%. Young children under the age of 5 years have early seizure rates of 7–9%. Early seizure rates are much higher in patients with more severe injuries. They are rare after injuries that cause no or brief loss of consciousness, except in children under 5 years of age. Prolonged unconsciousness, skull fractures, hematomas, hemorrhagic contusions and focal neurological signs—all are associated with increased risk of early post-traumatic seizures. About one third of early post-traumatic seizures begin within the first hour, one third between 1–24 hours and the remaining third between 1–7 days after injury, with adults having their first seizures somewhat later than children. Patients with intracerebral hematomas or hemorrhagic contusions tend to have early seizures after 24 hours more frequently than those without intracranial hematomas.

Late Seizures

Overall, about 2% of patients of head injury develop at least one late post-traumatic seizure. About 5% of hospitalized patients have late seizures; the highest risk of late post-traumatic seizures occurs following missile wounds. Risk factors are focal neurological signs, hematoma, presence of metal fragments and the location of the lesion. In blunt head injury, the main risk factors are hematomas, depressed fractures, focal signs and early seizures. In a study, low GCS, subdural hematoma and cortical contusion, each provided independent additional risk of late seizures, despite the inclusion of only high-risk cases. Seizure risk is initially great and decreases with time. About 60–70% of late post-traumatic seizures are generalized convulsive seizures, with or without focal onset. The remainder is simple or complex partial seizures. Other generalized seizures are virtually never seen.

ALCOHOL AND HEAD INJURY[2,65-68]

Alcohol intoxication is a compounding factor in up to three fourth of head injuries, with most reports documenting at least 25–50% of patients intoxicated at the time of injury. Alcohol use complicates head injury in several important ways. Intoxication increases the risk of all types of injury by impairing fine motor skills, reaction times and judgment. Ethanol also confounds the accuracy of diagnosis by lowering the level of consciousness, independent of head injury severity. Most individuals demonstrate a significant depression of the GCS when the blood alcohol concentration is over 200 mg/dl. Alcohol is assumed for altered GCS, if blood alcohol concentration (BAC) is above the mentioned limit and there is no history or signs of head injury and CT scan is unremarkable.

Pathophysiological consequences of acute and chronic alcohol consumption may also impact significantly on the outcome of head injury. Alcohol-induced exacerbation of trauma has been attributed to several effects of intoxication, including transient coagulopathy related to platelet dysfunction, blood-brain barrier impairment, increased free radical formation and cardiopulmonary depression. Chronic alcohol consumption can also impair normal hemostasis by inducing thrombocytopenia and by reducing production of clotting factors in the liver. Through these mechanisms, it is postulated that acute or chronic ethanol use can lead to increased hemorrhage, interstitial edema, cerebral ischemia and neuronal damage following trauma.

BATTERED BABY SYNDROME—NON-ACCIDENTAL HEAD INJURY

Child abuse is now well recognized as a major cause of serious head injury in children, and is second only to motor vehicle related injuries as a cause of traumatic mortality in the pediatric population (in western counties). The term child abuse refers to the deliberate infliction of injury rather than to neglect or inadequate supervision that leads to accidental injury. The true incidence of inflicted injuries remains unknown because of the nature of abuse, and many cases of abuse are unrecognized by health care providers and as such remain unreported. It has been postulated that many cases of unexplained developmental delay and retardation are the result of abuse-related head injuries sustained in infancy.

Shaken baby syndrome[69,70] can occur from as little as 5 seconds of shaking. When a baby is shaken, the brain bounces back and forth against the skull. This can cause bruising of the brain (cerebral contusion), swelling, increased pressure and subdural hematoma in the brain. The large veins along the outside of the brain may tear, leading to further bleeding, swelling and increased pressure. This can easily cause permanent brain damage or death.

It is most common in children younger than 3 years of age. Children with this syndrome are brought to medical attention for an unrelated problem or with a particular acute injury. When evaluated, they are noted to have signs of chronic abuse which may include poor hygiene, malnutrition, growth retardation, multiple cutaneous bruises of different ages, pattern injuries, burn marks and skeletal injuries at different stages of healing including skull fractures. Shaken baby syndrome does not result from gentle bouncing, playful swinging or tossing the child in the air or jogging with the child.

The triad of injuries includes encephalopathy, retinal hemorrhages and SDH. Encephalopathy include a range of clinical manifestations from poor feeding, lack of appetite, vomiting, extreme irritability, changes in behavior, pale or bluish skin, lethargy, sleepiness and grim-faced to seizures, decreased alertness, loss of consciousness or vision and fulminating cerebral edema. There may not be any physical signs of injury, such as bruising, bleeding or swelling. Rib fractures are common and can be seen on X-ray. SDH is the most consistent component of the triad and may be the first clinical sign identified on CT scan.

SPINAL INJURIES[70,71]

Spinal injuries are commonly associated with head injury and may cause significant amount of morbidity and socioeconomic burden. The annual incidence varies from 11.5–53.4 per million. There is a strong male preponderance and the incidence is high in the second and third decades, and in the elderly. Common causes are fall from height and RTAs. Bruises on the back or neck, neck pain or pain radiating to the arms are signs of cervical spine injury. Spinal immobilization via application of a cervical collar and possibly a long board should be done. If the neurological examination is normal, this may be reassuring. Reassessment is needed if there is a worsening headache, seizure, one sided weakness, or has persistent vomiting. About 60% of spinal injuries involve the cervical spine, most commonly at C5-6 level.

Most damage to the spinal cord arises from intrusion of some part of the spinal column into the canal, be it bony fragments or displacement, ligamentum flavum, disc annulus or extruded nucleus pulposum. There may be bleeding into the space outside the spinal dura causing a space-occupying lesion in the canal that can compress the cord, or bleeding may occur within the dura, either from ruptured vessels or from hemorrhage in the cord itself.

Damage to the cord may also occur in the absence of any apparent intrusion into the canal, in a manner similar to that seen in the brain in closed head injuries without a fracture. Hematomyelia and edema may develop without any obvious mechanical defect at that level in the spinal column. Such injuries must be attributed to some momentary collision of the cord against the wall of the canal or a transient deformity of the profile of the canal that did not exceed the threshold for fracture, dislocation or ligament rupture of the vertebral column. The damage in the cord may extend for several segments above and below the point of impact. Spinal injuries may be classified as:

- Incomplete
- Complete

Incomplete Lesion

It is defined as any residual motor or sensory dysfunction more than three segments below the level of the injury. Signs of incomplete lesion could be sensation (including position sense) or voluntary movement in the limbs, presence of sensation around the anus (sacral sparing), voluntary rectal sphincter contraction or voluntary toe flexion The level of injury is defined as the most caudal segment with motor function that is at least 3 out of 5, and if pain and temperature sensation is present. Various types of incomplete lesions are:

a. **Central cord syndrome:** Central cord syndrome (CCS) is the most common type of incomplete spinal cord injury syndrome. This is usually seen following acute hyperextension injury in an older patient with pre-existing acquired stenosis as a result of bony hypertrophy and in-folding of redundant ligamentum flavum, sometimes superimposed on congenital spinal stenosis. Translational movement of one vertebra on another may also contribute. A blow to the upper face or forehead is often disclosed on history or is suggested on examination (for e.g., lacerations or abrasions to face and/or forehead).

This often occurs in relation to RTAs or to a forward fall, often while intoxicated. Younger patients may also sustain CCS in sporting injuries.

The clinical syndrome is primarily motor weakness of upper extremities with lesser effect on lower extremities; varying degrees of sensory disturbance below level of lesion may occur with myelopathic or 'upper motor neuron' signs such as spasticity, hyperreflexia, clonus, Babinski and Hoffman signs, and bowel and bladder dysfunction (usually urinary retention). Hyperpathia to noxious and non-noxious stimuli is also common, especially in the proximal portions of the upper extremities, and is often delayed in onset and extremely distressing to the patient. *Lhermitte's sign* or electric shock-like feeling on flexing the neck occurs in few cases. There is often an initial phase of improvement when the lower limbs recover first, bladder function next; upper limb strength then returns with finger movements last to recover (sensory recovery has no pattern) followed by a plateau phase and then late deterioration. Recovery is usually incomplete, and the amount of recovery is related to the severity of the injury and patient's age. In patients with cord contusion without hematomyelia, 50% will recover enough leg strengths and sensation, and walk independently, although typically with significant spasticity. Recovery of upper limb function is usually not as good, and fine motor control is usually poor. Bowel and bladder control often recovers. Elderly patients with this condition generally have a bad prognosis.

b. **Brown-Sequard syndrome (cord hemisection):** It results from penetrating trauma, and seen in 2–4% of traumatic spinal cord injuries. This may also occur with radiation myelopathy, cord compression by spinal epidural hematoma, large cervical disc herniation, spinal cord tumors and cervical spondylosis.

   Classical form is rarely seen, contra-lateral findings include dissociated sensory loss, loss of pain and temperature sensation inferior to lesion beginning 1–2 segments below (spinothalamic tract), preserved light (crude) touch due to preserved ipsilateral and contralateral paths (anterior spinothalamic tracts). Ipsilateral findings include loss of posterior column function (proprioception and vibratory sense) and motor paralysis below lesion (due to corticospinal tract lesion). This syndrome has the best prognosis of any of the incomplete spinal cord injuries. Most of patients with this condition will regain the ability to ambulate independently, as well as anal and urinary sphincter control.

c. **Anterior cord syndrome:** It is caused by cord infarction in the territory supplied by the anterior spinal artery. This may result from occlusion of the anterior spinal artery, from anterior cord compression, by dislocated bone fragment or by traumatic herniated disc. Clinical features include paraplegia or quadriplegia (if higher than C7), and dissociated sensory loss below lesion:

   i. Loss of pain and temperature sensation (spinothalamic tract lesion)
   ii. Preserved two-point discrimination, position sense, deep pressure sensation (posterior column function).

   It has the worst prognosis of the incomplete injuries, as only 10–20% recovers functional motor control. Sensation may return enough to help prevent injuries (burns, decubitus ulcers).

d. **Posterior cord syndrome:** Is relatively rare, and produces pain and paresthesias (often with a burning quality) in the neck, upper arms and torso. There may be mild paresis of the upper limbs. Long tract findings are minimal.

Complete Lesion

Gross injury to the spinal column may be inflicted by a relatively high-speed motor vehicle or railway accident and the cord may be transected by a guillotine action of the two displaced fragments. This is most often seen on the upper or mid-thoracic region, from direct impact or gross 'whiplash' effects. The thoracic aorta at this level is often torn at the point where the descending arch meets the spine, even in the absence of a spinal fracture.

In this, there is no preservation of any motor and/or sensory function more than three segments below the level of the injury. About 3% of patients with complete injuries on initial examination will develop some recovery within 24 hours. The persistence of a complete spinal cord injury beyond 24 hours indicates that no distal function will recover.

In addition to loss of voluntary movement, sphincter control and sensation below the level of the injury, there may be priapism. Hypotension and bradycardia (spinal shock) may also present in spinal cord injury at or above C3 level. It may cause bulbar-cervical dissociation resulting in immediate cardio-pulmonary arrest. Death results if CPR is not instituted within minutes. Patients are usually quadriplegic and ventilator dependent, and develop ventilator associated complications and dependence.

SPINAL SHOCK[72]

This term may refer to hypotension (shock) that follows spinal cord injury (systolic BP is usually 80 mm Hg). It is caused by multiple factors:

i. Interruption of sympathetics leading to loss of vascular tone (vasoconstrictors) below the level of injury with unopposed parasympathetics causing bradycardia.
ii. Loss of muscle tone due to skeletal muscle paralysis below the level of injury resulting in venous pooling and thus a *relative* hypovolemia.
iii. Blood loss from associated wounds—true hypovolemia.

There is transient loss of all neurologic function (including segmental and polysynaptic reflex activity, and autonomic function) below the level of the injury. Flaccid paralysis and areflexia lasting varying periods usually 1–2 weeks, occasionally several months and sometimes permanently; the resolution of which causes spasticity below the level of the lesion. It is a poor prognostic sign. Spinal cord reflexes immediately above the injury may also be depressed.

Whiplash injury is currently defined as a traumatic injury to the soft tissue structures in the region of the cervical spine including cervical muscles, ligaments, intervertebral discs and facet joints due to hyperflexion, hyperextension or rotational injury to the neck in the absence of fractures, dislocations or intervertebral disc herniation. It is the most common nonfatal automobile injury. Symptoms may start immediately, but more commonly are delayed several hours or days. In addition to symptoms related to the cervical spine, common associated complaints include headaches, cognitive impairment and low back pain. About 80% patients recover by 2 years.

PEDIATRIC SPINAL INJURIES

Spinal cord injury is fairly uncommon in children, with the ratio of head injuries to spinal cord injuries being 30:1. Only 5% of spinal cord injuries occur in children. Due to ligamentous laxity together with a high head to body weight ratio, immaturity of paraspinal muscles and the underdeveloped uncinate processes, these tend to involve ligamentous rather than bony injuries. The cervical spine is the most vulnerable segment (with subaxial injuries being fairly uncommon), with 42% of injuries occurring here, 31% thoracic and 27% lumbar. The fatality rate is higher with pediatric spine injuries than with adults (opposite to the situation with head injury), with the cause of death more often related to other severe injuries than to the spinal injury.[73]

FRACTURE/DISLOCATION OF SPINE

Dislocation of cervical vertebra can occur under many conditions. An anterior dislocation can be caused by a fall onto the back of the head and a unilateral dislocation is common when a head strikes a windscreen. Posterior dislocation may be caused by blows to the jaw or face that jolt the head backwards with a hyperextension element. Falling onto the face, especially from a height (such as down a staircase) is a likely cause. Fracture of the odontoid process of the axis can occur from a variety of violent movements of the head on the neck, and is sometimes associated with fracture of the skull or mandible.

Atlas (C1) fractures: Acute C1 fractures account for 1–3% of all spinal injuries and 3–13% of cervical spine fractures. Commonest mechanism is axial loading. The fracture is classified as:

i. Type I: Fractures involving a single arch.
ii. Type II: Burst fracture (Jefferson fracture).
iii. Type III: Lateral mass fractures of the atlas.

In *Jefferson fracture,* there is usually no neurologic deficit, if isolated, due to large canal diameter at this level and tendency for fragments to be forced outwards. Posterior arch fractures are stable injuries but lateral mass fractures are unstable.

Axis (C2) fractures: It represents 10–20% of cervical spine fractures. There are two peaks—young adults (high speed trauma) and elderly. This can be classified as:

i. Type I is least common. Fracture line at the tip of dens, usually stable.
ii. Type II is most common, fracture line is at the base of dens.
iii. Type III is when the fracture extends to the base of dens.

Hangman's fracture is a bilateral fracture through the pars interarticularis of C2 with traumatic subluxation of C2 on C3, most often from hyperextension and axial loading. Traumatic atlantoaxial instability occurs as a result of ligamentous instability (transverse ligament) due to flexion injury. The normal atlanto-dens distance in adults is up to 3 mm.

Clinical presentation: Most are neurologically intact; those few with deficits are usually minor (paraesthesias, monoparesis), and many recover within one month. Almost all conscious patients will have cervical pain usually in the upper posterior cervical region, and occipital neuralgia is not uncommon.

C3–7 are referred to as subaxial cervical spine. They may be flexion injuries which constitute 15% of all cervical trauma and are caused by RTAs, falls and diving injuries (Fig. 13.17). They can be:

i. Flexion compression injuries
ii. Flexion distraction injuries
iii. Vertical compression injuries
iv. Extension

Investigation of Cervical Spine Injuries

Patients who have neck symptoms suggestive of possible injury, patients who are confused or intoxicated and those with other distracting injuries require cervical spine imaging.

There are four options for imaging of the cervical spine.

i. Plain X-ray: Three views should be obtained and be of sufficient quality for reliable interpretation.
ii. Lateral flexion/extension series—immediate and/or delayed.
iii. CT scan (localized or whole cervical spine including cervico-dorsal junction).
iv. MRI.

The current initial investigation of choice is the plain radiograph. However, in certain circumstances CT scan is preferred. MRI is indicated, if there is suspicion of vascular injury—subluxation or displacement of the spinal column, fracture through foramen transversarium or lateral processes and posterior circulation syndromes.

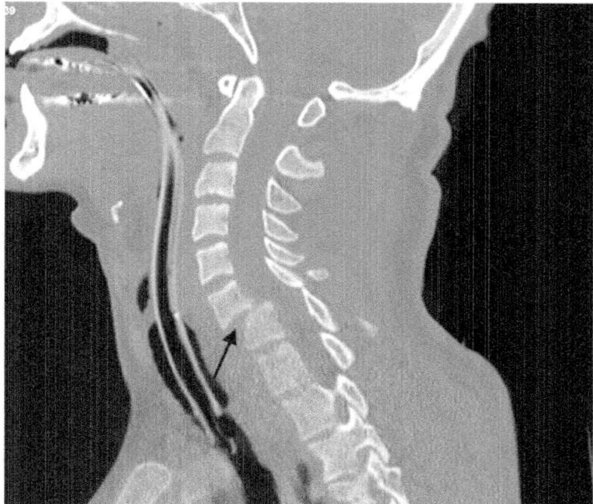

Fig. 13.17 CT spine showing anterolisthesis of C6 over C7 (arrow)

MEDICOLEGAL ISSUES

Medicolegal duties are part of the duty of the doctor to patient in the doctor-patient relationship. While dealing with a head injury patient, the medical practitioner comes across the following issues given in Box 13.4.[74,75]

Consent: Valid consent is obtained from the patient, and if minor—*loco parentis* (guardian) is applicable. In cases of emergency, Sec. 92 IPC gives implied consent for treatment.

Treatment: All relevant procedures should be noted and their progress out comes mentioned.

Prognosis: Appropriate counseling to patient/parent/guardian with regard to diagnosis, investigations, management, progress and possible outcome. After giving the required information, signature from the concerned parties is taken.

Medical records: Accurate documentation particularly with regard to external signs of injury is essential in cases of alleged assault. External signs of injury like bruising and lacerations heal with time, hence, photography of such injuries is recommended for a permanent record. Preserving the case-sheet and investigation reports is essential in order to prepare certificates and to prepare before attending the court of law. X-rays and CT scans provide evidence of the skull fractures and nature of cerebral injury.

Dying declaration: If the treating doctor after examining the patient feels that he/she is conscious, alert and oriented (compos mentis) to give a statement, then after certifying this fact, the statement or dying declaration may be recorded, preferably by a Magistrate. The treating doctor should also certify that after finishing of the statement, patient was in compos mentis. However, quite a few patients of head injury are unconscious, under the influence of alcohol, confused and disoriented. Under these circumstances, it is not possible to record any legally valid statement.

Box 13.4 Medicolegal issues in head and neck injured patient

- Dying declaration and compos mentis
- Lucid interval
- Focal lesions—clinical neurological deficits
- Recovery (total/partial)
- No recovery (prolonged coma/cerebral death/brain death/clinical death)
- Loss of life or loss of earning
- Inability to do routine work
- Compensation problems
- Industrial claims/occupational claims
- Concussion—transient unconsciousness
- Loss of consciousness
- Interventions—medical/surgical/both
- Completely bed ridden
- Incomplete recovery (disability—varying degrees: partial temporary or partial permanent)
- Tort cases
- Disability assessment
- Accident claims
- Criminal cases (assaults/RTAs)

MEDICOLEGAL REPORTS AND COURT ROOM QUESTIONS

Authorities requesting medicolegal reports include civil or consumer courts for personal injury claims, insurance companies for compensation, and the police and criminals courts for fixing the responsibility and punishment of the offender. Reports need to address the specific requirements of the requesting authority. An opinion on the degree of disability and whether it is likely to be temporary or permanent is required for insurance companies, whereas the nature and mechanism of injury is needed for the police.

Medicolegal injury reports usually require factual statement of the injuries, mechanism and nature of injury. Report need to provide a factual chronology of events, description of the presenting symptoms and examination findings. In addition to recording positive examination findings, relevant negative findings should also be noted. In the following paragraphs, the common queries that are sometimes required to be answered by the medical practitioner appearing as expert witness in a case of head injury are discussed.

One of the commonest questions is whether the alleged mechanism of injury is consistent with the nature of the injuries sustained. In assault cases, sometimes it is asked by the defense counsel as to whether the patient has sustained the injury himself at home after a fall? Answer to this depends upon the injury. It is very unlikely that injury has been caused by any other means but the possibility cannot be ruled out.

Another question frequently asked by the defense as to who has given the history? If patient is conscious and oriented in time place and person, then the history is usually given by the patient. If the patient is unconscious or unable to speak (for e.g., fractured jaw), the accompanying person furnishes the history. It should be mentioned in the file, whether the history is given by the injured person himself or by the accompanying person. The signature, address and relationship of the accompanying person who has given the history should be noted down in file.

Whether the condition of the patient can be due to any pre-existing illness? Quite unlikely but sometimes like in cases of epilepsy, patient may have a seizure while driving. Then, as per the medical history, an answer should be given.

Nature of Injury

This is undoubtedly the most important question that is asked by the court in criminal cases. Nature of injury in head and neck is sometimes difficult to opine for, and this should be decided based on clinical history, examination findings and radiology. Predicting outcome can be very difficult, particularly in the acute stages following injury. Guidelines for opining the nature of injury are given in Tables 13.6 and 13.7.

Scalp injuries are usually *simple injuries*. They are unlikely to endanger life, but if associated with bleeding from an artery like the superficial temporal may cause shock. Lacerations on forehead and face can cause disfigurement—grievous hurt.

Although the fractures are not dangerous to life by themselves, they are indicators of the severity of the head injury. Skull fracture without associated intracranial injury is considered to be a *grievous injury*. However, it may endanger

Table 13.6 Nature of head injury based on type of injury*

Type of injury	*Nature of injury*	*Remarks*
Superficial injury of head (abrasions and contusions) • Superficial injury of scalp • Contusion of eyelid and periocular area (black eye) • Superficial injuries of eyelid and periocular area • Superficial injury of nose • Superficial injury of ear • Superficial injury of lip and oral cavity • Multiple superficial injuries of head • Superficial injury of other parts of head	Simple	
Laceration of head	Simple	Grievous, if results in disfiguration
Fracture of skull and facial bones		
• Linear skull fracture	Grievous	In small children, it may be associated with seizures and can be dangerous to life even when CT head shows no parenchymal injury
• Depressed skull fracture – Simple – Compound	 Grievous Dangerous, if causing neurological deficit and requires surgical evacuation	 Compound fractures may endanger life with meningitis and seizures. If associated with underlying contusion with mass effect—dangerous to life
• Basal skull fractures	Grievous	There is a risk of CSF leak and meningitis—dangerous to life
Dislocation, sprain and strain of joints and ligaments of head	Grievous	
Injury of cranial nerves	Grievous	If there is loss of function
Intracranial injury		
• Concussion Grade I Grade II Grade III	Simple	

Contd...

Contd...

Type of injury	*Nature of injury*	*Remarks*
• Cerebral edema	Dangerous	Any amount of blood can be dangerous to life. The clot may enlarge; in SDH and intracerebral bleeds, the edema may be extensive causing herniation and death. Moreover there is risk of seizures
• Diffuse axonal injury Grade I Grade II Grade III	Dangerous, if causing neurological deterioration and needs ICU admission, because of loss of protective airway reflexes (cough reflex etc.); otherwise grievous	
• Contusion	Dangerous, if requiring surgical evacuation	
• Epidural hemorrhage	Dangerous	
• Subdural hemorrhage	Dangerous	
• Subarachnoid hemorrhage	Dangerous	
• Intracerebral hemorrhage	Dangerous	
• Intraventricular hemorrhage	Dangerous	
• Intracranial injury with prolonged coma	Dangerous	
Crush injury of head	Dangerous	
Traumatic amputation of part of head	Dangerous	
Other unspecified injuries of head		
• Injury of blood vessels of head, not elsewhere classified	Major vessels—grievous Minor vessels—simple	
• Injury of muscle and tendon of head resulting in loss of power	Grievous	
• Traumatic rupture of ear drum	Grievous	

*Head injury, if it causes neurological deterioration and requires neurosurgical intervention is dangerous to life. It is better to declare nature of injury after 72 hours of injury, as some intracranial injuries enlarge and may require neurosurgical intervention (dangerous to life).
†Dangerous injury means life is endangered.

Table 13.7 Nature of spinal injuries based on type of injury

Type of injury	*Nature of injury*	*Remarks*
Stable fracture without cord compression or dislocation	Grievous	
Unstable fracture along with cord compression	Grievous/ Dangerous	If causing compression above C5 along with neurological deficit – dangerous to life, since it may cause respiratory distress, quadriplegia, chest infections, sepsis and death; otherwise below C5 it is a grievous injury (loss of movement)
Incomplete and complete lesion	Grievous/ Dangerous	If lesion is above C5 level and there is involvement of phrenic nerve—dangerous to life
Epidural hematoma	Grievous/ Dangerous	If causing compression above C5 along with neurological deficit—dangerous to life; otherwise below C5 it is a grievous injury
Cord contusion	Grievous/ Dangerous	If causing compression above C5 along with neurological deficit—dangerous to life; otherwise below C5 it is a grievous injury
Vertebral artery injury	Dangerous	
Whiplash injury	Grievous/ Dangerous	If causing compression above C5 along with neurological deficit-dangerous to life, otherwise below C5 it is a grievous injury
Spinal cord injury without radiological association	Grievous/ Dangerous	If causing neurological deficit on clinical examination above C5-dangerous to life, otherwise below C5 it is a grievous injury

to life, if associated with seizures, depressed bone fragment. Skull fractures if associated with intracranial injuries are likely to be *dangerous to life*.

Any injury in which dura is breached, contusions have occurred or there is presence of intracranial bleeding (EDH, SDH, contusion, IVH, SAH causing neurological deterioration) is dangerous to life, i.e. life is endangered even if surgical intervention is not done. The nature of injury does not depend upon the volume of blood. Even small amount of blood seen on CT can be dangerous as it may enlarge, can cause edema, herniation and surgery may be needed later. More so, in areas like the brainstem, even very small contusion may cause damage to vital centers leading to coma and death. Any injury which poses an immediate danger to life is dangerous. A contusion in the frontal lobe which needs surgery poses immediate danger to life in the form of anesthetic and surgical complications. Moreover, seizure is always a risk and can cause death. A small extradural hematoma on initial CT scan may enlarge and require surgery. About 50% of EDH enlarges between 5–16 days.

Concussion implies that patient has a brief loss of consciousness and is fully conscious after that. However, a radiological assessment is needed to ascertain, if there is any structural damage to brain. Concussion injury with no abnormality on CT scan and GCS 15/15 is considered simple injury. Doctors need to be aware that people may demonstrate false symptoms of post-concussional syndrome to claim compensation.

Illustrative Cases

Case I

A 26-years-old male was brought to the emergency with alleged history of road traffic accident. History of loss of consciousness since accident was present. History of vomiting was present. There was no history of seizures. On examination, his GCS was E1, V1, M3. Pupils were bilaterally dilated, sluggishly reacting to light. Corneal, and gag reflex were present. Doll's eye was present. His blood pressure was 150/70 mm Hg, and pulse 90/min. Patient was intubated in emergency and put on ventilatory support. CT scan of head was done which showed right fronto-temporal contusion with SDH with diffuse SAH and cerebral edema (Fig. 13.18A). Patient's relative were explained about the high risk and prognosis, and written informed consent obtained for emergency operation. Patient was operated under GA in the form of right fronto-temporo parietal craniotomy with evacuation of SDH, fronto-temporal contusion with duraplasty was done on the same day (Fig. 13.18B). Postoperative, his neurological status did not improve. His GCS further deteriorated; pupils become bilaterally dilated, not reacting to light. Brainstem reflexes were absent. Patient had hypotension for which inotropes were started but blood pressure did not pick up. He had bradycardia followed by cardiorespiratory arrest. CPR was started immediately but patient could not be revived and was declared dead. *The injury was deemed as dangerous to life.*

Case II

A 16-year-old male was brought to the emergency with alleged history of assault by a group of unknown people. Brief history of loss of consciousness was present.

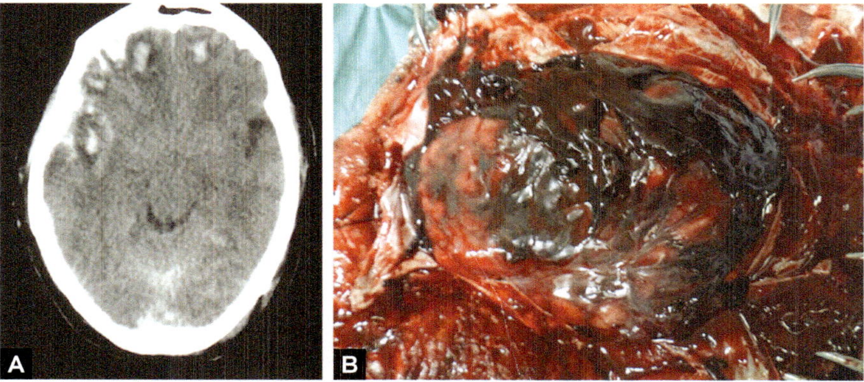

Figs 13.18A and B (A) CT head and; (B) Dura opened and SDH can be seen (intraoperative photograph)

No history of vomiting or seizures was present. On examination, his GCS was E4, V2, M6. Pupils were equal and reacting to light. There were multiple lacerated wounds over the left frontal, temporal and occipital region with fracture of the underlying bone. There was active bleeding also. This was confirmed on CT scan which showed fracture with frontal and occipital subdural hematoma. Bone window and 3D reconstruction showed frontal fracture with suture diastasis of the sagittal and left coronal suture (Fig. 13.19). Pneumocephalus was also present. Since the patient had come within 6 hours of injury, the wound was debrided (surgical intervention). SDH was conservatively managed and patient gradually improved and discharged. He was also put on antiepileptics.

The nature of injury was opined as *dangerous to life* as it caused altered sensorium/neurological deterioration (GCS=12/15) and could have caused infection, meningitis and death.

Case III

A 55-year-old male was brought to the emergency with history of assault in the market. On examination, there was a lacerated wound over the parieto-temporal region. On CT scan, there was no skull fracture, no midline shift but there was intraparenchymal hemorrhage with contusion underlying the injury. Patient remained admitted for three days in neurosurgery and was treated conservatively. His period of stay was uneventful.

This injury was opined as *dangerous to life*. Although patient was conscious, he had a temporal contusion which irrespective of the size is an immediate threat to life because of its vicinity to brainstem.

OTHER MEDICOLEGAL ISSUES

1. **Medical negligence:** The emergency medical doctor may discharge an apparently well patient with history of head injury or after the recovery of the transient concussion who later dies at home or is readmitted. The latent or 'lucid' interval in both EDH and SDH should be kept in mind which otherwise may lead to civil suits for negligence. Radiology of the skull is not mandatory,

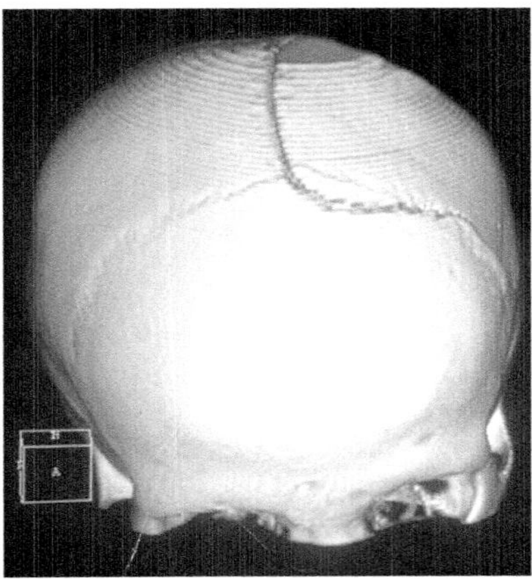

Fig. 13.19 CT head with 3D reconstruction

if the clinical indications are not present, but failure to X-ray/CT can be a legal hurdle for the defense.

2. **Dating of trauma:** In a person who has sustained SDH, question may be raised as to when the bleeding started and what prompted the bleed. Whether it was the alleged assault on such and such date and time or was it the fall caused by the RTA on such and such date and time, i.e., when it is being either maintained or denied that a particular episode of head injury caused the hematoma. In such cases, accurate dating of SDH becomes critical in both criminal and civil cases. Opinion can be given in terms of days, weeks or months which may be justified with CT findings. The possibility of a previous bleed being the precipitating factor in some later accidental injury, which then caused further bleeding must be kept in mind.
3. **Location of impact:** SDH commonly presents with an intact skull, though this is uncommon with EDH. An EDH is usually on the same side as the blow, but because of the distortion of the skull, the fracture that traverses the meningeal artery can be some distance from the point of impact. However, a reasonable opinion of the area (region) can be offered.

   Whereas SDH or SAH is concerned, it can be misleading to offer opinions about the nature and position of the impact, unless there is scalp or skull damage. Though sometimes it is clear from the presence of a scalp injury that the hemorrhage is either 'coup' or 'contrecoup', there are many exceptions when the bleeding is unrelated to the site of the blow that a firm opinion is not justifiable. Sometimes, it can be over-interpretation to use hemorrhage to localize an impact.
4. **Trauma and SAH:** Allegations of an injury leading to rupture of a pre-existing 'berry' aneurysm may have civil as well as criminal consequences. This may be the situation when an assault is rapidly followed by the signs of SAH. The question of causation then arises, the prosecution claiming that the head injury mechanically ruptured the aneurysm. Similarly, it is often difficult to determine whether spontaneous SAH immediately preceded and thereby caused a traffic accident or vice versa.

   There are no characteristic clinical or radiographical distinctions that might indicate whether the SAH is secondary to a ruptured congenital aneurysm or vascular malformation or traumatic in nature. However, it is hard to deny that a heavy blow to the head, jaw or neck could not rupture, split or weaken the fragile wall of a large, thin-walled aneurysm of the circle of Willis. However, in most assaults, both accused and victim are physically and emotionally charged-up, and catecholamines released due to adrenal response will increase muscle tone, heart rate and BP. Raised BP is far more potent reason for rupture of an already weak aneurysm than a blow on the head.

   It should also be considered that a person with an already spontaneously leaking aneurysm may have a rapidly developing neurological or behavioral abnormality that leads to a fight with another person or results in a fall or RTA. The aneurismal rupture may be blamed on the trauma instead of the reverse.

   Another factor that is suspected to increase the chance of rupture is alcohol, although there is no objective proof of this. A high blood alcohol concentration is said to facilitate bursting of an aneurysm because it dilates cerebral blood vessels, increases cerebral blood flow and raises BP. The latter is not true because alcohol does not raise systolic pressure, though the pulse pressure may widen. Pharmacologically, there is an insignificant effect of alcohol on the cerebral circulation. There is absolutely no evidence that alcohol is associated with a natural SAH from a ruptured aneurysm, though intense physical activity, such as sport or coitus, does predispose to rupture.

Where alcohol and ruptured berry aneurysm are concerned, the association is more of coincidental and not necessarily causative. Alcohol itself causes or contributes to unsteadiness, a fall or some other traumatic event which might lead to rupture of an aneurysm. Ataxia and hypotonia are features of acute drunkenness, and together with the aggressive behavior and alcoholic environment of most physical violence seem sufficient to account for their circumstantial association.

5. **Volitional activity:** A question may be asked from a doctor in a court trial about the volitional activity of a person can do after suffering from EDH or SDH. The person may talk, walk or do routine work, hours after an assault and may die at home later.
6. **Personal injury report:** Injury reports for compensation claims need to be comprehensive, covering a wide range of issues, of both fact and opinion. The mechanism of injury should be explained in detail and include the duration of loss of consciousness, retrograde and post-traumatic amnesia. Specific points, such as whether a seat-belt was in place may also need to be addressed. The main contention is what would have happened to the patient in the absence of the index event and what has happened to the patient as a consequence of the index event.

   Accurate documentation of pre-event history (neurological, psychological and psychiatric symptoms) and relationship with post-event symptoms is essential. The patient's past medical history, social and employment status should also be included. The acute symptoms experienced by the patient immediately after the injury such as dizziness, headache, focal deficits and psychological symptoms such as short-term memory problems and seizures should be documented in detail. These symptoms can then be compared with the current status of the patient. The treatment administered should be clearly described. Prognosis in terms of on-going symptoms and future pattern, and the effect on lifestyle is crucial. Recommendations for on-going treatment should be given, and finally a summary and opinion. If there is a range of medical opinion regarding the diagnosis, prognosis or significance of the injury to the constellation of symptoms and signs, it should be mentioned in the report.

   Specific concerns in terms of prognosis include risk of seizures and life expectancy. The risk of seizure depends on the severity of injury (GCS) and in addition, depressed skull fracture, intracranial hematoma and post-traumatic amnesia greater than 24 hours. The issue of life expectancy is often also very difficult to ascertain for an individual. It is well recognized fact that patients in vegetative state have reduced life expectancy.
7. **Restraint from driving:** The duration of restraint from driving following head injury depends upon features (post-traumatic amnesia, dural tear, focal signs and seizures) and clinical recovery. The current guidelines followed in the United Kingdom for light motor vehicles like car and motorcycle are given in Table 13.8. However, personal opinion for the individual case is required. For heavy goods vehicle such as bus, truck and coach, guidelines are far more stringent particularly with regards to the risk of seizures.

Table 13.8 Recommendations for driving off period after head injury

Type of Injury	*Driving off period*
Loss of consciousness with no history of intracranial hematoma, depressed fracture or seizures and recovery is complete	May resume driving
Serious head injury and no neurosurgical intervention, free from seizures	Up to 6 months
EDH requiring craniotomy but with no cerebral damage, acute SDH and ICH treated with burr hole drainage	6 months
Serious head injury with a compound depressed fracture requiring surgical treatment	6–12 months
EDH with cerebral damage requiring craniotomy, acute SDH and ICH treated with craniotomy	1 year
Chronic SDH treated surgically	May resume driving on recovery

MALINGERING

Malingering is the intentional production of false or grossly exaggerated physical or psychological symptoms, motivated by external incentives. In practice, malingering must be differentiated from factitious disorder which also involves intentional production of symptoms. In factitious disorders, the patient's motivation is to assume the sick role which can be thought of as an internal or psychological incentive. There have been no studies giving consistent result, and clinicians should mostly use open-ended questions. Inquiries should be phrased without giving clues, and the more prolonged the interview, the more difficult it is for the malingerer to maintain a counterfeit account (Box 13.5).[76-78]

Box 13.5 Pointers to a malingerer

- Exaggerated story
- Flamboyant presentation
- Incongruity between patient's claimed distress and objective findings
- Vague answers to questions when the answers should be clear which is seen when the patient is unsure which of the answers would signify psychopathology
- Easy suggestibility and induction to add absurd or bizarre elements to the story
- Nonconformity with orthodox psychopathologic experiences, for e.g., continuous rather than intermittent hallucination
- Lack of knowledge about whether extraneous events like sleep or noise could affect symptoms, for e.g., voices that persist even during sleep
- Tendency to favor command hallucinations which in the forensic setting may be exculpatory, or in the emergency room may facilitate hospitalization.
- Hostility and intimidation of the clinician, especially when the clinician displays obvious scepticism

Possible Settings of Malingering

Malingering should be suspected if there is:

- Lack of cooperation with diagnostic evaluation and lack of compliance with prescribed treatment regimen
- Presentation within a medicolegal context
- Foreseeable external gain like avoidance of military duty or financial compensation
- Presence of antisocial personality disorder
- Drug seeking behavior.

Possible External Gains

- Food and shelter, especially during winter periods
- Narcotic medications
- Financial gain in the context of compensation, social security benefit
- Avoidance of jail, work, military or family responsibility
- Damages for alleged psychological injury
- Transfer to psychiatric hospital to avoid arrest
- Criminal setting to avoid standing trial or to mitigate sentence

Some tests to detect malingering:[76-78]

1. **The Structured Interview of Reported Symptoms** (SIRS) consists of 172 items organized along a number of scales. It permits symptom phenomena to be judged as exaggerated, over-reported, atypical or absurd. It demonstrated solid sensitivity and specificity. In 1992, Rogers and colleague tested the effectiveness of the SIRS to detect feigning of three diagnostic groupings, schizophrenia, mood disorders and PTSD on 45 psychologically knowledgeable correctional residents. They found that the SIRS maintained its powers of discrimination with respect to clinical samples. There is an abbreviated version adapted as a screening measure of malingering in a correctional setting.
2. **The Miller Forensic Assessment of Symptoms Test** (M-FAST) was developed as a brief, reliable and valid screen for malingered mental illness. In 2004, Miller examined the initial validity of the M-FAST in a sample of 50 criminal defendants found incompetent to stand trial because of a mental illness. The M-FAST total score and items were compared with the SIRS and the fake-bad indicators of the MMPI-2. Results indicated good evidence of construct and criterion validity as well as high correlations between the M-FAST, SIRS and the fake-bad indices on the MMPI-2.
3. **The Victoria Symptom Validity Test** (VSVT) is computerized and consists of 48 trials, subdivided into 3 blocks of 16 trials a-piece. Each block contains 8 'easy' and 8 'difficult' items. The VSVT analysis provides details of the total errors, errors on easy versus difficult items and reaction times on easy versus difficult items. The test requires approximately 15 minutes to administer. The computer program performs all relevant calculations, determines the relationship of this performance to chance levels, and organizes this information into a printed report.
4. **Minnesota Multiphasic Personality Inventory:** The largest body of research on detection of feigning using self-report inventories has focused on the

Minnesota Multiphasic Personality Inventory (MMPI) and its successor, the MMPI-2. Meta-analyses on the detection of feigned symptoms have indicated that validity scales from the MMPI and the MMPI-2 are quite sensitive to 'faking bad' at the group level. Some studies further found that the optimal scales for detection of faking are the dissimulation subscales. A specialized validity scale on MMPI-2, referred to as the malingered depression scale, consists of 32 items that detected malingered symptoms of depression. Elhai and colleagues compared 64 adult PTSD outpatients at a child sexual abuse survivor treatment program with 85 adult college students instructed and trained to malinger PTSD. They found that MMPI-2 contains indices that adequately predicted malingering with strong cross-validation.

CONCLUSION

Head and spine injuries in our country have multiple aspects and causes. There is a need to have clear cut guidelines regarding the nature of injuries enabling the judiciary to impart punishment to those guilty in an impartial and scientific manner. This review is an attempt to classify nature of head and spine injuries for medicolegal purposes.

REFERENCES

1. Jennett B. Epidemiology of head injury. *J Neurol Neurosurg Psychiatry* 1996; 60: 362-69.
2. Gururaj G. Road traffic deaths, injuries and disabilities in India: current scenario. *Natl Med J India* 2008; 21: 14-20.
3. Gennarelli TA. Mechanisms of brain injury. *J Emerg Med* 1993; 11: 5.
4. Graham, DI, Adams JH, Gennarelli TA. Pathology of brain damage in head injury. In: Cooper P (ed). Head injury. Baltimore: Williams and Wilkins; 1987. p. 72-88.
5. Biswas G. Regional injuries. Review of forensic medicine and toxicology. 2nd edn. New Delhi: Jaypee brothers; 2012. p. 204-31.
6. Doberstein CE, Hovda DA, Becker DP. Clinical considerations in the reduction of secondary brain injury. *Ann Emerg Med* 1993; 22: 993-97.
7. Felten DL, Shetty AN. Netter's atlas of human neuroscience. 2nd edn. Philadelphia: Saunders, Elsevier; 2009.
8. Langlois JA, Rutland-Brown W, Thomas KE. Traumatic brain injury in the United States: emergency department visits, hospitalizations, and deaths. Atlanta: Centers for disease control and prevention. National Center for Injury Prevention and Control; 2004.
9. Critchley G, Memon A. Epidemiology of head injury. In: Whitfield PC, Thomas EO, Summers F, Whyte M, Hutchinson PJ (eds). Head injury: a multidisciplinary approach. Cambridge: Cambridge university press; 2009. p. 1-11.
10. Teasdale G. Neurological management: head injury. *J Neurol Neurosurg Psychiatry* 1995; 58: 526-39.
11. Slein SC. Classification of head injury. In: Narayan RK, Wilberger JE, Povlishock JT. Neurotrauma. New York: McGraw Hill; 1996. p. 31-41.
12. Steinbok P, Flodmark O, Martens D, Germann ET. Management of simple depressed skull fractures in children. *J Neurosurg* 1987; 66: 506-10.
13. Gurdjian ES, Webster JE, Lissner HR. The mechanism of skull fracture. *Radiology* 1950; 54: 313-39.
14. Pekka S, Knight B. Head and spinal injuries. Knight's forensic pathology. 3rd edn. London: Arnold; 2004. p. 174-221.

15. Gennarelli TA, Thibault LE. Biomechanics of acute subdural hematoma. *J Trauma* 1982; 22: 680-86.
16. Gennarelli TA. Mechanisms and pathophysiology of cerebral concussion. *J Head Trauma Rehabil* 1986; 1: 23-29.
17. Madikians A, Giza CC. A clinician's guide to the pathophysiology of traumatic brain. *Indian Journal Neurotrauma* 2006; 3: 9-17.
18. Doczi T. Volume regulation of the brain tissue-a survey. *Acta Neurochir* 1993; 121: 1-8.
19. Bergsneider M, Hovda DA, Shalmon E, Kelly DF, Vespa PM, Martin NA et al. Cerebral hyperglycolysis following severe traumatic brain injury in humans: a positron emission tomography study. *J Neurosurg* 1997; 86: 241-51.
20. Dingman RO, Argenta LA. The surgical repair of traumatic defects of the scalp. *Clin Plast Surg* 1982; 9: 131-44.
21. Hennessy RJ, Persing JA, Morgan RF. Scalp injuries and their management. In: Youmans JR (ed). Neurological surgery. Philadelphia: WB Saunders; 1990. p. 2352-65.
22. Tandon PN, Ramamurthi R. Scalp injuries. Ramamurthi and Tandon's textbook of neurosurgery. 3rd edn. New Delhi: Jaypee brothers; 2012. p. 422-4.
23. Nicolas Hardt, Johannes Kuttenberger. Craniofacial trauma: diagnosis and Management. 1st ed. Springer; 2009.
24. Bullock MR, Chesnut *R*, Ghajar J, Gordon D, Hartl R, Newell DW et al. Surgical management of depressed cranial fracture. *Neurosurgery* 2006; 58: S56-60.
25. Bullock R, Maxwell WL, Graham DI, Teasdale GM, Adams JH. Glial swelling following human cerebral contusion: an ultrastructural study. *J Neurol Neurosurg Psychiatry* 1991; 54: 427-34.
26. Bullock MR, Chesnut RM, Ghajar J, Gordon D, Hartl R, Newell DW, et al. Surgical management of traumatic parenchymal lesions. *Neurosurgery* 2006; 58: S25-46.
27. Pang D, Horton JA, Herron JM. Wilberger JE, Vries JK. Nonsurgical management of extradural hematomas in children. *J Neurosurg* 1983; 59: 958-71.
28. McKissock W, Taylor JC, Bloom WH, Till K. Extradural hematoma: observations on 125 cases. *Lancet* 1960; 2: 167-72.
29. Aoki N, Oikawa A, Sakai T. Symptomatic subacute subdural hematoma associated with cerebral hemispheric swelling and ischemia. *Neuro Res* 1996; 18: 145-49.
30. Sean S, Armin, Austin RT, Colohan, John H, Zhang. Traumatic subarachnoid hemorrhage: our current understanding and its evolution over the past half century. *Neurological Research* 2006; 28: 445-52.
31. Baraatham G, Dennyson WG. Delayed traumatic intracerebral hemorrhage. *J Neurol Neurosurg Psychiat* 1972; 35: 698-706.
32. Bullock, M Ross, Chesnut, Randall, Ghajar. Post-traumatic mass volume measurement in traumatic brain injury patients. *Neurosurgery* 2006; 58: S16-24.
33. Mahapatra AK, Kumar R, Kamal R (eds). Textbook of traumatic brain injury. 1st edn. New Delhi: Jaypee Brothers; 2012.
34. Berry K, Rice J. Traumatic tear of tela choroidea resulting in fatal intraventricular hemorrhage. *Am J Forensic Med Pathol* 1994; 15: 132-37.
35. Jayakumar PN, Sastry-Kolluri VR , Basavakumar DG. Prognosis in traumatic intraventricular hemorrhage. *Acta Neurochir* 1990; 106: 48-51.
36. Lee JP, Lui TN, Chang CN. Acute post-traumatic intraventricular hemorrhage analysis of 25 patients with emphasis on final outcome. *Acta Neurol Scand* 1991; 84: 85-90.
37. LeRoux PD, Haglund MM, Newell DW, Grady S, Winn HR. Intraventricular hemorrhage in blunt head trauma: An analysis of 43 cases. *Neurosurgery* 1992; 31: 678-84.
38. Quality Standards Subcommittee of the American Academy of Neurology: Practice parameter: the management of concussion in sports. *Neurology* 1997; 48: 581-85.
39. Cantu RC. Guidelines for return to contact sports after a cerebral concussion. *Physician Sports Med* 1986; 14: 75-83.
40. Cantu RC. Head injuries in sports. *Br J Sports Med* 1996; 10: 289-96.

41. Adams JH, Graham DI, Murray LS, Scott G. Diffuse axonal injury due to non-missile head injury in humans: An analysis of 45 cases. *Ann Neurol* 1982; 12: 557-63.
42. Gennarelli TA, Thibault LE, Adams JH, Graham DI, Thompson CJ, Marcincin RP. Diffuse axonal injury and traumatic coma in primate. *Ann Neurol* 1982; 12: 564-74.
43. Strich SJ. Shearing of nerve fibre as a cause of brain damage due to head injury. *Lancet* 1961; 2: 443-48.
44. Murr R, Berger S, Schurer L, Kempski O, Staub F, Baethmann A. Relationship of cerebral blood flow disturbances with brain oedema formation. *Acta Neurochir* 1993; 59: 11-17.
45. Shapira Y, Setton D, Artru AA, Shohami E. Blood-brain barrier permeability, cerebral edema, and neurologic function after closed head injury. *Anesth Analg* 1993; 77: 141-48.
46. Benzel EC, Day WT, Kesterson L, Willis BK, Kessler CW, Modling D et al. Civilian craniocerebral gunshot wounds. *Neurosurgery* 1991; 29: 67-72.
47. Steinberg CM, Jahrsdoerfer RA, Gillenwater A, Joe SA, Alcalen SV. Gunshot wounds to the head and neck. *Arch Otolaryngol Head Neck Surg* 1992; 118: 592-7.
48. Copley IB. Cranial tangential gunshot wounds. *Br J Neurosurg* 1991; 5: 43-53.
49. Jeyaretna DS, Whitfield PC. Clinical assessment of head injured patient: an anatomical approach. In: Whitfield PC, Thomas EO, Summers F, Whyte M, Hutchinson PJ (eds). Head injury: a multidisciplinary approach. Cambridge: Cambridge university press; 2009. p. 28-35.
50. The Royal College of Surgeons of England. Head Injury: triage, assessment, investigation and early management of head injury in infants, children and adults. National collaborating centre for acute care; 2003.
51. Quality Standards Subcommittee of the American Academy of Neurology: Practice parameters for determining brain death in adults. *Neurology* 1995; 45: 1012-14.
52. Grewal A, Kaul TK, Grewal SS. Brain Death. *J Anaesth Clin Pharmacol* 2006; 22: 115-38.
53. Doble JE, Haig AJ, Anderson C, Katz. Impairment, activity, participation, life satisfaction, and survival in persons with locked-in syndrome for over a decade. *J Head Trauma Rehabil* 2003; 5: 435-44.
54. Smith WS, Johnston SC, Skalabrin EJ, Weaver M, Azari P, Albers GW, et al. Locked-in syndrome. *Neurology* 2008; 60: 1424-28.
55. Jennett B, Plum F. Persistent vegetative state after brain damage. A syndrome in search of a name. *Lancet* 1972; 1: 734-37.
56. The multi-society task force on PVS. Medical aspects of the persistent vegetative state. *N Engl J Med* 1994; 330: 1499-1508.
57. Rutherford WH, Merrett JD, McDonald JR. Symptoms at one year following concussion from minor head injuries. *Injury* 1979; 10: 225-30.
58. Goldstein J. Posttraumatic headache and the post-concussion syndrome. *Med Clin North Am* 1991; 75: 641-51.
59. Montgomery EA, Fenton GW, McClelland RJ, MacFlynn G, Rutherford WH. The psychobiology of minor head injury. *Psychol Med* 1991; 21: 375-84.
60. Russell WR. The traumatic amnesias. London: Oxford university press; 1961.
61. Ewing-Cobbs L, Levin HS, Fletcher JM, Miner JM, Eisenberg HM. The children's orientation and amnesia test: relationship to severity of acute head injury and to recovery of memory. *Neurosurgery* 1990; 27: 683-91.
62. Lee ST, Lui TN. Early seizures after mild closed head injury. *J Neurosurg* 1992; 76: 435-39.
63. Temkin NR, Dikmen SS, Wilensky AJ, Keihm J, Chabal S, Winn HR. A randomized, double-blind study of phenytoin for the prevention of post-traumatic seizures. *N Engl J Med* 1990; 323: 497-502.
64. Kraus JF. Epidemiology of head injury. In: Cooper R (ed). Head Injury. 3rd edn. Baltimore: Williams and Wilkins; 1993. p. 1-25.

65. Ruff RM, Marshall LF, Klauber MR, Blunt BA, Grant I, Foulkes MA et al. Alcohol abuse and neurological outcome of the severely head injured. *J Head Trauma Rehabil* 1990; 5: 21-31.
66. Waller PF, Stewart JR, Hansen AR, Stutts JC, Popkin CL, Rodgman EA. The potentiating effects of alcohol on driver injury. *JAMA* 1986; 256: 1461-66.
67. Jagger J, Fife D, Venberg K, Jane AJ. Effect of alcohol intoxication on the diagnosis and apparent severity of brain injury. *Neurosurgery* 1984; 15: 303-6.
68. Caffey J. On the theory and practice of shaking infants, its potential residual effects of permanent brain damage and mental retardation. *Am J Dis Child* 1972; 124: 161-9.
69. Hadley MN, Sonntag VKH, Rekate HL, Murphy A. The infant whiplash-shake injury syndrome: A clinical and pathological study. *Neurosurgery* 1989; 24: 536-40.
70. White AA, Panjabi MM. The problem of clinical instability in the human spine: A systematic approach. Clinical biomechanics of the spine. 2nd edn. Philadelphia: JB Lippincott; 1990. p. 277-378.
71. Waters RL, Adkins RH, Yakural J, Sie I. Profiles of spinal cord injury and recovery after gunshot injury. *Clin Orthop* 1991; 267: 14-21.
72. Atkinson PP, Atkinson JLD. Spinal shock. *Mayo Clin Proc* 1996; 71: 384-9.
73. Hamilton MG, Myles ST. Pediatric spinal injury: review of 174 hospital admissions. *J Neurosurg* 1992; 77: 700-04.
74. Hutchinson PJ, Whitfield PC. Medicolegal aspects of head and neck injury. In: Whitfield PC, Thomas EO, Summers F, Whyte M, Hutchinson PJ (eds). Head injury: a multidisciplinary approach. Cambridge: Cambridge university press; 2009. p. 288-98.
75. Subrahmanyam BV, Agrawal A. Medicolegal issues in patients of traumatic brain: Indian Perspective. *Indian Journal Neurotrauma* 2012; 9: 117-22.
76. Cunnien AJ. Psychiatric and medical syndromes associated with deception: In: Rogers R (ed). Clinical assessment of malingering and deception. 2nd edn. New York: Guildford press; 1997. p. 23-46.
77. Cornell DG, Hawk GL. Clinical presentations of malingerers diagnosed by experienced forensic psychologist. *Law Hum Behav* 1989; 13: 375-83.
78. Slick DJ, Sherman EMS, Iverson GL. Diagnostic criteria for malingered neurocognitive dysfunction: proposed standards for clinical practice and research. *Clinical Neuropsychologist* 1999; 13: 545-61.

An Approach to a Case of Near-hanging/ Attempted Strangulation

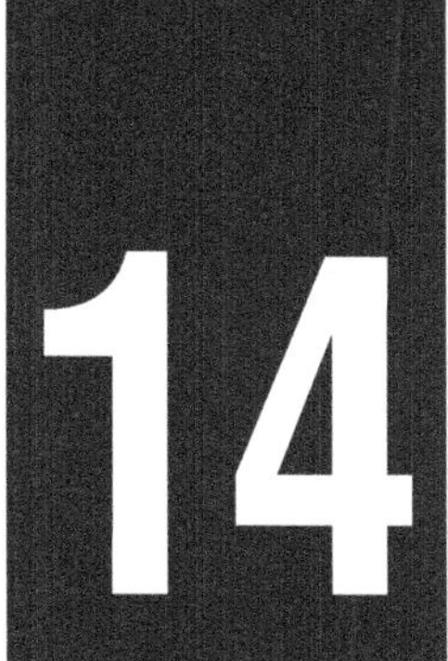

Bhupesh Khajuria

'Your opinion is not my reality.'
Steve Maraboli (Motivational speaker and author)

ABSTRACT

Victims of near-hanging and attempted strangulation are being increasingly seen in emergency department. Manual strangulation has been identified as one of the most lethal forms of domestic violence since the neck is uniquely vulnerable to life-threatening injuries. Near-hanging is also not uncommon and represents calls for help or parasuicide attempts. Injuries sustained in hanging and strangulation are well documented in autopsy studies. However, patients who survive such incidents are documented mostly as case reports and very few studies characterize these injuries.

All such cases should be actively and vigorously resuscitated, as initial presenting features bear a poor correlation to eventual outcome.[1] Management should be based as per the Advanced Trauma Life Support (ALTS) guidelines, primarily including cervical spine immobilization, securing airway by endotracheal intubation, positive pressure ventilation, maintenance of fluid, electrolyte balance, euglycemia, and normocarbia along with X-rays and CT scans. Complications involving the mental status or behavioral changes and acute respiratory complications may arise in days or weeks in victims who survive such attempts. This chapter reviews demographics, injury patterns, management guidelines and prognostic factors in unsuccessful strangulation and hanging victims. Moreover, accurate documentation in the medicolegal report is essential to substantiate the victim's account of such incident and subsequent prosecution of the alleged perpetrator.

Keywords: Asphyxia, manual strangulation, domestic violence, dysphonia, ligature mark, carotid artery rupture.

INTRODUCTION

Cases of Interest

- **Domestic violence:** A 29-year-old lady was admitted in the emergency of Govt. Medical College, Jammu as a suspected case of poisoning with history of found unconscious at her residence after taking some drugs (as alleged by her husband). On examination, the lady was cyanosed. She was managed and treated as a case of suspected poisoning. Next day, the department of Forensic Medicine was approached for review of the case and on thorough examination, a ligature mark was found all around the neck which was circular, and horizontally placed below the level of thyroid cartilage. The patient was immediately shifted to ICU, since the patient had developed pulmonary edema. On detailed investigation by the investigating officer, it was confirmed that the husband had tried to strangulate her over some family dispute but could not succeed.

- **Sexual assault with manual strangulation:** A 13-year-old young girl was found from a desolated street in semiconscious condition. She was shifted to Govt. Medical College, Jammu for treatment. During examination, crescentic abrasions along with multiple oval shaped bruises were found over the neck and nasal region. Two days later when she regained full consciousness, her statement was recorded by the police. It was revealed that she was kidnapped by her close relative who tried to sexually assault her and when she tried to shout for help, she was throttled and smothered by the accused, thereafter she fell unconscious.
- **Traumatic asphyxia:** A truck conductor was brought to the emergency in Govt. Medical College, Jammu in semiconscious condition with labored breathing, intense cyanosis and tachycardia. The history revealed (by the police) that he was helping the driver to park and was standing behind the truck. However, the driver could not control the truck while reversing that lead to fixation of the conductor in between the back of truck and the wall resulting in traumatic asphyxia. On examination, multiple bruises and contusions over the chest with fracture of ribs were found. Patient was immediately shifted to ICU but could not survive and died after two days

The underlying cause in all the above mentioned cases was asphyxia. As outlined above, most of the patients presenting in the emergency may not have any physical findings on examination with very few patients having only minor findings. Thus, the medical officer may have to depend entirely on the history provided and search for secondary signs of injury.

As we are all aware that the neck is exceptionally vulnerable to injury with its relatively small diameter, lack of bony protection and close relationship of the airway, vascular supply to the brain, spinal cord and other vital nerves, and the cervical vertebral column (Fig. 14.1). Any external force can injure any of these important structures. The trachea is attached at its superior end by the thyroid cartilage and the hyoid bone. Fractures of both structures may occur from manual strangulation and suicidal hanging. With fractures, hemorrhage and edema may develop to obstruct the airway.

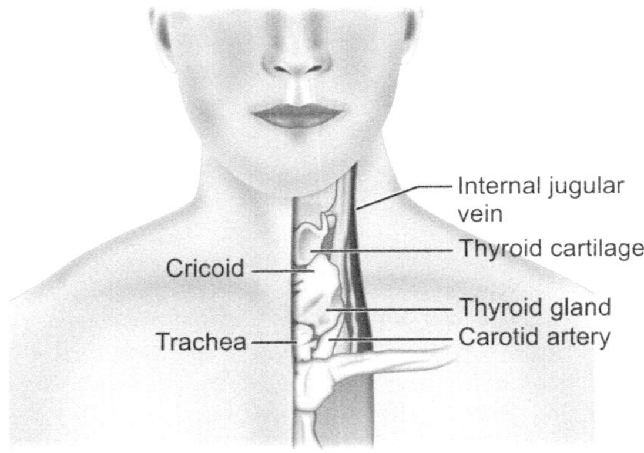

Fig. 14.1 Normal anatomy of neck

Hanging is one of the common mode of suicide across the world. Survival after attempted hanging is very rare with death usually ensues within few minutes to 24 hours. If the person survives the initial trauma, he/she may die subsequently due to the initial hypoxic and ischemic brain damage. Survival from hanging is often associated with various complications including a large variety of neurological consequences.[2]

Strangling injuries are common, as the essential weapons are as close as the assailant's own hands. An estimated 5–10% of urban assaults involve manual or ligature strangulations. Studies also indicate that 23–68% of female domestic violence victims experienced at least one strangulation-related incident from their abusive husband/male partner during their lifetime.[3] Strangulation is a well-recognized event in the practice of forensic medicine and much of the knowledge on strangulation injuries has been gathered from homicide victims. Most forensic medicine textbooks extensively describe the severe damage to the vital structures in the neck which are commonly seen in homicide cases. They provide little information and guidance to evaluate the patients who present to the emergency department with attempted hanging or strangulation injuries. It is also important to note that there are important differences between manual strangulation and hanging, so at times the presentation may be different.[4]

DEFINITIONS

Some definitions which a medical practitioner must know while dealing with such cases:[4-6]

- **Asphyxia:** Restriction of oxygen due to mechanical interference with respiration.
- **Suicide:** The act of intentionally causing one's own death.
- **Failed suicide attempt**: A suicide that did not result in death. Some may not be true attempts at all, but rather parasuicide.
- **Hanging or 'self-suspension':** Asphyxia caused by suspension of the body by a ligature which encircles the neck, the constricting force being at least part of the weight of the body. It may be either complete (feet not touching the ground) or partial (feet touching the ground).
- **Near-hanging:** Patients who survive a hanging injury long enough to reach the hospital.
- **Strangulation:** Asphyxia caused by mechanical disruption of blood flow through the vessels of the neck and/or blockage of air passage through the trachea by means of a ligature or by any means *other than suspension of the body.*

Classification

i. **Ligature strangulation:** When ligature material is used to compress the neck. It includes the use of any object, such as an electrical cord, purse strap, articles of clothing, phone or cable cords, ropes and belts or seat belts, *'chunni' or 'dupatta'* or scarf.
ii. **Manual strangulation or throttling:** When fingers, palms, hands or forearms are used to compress the neck.
iii. **Mugging:** Strangulation caused by holding the neck of the victim in the bend of elbow (i.e. the 'sleeper hold') or knee of the assailant.

iv. **Garroting:** Strangulation is caused by compression of the neck by a ligature which is quickly tightened by twisting it with a lever (rod, stick or ruler), resulting in sudden loss of consciousness and collapse.

- **Positional/postural asphyxia:** Airway obstruction due to peculiar body position or body weight over an object that results in inadequate gas exchange. This may be seen infants, alcoholics or addicts or in *hogtying.*
- **Drowning:** The process of experiencing respiratory impairment from submersion/immersion in liquid.
- **Suffocation:** Asphyxia caused by mechanical obstruction to the passage of air into the respiratory tract *by means other than constriction of neck or drowning.*

Classification

i. **Smothering:** It is caused by mechanical occlusion of external air passages, i.e. the nose and mouth from outside by hand, cloth, pillow, plastic bag or other material.
ii. **Choking:** It is caused by an obstruction within the trachea, either partially or completely, from inside by a foreign body, like coin, fruit seed, toffees, candies, fish or any other material.
iii. **Gagging:** It results from pushing a gag (rolled up cloth or paper balls) into the mouth, sufficiently deep to block the pharynx. It combines the features of smothering and choking.
iv. **Overlaying:** It results from compression of the chest, nose and mouth so as to prevent breathing (common in neonates).
v. **Traumatic/crush asphyxia:** It results from respiratory arrest due to mechanical fixation of chest so that the normal movements of chest wall are prevented.
vi. **Confined space entrapment:** It occurs when there is inadequate oxygen in the enclosed space due to consumption or displacement by other gases.
vii. **Burking:** It is a combination of homicidal smothering and traumatic asphyxia.

EPIDEMIOLOGY

- The rate of suicide is far higher in men than in women (3-4: 1) with suicidal hangings more common. However, recent trends suggest that women are gradually using hanging than other methods of suicide.
- Women are more likely than men to be victims of strangulation (domestic violence or sexual assault).[7]
- Nearly all reported autoerotic hanging incidents involve men.[7]
- Accidental strangulation may occur in both men and women.

Causes

Several populations are at risk of hanging or strangulation.[4-8]

- *Toddlers*: The neck may get caught and strangled in ill-constructed cribs as they put their heads out. Window cords have also been implicated in such deaths. Children < 1-year-old are particularly vulnerable.
- *Adolescents*: Incidence of accidental hanging, throttling or strangulation due to 'choking game' (voluntary asphyxia or self-induced hypoxia in order to enjoy the altered sensations due to cerebral hypoxia) has been reported. Playground

slide tie rope has been implicated in accidental strangulation. Emulating TV shows and depression can also lead to hanging.

- *Adults*: Autoerotic accidents, assaults (sex-related offences such as rape, attempted homicide and cases of domestic violence), and suicidal depression are common causes (for e.g., in prisons, where hanging is easier and available method). Accidental strangulation from scarfs and '*chunni*' (in females) and by cotton cloth entangled in the rotor of a machine (in males) have been reported. Rarely, the gauze used to secure endotracheal tube may leave behind a ligature mark which may create a suspicion of foul play (Figs 14.2A to C).
- *Elderly:* Depression can lead to hanging.

Isadora Duncan syndrome: The world famous dancer Isadora Duncan died on 14th September 1929 as a result of her long scarf which she was wearing got caught in the wire wheels of her Buggati car. She died at the scene and was later found to have sustained a fractured larynx and carotid artery injury.[9]

PATHOPHYSIOLOGY

The mechanism of injury in judicial hanging where the body drops to a distance equal to or greater than the height of the individual is due to hangman's fracture,

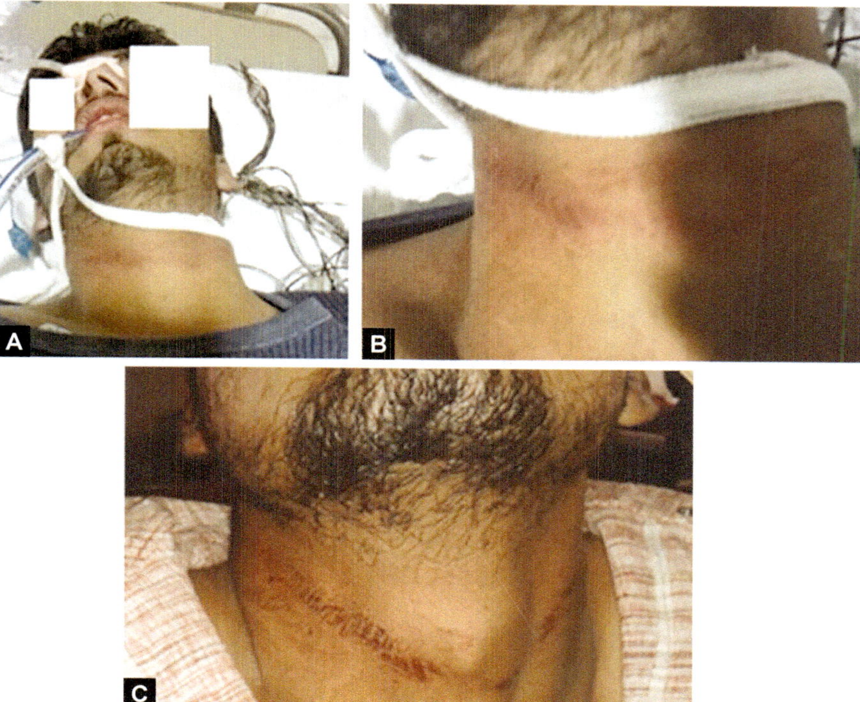

Figs 14.2A to C Accidental ligature mark caused by the gauze used to secure the endotracheal tube. (A and B) At the time of admission; (C) 36 hours after admission (*Courtesy:* Dr Parmod Goyal, Prof. and Head, FMT, Adesh Institute of Medical Sciences and Research, Bathinda)

spinal cord transection or asphyxiation, and subsequent death. The proposed mechanism in most of the other asphyxial conditions [whether by near-hanging (drop from no or minimal height, usually < body height), manual strangulation, application of ligature, or postural asphyxiation (in children whose necks are caught in an object such as a crib)] are the following:[1,10-12]

- **Venous obstruction:** It occurs if ligature is made up of broad and soft material. This may lead to cerebral congestion, hypoxia and unconsciousness which in turn produces loss of muscle tone leading to airway obstruction. For manual strangulation and suicidal near-hanging victims, it is a significant factor that produces loss of consciousness.
- **Arterial blockage:** It occurs when ligature is made of thin cord which puts pressure on carotid artery. This may lead to cerebral anemia and collapse, due to low cerebral blood flow.
- **Reflex vagal inhibition:** It is caused by pressure to the carotid sinuses and increased parasympathetic tone leading to sudden cardiac arrest (less common).

The incidence of cervical spine injuries in near-hanging has been reported to be low or nonexistent.[11-13] However, Salem et al found cervical spine injuries in 5% of cases in their study of 63 patients of near-hanging.[10] Most experts agree that regardless of the events occurring in any given hanging or strangulation, death ultimately occurs from cerebral hypoxia and ischemic neuronal death. Notably, none of the proposed mechanisms advocates airway blockage as the immediate cause of signs and symptoms observed in such cases. Although mechanical airway compromise occurs subsequently and eventually complicates patient management, it appears to play a minimal role in the immediate death of victims.

EFFECTS OF ASPHYXIA

Clinical effects of asphyxia are shown in Flow chart 14.1. The triad of asphyxial stigmata that may be seen are:[5]

i. *Cyanosis:* Bluish discoloration of skin, face (particularly in the lips, tip of nose, ears lobules), nailbeds and mucous membranes (Fig. 14.3).

Flow chart 14.1 Clinical effects of asphyxia

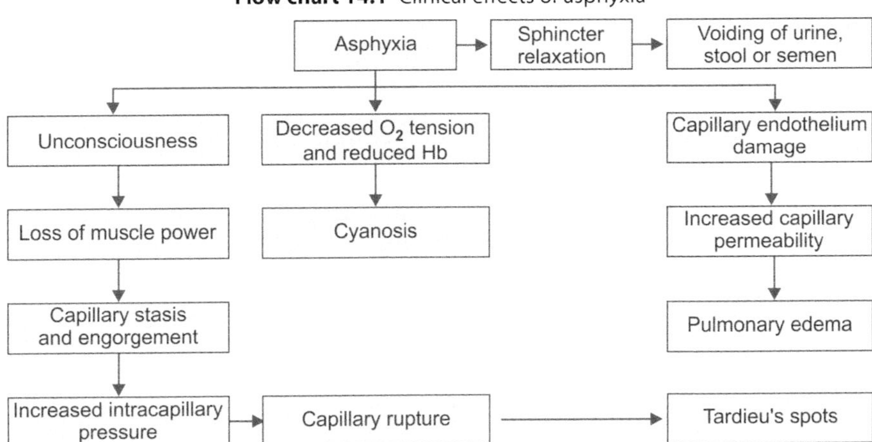

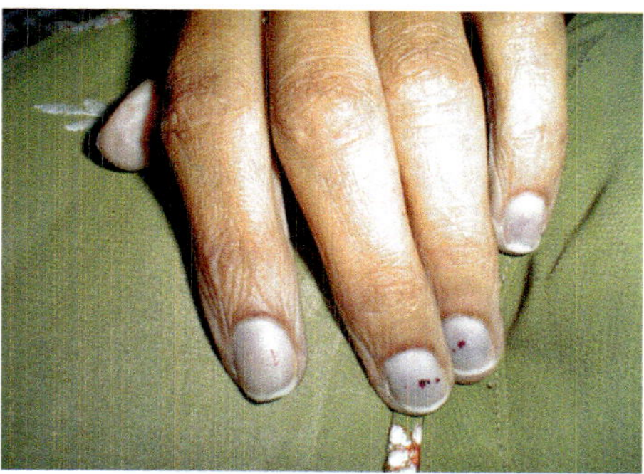

Fig. 14.3 Cyanosis of nailbeds

ii. *Petechial hemorrhages* (Tardieu's spots) are found in those parts where capillaries are least supported, for e.g., conjunctiva, epiglottis or on the face. They tend to be better made out in fair skinned persons.
iii. *Congestion and edema of the face* due to raised venous pressure.

EVALUATION AND DOCUMENTATION

History

The manually strangled or near-hanging victims are usually brought to the emergency department in unconscious state after being found by friends, family members, strangers, or sometimes, police. On many occasions, the exact history may not be disclosed by the relatives or it may be vague or cooked up. In such cases, the doctor must try to extract the history from different sources available.[4,14]

Even if the victim is conscious, she may not always report the attempted strangulation episode. As is common with cases of domestic violence, the victim may be hesitant to fully describe what happened or will minimize the severity of the attack. Moreover, visual evidence of force applied to the neck during such incident is often absent or minimal on initial medical evaluation (since bruises takes time to develop). The lack of physical findings may lead authorities to disbelieve the patient's report. Hence, specific questions often are required to elucidate the history.[14]

In strangulation victims, they should be asked about the position, method or manner of strangulation; whether hands, elbow or forearm or any ligature or any other method was used. The number of such episodes, whether single, multiple or repeated with different methods. Other circumstances should also be enquired like whether the victim was smothered, shaken, knocked or pounded into a wall or on the ground? Was the victim physically and/or sexually assaulted? This will help determine mechanism and predict potential injuries. Whether the victim has consumed any alcohol, drug or any other poison (any smell from breath)? Whether she is pregnant?[4,6]

Hanging victims are more likely to arrive in the emergency department with a depressed level of consciousness than are victims of manual strangulation. This is due to the more intensive and prolonged compressive force applied to the neck due to hanging than is seen with manual pressure. Whether the victim attempted hanging? The height, position of knot and ligature material used should be enquired. Attempts to determine the height of the drop in near-hanging victim is important, since the pattern of injury may differ as the drop height increases. If the drop is greater than the height of the patient, then there is a high probability of cervical spine injury.[1,6,10]

The practitioner has to enquire about specific symptoms like whether the victim lost consciousness, if there is any neck pain, any difficulty in breathing or swallowing, any change of voice, or headache, and if there was any urinary and/or fecal incontinence.[4]

CLINICAL PRESENTATION

In nonlethal strangulation, the victim may present with seemingly harmless signs and symptoms with no or minimal external signs of soft tissue injury, because of the slowly compressive nature of forces involved. The upper airway may also appear normal beneath intact mucosa, despite hyoid bone or laryngeal fractures. It takes time for hemorrhage and edema to develop after compressive injuries (may take up to 36 hours post-incident) and the patient can develop edema of the supraglottic and oropharyngeal soft tissue, leading to airway obstruction.

Signs and Symptoms (In Surviving Victims)

The clinical presentations can vary according to the age and sex of the victim, and the method, force and duration of asphyxiation. The following specific clinical manifestations are usually encountered in asphyxiation victims:[1,4,6,8,11,13,14]

i. **Dysphonia or hoarseness of voice:** It is commonly seen. Patient may sometimes present with aphonia.

ii. **Dysphagia or difficulty in swallowing:** It may occur due to injury to larynx or hyoid bone which is not common symptom on initial assessment, but may be reported within 2 weeks (Fig. 14.4). Sometimes it may be painful (odynophagia).

iii. **Dyspnea:** It is very common, but often a late development. Respiratory distress is seen in 2 weeks which may be due hyperventilation or psychogenic (anxiety, fear or depression). Difficulty in breathing can also be due to laryngeal edema or hemorrhage, although these injuries are less common in surviving victims.

iv. **Pain and swelling in the throat or neck:** It is common after attempted strangulation. The patient may be able to localize it to a specific area of injury, or it may be diffuse and poorly localized. Edema may be caused by internal hemorrhage, injury to underlying neck structures or fracture of the larynx. Laryngeal fracture can manifest as severe pain on gentle palpation of the larynx, or subcutaneous emphysema over or around the laryngeal cartilage (Fig. 14.4).

v. **Altered mental status:** Restlessness, confusion, loss of orientation or combativeness due to cerebral hypoxia or from concomitant intracranial injury or ingestion of drugs or ethanol.

vi. **Neurologic symptoms:** These include changes in vision, tinnitus, ptosis, facial droop, or unilateral weakness, paralysis or loss of sensation. In many patients, the findings are transient and believed to be caused by focal cerebral ischemia produced by the strangulation process that resolves with time. In

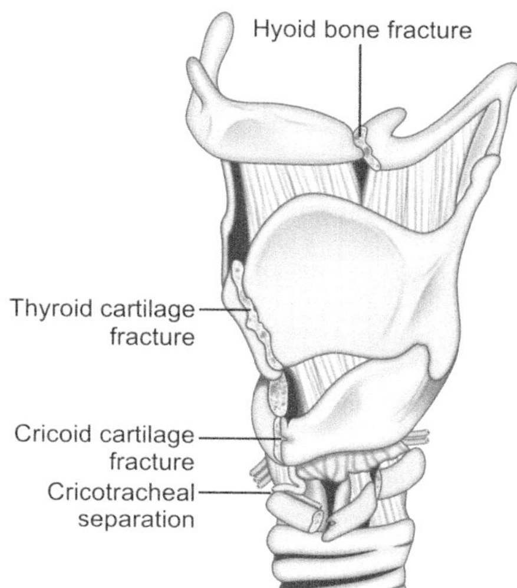

Fig. 14.4 Injuries possible in attempted strangulation and near-hanging

rare cases, damage to the internal carotid artery may induce thrombosis with a delayed neurologic presentation.

vii. **Petechiae:** It can occur at or above the area of compression, and are most frequently seen on the face, periorbital region, eyelids, scalp and conjunctiva. Facial and conjunctival petechiae are evidence of prolonged gripping of the neck resulting in elevated venous pressure. It has been found that the jugular vein needs to be occluded for at least 15–30 seconds for the development of facial petechiae. Subconjunctival hemorrhage is usually seen after a vigorous struggle between the victim and assailant (Fig. 14.5).

viii. **Neck:** Injury to the soft tissues in the neck may manifest with abrasions (scratches), hyperemia, ecchymoses and edema. The hyperemia may be transient and may not visible at the time of assessment. Similarly, ecchymoses and swelling may take time to develop and may not be visible on initial assessment.

Attempted manual strangulation: Fingertips may produce faint oval or discoid bruises 1.5–2 cm in size (may be more in case of continued bleeding or confluent bruises). A grip from right hand produces a bruising due to bulb of pressing thumb over the cornue of hyoid/thyroid on anterolateral surface of right side of victim's neck, and several fingertip bruising marks and overlying nail scratch abrasions (crescent shaped) over left side. A single bruise on the victim's neck is most frequently caused by the assailant's thumb as bruises made by tips of thumbs are more prominent than with other fingers.[5,15]

Multiple abrasions on the neck may be defensive in nature from use of victim's own fingernails in an effort to dislodge the assailant's grip, but commonly are a combination of lesions caused by both the victim and the assailant's fingernails.

Chin abrasions may also occur from the defensive actions as the victim tries to protect their necks from the manual strangulation of the assailant.

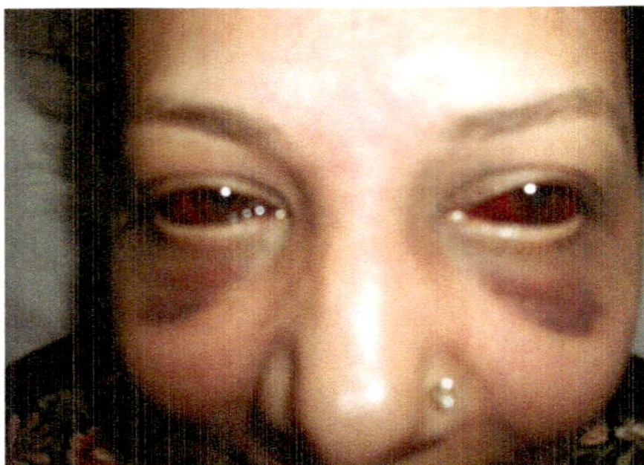

Fig. 14.5 Subconjunctival and periorbital hemorrhages

Attempted ligature strangulation or hanging: Ligature marks may be subtle or hidden within the natural skin folds of the neck (Fig. 14.6). It may be missed on quick examination, especially if the cervical collar (if present) is not removed and good lighting is not used. The appearance of marks on the skin is influenced by the nature of the ligature (width, roughness and surface pattern), the force and duration of the strangulation, and the interaction with a resisting victim (displacement of the noose in attempts to remove it).[15] Congestion and petechial hemorrhages above the ligature are usually more remarkable than in throttling victims (Fig. 14.6). Similarly, hanging mark is influenced by the nature of the ligature material, duration of hanging, type and placement of the knot, and height of drop. The pattern of ligature mark is different in strangulation and hanging as given in Table 14.1 (Figs 14.6 and 14.7A and B).[5,15]

ix. **Lungs:** Aspiration pneumonitis may occur due to inhalation of vomitus. Pulmonary edema is common in comatose hanging victims. The cause of the pulmonary edema can either be due to anoxic injury to the central nervous system (neurogenic pulmonary edema) or from obstructive pulmonary edema. The mechanism of *obstructive pulmonary edema* is thought to be complex of negative intrathoracic pressure (when the victim struggles to breathe in against an occluded airway), increased left ventricular afterload and massive sympathetic outflow resulting in pooling of blood in the pulmonary capillaries—pulmonary edema.[12,16]

x. Involuntary urination or defecation, expulsion of fetus (if pregnant) may occur.

Fractures of the thyroid cartilage or hyoid bone in victims of accidental strangulation, and direct injury to the trachea is uncommon with strangulation. Fracture of hyoid bone is often associated with injuries to vascular and airway structures.[8] Carotid artery injury is also uncommon after attempted hanging and strangulation but has been reported in some cases.[17]

Injury to other organ systems from strangulation is rare and mostly described in some case reports. Case reports of diaphragmatic injury, multiple organ failure and thyroid storm after attempted strangulation; cricotracheal separation and common carotid artery dissection and laryngotracheal separation after attempted hanging; and laryngeal rupture and carotid artery stenosis after accidental strangulation are all documented in the medical literature.[9,18,19]

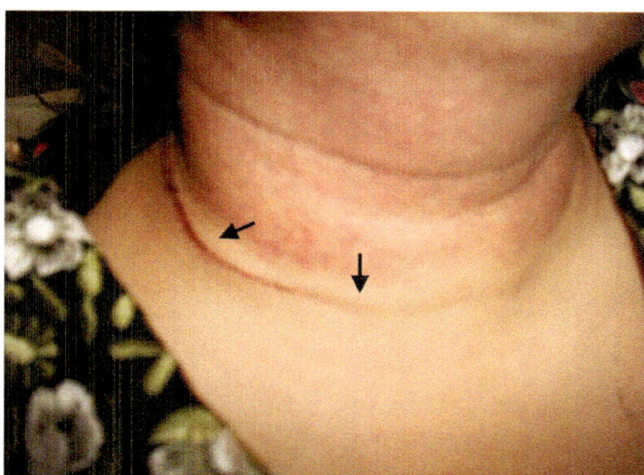

Fig. 14.6 Survived victim of chain-snatching. The ligature mark corresponds to the chain she was wearing (arrows). Note the congestion and petechial hemorrhages above the ligature mark

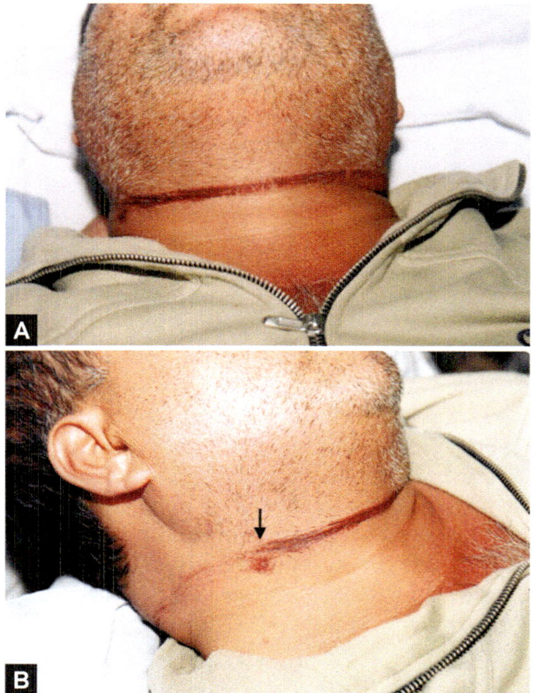

Figs 14.7A and B Near-hanging. The victim was found with legs supported on the floor. Note the site of knot (arrow)

The clinical features of dysphagia, hoarseness and dyspnea are related to edema and/or the distortion of the laryngeal structure including fracture of the hyoid and/or dislocation of the arytenoids cartilages.[9]

Examine for other associated injuries in cases female patients regarding injuries on lips, face, cheeks, abdomen, back, genital organs and breast (if there

Table 14.1 Ligature mark (furrow) in attempted hanging and strangulation

S. No.	Features	Hanging	Strangulation
1.	Direction	Oblique	Transverse
2.	Continuity	Noncontinuous	Continuous
3.	Level in the neck	Above thyroid	At or below thyroid
4.	Base	Pale, hard, parchment-like	Soft and transverse streak-like reddening

is any history suggesting sexual abuse). In such cases, complete examination of genital organs is of critical importance.

However, some victims may not show any external evidence, although there is history suggestive of attempted strangulation. This is possible when the palm or forearm was placed over the neck or when a soft object, such as a garment or a pillow was put in while applying pressure.[6,15] At times, the injuries may not have developed at the time of examination. Hence, re-examination after 24 hours is recommended in such cases.

Diagnosis

The majority of the victims present with some common features, a combination of these findings should be taken into consideration for diagnosis:[16]

- Hyperemia and/or ecchymosis
- Facial or conjunctival petechiae
- Change of voice or difficulty in breathing
- Marks on the neck
- Loss of consciousness or altered mental status

In *suspected assailants,* examination may be indicative of having been the offender in an attempted strangulation. It is better to examine the accused after examination of the victim and to look specifically for any injuries which she/he allege to have inflicted. The most frequent injuries seen are nail marks inflicted by the victim. Nail marks have been classified morphologically into three types: impression marks, claws and scratches. The majority of the skin lesions are located on the dorsal aspects of the forearms and hands, face, neck, shoulders and anterior chest wall. Bite marks on the hands is another characteristic injury seen in such cases. The assailant may also sustain nonspecific blunt trauma from blows which she may inflict in self-defense or from grappling with the victim in case of any struggle.[15]

DIAGRAMS AND PHOTOGRAPHS

It is important to document the injuries through diagrams and photographs (if facility is available) that may be seen at the time of examination for evidence purpose. The injuries should be mentioned in the pictograph given along with the medicolegal report. The following photographs may also be taken:[12]

- *Distance photo:* Full body photograph to identify the victim and location of the injury.

- *Close-up photo:* Photographs of injuries along with a measuring scale from different angles to maximize visibility and to document the size.
- *Follow-up photo:* As the injuries may take time to develop, taking follow-up photographs at different time intervals will document injuries as they evolve.

LABORATORY AND IMAGING

The following investigations are recommended to assess the patient, depending on their clinical presentation:[4,6,8,12,16]

i. **Arterial blood gases (ABGs) analysis:** It should be done in all patients who require intubation, for subsequent ventilator management.
ii. **Pulse oximetry:** It is indicated in patients with altered mental status and respiratory distress. It also makes ABGs unnecessary in patients who do not require endotracheal intubation.
iii. **Neck X-ray:** It should be done in all strangulation and hanging victims. It is useful to detect fractured hyoid bone and for evaluation of subcutaneous emphysema due to fractured larynx. The incidence of such fractures is correlated with the extent of ossification, depending on the age and sex of the person. Generally, a fractured hyoid bone indicates a severe, occult soft-tissue injury, even in a patient whose medical condition is otherwise stable. Fractures of the cervical vertebrae are extremely rare in strangulation and hanging injuries unless there has been a hanging with a free-fall drop (long drop) of the body.
iv. **Chest X-ray:** It is indicated after endotracheal intubation for placement confirmation, diagnosis of pulmonary edema, aspiration pneumonitis and acute respiratory distress syndrome (ARDS).
v. **CT scan:** It is indicated to detect hyoid bone and laryngeal fractures, injury to carotid arteries and other soft-tissue abnormalities that may not be apparent on plain radiographs. CT head is done to evaluate neurological status. CT is more sensitive for bony injuries, subcutaneous emphysema, soft-tissue edema and internal hemorrhage.
vi. **Doppler vascular imaging, CT angiography or arteriography:** It is useful to detect injury to the carotid arteries (in patients with unilateral neurological findings). The current 'gold standard' for blunt carotid artery injury is four-vessel selective angiography.
vii. **MRI:** It is the most useful imaging modality for the majority of such victims because of its highest sensitivity for deep soft-tissue injury including the larynx and vessels. Hypoxic brain damage may result in changes mainly in the globus pallidus, caudate nucleus and thalamus.[20]
viii. **Fiberoptic laryngoscopy:** It is indicated for visualization of the laryngeal structures (vocal cords) and adjacent structures for edema and hemorrhage.

The choice and sequence of imaging is dependent on patient's clinical condition, suspected injuries and availability of the specific modalities in that set-up. Usually, radiological evaluation, including CT scan of head and neck are done after the patient is stable hemodynamically and if there is no neurological improvement within 24 hours of admission. An ENT consultation can establish both the need for, and the timing of these studies.

MANAGEMENT

Like any other traumatic injuries, the victim is managed as per recommendations of advanced trauma life support (ATLS) guidelines:[1,6,8,11]

i. The management of a victim starts with the ABCs—airway, breathing and circulation. Fluid resuscitation must be done judiciously as there is risk of subsequent ARDS and cerebral edema.
ii. Cervical spine stabilization should be done and maintained, until such injury is excluded, although the likelihood of spinal cord injury is rare in strangulation victims. The risk of such injury increases substantially in hanging victims whose drop was equal to or greater than their height.
iii. Orotracheal intubation should be done preferably by an anesthetist. It can be difficult, if laryngeal edema is present or if direct traumatic disruption of the larynx has occurred. Cricothyroidotomy is indicated for any patient with severe respiratory distress and completely obstructed airway. If associated neck injuries make cricothyroidotomy difficult, percutaneous translaryngeal ventilation may be used to temporarily oxygenate a patient.
iv. The definitive airway management is laryngotomy which must be done at the earliest.
v. Fluids are restricted, and diuretics with or without mannitol or hypertonic saline may be indicated.
vi. Elevated blood pressure is managed with short acting sympatholytic or centrally acting agents, and vasodilating agents are avoided.
vii. Sedation and neuromuscular block, if indicated.

COMPLICATIONS

The complications make develop immediately or may develop subsequently in few days. The patient needs to be reassessed and observed for these complications before being discharged:

- *Respiratory system:* Aspiration pneumonia, bronchopneumonia and ARDS may develop; tracheal stenosis in case of rupture.[11,12]
- *Neurologic sequelae* including muscle spasms, transient hemiplegia, central cord syndrome and seizures. Long-term paraplegia or quadriplegia and short-term autonomic dysfunction may be seen in spinal cord injury.[20,21]
- *Psychiatric symptoms:* Encephalopathy, insomnia, nightmares and anxiety and an inclination for violence are seen in such victims. Psychosis, depression, suicidal ideation, Korsakoff syndrome, amnesia and progressive dementia may develop.[1,6,16,22]

PROGNOSIS

The prognosis for survivors of hanging and strangulations arriving to the emergency department is widely variable (Table 14.2).[10-12] However, with aggressive resuscitative measures and management, overall survival rates in patients with near-hanging have been reported to be 70–100%.[1,2,11,23]

The outcome is mostly determined by the presence of cardiopulmonary arrest (as indicated by a requirement for cardiopulmonary resuscitation and/or invasive airway management) and degree of anoxic brain injury [low Glasgow Coma Score (GCS) and cerebral edema on initial CT scan].

Table 14.2 Factors associated with poor outcomes

Circumstantial factors	*Admission conditions*	*CT findings*
Extended hanging time	Systolic BP < 90 mm Hg	Anoxic brain injury
Contact with ground	GCS ≤ 8	Cerebral edema
Circumferential marks	Injury severity score > 15	Cervical spine injury
Drop > body height	Cardiopulmonary arrest needing resuscitation Presentation > 4 hours Need for airway control PaO_2/FiO_2 ratio < 100	

The duration of hanging and type of ligature mark also correlates with outcome. Hanging times of less than 5 minutes predicts good outcome. Circumferential marks vs. partial marks indicate severe arterial occlusion and cerebral anoxia and may be associated with poor outcomes.

In general, admission criteria in emergency room are primarily determined by their clinical condition and evidence of injury to the deep neck structures.[4,6]

- *Patients requiring ICU admission*: comatose, persistently altered mental status, ventilatory and/or cardiovascular support, laryngeal fracture, hyoid bone fracture or carotid artery injury.
- *Patients requiring admission for at least 12–24 hours*: history of unconsciousness, evidence of vascular obstruction with facial or conjunctival petechiae, signs or symptoms of soft-tissue injury to the neck. While they may be breathing normally, soft-tissue swelling and/or bleeding is likely to get worse. Also, victims who are intoxicated from ethanol or drugs should be observed until the effect of those agents has dissipated.
- *Patients that can be discharged*: No history of unconsciousness, minimal or no physical evidence of soft-tissue injury to the neck, completely normal neurologic examination; responsible adults who can watch for the late development of complications.

Anyone presenting with attempted hanging should be evaluated by a psychiatrist once medically stable.[6,16]

MEDICOLEGAL ASSESSMENT

Medical practitioners who examine such cases in the emergency have to follow a protocol regarding the documentation of medicolegal formalities, besides imparting treatment in order to save the life of patient. Injuries due to assault are required to be informed to the police (if police is not accompanying) to ensure safe disposition of the patient. In case of suspected child abuse, child protective agency should be notified.

LEGAL PROVISIONS

In India, attempt to commit suicide is an offence punishable under Sec. 309 IPC. It states that whoever attempts to commit suicide and does any act towards the commission of such offence, shall be punished with simple imprisonment for a term which may extend to 1 year or with fine, or with both.

Abetment of suicide: As per Sec. 306 IPC, any person who abets the commission of suicide shall be punished for a term which may extend to 10 years imprisonment and also liable to fine.

The Protection of Women from Domestic Violence Act, 2005

Salient features of the Act:[24]

- The term 'domestic violence' covers all forms of physical, sexual, verbal, emotional and economic abuse that can harm, cause injury to, endanger the health, safety, life, limb or well-being, either mental or physical of the aggrieved person.
- 'Aggrieved' person' is not just the wife but a woman who is the sexual partner of the male irrespective of whether she is his legal wife or not. It includes daughter, mother, sister, child (male or female), widowed relative, or any woman residing in the household who is related in some way to the respondent.
- 'Respondent' is any male, adult person who is, or has been, in a domestic relationship with the aggrieved person that includes his mother, sister and other relatives; the case can also be filed against relatives of the husband or male partner.
- **Information to Protection Officer:** The information regarding any acts of domestic violence does not necessarily have to be lodged by the aggrieved party but by any person who has reason to believe that such an act has been or is being committed. Any medical officer, neighbors, social workers or relatives can all take initiative on behalf of the victim.
- **Duties of medical facilities**: If an aggrieved person or a Protection Officer or a service provider requests the medical practitioner to provide any medical aid to the victim, the doctor should provide medical aid to the aggrieved person in the medical facility.
- **Penalties**: The Magistrate can impose a penalty of up to 1 year of imprisonment and/or a fine of up to ₹ 20,000/- for an offence under this Act. The offence is also considered cognizable and nonbailable. The decision can be taken under the sole testimony of the aggrieved person; the court may conclude that an offence has been committed by the accused.

The Magistrate can impose monetary relief and monthly payments of maintenance. The respondent can also be made to meet the expenses incurred and losses suffered by the aggrieved person as a result of domestic violence, and can also cover loss of earnings, medical expenses, loss or damage to property and can also cover the maintenance of the victim. The Act also allows the Magistrate to make the respondent pay compensation and damages for injuries including mental torture and emotional distress caused by acts of domestic violence.

Key Elements of Strangulation and Suffocation Statute in the US

The Strangulation and Suffocation Law in the US defines and provides penalties for a person who engages in intentional strangulation and suffocation.[25] The states of Iowa, South Dakota, California, Wisconsin, Tennessee, Virginia and

New York have passed laws making it a felony (a crime punishable by death or imprisonment in excess of 1 year) under certain conditions to knowingly impede someone's breathing. Under this law 'dangerous weapons' and 'substantial bodily harm' have been defined as:

- 'Dangerous weapon' means any firearm, whether loaded or unloaded; any device designed as a weapon and capable of producing death or great bodily harm; any ligature or other instrumentality used on the throat, neck, nose, or mouth of another person to impede, partially or completely, breathing or circulation or blood; any electric weapon, or any other device or instrumentality which, in the manner it is used or intended to be used, is calculated or likely to produce death or great bodily harm.
- 'Substantial bodily harm' means bodily injury that causes a laceration that requires stitches, staples or a tissue adhesive; and fracture of a bone, broken nose, burn, petechia, temporary loss of consciousness, sight or hearing, concussion, or loss or fracture of a tooth.

CONCLUSION

Near and accidental hanging, and attempted strangulation injuries are becoming more prevalent in urban areas. Many survivors of strangulation or hanging may not volunteer information. These survivors may have minimal visible external signs of injury. However, there may be signs of bruising around the neck and petechia above the point of the ligature.

Victims of near hanging and attempted strangulation require emergent evaluation, since the vital structures in the neck may have sustained injury. All such patients even with initial neurological deficits and/or respiratory distress should be aggressively managed, since the recovery is often complete. All survivors of hanging should receive support and follow up after discharge from hospital. With proper training and education, the emergency medical doctor can also improve the medicolegal documentation which in turn will make such cases prosecutable and the alleged perpetrator can be brought to justice.

REFERENCES

1. Howell MA, Guly HR. Near hanging presenting to an accident and emergency department. *J Accid Emerg Med* 1996; 13: 135-36.
2. Kodikara S. Attempted suicidal hanging: an uncomplicated recovery. *Am J Forensic Med Path* 2012; 33: 317-18.
3. Fact sheet: Strangulation assaults in domestic violence cases. Available from: http://www.sp2.upenn.edu/ortner/docs/factsheet_strangulation.pdf.
4. Stapczynski JS. Strangulation injuries. *Emergency Medicine Reports* 2010; 31: 193-203.
5. Biswas G. Asphyxia. Review of forensic medicine and toxicology. 2nd edn. New Delhi: Jaypee Brothers; 2012. p. 138-64.
6. Della-Giustina D, Laselle BT. Neck injury by strangulation/hanging. In: Schaider JJ, Barkin RM, Hayden SR, Wolfe RE, Barkin AZ, Shayne P, Rosen P (eds). Rosen and Barkin's 5-minute Emergency Medicine Consult. 4th edn. Philadelphia: Lippincott Williams and Wilkins; 2010. p. 732.
7. Ernoehazy W. Hanging injuries and strangulation. Available from: http://emedicine.medscape.com/article/826704.
8. Sajed D. Strangulation trauma. In: Shah K, Egan D, Quaas J (eds). Essential emergency trauma. 1st ed. Philadelphia: Lippincott Williams and Wilkins; 2010. p. 155-58.

9. Gowens PA, Davenport RJ, Kerr J, Sanderson RJ, Marsden AK. Survival from accidental strangulation from a scarf resulting in laryngeal rupture and carotid artery stenosis: the 'Isadora Duncan syndrome'. A case report and review of literature. *Emerg Med J* 2003; 20: 391-93.
10. Salim A, Martin M, Sangthong B, Brown C, Rhee P, Demetriades D. Near-hanging injuries: A 10-year experience. Injury, *Int J Care Injured* 2006; 37: 435-39.
11. Gandhi R, Taneja N, Mazumder P. Near hanging: Early intervention can save lives. *Indian J Anaesth* 2011; 55: 388-91.
12. Nair S, Jacob J, Aaron S, Thomas M, Joseph M, Alexander M. Pulmonary distress following attempted suicidal hanging. *Indian J Med Sci* 2009; 63: 53-57.
13. Davidson JA. Presentation of near-hanging to an emergency department in the Northern Territory. *Emerg Med* 2003; 15: 28-31.
14. Funk M, Schuppel J. Strangulation injuries. *Wisc Med J* 2003; 102: 41-45.
15. Pollak S, Saukko PJ. Clinical forensic medicine: overview. In: Siegal J, Knupfner G, Saukko P (eds). Encyclopedia of Forensic Sciences. 1st edn. New York: Academic press; 2000. p. 362-68.
16. Bisanzo M, Bhatia K, Filbin MR (eds). Penetrating neck injury. Emergency management of the trauma patient: cases, algorithms. 1st edn. Philadelphia: Lippincott Williams and Wilkins; 2007. p. 30-39.
17. Hausmann R, Betz P. Delayed death after attempted suicide by hanging. *Int J Legal Med.* 1997; 110: 164-66.
18. Linnau KF http://www.ajronline.org/content/ 178/1/214.full - aff-1, Cohen WA. Radiologic evaluation of attempted suicide by hanging. Cricotracheal separation and common carotid artery dissection. *AJR* 2002; 178: 214.
19. Deshpande S. Laryngotracheal separation after attempted hanging. *Br J Anaesth* 1998; 81: 612-14.
20. Kalita J. Clinicoradiological observation in three patients with suicidal hanging. *J Neurol Sci* 2002; 198: 21-24.
21. Hausmann R, Betz P. Delayed death after attempted suicide by hanging. *Int J Legal Med* 1997; 110: 164-66.
22. Medalia AA, Merriam AE, Ehrenreich JH. The neuropsychological sequelae of attempted hanging. *J Neurol Neurosurg Psychiatry* 1991; 54: 546-48.
23. Richards CE, Wallis DN. Asphyxiation: a review. *Trauma* 2005; 7: 37-45.
24. Protection of Women from Domestic Violence Act, 2005. Available from: http://www.wcd.nic.in/wdvact.pdf.
25. Strangulation and suffocation statute. Available from: http://www.wcadv.org/sites/default/.../Wisconsin_Strangulation_Suffocation_Law.

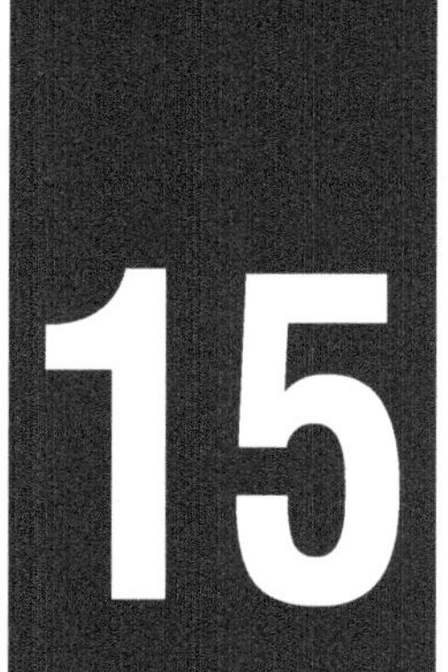

Emerging Issues in Sex Verification

Jagadeesh Narayanareddy

'I think what you're seeing is a profound recognition on the part of the American people that gays, lesbians and transgender persons are our brothers, sisters, children, cousins, friends and co-workers, and that they've got to be treated like every other American. And I think that principle will win out.'

Barack Obama (President of the United States)

ABSTRACT

Sex verification to identify an individual as 'male' or 'female' is often easy, barring the cases of disorders of sexual development (DSD). Although there are many biological markers of sex—chromosomes, gonads, external and internal genitalia and secondary sexual characteristics, but none is conclusive. In sports, tests to verify 'sex' have evolved from the days of 'nude parading', 'sex chromatin identification', 'karyotyping', 'hormonal assay', to a combination of these tests, to a 'team of experts in the field' opining. The failure of the methods is because of the assumption that any singular marker of sex is adequate to classify people into a two sex system. With not enough scientific research evidence to verify 'sex' in absolute terms, many recommendary bodies/agencies encourage to accept these DSD as deviations of normal and identify them with their preferred sex identity, provided they fulfill the guidelines of those recommendary bodies/agencies. This chapter presents a general overview of the basic ethical and legal issues concerning individuals with DSD.

Keywords: Sex verification tests, gender, disorders of sexual development (DSD), identification, transgender, rape, SRY gene.

INTRODUCTION

Many a time lay people wonder, what is this fuss all about identifying the biological sex of an individual. They would recall a granny or midwife immediately after delivery, even in the dim midnight, declaring with ease that it is a girl or a boy to the rejoicing crowd waiting eagerly outside the delivery room. When it is so simple, why are the doctors, sports administrators and investigators making such a hue and cry? How do we identify the biological sex of an individual? What is this fuss about sex verification tests? Are they same as gender verification tests? What are the ethical, legal and social concerns of these sex verifications?

Sex determination has been and continues to be problematic because there is no single physiological or biological marker that allows for the classification of people into either male or female. The verification of the sex of athletes has been an issue for many decades. Sex verification of female athletes began primarily as means to prevent gender fraud (men masquerading as females), with a secondary task of ensuring fair competition by excluding persons with intersex medical conditions that might confer physical advantage. The purpose of this chapter is to enable the reader understand the various changes that have evolved over the years in the 'tests to verify sex', their advantages/disadvantages and limitations. This chapter also focuses on the ethical, legal and social concerns of such sex verifications with suitable case examples.

DEFINITIONS

- **Sex:** It is the biological term denoting the genetic, physiologic and anatomical characteristics of an individual, based on which we can identify ourselves into 'males' and 'females'.[1]
- **Gender:** It is a sociological construct that denotes how an individual identifies according to social norms (social roles, position and behavior), based on which an individual exhibits 'masculine' or 'feminine' qualities.[1] It is the sexual identity of an individual from birth to puberty and adulthood.

  So when we have to identify whether an individual is 'male' or 'female', the correct word should be 'sex verification tests' and not 'gender verification tests' or 'femininity testing' as reported in lay press as well as in some publications.[2-4] The common person's view is that biological and social features are concordant. They regard that the outward signs of gender (how someone acts, behaves, dresses) tells us about that person's biology—about their sex.
- **Intersex:** There is an intermingling of sexual characters of either sex in one individual to a varying degree including the physical form, reproductive organs and sexual behavior.[5]
- **Pseudohermaphrodite:** In this, gonadal tissue of only one sex is seen internally, but external appearance is that of opposite sex.[5]

NEED FOR SEX VERIFICATION TESTS

Sex determination is required for following reasons:[5]

- *Identification in living:* Sex, age and stature are said to be the primary characteristics of identification. Sex is important in any chain of identity data and determination of the individuality of a person.
- *Participation in sports:* Sex segregation in sports is based on the long-term endogenous androgen exposure of men at puberty that lead to the physiological gap with women.
- For deciding whether an individual can *exercise certain civil rights* extended to one sex only.
- For deciding questions relating to legitimacy, divorce, paternity, marriage, impotence, rape and affiliation.

At present, there are three frequent circumstances wherein determination of sex has become necessary—sports, pre-employment and sex specific crimes which require us to know whether the individual is a male or a female.

In sports, the competitions are mostly held in different categories for males and females, and thus there is a need to segregate the individuals into these sexes to avoid undue advantage. Consequently, all athletes including intersex and transgender individuals are assigned to compete in one or other category.[6] Though some sporting events like boxing and wrestling are held based on segregation on weight of the individual also; there is an increasing demand to segregate based on height of the individual, hormonal levels, strength and power to avoid undue advantage in the sport arena rather than only on segregation based on sex. Of late, we notice in sports like equestrian, badminton and tennis, both males and females compete with each other together.

If the employments are reserved for a particular sex, then there is a need for identifying the sex of an individual. Several employments in garment manufacturing sector and hospitality industry are reserved for females. There is also particular percentage of posts reserved for female applicants only in many other sectors of employments.

In sex specific crimes like rape, adultery and kidnapping, there is a need to identify the sex of the accused and victim. If we consider Sec. 375 IPC, still only a man can rape a woman. For an offence of adultery, only the male is the accused. The age for considering the offence of kidnapping is different for a male victim (16 years) and for a female victim (18 years).

HISTORY

The need for sex verification tests were first noticed in the sports arena as there were several examples of individuals who had competed as females and were later identified to be males or individuals with disorders of sexual development (DSD) that might have given them undue physical advantage. Some reports are cited below:[6,7]

- Stella the Fella—the 100 m women's sprint champion of the 1932 Olympic Games, whose autopsy in 1980 discovered to have ambiguous genitalia.
- Dora Ratjen—at the 1936 Berlin Games, through loyalty to the Hitler Youth, bound his genitals and competed as a woman—only to be discovered when he revealed this to a journalist in 1950.
- A runner, who broke the female world track records in the 400 m and 800 m events in 1964 was later discovered to be a male.
- The winner of the 1966 women's world downhill ski title retired after receiving a medical examination in 1967. After undergoing surgery, the athlete was pronounced a male, and later married and fathered a child.

Under these circumstances, there was mistrust and ambivalent attitude towards women in sport, particularly those with outward signs that many read as 'masculine'—lack of makeup, impressive musculature, closely cropped hair and tall stature. The traditional cultural stereotype of femininity was challenged, although this may be due to vigorous training programs that may lead to the development of muscular bodies. Women who excelled in sports were pressured to actually prove that they were women, and not men in masquerade.

CASE REPORTS

Case 1: Maria Jose Martinez-Patino's Case

Maria Jose Martinez-Patino from Spain was a national champion hurdler. She had obtained the certificate of femininity by passing the sex verification test (sex chromatin test) in 1983. But when the test was repeated in the year 1985, she failed in the test. Shockingly, the test results were disclosed in front of her team mates by the team doctor, who asked her to undergo further testing by getting her karyotyping done. She was also asked to fake an injury to prevent others from knowing the truth. Without having any choice, she silently had agreed for the same. Two months later, when the results of the karyotyping analysis came, it showed as 46XY AIS. Without the stimulation provided by the masculine hormone, her body developed a female phenotype but did not have any competitive advantage. In 1986, when she was again asked to feign an injury and withdraw herself from the race, she refused only to get her story leaked to the press. She was expelled from her athlete's residence, her sports scholarship revoked and all her running times were erased from her country's athletic records.[8]

She felt ashamed and embarrassed. She questioned herself whether her genetic difference in anyway gave her any unfair physical advantage? She could not pretend to be a man as she always had her breasts and vagina. She fought for her disqualification. Later, a Finnish geneticist and an American journalist presented her case in the press, and in 1988 to the Medical Chairman of the International Federation of Athletics which triggered the end of chromosomal based testing, and also gave her the license to run again. She had paid a huge price to get back her license. Her story was told, dissected and discussed in a very public way, though her victory was bitter sweet.[8]

Case 2: Caster Semenya Case

Mokgadi Caster Semenya is a South African middle-distance runner and world champion. The International Association of Athletics Federations (IAAF) says it was 'obliged to investigate' after she made improvements of 25 seconds at 1500 m and eight seconds at 800 m at the 2009 World Championships—'the sort of dramatic breakthroughs that usually arouse suspicion of drug use'. The IAAF also asked Semenya to undergo a sex test after the win. The IAAF's handling of the case spurred many negative reactions. Prominent South African civic leaders, commentators, politicians and activists described the controversy as racist, as well as an affront to Semenya's privacy and human rights. The IAAF said it only made the test public after it had already been reported in the media, denying charges of racism and expressing regret about 'the allegations being made about the reasons for which these tests are being conducted'. The federation also explained that the motivation for the test was not suspected cheating but a desire to determine whether she had a 'rare medical condition' giving her an unfair competitive advantage. The 'condition' was reported to be hermaphroditism.[3]

Athletics South Africa (ASA) President Leonard Chuene admitted to having subjected Semenya to sex determination tests. He had previously lied to Semenya about the purpose of the tests and to others about having performed the tests. He ignored a request from ASA team doctor Harold Adams to withdraw Semenya from the world championships over concerns about the need to keep her medical records confidential. On 6th July 2010, the IAAF cleared Semenya to return to international competition. The results of the tests, however, were not released for privacy reasons. Caster Semenya was chosen to carry the country's flag during the opening ceremony of the 2012 Summer Olympics.[3]

Case 3: Pinki Pramanik Case

The arrest and subsequent humiliation of Indian athlete and international medal winner Pinki Pramanik that violated her right to privacy, bodily integrity and basic human dignity raised important and often sidelined questions about gender, sports and the way the world is organized. Twenty-six-year-old Pramanik was accused by her live-in partner of repeated rape and torture, and of being a man. She was arrested on 14th June 2012 and was not granted bail for 26 days. She had to spend the entire period in a male cell in a West Bengal jail, and had to undergo three sex determination tests at different state hospitals, because the necessary facilities were not available at a single hospital. An MMS clip, showing her in the nude while undergoing one of the tests was leaked online and went viral. The District and Sessions Judge, while granting Pramanik bail on 11th July held that she was physically incapable of rape and that the petitioner who alleged rape had been in a consensual live-in relationship with Pramanik for nearly 3 years. Pramanik was suspended from her job as a ticket collector with the Eastern railways; the suspension was revoked after her bail. She alleged that in police custody, sex determination tests were forcibly carried out on her after drugging and tying her hands and feet.[9]

In November 2012, the West Bengal police submitted a charge-sheet before the district court in which, citing medical reports, they alleged that Pramanik is indeed male, and charged with rape. Later, the doctor who headed the medical investigation in her sex determination clarified that Pramanik suffered from a disorder of sexual development, which may be described as male pseudohermaphrodite. Pramanik has responded by saying she feels 'like a joker in a circus', and is being driven by the police to think of suicide. According to some reports, she has planned to file a defamation case against the police and the public prosecutor, and asked the West Bengal Chief Minister and the Union Sports Ministry to intervene in her case.[9]

Case 4: Santhi Soundarajan Case

Santhi Soundarajan was stripped of her 800 m silver medal after failing a sex verification test at the 2006 Doha Asian Games. She was later forced to work as a laborer in a brick kiln, before the government recently gave her an opportunity to become a qualified athletics coach. The government has removed its rider of ascertaining her sex before allowing her to pursue the diploma course in Patiala. There was a delay in getting the letter since Sports Authority of India (SAI) took a different view on the matter. Santhi's sex became the focal point, as the government agency summoned her for tests at the All India Institute of Medical Sciences on a couple of occasions. Santhi refused, wondering why she had to submit to tests if her aim was to become a coach.[10]

The situation was unprecedented as the course rules do not specify sex tests for admission. SAI explained that they were insisting on the tests as it would have helped in clearing the air, since they anticipated some discomfort in the hostels. But later on, SAI took a refreshingly different view on the matter and informed that there was no need for a sex test. They found no logic behind such a test when women are essaying major roles in men's teams and men coaching women's teams. SAI's Director General too said he was against the sex determination test. Santhi got the letter stating that 'sex verification may be relaxed' for admission to the course. She would also be given a separate room to stay at the campus.[10]

DETERMINATION OF SEX

In normal cases, the assumption is:[5]

- **Most certain evidence of sex:** Possession of ovaries in females and testes in males.
- **Highly probable evidence of sex:** Possession of secondary sexual characters, for e.g., developed breasts and vagina in females, and male distribution of hair and penis in males.
- **Presumptive evidence of sex:** Outward appearance of individual features, contours of face, clothes, voice and figure.

Routinely at birth, identifying biological sex of an individual is based on '*external genitalia*' (phenotype sex), i.e. whether it is penis and scrotum (in males) or vulva and vagina (in females). Identification of 'sex' of an individual may become problematic in:[5,11]

i. **Intersex:** They can be natural or acquired ('*hijras*' are castrated before puberty and '*zenanas*' are castrated after puberty). They may have features resembling one sex and the internal gonads could be of other sex or of both sexes (true hermaphrodite).
ii. **Transvestism:** Individuals who cross dresses for sexual gratification.
iii. **Transgender:** It is denoting or relating to an individual whose self-identity does not conform unambiguously to conventional notions of male or female gender. It is a state of one's gender identity or gender expression not matching one's assigned sex.
iv. **Transsexualism:** Individuals who have undergone sex change surgeries or sex reassignment (male-to-female or female-to-male).
v. **Concealed sex:** Individuals who hide their real sex for a motive by cross dressing.

In this context, it can be argued that majority of people with intersex conditions may identify themselves as male or female, rather than transgender or transsexual. However, some people who have intersex conditions may decide to change sex at some point in their life, so some people with intersex conditions might also identify themselves as transgender or transsexual.

Identification of biological sex in concealed sex and transvestism can be easily done by physical examination, but difficulty arises in cases of ambiguous genitalia wherein the external genitalia are a combination of both sexes. In such cases, the detection of '*internal gonads and sex chromosomes*' (genotype sex), i.e. the identification of testes and XY sex chromosomes (in males), or ovary and XX sex chromosomes (in females) solves the problem to a certain extent. Suspicion is then cast on them that they deliberately hid their real sex identity to gain advantage and are then forced towards compulsory sex verification tests. Is informed consent sought before these tests? Do they explain the limitations of these sex verification tests? Like in Pinki Pramanik case, when somebody is accused of a particular crime—is informed consent overlooked sighting Sec. 53 CrPC (medical examination of an accused of a crime)? Are we ethical in performing such tests against the wishes of an individual, even though Sec. 53 CrPC allows reasonable force in performing medical examination of an accused of a crime?[11]

DISORDERS OF SEXUAL DEVELOPMENT

The disorders of sexual development (DSD) usually pose significant problems in sex verification tests because of the ambiguity between genotype sex and phenotype sex of the individual. At 5 weeks of intrauterine development, if the Y chromosome is present, the gonads are signaled to develop into testes which produce testosterone and other male hormones. This ultimately results in the development of male reproductive organs, and at puberty, development of secondary sexual characteristics, such as increased musculature, increased skeletal muscle mass and hair growth (in face, chest and underarms).*[6]

Disorders of sexual development is a broad term encompassing any condition where external genitalia are atypical in relation to chromosome and gonads. Nowadays, this term is used to substitute the obsolete nomenclature of 'intersex', 'hermaphrodite' and 'pseudohermaphrodite', since they are based only on identifying the gonads and they fail to take into consideration whether those gonads are functioning or not. The new terms and possible diagnosis is such cases are given in Table 15.1.[6,7,12]

Table 15.1 Classification of disorders of sexual development (DSD)

Old name	*New name*	*Possible diagnosis*
True hermaphrodite	Ovotesticular DSD	46XX/46XY 45X/46XY (mixed gonadal dysgenesis)
Male pseudohermaphrodite Undervirilization of an XY male Undermasculinization of an XY male	46XY DSD	Androgen insensitivity syndrome (partial or complete) 5-α-reductase deficiency
Female pseudohermaphrodite Over virilization of an XX female Masculinization of an XX female	46XX DSD	Congenital adrenal hyperplasia
XX male or XX sex reversal	46XX testicular DSD	
XY sex reversal	46XY complete gonadal dysgenesis	
Gonadal dysgeneis	Sex chromosome DSD	45XO Turner 47XXY Klinefelter

*Although Y chromosome is the principal decisive factor in human sexual differentiation, prominent exception is 46XY females with complete androgen insensitivity syndrome (cAIS).

Different kinds of DSD have been classified. Some of these are briefly described below:[11,13,14]

1. **Ovotesticular DSD (true hermaphroditism):** It is a rare condition; also known as double-sex or bisexual. Both ovarian and testicular tissues are present. External genitalia of both sexes exist in one individual, but sex chromatin may be either male or female pattern (46XX or 46XY or mosaics). True hermaphroditism is very similar to mixed gonadal dysgenesis. The karyotype could be 46XX/46XY or 46XX/47XXY.
2. **Gonadal dysgenesis:** It refers to a defect in gonad formation that is characterized by a progressive loss of primordial germ cells in the developing gonads of an embryo with consequent formation of hypoplastic and dysfunctioning gonads composed mainly of fibrous tissue—*streak gonads*. External sexual characters are present, but testes or ovaries fail to develop at puberty. This is seen in Klinefelter syndrome, Turner syndrome and its variants (i.e. mosaicism), XX gonadal dysgenesis (pure gonadal dysgenesis 46XX), Swyer syndrome (pure gonadal dysgenesis 46XY), Perrault syndrome (XX gonadal dysgenesis with sensorineural hearing loss) and mixed gonadal dysgenesis.
    i. **Klinefelter syndrome:** It is male hypogonadism, with two or more X chromosomes and one or more Y chromosomes, most common presentation being 47XXY karyotype. Characteristic features being eunuchoid body, long legs, gynecomastia, small atrophic testes, small penis and absence of secondary male sexual characteristics. These individuals fail in external examination of genitals but would have false positive Barr body testing (as they have two X chromosomes).[15]
    ii. **Turner syndrome:** It is female hypogonadism with 45XO karyotype. Characteristics include short stature, low posterior hair line, webbing of neck and broad chest with widely spaced nipples. These individuals pass in external examination of genitals, and also have false negative Barr body testing (as they have one X chromosome).[15]
    iii. **Swyer syndrome**: The individuals with pure gonadal dysplasia and a 46XY karyotype will display variable degrees of undermasculinization, dependent upon the amount of testicular dysplasia. Both XX and XY gonadal dysgenesis are due to mutation or deletion of part of the sequence of the SRY gene. Surgery is possible to redirect external genitalia to female or male 'normal' structures.
    iv. **Mosaicism:** It is a genetic abnormality with mixture of cells with XX and XY, or X and XY sex chromosomes.[1] Accordingly we may have false positive or false negative Barr body tests depending on number of X chromosomes. In 1967, Polish sprinter Ewa Klobukowska was diagnosed as a case of mosaicism with abnormal genitalia, after being submitted to a nude parade, external genitalia examination and a chromosome analysis. Although, she passed the phenotype tests, the chromosome analysis revealed a XX/XXY mosaicism, so that she was considered as a man and banned from competitions (first individual to fail an Olympic sex test).
    v. **Mixed gonadal dysgenesis:** It is a partial gonadal dysgenesis variant of the Y chromosome mosaicism and the subjects have 45XO/46XY karyotype being characterized by unilateral testis, a contralateral streak gonad, persistent müllerian ductal structures ipsilateral with the streak gonad and

varying levels of external genitalia undervirilization. Most of the patients are reared as females while those who are highly masculinized are reared as males with testis preservation.

3. **Androgen receptor deficiency:** Androgen insensitivity is caused by receptors that are insensitive to androgens, particularly testosterone. The basic etiology is mutation in the androgen receptor gene. As a result, the individual even though genetically male (XY) and possess testes would fail to develop male characteristics.[1] These individuals would develop as female but would fail the Barr body test as they have only one X chromosome (case of Maria Patino).[8] These individuals are born and raised as girls and have female gender identity. It can be:
   i. **Complete androgen insensitivity syndrome** (cAIS), previously known as *testicular feminization,* is an X-linked recessive condition resulting in failure of normal masculinization of the external genitalia in genetically male (XY) individual. They have female external genitalia with normal labia, clitoris and vaginal introitus.

      In sports, 46XY DSD (cAIS) can be expected to have disadvantage compared to 46XX women with a functional androgen receptor, the latter benefitting from the stimulation of muscle strength by circulating testosterone (albeit low concentration). In this context, it may be argued that the presence of a uterus categorizes an individual as female. However, a woman who has undergone a hysterectomy has no uterus in the same way a woman with cAIS has no uterus, yet no questions is asked about the sex of the former.

   ii. **Incomplete androgen insensitivity:** The phenotype of individuals with partial androgen insensitivity syndrome may range from mildly virilized female external genitalia (clitorimegaly without other external anomalies) to mildly undervirilized male external genitalia (hypospadias and/or diminished penile size) with gynecomastia. They tend to be tall. Since there is some responsiveness of testosterone, they may have more muscle mass/ body weight and aggressiveness—more successful in sports.

      In either case, affected individuals have normal testes with normal production of testosterone and normal conversion to dihydrotestosterone (DHT), which differentiates this condition from 5-alpha reductase deficiency.

4. **5-α reductase deficiency (5-ARD):** This is an autosomal recessive sex-limited condition resulting in the inability to convert testosterone to the more physiologically active dihydrotestosterone (DHT). Since DHT is required for the normal masculinization of the external genitalia in utero, genetic males with 5-ARD deficiency are born with ambiguous genitalia. The individual presents with a clitoral-like phallus, markedly bifid scrotum, pseudovaginal blind-ending introitus with perineoscrotal hypospadias and a rudimentary prostate. The uterus and fallopian tubes are absent. Testes are intact and are usually found in the inguinal canal or scrotum or occasionally in the abdomen. At puberty, musculature, body and facial hair develop owing to normal levels of testosterone.[1] These individuals fail in external examination of genitals and fail in Barr body testing.

   Females homozygous for 5-ARD may present with delayed menarche, minimal acne and minimal body hair. Fertility is normal in such females.

5. **Congenital adrenal hyperplasia (CAH):** It is a condition wherein adrenal glands produce excessive amounts of testosterone in females. These individuals can develop secondary male characteristics but are genetically female (46XX, DSD), lacking testes and male reproductive organs (masculinized females).[1] Among the various forms of CAH, the 21-hydroxylase deficiency resulting from mutations or deletions of CYP21A, is most common but sexual ambiguity can also be seen in defects in 17-hydroxylase, 3β-hydroxysteroid dehydrogenase, 17-ketosteroid reductase and 11β-hydroxylase. Females appear phenotypically female at birth, but do not develop breasts or menstruate in adolescence; they may present with hypertension. Genital anomalies range from complete fusion of the labioscrotal folds and a phallic urethra to clitoromegaly, partial fusion of the labioscrotal folds, or both. These individuals fail in external examination of genitals but would have positive Barr body testing (as they have two X chromosomes).

   Males with 21-hydroxylase deficiency have normal genitalia. However, males with steroidogenic acute regulatory (StAR) deficiency, 3-β-hydroxysteroid dehydrogenase deficiency, or 17-hydroxylase deficiency may have ambiguous genitalia or female genitalia. They may be raised as girls and seek medical attention later in life because of hypertension or a lack of breast development.

TESTS TO VERIFY SEX IDENTITY

In sports, prior to 1960, an athlete needed a medical certificate signed by a doctor in their own country to verify their sex. To overcome the inherent bias in such certificates, official sex verification testing in sports started in 1960. In this procedure, '*nude parading*' of female competitors before a panel of judges (female doctors) which included 'manual inspection of the external genitalia' started, only to result in resentment, embarrassment and high risk of incorrect evaluation (for the reasons explained above).[1] Such crude tests were subsequently not accepted which were demeaning, and blatantly violate the dignity and privacy of an individual.[6,11]

This was replaced by '*nuclear sexing or microscopic test or sex chromatin test*' (in 1967) wherein buccal epithelial cells or hair follicle cells were sampled and examined microscopically to detect the presence of '*Barr body*'. If Barr bodies were detected then a certificate of 'femininity' was being issued.[1] Thus, in males (XY) possessing only one X chromosome would produce negative Barr body test. But this testing also has its problems in cases of AIS, 5-α-reductase deficiency and Turner's syndrome. Women with Turner syndrome (XO) would 'pass' the anatomically based tests but 'fail' the sex chromatin test. Conversely, men with Klinefelter syndrome (XXY) would 'fail' the anatomically based test but 'pass' the sex chromatin test as their second 'X' would be inactivated and forms a Barr body. Women with AIS (complete or partial) will not have Barr body and thus fail in sex chromatin test. The chromatin test has its own limitations since Barr bodies are not detected in every cell, and so are chances of false negative conclusions (20% uncertainty).[6,11]

Subsequently, the sex chromatin test was replaced by the gene-based test. The use of polymerase chain reaction (PCR) for the detection of SRY gene (sex-determining region of the Y-chromosome) and/or the DYZ1 region of

Y chromosome became diagnostic.[1] SRY gene is expressed in a small group of somatic cells of the developing gonads, and it is responsible for the expression of a male-specific cell membrane component (the H-Y antigen) and induces them to become Sertoli cells. In this, a sample is obtained (any cell, including blood) and the DNA is extracted. The diagnostic regions of the gene are amplified using PCR. The amplification product can be isolated by size by running through the electric field and visualized with a DNA-staining dye. The presence of an amplification product was evidence of an XY genotype. This test correctly diagnosed Turner and Klinefelter individuals but not able to solve the troublesome problem of AIS women, as they are genetically male and therefore have diagnostic SRY gene and DYZ1 region.[6,11]

The molecular test also had difficulties—chromosomal abnormalities can cause inactivation or deletion of the sex-determining SRY region leading to sex-reversed XY women, who might pass the test for SRY region but fail for the test for DYZ1. Moreover, SOX 9 can mimic SRY and is essential for male development, so the presence of SRY alone is not a definitive molecular marker of maleness.[11]

Accuracy of the test was an issue too. Although the PCR technique was supposed to identify uniquely male DNA sequences, further investigation revealed that it also had false positive test results.[3] Subsequently, a *combination of all these tests* including *chromosomal studies* and *hormonal assays* were carried out to determine the 'sex' of the individual.

Now IAAF have proposed that *assay of testosterone levels* will help in differentiating the sex of an individual. For females, they should have levels less than 10 nmol/l (lower than the lower limit of normal for male). Only female athletes who have testosterone levels below the 'normal male range,' or who have an androgen resistance condition, are permitted to participate in women's competitions. This may sound great, but it has its own demerits. Though this may easily segregate those with synthetic supplements of testosterone and also detect those cases of high natural testosterones of adrenal hyperplasia wherein they may have beneficial effects (increased musculature, power and strength), it may falsely implicate those cases of cAIS wherein even though there are high levels of testosterones, these individuals cannot make use of this hormone. Moreover, the female's testosterone level vary on circadian rhythm (time of day, month and life), tissue responses that vary across individuals due to differences in hormone receptors, and laboratory testing methodology.[16-18]

CURRENT STATUS OF SEX VERIFICATION TESTS

In sports, the compulsory testing of all female competitors (in an effort to prevent male imposters) was banned in 1992. It was irony to test all females, when the real culprits were males who were posing as imposters and the illogic compulsory testing continued for decades in this male dominated society. Currently, the International Olympic Committee's (IOC) policy is, a female athlete is considered for sex determination and evaluation in the following conditions:[16-18]

1. If a female athlete already has been diagnosed with hyperandrogenism, she is required to notify and undergo evaluation (Box 15.1).
2. If there are reasonable grounds for believing that a case of hyperandrogenism may exist in any female athlete, evaluation may be initiated by concerned official (suspicion-based testing).

Box 15.1 Conditions leading to hyperandrogenism in women (first six are DSD conditions)

i. Congenital adrenal hyperplasia (CAH): 21-hydroxylase or 11β-hydroxylase deficiency
ii. 3β-hydroxysteroid dehydrogenase deficiency
iii. 5α-Reductase type 2 deficiency
iv. Androgen insensitivity syndrome (AIS)
v. Ovotesticular DSD
vi. 17β-hydroxysteroid dehydrogenase type 3 deficiency
vii. Polycystic ovary syndrome
viii. Adrenal carcinoma
ix. Luteoma of pregnancy

Today, the sport's governing bodies adopt more comprehensive medical evaluation by a team of experts including gynecologist, endocrinologist, internal medicine expert, geneticist, and an expert on gender/transgender issues (expertise in hyperandrogenism).[12] The concerned person has to undergo a combination of three types of examinations:[16-18]

i. Clinical examination;
ii. Endocrine examination (testing urine and blood for hormone levels); and/or
iii. Full examination (which may include genetic testing, imaging and psychological evaluation).

The expert panel will then examine all available information and establish:

i. Whether the investigated athlete's androgen level, measured by reference to testosterone levels in serum is within the female range,
ii. Whether hyperandrogenism (if present) is functional or not.

In order to help protect the dignity and privacy of the athlete concerned, requests for investigations, information gathered during investigations, results of investigations and decisions regarding a case (or potential case) of female hyperandrogenism should be kept confidential and not released or made public.

Following evaluation, if she 'fails', then a final diagnosis and 'therapeutic proposal' is issued to her in writing. She is banned from competitions till her testosterone is within the approved levels. If she follows the 'prescribed medical treatment', she may be reassessed for possible participation in future women's competitions. The treatment includes either pharmaceutical intervention and/or gonadectomy.

The sole aim of such an evaluation being, that there should not be any unfair advantage by virtue of increased androgen levels and increased skeletal musculature as a result of DSD; or no unfair height as a result of increased growth hormones following estrogen hormonal supplements post sex-change surgeries. Though there is a theoretical possibility of above assumption, with lack of research evidence, it remains difficult to disqualify individuals of DSD due to their increased androgen levels and increased skeletal musculature or increased height post estrogen therapy, and categorically say they cannot compete as female competitors. Treatment decisions should be individualized and to what extent it is safe and effective is a matter of debate. Moreover, anti-androgens used to treat can have potentially debilitating side-effects for an athlete.

The Canadian Academy of Sports Medicine recommends that 'individuals raised as females and are psychologically and socially females from childhood should be eligible to compete in women's competition regardless of their chromosomal, gonadal and hormonal sex'.[2]

GUIDELINES FOR INDIA

At present, we do not have any guidelines from either Medical Council of India (MCI) or Indian Council of Medical Research (ICMR). Hence, good practice guidelines from the IOC/sports field can be followed.

ETHICAL ISSUES

- Sex verification testing is often done compulsorily which ought to have been voluntary (autonomy of the person).
- It is discriminatory as only females are tested, and also as athletes are unfairly disqualified for genetic abnormalities which do not give them unfair advantage.
- It is regarded as invasive and abusive, and disregard of autonomy of female athlete. The testing is performed during sports competitions, once the athlete has arrived at an international competition site, away from home and without her personal support group. The opinions of athletes are not considered in the debate on sex testing.[19]
- Sex verification testing of athletes should be considered as human rights violation and eliminated from all levels of sport.[20]
- These tests are unfair, unscientific and possibly discriminatory against woman who may not meet the traditional notions of femininity.[21]
- The limitations of the sex verification tests are never brought to the knowledge of the person undergoing the tests.
- The results of these tests should be confidential and not available for public and/or media scrutiny; but in reality it is the converse.
- Now that the sport's governing bodies are asking for mandatory treatment of a sportsperson if their testosterone levels are abnormal (before they wish to compete again)—it definitely violates the autonomy of a person.
- Doctors treating sportspersons also face dilemma whether to consider long-term health consequences or short-term gains in them (as sports person) whenever they supplement hormones in sex reassigned sports persons.

LEGAL ASPECTS

The law regarding intersexuality is largely underdeveloped or ignored in most of the countries. In the US, intersexuality has been explored in the area of marriage, employment, criminal justice, and human rights—with all case law holding that the law does not provide protection to those with intersex status. Columbia and Australia seem to be the only countries that have begun to give some protection to intersex individuals. In one Australian province, 'legislation regarding police searches also includes intersex.' The law allows for intersex individual to request either a male or female to conduct a clothing or body search—a first in criminal law towards recognition of intersex. In Columbia, the Constitutional court has issued directives for the protection of human rights of intersex individuals, and limited the authority of both parents and doctors to authorize medically unnecessary genital plastic surgery—they considered the social and psychological impacts due to intersex, if they assign wrong sex to the child. The legal issues pertaining to transgender and sex verification tests are discussed below:[3,9,11,22,23]

- **Informed consent:** Often the sex verification tests are done compulsorily or in a situation where the examinee is not having any choice to decide. If at all consent is obtained it may not be an informed one (like in sports competitions). In case of an examination of a person accused of crime, often it is presumed that consent is not needed if a requisition is received under Sec. 53 CrPC (like in Pinki Pramanik case). But Sec. 53 CrPC only authorizes use of reasonable force! And nowhere it mentions examination should be done without consent. Ideally speaking, the doctor should provide all the information on the sex verification tests including its inferences and limitations and then seek consent. Only such informed consent is valid in the eyes of law.
- **Privacy and confidentiality:** The leaking of the nude photos of Pinki Pramanik while undergoing medical examination speaks volumes about the violation of privacy and confidentiality. Even in sports competitions, the results of such sex verification tests should be kept confidential. If a sports person is disqualified on not meeting the qualifying criteria on sex verification tests, she should be given an opportunity to withdraw from the competition rather than disclosing the test results to public and/or media. Otherwise, every person undergoing such a humiliation would not hesitate to file a defamation suit as is the case of Pinki Pramanik.
- **Contract:** Sex verification in employments (military), professional beauty pageant contests depend on their policies of contract; however no sex verification tests could be unscientific, inhuman, unethical or irrational or forced on an individual against their will.
- **Marriage:** Even Sec. 4 of the Special Marriage Act, 1954 mentions about a male and a female can only marry. So, if an intersex person has married without bringing it to the knowledge of the other partner (information about the condition), then that marriage could be nullified, if the aggrieved challenges it in the court.
- **Employment:** If a post is reserved for a particular sex, for e.g. female, and if a DSD person gets that post, it can be definitely challenged by the aggrieved female who is next in the waiting list and could have got the post as it was exclusively reserved for females.
- **Inheritance of property:** Today, even religious laws also recognize the right of a female to get property inherited from the ancestral property. But in a situation of self acquired property, if the bequeather stipulates condition that the property should be inherited by either a male or a female, then definitely an intersex person loses the right, if there is an aggrieved male or a female (depending on the situation) challenging it.
- **Civil rights and human rights:** The Declaration of Human Rights from the United Nations ensures these rights for everyone. Thus, even the intersex persons are also included. This is the basis for the successful legal battles of those aggrieved (Maria Patino or Caster Semenya or Pinki Pramanik) in any country. The Guidelines from International Olympic Association/ International Amateur Athletics Federation also are in this regard guaranteeing fairness, rights and privacy. Countries like Australia and Germany have already recognized the third sex, thus putting an end to the issues of marriage,

employment and inheritance of property in their countries. India till now allowed the option of third sex entry in some of the official documents like the voter's card and Aadhar card. However, in a landmark judgment, the Supreme Court directed the federal and state governments to include transgender people in all welfare programs for the poor, including education, health care and jobs to help them overcome social and economic challenges. The court noted that it is the right of every human being to choose their gender while granting rights to those who identify themselves as neither male nor female. All documents will now have a third category marked 'transgender.' The court's decision would apply to individuals who have acquired the physical characteristics of the opposite sex or present themselves in a way that does not correspond with their sex at birth. The Supreme Court specified its ruling would only apply to transgender people but not to gays, lesbians or bisexuals. The court ruled that transgender people would have the same right to adopt children as other Indians. The court said any person who underwent surgery to change his or her sex would be entitled to be legally recognized as belonging to the gender of their choice.[24]

- **Investigations of a crime:** Sex verification in crime cases (Pinki Pramanik) depend on the charges leveled against the accused. In this case, charge of rape (Sec. 375 IPC) had to be decided by confirming whether Pinki Pramanik was indeed a male. In Indian legal system, the investigating officers are empowered to do everything possible to investigate a case (including sex verification tests). In such sex specific offences, often they claim that there is no alternate choice. What remains is how scientifically we can conclude such sex verification tests with proper reasoning. In this era of media trails (rational or not?) and with unethical corrupt practices, the accused is painted as culprit even before being properly heard in the courts (as in Pinki Pramanik case). Ultimately, if the accused is indeed an innocent person, who is accountable for all the mental agony, defamation and losses/damages suffered?

Pinki Pramanik's ordeal and its media coverage have had ripple effects, voyeurism aside. There are two charges leveled against her, connected in some ways, but should not be conflated. One is the question of whether Pramanik raped and tortured her partner, and the second is the question of whether she is a man. Both questions may confuse. But her absolution from one does not necessarily imply absolution from the other. And yet, in the media, only one question was standing in for all the charges against Pramanik, as though her femaleness, if proven, would subsume within it any possibility of sexual assault, and mental or physical torture, *particularly against another woman*. This betrays the easy and utterly homogenized idea in the public imagination that only two gender identities, with only one kind of (hetero)sexual relationship between them are possible and legitimate. And this kind of polarized media representation—symptomatic of the larger gender politics that erases plurality, and disallows more considered and nuanced discussions—did not end here. The more Pramanik's humiliation at the hands of legal and medical authorities outraged us, the more the space to consider the other, unrelated question of whether Pramanik was guilty of sexually assaulting her partner shrank, and became impossible to address. In our liberal imagination that follows the agent/victim binary, Pramanik had become, and not wrongly so, the victim.

Rape is defined too narrowly in India, wherein only a man can be charged with rape. Pramanik could not have raped another woman, if she is proven to have female genitalia. Yet, it is a well documented fact that like any other intimate relationship, same sex relationships do not enjoy immunity from power-play, violence and sexual assault. Hence, the following considerations emerge: rape needs to be understood and redefined as an experience of subjugation and violation that can occur not just in a heterosexual setting. Also, same sex relationships carry the same potential for abuse as any other intimate relationship. Consent for sex is required even in a consensual relationship and no matter how many 'yeses' preceded it, a 'no' is always a 'NO'. If sexual violence has taken place in a relationship between two women, it merits scrutiny, even though due process may have to differ for certain reasons.

POSTMORTEM FEATURES

Identification of sex of an individual is one of the objectives of medicolegal autopsy. In fresh cases, external physical characteristics and genital characteristics help in identification of sex of the individual (Box 15.2). Internal gonads help in confirming the sex of the individual. There are no such reports of genetic studies, chromosomal analysis and hormonal assays being done in medicolegal cases for identification of sex of the individual. Identification of sex of an individual in burnt and decomposed bodies, and mutilated remains poses a significant challenge wherein use of DNA analysis to identify sex of an individual is in vogue.

RECOMMENDATIONS

- Seek informed consent before performing the sex verification tests.
- Maintain privacy and confidentiality of all the information.
- Perform a combination of tests to verify the sex of an individual preferably by a team of doctors including gynecologist, endocrinologist, internal medicine expert, geneticist, and an expert on gender/trans gender issues. The forensic medicine specialist should also be part of the team to look into medicolegal issues.

Box 15.2 Transexual autopsy case

Case Report

A 24-year-old transexual was found hanging in her bedroom. The ligature material used was a saree which was tied to the metal hanger of the ceiling roof. The dead body was of length 170 cms, weight 58 kg and moderately built individual. When the autopsy was conducted apart from the ligature mark on the neck and features of asphyxia, there were signs related to her identity as transexual. Face was clean shaven. In front of the chest, on both inframammary areas, there were surgically sutured scar marks. On dissection underneath, breast silicone implants were found indicating breast augmentation surgery done on both the sides. Nipple and areola were relatively small. The genitals showed pubic hair distribution more inclined towards a male pattern. The external genitalia appeared to be towards female type with sex reassignment surgery done with an opening for urethra, feminizing genitoplasty and penectomy. On internal examination, there were no ovaries or uterus or testes (Figs 15.1 to 15.5).

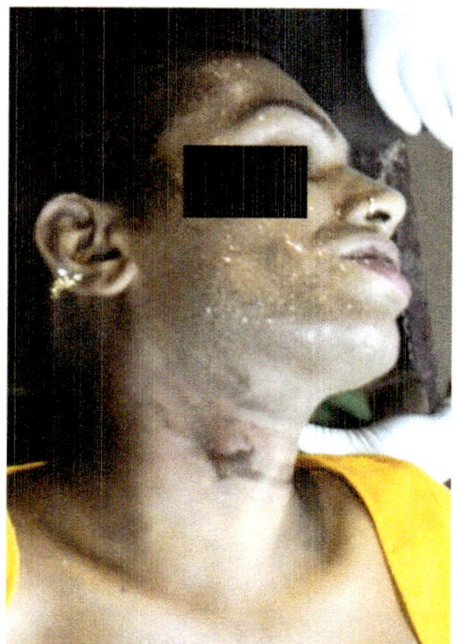

Fig. 15.1 Prominent adams apple, chin and mustache (appeared to be shaven with tiny hair buds of 1 mm) and ligature mark over the neck

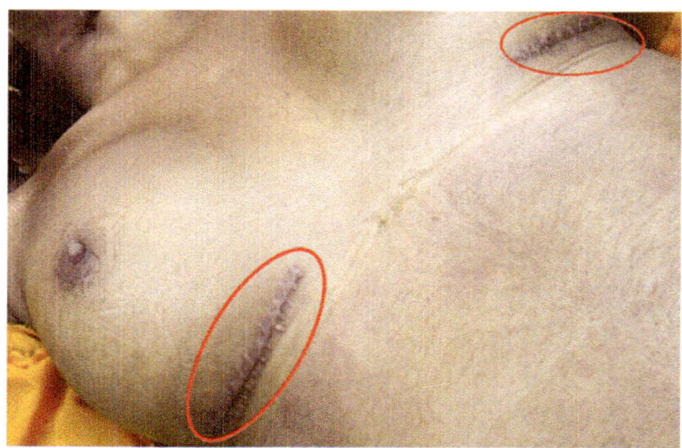

Fig. 15.2 Inframammary surgically sutured scar mark indicating breast augmentation surgery done on both the sides

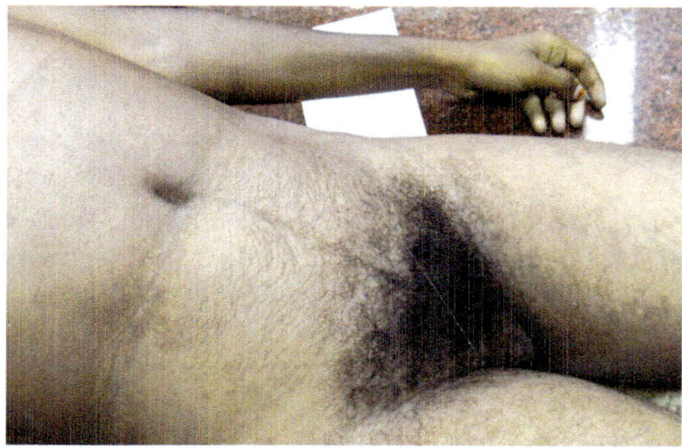

Fig. 15.3 Male pattern of hair distribution in abdomen and pubic regions, with feminine looking external genitalia

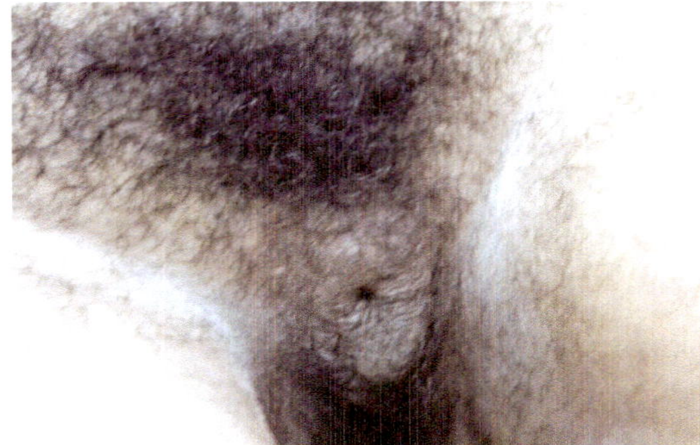

Fig. 15.4 Sex reassignment surgery done with an opening for urethra, feminizing genitoplasty and penectomy

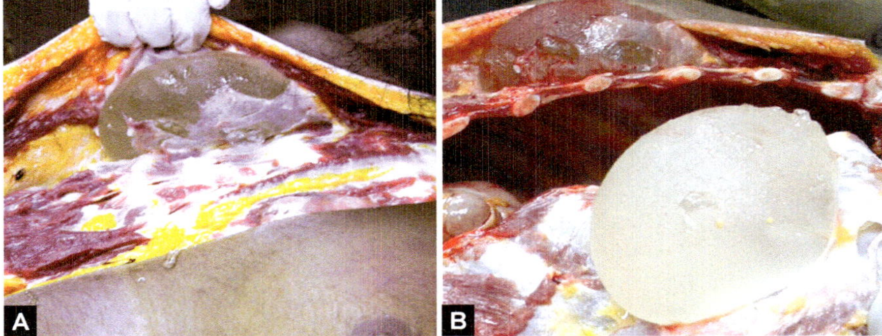

Figs 15.5A and B Breast silicone implant seen on reflection of chest

- Perform external physical and genital examination, internal gonadal examination and hormonal assay, and if needed, chromosomal assay.
- Perform all these tests following all ethical principles and laws of the land.
- The causes and consequences of hyperandrogenism should be dealt with in private, not in public and without questioning gender identity.

CONCLUSION

When today's scientific community does not have a single test to provide accurate answer for all cases of sex verification, can we consider our grannies are passing wrong verdicts on such sex verifications with ignorance? With such ignorance if some innocent individual is raised till puberty and adulthood with wrong sexual identity; is our society conducive to answer the needs/rights of such individuals? Are we not violating the rights of those individuals who want to recognize themselves with 'a' particular sexual identity? With the recent Supreme Court judgment paving way for the recognition of transgender in passports, driving licenses, PAN cards, ration cards and bank accounts; it is also eagerly anticipated to end the misery of all those intersex persons in availing legal benefits related to marriage, adoption, divorce, succession and inheritance of property.[24]

The issues related to individuals who undergo deliberate sex change surgeries (pre-pubertal or post-pubertal) as a 'right' to identify themselves with other sexual identity of their choice (which is other than their birth sex) are least understood. Only time should provide answers to the ethical, legal and social issues related to deliberate sex change surgeries.

Sex verification tests, though accepted by society, should not be forced on any individual against their consent nor performed violating privacy or dignity of the individual. With the inherent limitations of the accuracy of the results, utmost confidentiality has to be maintained in disclosing the results. The consequence of false positives is immense. Harm is documented in a number of cases including unjustified disqualifications or banning from competitions (in sports). With lot of intricacies involved in clear understanding of the conditions causing ambiguity in sexual identity, the society and the media should always have restraint in being judgmental before understanding the nitty-gritty of the situation.

After so many decades of sex verification tests done in international sport competitions, there were only few instances wherein a man has been caught masquerading as a female. In most instances, sex determination tests have mostly 'caught' women with DSD. If the abnormal results are made public, there may be long lasting psychological damage. This includes humiliation, embarrassing scrutiny of their sexuality, sex and gender identity crisis, sarcasm, demeaning reactions, social isolation depression and suicide. The only valid reason for conducting such tests would be that the individual gets the medical attention and psychological support she needs. Even with so much of scientific development today, we have limited solutions for all the ethical, legal and social concerns of these sex verification tests.

ACKNOWLEDGMENT

The author would like to thank Dr Shobana SS, Assistant Professor, Forensic Medicine and Toxicology, Vydehi Institute of Medical Sciences and Research Centre, Bangalore for sharing the photographs of the autopsy case.

REFERENCES

1. Tucker R, Collins M. The science of sex verification and athletic performance. *Int J Sports Physiol Perform* 2010; 5: 127-39. Available from: http://www.adas.org.rs/.../doping-The-science-of-sex-verification-and-athle...
2. Tucker R, Collins M. The science and management of sex verification in sport. *S Afr J SM* 2009; 21: 147-50. Available from: http://www.sajsm.org.za/index.php/sajsm/article/download/147/129.
3. Wiesemann C. Is there a right not to know one's sex? The ethics of 'gender verification' in women's sports competition, *J Med Ethics* 2011; 37: 216-20. Available from: http://jme.bmj.com/content/37/4/216.abstract.
4. Reeser JC. Gender identity and sport: is the playing field level? *Br J Sports Med* 2005; 39: 695-99. Available from: http://bjsm.bmj.com/content/39/10/695.full.
5. Biswas G. Identification-I. Review of forensic medicine and toxicology. 2nd edn. New Delhi: Jaypee Brothers; 2012. p. 45-69.
6. Rupert JL. Genitals to genes: the history and biology of gender verification in the Olympics. *Can Bull Med Hist* 2011; 28: 339-65.
7. Martínez-Patiño MJ, Mateos-Padorno C, Martínez-Vidal A, Sánchez AM, García JL, Díaz MP, Touriño CF. An approach to the biological, historical and psychological

repercussions of gender verification in top level competitions. *J Hum Sport Exerc* 2010; 5: 307-21.
8. Patino MJM. Personal account a woman tried and tested. Lancet. 2005; 366: S38. Available from: http://www.thelancet.com/journals/lancet/article/PIIS0140-6736(05)67841-5/fulltext.
9. Marwah V. Gender bending, gender testing: reflections on the Pinki Pramanik case. *Indian J Med Ethics* 2013; 10: 45-48.
10. Narayan Swamy V. Door opens for Santhi Soundarajan after gender humiliation. Times of India [Internet]. 2013, March 29. Available from: http://articles.timesofindia.indiatimes.com/2013-03-29/others/38125168_1_nis-patiala-gender-test-santhi-soundarajan.
11. Jagadeesh N. Sex verification tests: ethical, legal and social aspects. *Indian J Med Ethics* 2013; 10: 49-51.
12. Huges IA, Houk C, Ahmed SF, Lee PA. Consensus statement on management of intersex disorders. *Arch Dis Child* 2006; 91: 554-63.
13. Hutcheson J. Ambiguous genitalia and intersexuality. http://emedicine.medscape.com/article/1015520-overview.
14. Öçal G. Current concepts in disorders of sexual development. *J Clin Res Pediatr Endocrinol* 2011; 3: 105-14.
15. Bhuvaneshwari S. Identification. In: Pillay VV (ed). Textbook of forensic medicine and toxicology. 16th edn. Hyderabad: Paras medical publisher; 2011. p. 52.
16. Xavier NA, McGill JB. Hyperandrogenism and intersex controversies in women's Olympics. *J Clin Endocrinol Metab* 2012; 97: 3902-07.
17. Ballantyne KN, Kayser M, Grootegoed JA. Sex and gender issues in competitive sports: investigation of a historical case leads to a new viewpoint. *Br J Sports Med* 2012; 46: 614-17.
18. Karkazis K, Jordan-Young R, Davis G, Camporesi S. Out of bounds? A critique of the new policies on hyperandrogenism in elite female athletes. *Am J Bioethics* 2012; 12: 3-16.
19. Canadian Academy of Sports Medicine. Position statement, Sex testing (Gender verification) in sports. Available from: http://www.casm-acms.org/forms/statements/GendereVerifEng.pdf.
20. Promising practices: working with transitioning /transitioned athletes in sport project. http://www.transgenderlaw.org/resources/InclTransitioning.pdf.
21. Is the International Olympic Committee's policy governing sex verification fair? http://scopeblog.stanford.edu/2012/06/25/is-the-international-olympic-committees-policy-governing-sex-verification-fair/.
22. Larson S. Intersexuality and gender verification tests: The need to assure human rights and privacy. *Pace International Law Review* 2011; 23: 215-48. Available from: http://digitalcommons.pace.edu/pilr/vol23/iss1/6.
23. Bhan G. The right to our bodies. The Times of India [Internet]. 2012 July 9. Available from: http://articles.timesofindia.indiatimes.com/2012-07-09/edit-page/32589114_1_gender-identity-pinki-pramanik-gender-test.
24. Supreme Court recognizes transgender as third gender. The Times of India, epaper. Available from: http://timesofindia.indiatimes.com/india/Supreme-Court-recognizes-transgenders-as-third-gender/articleshow/33767900.cms.

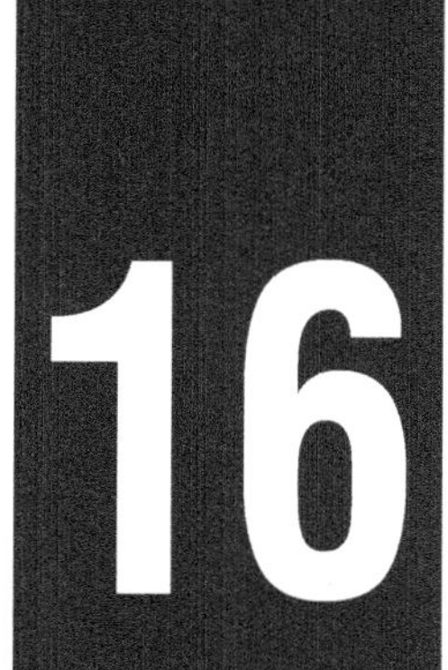

Victim Identification in Mass Disasters

Suresh K Dhattarwal

'The boundaries which divide life from death are at best shadowy and vague. Who shall say where one ends, and the other begins?'
Edgar Alan Poe (American author, poet and literary critic)

ABSTRACT

A disaster is an occurrence disrupting the normal conditions of existence and causing a level of suffering that exceeds the capacity of adjustment of the affected community.[1] Mass disasters are global occurrence and India is no exception with floods, droughts, cyclones, earthquakes and landslides being recurrent phenomena. Mass disasters not only results in loss of human lives, but economic loss as well. Law enforcement and/or public safety and health officials often have the responsibility of identifying the human remains found at the scene, so they can be returned to their families. The recovered human remains range from being relatively intact to highly degraded and dismembered body parts. The various means of identification are visual identification, fingerprint analysis, DNA, dental analysis, physical characteristics, personal belongings and clothing.[2]

The most common role of the forensic odontologist is the identification of deceased individuals. Since, dental tissues are resistant to environmental assaults such as incineration, immersion, trauma, mutilation and decomposition, teeth represent an excellent source of DNA material. DNA-based identity testing is a powerful tool and the data are not restricted to any particular one-to-one body landmark comparison. DNA profile comparisons can be used to associate separated remains or body parts. Even though DNA typing is straightforward, a disaster is a chaotic environment that can complicate effective identification of the remains. With some planning and preparedness, and approaching the situation as per the 'standard protocols', an early and accurate identification of the deceased can be achieved. In our country, in many of these 'standard' mass disaster plans, the role of forensic pathologist is often ignored or even if it is mentioned, provision of logistic support is never a priority for the policy makers with obviously no thought as to how crisis could be managed with the hands tied. This chapter outlines the effective management and early identification of victims in mass disaster situation.

Keywords: Natural disasters, loss analysis, risk reduction, DNA, mass disaster, missing person, human remains, identification, PM odontogram.

INTRODUCTION

Mass disasters have been variously defined in the literature, but a common theme is serious disruption of the functioning of a community or a society causing widespread human, material, economic or environmental losses which exceed the ability of the affected community or society to cope using its own resources.[3] The overwhelming nature of this kind of situation often requires the importation of forensic and policing expertise from other jurisdictions in order to cope effectively.[4]

In the modern world, weapons of mass destruction (for e.g., biological, chemical) are increasingly becoming cause of mass disaster, both in an armed conflict and a terrorist act. The others can be considered as civilizational disasters which may be due to technological progress like the recent 'Himalayan Tsunami' at Uttarakhand.

One of the key issues during the disaster response is the need to identify victims. Disaster victim identification is done by employing all possible methods—visual identification, collection of fingerprints, dental data, hair, physical identification of documents, jewellery and other belongings.[5] Moreover, with globalization of the world, mass disasters these days often involve victims of many different nationalities, requiring the assistance of DVI teams from various countries.[6] Every natural or man-made disaster presents a different set of circumstances and, consequently, each event results in new challenges for identification teams. This chapter discusses the systematic approach in cases of mass disaster which may ultimately help in early identification of the victims and repatriation to their families.

DEFINITIONS

- **Disaster:** A sudden ecological phenomenon of sufficient magnitude to require external assistance (WHO).[5]

  The term *disaster* owes its origin to the French word *desastre*, which is a combination of two words *des* meaning 'bad' and '*aster*' meaning 'star'. In earlier days, disasters were considered to be an outcome or outburst of some unfavorable star.[1] The distinction should be drawn between *mass disasters* and *multifatality incidents*—those in which local personnel and infrastructure are adequate for the task of timely and sufficiently comprehensive medicolegal death investigation, as opposed to a disaster situation which by definition, overwhelms the capacity of local agencies.
- **Disaster victim identification (DVI):** Process and procedures for recovering and identifying deceased people and human remains in multifatality incidents.
- **Forensic anthropology** is the application of the science of physical anthropology to identify human remains and to assist in the detection of crime.[7]
- **Forensic odontology** deals with the application of dentistry to aid in the identification of unknown bodies through dental records.[8]

CLASSIFICATION

Mass disaster can be broadly classified into natural and human-generated.

Natural disasters: The Center for Research on the Epidemiology of Disasters (CRED), located in Brussels, Belgium, maintains the official international disaster registry. Whenever a disaster occurs anywhere in the globe, the event is reported to CRED and logged into the disaster database. CRED classifies natural disasters (acts of nature) into four sub-categories:[9]

i. *Hydrometeorological disasters* include weather-related events such as tropical cyclones (hurricanes, typhoons and cyclones), windstorms, winter-storms, tornadoes and floods.
ii. *Geophysical disasters* are seismic events related to the motion of the earth's tectonic plates. Prominent among geophysical events are earthquakes, tsunamis and volcanoes.
iii. *Droughts* are grouped with additional events including extreme hot and cold temperatures, wildfires, forest fire and insect infestations.
iv. *Pandemic diseases* are distinguished by the global spread of newly-emerging infectious diseases or uncharacteristically virulent strains of well-known foes such as influenza.

Human-generated disasters include various forms of 'technological' disasters. This can be further subdivided into:

a. Non-intentional
b. Intentional events

Human-Generated: Non-intentional

Failures of human technologies are rarely intentional. However, poor judgment or human neglect may be precipitating or contributory factors.

i. Transportation/vehicle accidents: Air/space, rail, road/highway.
ii. Miscellaneous
    - *Structural collapse:* Building, bridge, dam, tunnel
    - *Fire/incineration:* Structure fire, explosion
    - *Hazardous materials release/spill:* Chemical, gas/aerosol, radiation, biological agent.
iii. Ecological/environmental destruction.

Human-Generated: Intentional

Intentional acts of 'mass violence' occur as an outcome of acts of terrorism, declared war, civil strife and ethnic conflict, and may also eventuate from mass gatherings and demonstrations.[10]

i. Race/ethnic conflict
ii. Violent mass gatherings
iii. Terrorism
    - *Biological:* Aerosol anthrax, smallpox, pneumonic plague, food contamination
    - *Chemical:* Blister agent, nerve gas, chlorine gas, toxic industrial chemical
    - *Nuclear:* Improvised nuclear device, radiological dispersal device (dirty bomb)
    - *Conventional:* Improvised explosive device.

HISTORY AND EPIDEMIOLOGY

The earliest recorded natural disaster—the eruption of Santorini in the Aegean Sea was in 1628 BC. Another catastrophe was in 79 BC, which resulted in death of thousands of victims at Pompeii and Herculaneum. In the next 2,000 years, various types of disasters were recorded, notably among them was the plague epidemic which claimed 75 million lives in the years 1347-51; explosions of volcanoes in Indonesia in 1815 and 1833 with 90,000 and 40,000 deaths respectively; events in China, like flooding along the river Huang-Ho in 1887 (one million victims), landslides in the province of Kansu in 1920 (180,000 killed) or the blowing up of a dam on the Yang-tse-kiang in 1938 (890,000 deaths); the cyclone in Bangladesh in 1970 (300,000 victims); the earthquake in Tangsham, China in 1976 (750,000 deaths) and the earthquake in Haiti in January 2010 (230,000 deaths). Recently, in Japan (2011), an earthquake followed by a tsunami resulted in 28,000 deaths. Other man-made disasters include the explosion of the Chernobyl nuclear reactor in Ukraine in 1986 (between 31,000 and 75,000 killed) and the terrorist attack on the Twin Towers of the World Trade Center in New York City in 2001, which killed nearly 3,000 people.[5]

India too is vulnerable, in varying degrees, to a large number of natural as well as man-made disasters. About 60% of the landmass is prone to earthquakes of moderate to very high intensity, over 40 million hectares (12% of land) is prone to floods and river erosion; of the 7,516 km long coastline, close to 5,700 km is prone to cyclones and tsunamis; 68% of the cultivable area is vulnerable to drought and hilly areas are at risk from landslides and avalanches. Vulnerability to disasters of chemical, biological, radiological and nuclear (CBRN) origin also exists. A chemical disaster happened in Bhopal in 1984, wherein 3,500 were killed. Heightened vulnerabilities to disaster risks can be related to expanding population, urbanization and industrialization, development within high-risk zones, environmental degradation and climate change. In June, 2013, about 5,000–10,000 people died and thousands of people went missing following the floods and landslides in Uttarakhand (Fig. 16.1). Environmentalists and experts consider it a man-made disaster, since they attribute this to unplanned development and deforestation as a chief cause for the disaster. Data related to human and economic losses from disasters that have occurred between 1980 and 2010 is given in Table 16.1.[11]

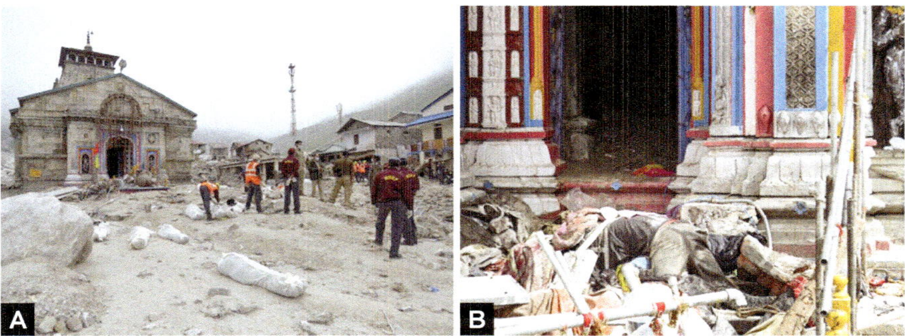

Figs 16.1A and B Recent mass disaster in Uttarakhand (Kedarnath) (*Courtesy:* Dr Sanjoy Dass, Prof. and Head, FMT, Himalayan Institute of Medical Sciences, Dehradun, Uttarakhand, India)

Table 16.1 Human and economic losses from disasters (1980–2010)

Number of events	431
Number of people killed	143,039
Average killed per year	4,614
Number of people affected	1,521,726,127
Average affected per year	49,087,940
Economic damage (US$ X 1,000)	48,063,830
Economic damage per year (US$ X 1,000)	1,550,446

OBJECTIVES OF DISASTER MANAGEMENT

The main objectives of mass disaster management are the following:[12]

1. Promoting a culture of prevention, preparedness and resilience at all levels through knowledge, innovation and education.
2. Encouraging mitigation measures based on technology, traditional wisdom and environmental sustainability.
3. Mainstreaming disaster management into the developmental planning process.
4. Establishing institutional and technolegal frameworks to create an enabling regulatory environment and a compliance regime.
5. Ensuring efficient mechanism for identification, assessment and monitoring of disaster risks.
6. Developing contemporary forecasting and early warning systems backed by responsive and failsafe communication with information technology support.
7. Promoting a productive partnership with the media to create awareness and contributing towards capacity development.
8. Ensuring efficient response and relief with a caring approach towards the needs of the vulnerable sections of the society.

DISASTER VICTIM IDENTIFICATION (DVI)

The proper identification of a deceased individual is not only important for humanitarian and emotional reasons for the next-of-kin, but also for legal and administrative purposes. However, this identification issue that can withstand legal scrutiny, represents one of the most difficult medicolegal and anthropological tasks. All possible means must be applied to achieve a scientific identification which is sometimes extremely difficult, particularly in mass disaster situations or in matters of genocide crimes.[7] The primary and most reliable means of identification are visual identification, fingerprint analysis, comparative dental analysis and DNA analysis.[13] The secondary means of identification include personal description, medical findings as well as evidence and clothing found on the body. These means of identification serve to support identification by other means and are ordinarily not sufficient as a sole means of identification.[2]

Visual Identification

Visual identification is the most frequently used method of identification. Whenever a dead body is found or before starting of autopsy, this is attempted by involving person(s) (friends or relatives) familiar with the deceased stating that the victim is a particular person. Visual identification can be corroborated by viewing of property, such as clothing, documents or jewellery found on the body. This is a preferred method, since it is an inexpensive, quick and easy. However, in some circumstances, such as postmortem animal predation, putrefaction, facial trauma or disfigurement, burn or skeletonization may make visual identification unacceptable. In situations of multiple fatalities from the same family, there may be nobody to view the body and conduct a visual identification. Sometimes, families are extremely distressed about the death of a relative and may find it hard to identify a body positively. In these instances, other methods of identification are attempted. Even if the victim is identified by relatives, the body is subjected to autopsy to address the other issues concerned.

The protocol of the disaster victim identification described below is to be followed especially for unidentified bodies.

Disaster victim identification (DVI) is a demanding task that can only be brought to a successful conclusion, if properly planned by selecting the appropriate forensic diagnostic tools and involving a team of well-trained key experts.[6] This is basically a team work consisting of police, army, homeguards, civil authorities and medical experts like forensic pathologist, forensic odontologist, forensic anthropologist, fingerprint expert, and/or ballistic expert. DVI guidelines were issued in 1984 by the Interpol DVI Standing Committee to emphasize the multidisciplinary approach of victim identification. Standard Operating Protocols (SOPs) for antemortem (AM) and postmortem (PM) procedures were established for fingerprinting, forensic pathology, forensic odontology and DNA profiling. The use of standardized AM and PM forms is to be used across personal and national preferences in all member countries. Such protocols have been found crucial in the quality of the entire DVI process, especially in case of rapidly decomposing bodies.[6] The Interpol AM and PM forms are completed separately. These data are entered into a computer database that will ultimately search for best possible matches (Flow chart 16.1).[2,7,14] Examples of the most common computer applications are DVI System International from Plass Data® (approved and used by Interpol), 2 WinID® (North America) and DAVID® (Australia).[6] Since, it is impossible to know in advance what data can be obtained from bodies and what information can be obtained for purposes of comparison at the victim's place of residence, all available information (both AM and PM) must be collected and documented.[2]

Ideally, a DVI team should compose of:[7]

i. Individuals specialized in recovery/exhumation, logistics and/or administration, scientific laboratory and photography.
ii. Forensic medicine experts (preferably with knowledge of forensic anthropology and genetics).
iii. Forensic odontologists.
iv. Members of a civil protection unit for body care and transport, and for assisting with the deployment and use of heavy equipment or machinery.
v. A psychologist trained in post-traumatic stress disorder (PTSD).
vi. A medical doctor and a nurse to attend to all team members' medical needs.

Subteams are formed comprising of:[6,7]

a. Recovery or 'necrosearch' team
b. Antemortem (AM) team
c. Postmortem (PM) team
d. Logistics support (identification) team

Hence, the overall identification process involves recovery-, AM-, PM- and identification teams (Flow chart 16.1).[14]

RECOVERY TEAM

Body recovery and search teams are the first link in the identification process. The recovery team has the important task to collect evidence, such as bodies and

Flow chart 16.1 DVI protocol

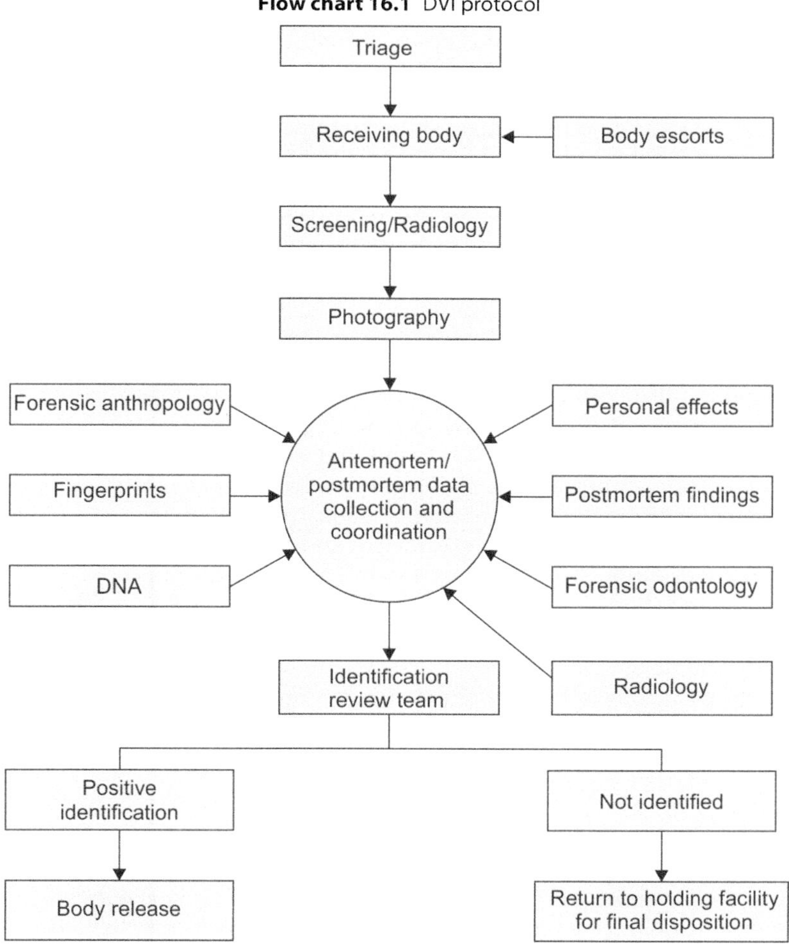

body parts, personal property from the disaster scene and to record the findings accurately.[6] The recovery team is involved in:

i. Identification of the site of occurrence and prepare a sketch diagram showing geographical location.
ii. Reaching the spot along with the team and necessary equipment.
iii. Immediate isolation, demarcation and protection of the site.
iv. Identifying and isolating cases according to seriousness of injuries for first-aid and referral treatment by color coding system (triage). Medical responders classify the injured according to severity and evacuation priority.
v. Arranging transport facilities for both—alive for treatment purposes to hospital and dead to mortuaries. Deceased persons are separated from the injured and moved to a separate area for dispatch. No person is considered deceased, until there is a formal certification by an authorized person, no matter how obvious death might be. Those who die *en route* to hospital or in hospital after a disaster are transferred to the morgue, even if there is no problem of identification.
vi. Each unknown body found is given a number. Body numbering in case of multinationality fatality is done according to Interpol guidelines and has to be applied by all teams to avoid errors and creation of even more chaos. The given body numbering system—international country telephone code, site number and body number as applied. This unique body number has to stay with the body during the subsequent stages of the identification process and will be visible on all related documentation (forms, photographs).[6]
vii. The bag in which the body is removed should also bear the same number. The personal belongings should be labeled and bagged separately, and if necessary the location from which they were recovered should be marked with a number. Separate property recovery teams must be formed to operate in a similar way to body recovery teams. The personal effects can often be an aid to victim identification and should be kept available for examination.
viii. Photography of the site from various angles. Photographers should be attached to search and recovery teams and work in conjunction with them. The importance of photographs, films and videos cannot be overemphasized. Photographic and video recording of bodies at the disaster site and within the mortuary is important for evidence and identification purposes. Body reference numbers must be clearly visible on each exposure.
ix. The Morgue Station is a temporary holding area for bodies and body parts until transport can be arranged and the mortuary is ready to receive them. The Morgue Station will keep its own record of bodies received and stored, listing each body reference number, the date and time of receipt, from whom received and where stored. Subsequently, details of the transfer should be recorded.

AM TEAM

The work of the AM teams starts with obtaining missing persons lists from each country and entering this information into a missing person database.[6] The antemortem material is collected by medical personnel, psychologists, Red Cross members, police officers, home guards and social assistants who will try to obtain information from the missing person's families.[7] This information can be collected at their home or at a place where the family members may have gathered. More specific information may be collected from friends and acquaintances, the missing person's employer, doctor or dentist. All available material (dental records, X-rays, CT scans, dental models and full face photographs) should be collected, with respect for the patient's rights to professional secrecy.[6,7,15]

Hair samples, toothbrushes, mouth guards or other personal belongings of the missing person that can be useful to determine a DNA profile should be searched for, and collected. In case DNA analysis, the family lineage need to be established to determine from which relative's blood or saliva samples must be collected.

Antemortem fingerprints are collected at the homes of the presumed victims from objects that might have been touched by them only (for e.g., a perfume bottle for women or an aftershave bottle for men). The records (personal, medical, dental, DNA and fingerprints) forwarded by the specialists of countries with missing citizens are also entered.[6]

The AM forms (yellow) are then completed by the team incorporating the following:[7]

i. Medical and surgical antecedents.
ii. Morphological characteristics.
iii. Professional antecedents and characteristics that result from these.
iv. Dental information.
v. Description of clothing, jewellery and other personal objects worn by the missing person.
vi. Missing person's pictures.

PM TEAM

Setting up of Temporary Mortuary

A temporary mortuary is established with best possible facilities under the circumstances. Ideally, there should be facilities to keep bodies refrigerated, and not frozen. Dry ice is used but should not be placed in direct contact with bodies as it causes skin burns. This building should cater for the needs of various other sections involved in identification like fingerprint experts, property and personal effects section, medical and dental personnel, documentation facilities, X-rays and photography. The benefits of working in a well-equipped mortuary, even a temporary one, have always proved to be most useful for identification.[2]

Overview of Examination Procedure (Flow chart 16.2)

In the mortuary, the body is thoroughly examined by a multidisciplinary team of specialists and all useful elements for identification are noted systematically on the pink PM Interpol forms.[6,7] The PM identification is divided into four work stations: fingerprinting, autopsy, DNA sampling and odontological examination. This can be very intense, not only because of the number of victims but also because of time restrictions for such examination.[7] All data obtained during autopsy are evaluated with reference to information obtained on missing persons.

Flow chart 16.2 Schematic representation of PM line

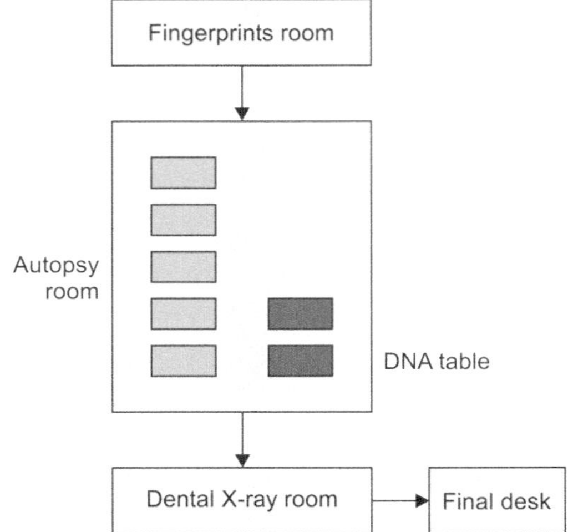

The protocol followed in autopsy room is as follows:[2,7,14,15]

i. Following receipt of the body and the recovery record, the body is placed on an autopsy table.
ii. The body registrar issues one unique number (if it isn't issued so far) and records it on a blank PM form. If a specific recovery number has been assigned, this number is also recorded on the PM form. He/she then gives the PM form to the autopsy recorder. The body registrar enters the PM number on the recovery report and gives any existing belongings in evidence bags to the property processor.
iii. If possible, before start of the autopsy, full body X-rays or CT-scans should be made to find pacemakers, implants and fracture sequelae.
iv. Then, collection of fingerprints, palm prints and footprints (as needed) is done by fingerprint expert.
v. The photographer photographs the clothed and unclothed body bearing the same PM number.
vi. The external and internal examination of the body is performed and DNA samples are collected by forensic pathologist, autopsy assistant and autopsy recorder. The photographs of important identifying features are also taken.
vii. Assessment of dental status is done by forensic odontologist, dental recorder and dental X-ray assistant; photograph is also taken of odontological identifying features.
viii. The final desk manager has to make sure that the PM folders are complete and correctly numbered, including the femoral or teeth sampling for DNA.

Each body to be moved into the examination room for autopsy should be placed under custody of a PM records officer, who follows the body through all the examination stages, until it is returned for storage. The PM records officer should be in possession of all PM DVI forms for each body.[6] The possibility of cross-contamination between remains must be taken into account both at the disaster site and at the autopsy station, which is why every individual body or body part must be assigned a separate number. The remains should not be matched or placed together with other remains simply on the basis of external appearance.

Fingerprints

The easiest and most accurate means of identification is by fingerprints. Fingerprints are unique to every person. If fingers are available with the body, they constitute the safest and fastest identification means available, provided antemortem prints can be obtained for comparison. Now, many countries are maintaining large databases of fingerprints of various categories of people. The finger/palm prints from the victims is taken by fingerprint specialists. The recovered fingerprints are then entered into the Automated Fingerprint Identification System (AFIS) for comparison with existing antemortem data.[6] The number of comparisons acceptable for positive identification differs—for criminal cases a 16 point match is needed, while in civil cases, a 10 point match is acceptable.

At times, fingerprinting can be very difficult due to the mutilated condition of the bodies but specialized techniques may have to be used. Finger skin can be removed by 'degloving' and placed on the fingertip of one of the autopsy assistants. After inking, the fingerprints can then be transposed onto paper.[7]

In some cases where fingerprints are not possible, palm, foot, ear and lip prints can be examined and compared in a similar manner, since these are also unique among individuals.

Personal Effects

In the next step, the body is photographed, followed by an extensive external description of the body, clothing and personal belongings.[6] The photographer should always take full body and full-face pictures, as well as close-ups of specific external findings. The autopsy assistant removes the clothing from the body systematically, and cleans the clothing and other personal items of evidence. All these items are photographed, preferably in color alongside a metric scale with the reference body number clearly visible.

Personal effects such as clothing, jewellery, mobile, watch and pocket contents including key rings, wallet with documents may constitute valuable circumstantial evidence of identity, but not considered absolute proof (Box 16.1). They must be combined with other evidence to conclude to a positive identification.[6,7] It is important to consider that certain items of evidence may not actually belong to a given body (for e.g. identity papers may be carried by a different person; items of jewellery or clothing may have been looted or lent intentionally to another individual; and sometimes during retrieval, items may have inadvertently been placed in one body bag).[2,14]

Documentation of clothing, jewellery and other personal effects is done by evidence processor and photographer. Evidence is placed in separate evidence bags. The evidence processor must also document the locations at which each item of evidence was found.[6] After completion of examination, clothing is placed in a clear bag and inserted into the body bag. Items of identification, objects of value and jewellery are taken to an evidence storage room.

Box 16.1 Personal effects in victim identification

- **Clothing:** Clothing itself and the clues in the clothing such as the maker's tag, laundry marks or dyer's mark help in identification of individual. Labels can be examined for the location of manufacturer or purchase. Uniforms can provide information on the rank of an individual. The size of clothing can give an estimation of stature and body build. If footwear is present, it might give indications of unusual wear patterns resulting from differences in gait. Occupational residues, such as oil and paint may also be present and may assist with identification. However, clothing may be lost, burnt in fires or damaged by the time a body is found, although remnants can often be found in the axilla and groin. This can be examined for an indication of fabric and color.
- **Currency** can provide information on the person's country of origin or their holiday destination. Coins may survive fires. Similarly, postage stamps may also indicate nationality.
- **Jewellery** worn for decoration is highly individualistic and females tend to have more jewellery than males. It can be found on fingers, toes, wrists, ankles, neck, around the waist and in the hair, as piercings, or on clothing. Some jewellery resists fires and damage, and depending on its location, may not be torn from the body in situations of trauma. Items of jewellery have a higher identification value if they are firmly attached to a victim's body (for e.g., piercing plugs or 'ingrown' wedding rings).[2] Engraved items of jewellery may also provide important clues to the identity of a victim.
- **Documents** may include passports, driver's license, credit or bank cards, aadhar or voter's card, receipts, cheque books, visiting cards or any other piece of paper. It can provide personal information about the bearer, or at least some information linking them with a particular country or government. Documents containing photographs of the bearer are particularly valuable.
- **Lottery tickets** can often be traced to the country of purchase and also to the location of sale, as most national lottery tickets contain a retailer code. Since it can be deduced that the bearer probably bought the ticket close to their home or work, the list of possible missing people can be narrowed accordingly.
- **Mobile phones** are often registered to a single user, with name and address details held by the service provider. It can be used as a guide to identification since the mobile number is unique. Some phones also have code numbers on the body or other identifying features. The chip inside the phone can withstand fire and trauma, and the information may be retrieved to assist identification, such as the last number dialed and stored numbers of relatives and friends. Occasionally, fingerprints may also be present on the body of the phone. The network provider of the phone can also be displayed by the phone, which may assist in determining the country of origin of the owner.
- **Spectacles and contact lens** are worn by an increasing number of the population. Spectacles found on a person's face are much more likely to belong to that person than those found next to or near a body, in which case, they may have originated from a different person. Intraocular lens may also help in this regard.

Postmortem Examination

The forensic medicine expert should do an external and internal examination and take DNA samples. He/she then enters the data in the blocks provided in the PM record. A forensic anthropologist (if available) can provide critical information for a biological profile of a given deceased person, for e.g., age, gender, ethnic affiliation, stature and individual identifying features. These parameters can be assessed on the basis of analyses of body structure and body size.[2]

It should be standard practice to perform full autopsies on all disaster victims not only for identification and cause of death purposes, but also to assist in preventing or minimizing the effects of similar incidents in the future (Box 16.2).[6,7] However, it is not necessary to open the cranium for identification purposes.

The main objectives of the PM examination are:[2]

- Cause, manner, mechanism of death (simple or combined).
- Survival time.
- Identification.
- Documentation of injuries and evidences for the benefit of investigators.

Details of Examination

If for whatever reason the body cannot be identified by visual examination, there are a number of potentially unique characteristics that can be looked for during autopsy that can assist with the identification.

External Findings

i. State of body—entire, mutilated or frag-mentary remains.
ii. Height and weight. In the case of mutilated and fragmentary remains, the actual measurement of the parts and the nature of mutilation should be recorded.
iii. Presence or absence of specific cadaveric changes—rigor mortis, postmortem staining and cadaveric spasm.
iv. Putrefactive changes—nature and extent.
v. Color of eyes.
vi. Hair—color, length and other features (for e.g., exceptional hair growth) with regard to both scalp and body hair.
vii. Identification marks—scars (appendectomy/cesarean), moles, tattoo-marks, deformities and disfiguration.
viii. Injuries: Site, number, nature and special features, if any (Figs 16.2A and B).

Internal Findings

The procedure of internal examination remains the same as that of any routine autopsy. Sometimes, for identification purpose and excessive workload, the internal autopsy may be limited to the abdominal cavity. The following points need special attention and recording:

i. State of putrefaction of the internal organs.
ii. Any surgical absence of an internal organ (appendix, spleen or tonsil).

Box 16.2 Methodology applied

- Complete autopsies (homicide, unknown cause, and unidentified remains).
- External injuries, position of injuries and burns (as applicable).
- Description of trauma, fractures, internal bleeding.
- Description upper respiratory tracts (trauma, soot particles).
- Old surgical procedures and internal implants: silicone breast implant, pacemaker, IUD, and prosthetics*.
- Listing of anatomical particularities, description of tattoos, scars, congenital abnormalities, amputations
- Systematic samples for toxicology and DNA.

*Unique numbers found on heart pacemakers and prosthetic devices are reliable identifying features.

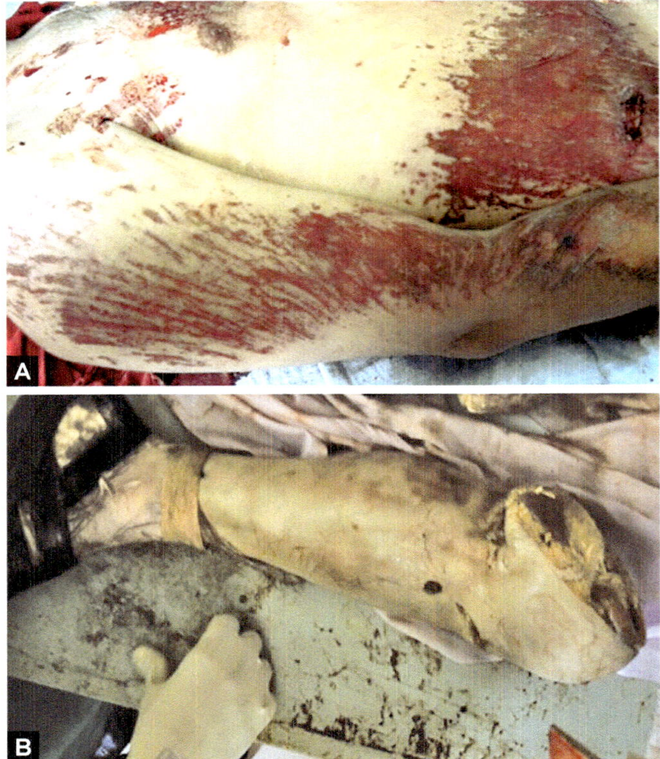

Figs 16.2A and B Pattern of injuries

iii. Any evidence of pre-existing disease (for e.g., biliary or renal calculi, uterine fibroid, absence of genitalia or old fractures).
iv. Any abnormal anatomic findings are further investigated with more extensive examination (for e.g., dissection of a uterine tumor, description of tubar clips or intrauterine devices).[7]
v. Internal injuries—nature, extent and specific organ involved.
vi. Any evidence of organic disease suggesting sudden death—coronary occlusion, cere-brovascular accident, ruptures or aneurysm.
vii. Any evidence of poisoning.

Physical Characteristics

The most common physical characteristics used to describe missing people include race, sex, age, height, weight, eye color, hair color, skin color, body build and any distinguishing marks such as scars, tattoos, or birthmarks.

A. **Race:** If soft parts are available, the deter-mination of race is possible on careful examination of clothes, complexion, hairs, eyes and lips. In absence of such data, it may be possible to determine the race from examination of the skull, mandible and teeth, and relative measurements of limb bones in broad categories of appearance such as caucasoid, mongoloid or negroid.[16] However, the biological variability of physical characteristics must also be considered. Other indications of racial or population origin could be determined from property such as clothing and ornaments, or particular physical characteristics such as body piercing or tattoos; however, these should not be substantially relied upon.

B. **Sex:** In case of mutilated remains, identity is simple when those parts bearing sexual characters are available. The normal nonpregnant uterus resists putrefaction longer and its identification is proof of female sex. The prostate gland likewise resists putrefaction and its presence indicates male sex. The general appearance of the parts, the disposition of the hair, the presence of hair on face and any parts of the external genitals are helpful in identification of sex. When sexual characteristics of the soft parts are not available, the diagnosis of sex can be based on the characters displayed by the skeleton. The important bones for this purpose are pelvis, skull, mandible, sternum and long bones.[16] Distinction between gender and anatomical sex should also be sought.

C. **Stature:** Stature may be shortened by flexure of muscles due to rigor mortis or exposure to heat, and lengthened due to flaccidity or with decomposition. Incomplete bodies or body parts can also lead to an error in stature estimates. If a complete skeleton is available, stature is determined by the length of the skeleton plus 2.5 cm for thickness of soft parts. If the body is mutilated, the stature is determined using the following data:[16]
   - It is approximately equal to length from tip of the middle finger to the tip of the opposite middle finger when arms are fully extended.
   - From 20th or 25th year onwards, stature is twice the length from the vertex or heel to the top of the symphysis pubis.
   - The height can be ascertained from one arm by multiplying its length by 2 and adding 34 cm.
   - The length of forearm measured from tip of olecranon process to the tip of middle finger is equal to 5/19 of stature.
   - The length from the sternal notch to pubic symphysis is 1/3 of stature.
   - The vertical distance from the top of the head to the tip of chin is about 1/7 of stature.

D. **Age:** The age of an individual can be determined with a certain degree of accuracy from a combination of data provided by teeth, bones, height and weight and miscellaneous particulars like birth record, changes occurring at puberty and changes due to old age.[15] Broad age categories such as infant, juvenile, adolescent and early/middle/late adulthood are easier to determine. In general, the younger person, more accurate is the age estimation. This is because there is increasing individual variation in biological characteristics with advancing age, especially after the first three decades.

E. **Appearance**
   a. **Hair:** A description of color (scalp hair color and thoracic, axillary, arm and pubic hair), length and waviness of hair offers useful contributory evidence in identification. The pattern of baldness or hair distribution is generally persistent, and similarities between antemortem and postmortem appearances can be described.
   b. **Deformities, birth marks, occupational marks, scars and tattoo marks:** These may be helpful in the establishment of identity to a certain extent,

since they are often recognized and remembered by family, friends and relatives as identifying features. In some cases, due to decomposition, the search for scars may prove to be inadequate, but tattoos can be more easily detected and of great value (Fig. 16.3 and Box 16.3).

Serology of the victim's blood type can help narrow down the search for a missing person. If the blood type of both biological parents is known, determination of a victim's serology can help exclude them from a match. The most commonly known blood groupings are the ABO and rhesus (Rh) group, the frequencies of which vary between populations.

DNA Sampling

For a DNA profile, the sample is taken from the deceased body or body parts and from the references [relatives, self-samples or belongings (stored blood, hairbrush, toothbrush, towels, clothing, cervical smear or biopsy)]. DNA matching is the only method for primary identification independent from direct comparison (fingerprint or dental record).[2] However, DNA testing is both expensive and time consuming.

The environmental conditions of a mass disaster often result in severe fragmentation, decomposition and intermixing of the remains of victims. In such

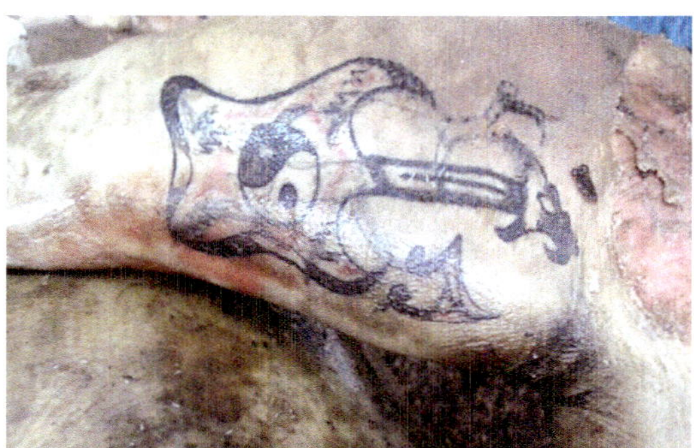

Fig. 16.3 Tattoo mark can help in identification

Box 16.3 Individual peculiarity in victim identification

- **Birthmarks and moles:** The commonly seen birthmarks include salmon pink patch, strawberry nevus, portwine stain and cavernous hemangioma.
- **Scars** can be accidentally or intentionally inflicted. Surgical scars can provide information on medical history. Self-inflicted scars may indicate previous suicide attempts or self-mutilation, while other scars may provide information on cultural or social persuasions.
- **Body piercing** is commonly seen in many cultures, and in both sexes. Typical areas of the body for piercing are the ear, face, nipples, navel and genitals.
- **Tattoos** are accidentally or intentionally obtained. Some tattoos may have names, religious symbols, dates, blood types or medical conditions. They can also persist in immersed bodies and superficial burns. People often have multiple tattoos which greatly assists identification. Local auxiliary personnel can help in interpreting or translating some of the tattoos.[7]

cases, traditional identification based on the anthropological and physical characteristics of the victims is frequently inconclusive. This is the reason why DNA profiling has became the gold standard for victim identification in mass disasters.[5]

The samples should be sent to a laboratory and analyzed according to international standards and the profiles matched with respect to the source of reference.[2] The actual Interpol forms also contain an important DNA document, indicating the methods and the markers to be used, in order to allow a uniform comparative application at an international level.[7]

During sample collection, the forensic pathologist should have a basic knowledge of forensic genetics to provide guidance for DNA sample collection (Table 16.2).[2] It is recommended that a sampling of the femoral shaft can be carried out because of the rapid decomposition and subsequent muscular alterations.[7] The recorder and sampler should verify the placement of the sample in a properly labeled tube and the entry of the corresponding data in a sample log. The sampler then needs to dispose off the scalpel blades and rotary bits. He/she cleans the cutting surface, scale, Stryker saw, rotary instrument, forceps and hemostats with a 10% bleach solution, then wipes all surfaces down with ethanol before taking the next sample.[14]

Dental Examination

Dental age estimation is a major component of the identification process.[6] The body is transferred to the next room, where the forensic odontologists can examine and take dental radiographs (bite wing radiographs, and X-rays of individual dental particularities).[7] All dental related data are entered on the PM F1/F2 Interpol forms. As a general rule, jaws should not be removed by dental experts unless a more specific examination is mandatory.[6]

To create more access to the dentition, a non-destructive method of mandibular dissecting technique may be followed. This allows an easy access to both maxilla and mandible and enable a complete repositioning of the facial tissue after autopsy, so that the body can still be shown to relatives if required. All dental characteristics should be recorded by color photography too.[6]

Table 16.2 Collection of samples for DNA[2,6,14]

Condition of body	*Recommended sample*
Complete, non-decomposed body	Blood (on FTA paper or swab) and buccal smears
Mutilated, non-decomposed body	If available: blood and deep-seated skeletal muscle tissue (about 10-15 g)
Complete, decomposed body or mutilated remains	Sample from long, compact bones (4-6 x 1-2 x 0.5-1 cm sections, window section, without shaft separation), or healthy teeth (preferably molars, upper or lower canine), or any other available bone (preferably cortical bones with dense tissue)
Severely burnt body	All samples listed above and impacted teeth or tooth roots if present, or smears from the bladder

Postmortem dental age estimation allows forensic odontologists to focus on the search for a matching antemortem file on a specific age range among the possible candidates for identification from the missing persons list. Age estimation is based on the eruption and tooth development in children and adolescents or morphological changes in adults (enamel wear, cementum incremental lines, root translucency or secondary dentine formation). This is an advantage compared with the age estimation of living individuals, where the methods of age assessment involving tooth extraction have to be excluded.[6]

After postmortem examination, at the final desk, there is (i) checking, whether all examinations were carried out; (ii) checking correspondence of all numbered samples with the given body number; (iii) ensuring exploitable quality of all the X-rays after development.[7]

Identification Center (Comparison of Record)

The Identification Center handles and compares AM and PM documents forwarded from the AM and PM teams. This center should have availability of experts in fingerprint identification, property comparison, photography, forensic experts, dental experts and radiologist. All collected AM data - even partial-are transmitted to the Identification Section and transcribed into the computer data file.[7] In the different sections of this center, the quality controls and the transcription of the AM and PM documents take place.[6]

During the reconstructive identification process, all information gathered from the unknown body is entered in computer database. The identification software runs an automatic comparison and matching between the ante- and postmortem data in both directions: AM to PM or *vice versa*.[7]

The correspondences suggested by the computer between an unidentified body and a missing person facilitate a more specific manual control and comparison of the corresponding AM and PM data by a team of specialists.The matches is then verified by the different experts on the Reconciliation Board. The final judgment is made by professional experts and based on personal evaluation of the evidence. Once identification was confirmed, a death certificate is issued and the body released. The national authorities of the victim's country are contacted so that the victim's family could be informed about the positive identification, and then the repatriation process could begin.[7]

DNA IN MASS DISASTER

Genetic identification techniques provide a powerful tool in the identification of disaster victims. DNA analysis techniques, currently in use, complement other methods commonly used in DVI, especially when a body has been severely mutilated.[6] Even when a victim has been identified on the basis of other methods, a DNA sample should be taken for the purpose of matching or ruling out matches between body parts and to facilitate the identification of other missing persons.[2] Samples should be sent for analysis as soon as possible. In the meantime, from collection till it is sent, it should be kept cool and shaded from daylight.[2]

Early molecular biology procedures used for DVI were based on the analysis of protein or blood group polymorphisms. Most of these systems (with the exception of human leukocyte antigen [HLA typing]) have a low degree of discrimination.

Their use was also limited by an insufficient amount of genetic information in many tissues and low stability in biologically degraded forensic samples. With the breakthrough of DNA fingerprinting, developments started for more specific and more sensitive methods, allowing identification based on less material of lower quality. The introduction of polymerase chain reaction (PCR)-based techniques allowed the targeting of a variety of genetic markers, from single-nucleotide polymorphisms (SNP) to variable number of tandem repeats (VNTRs); VNTRs include minisatellites (repeated motif of 6–100 bp) and microsatellites (repeated motif of 1–5 bp), often referred to as short tandem repeats (STRs) or simple sequence repeats (SSRs). The current methodology in genetic identification relies on the use of direct analysis of the DNA sequence and the availability of numerous genetic databases.[5]

Any type of biological remains (including soft tissue, bone, saliva and hair) can be used as a source of genetic material for DNA profiling. However, the quality of the genetic material to be analyzed is strongly influenced by the time since death and environmental conditions. Factors such as high temperature, contamination of remains with dirt or jet fuel, the putrefaction process or microbiological infestation, may significantly impair DNA quality. When using degraded and limited samples, extraction methods have to be optimized for maximum yield and typing success.[5]

In the case of sample collection, procedures that take several weeks or longer to complete or unfavorable weather conditions, whole blood from the core of the body, deep muscle tissues, bones or teeth are the most reliable sources of DNA.[2,5] In comparison to soft tissues, hard tissues are greatly resistant to autolysis and decay caused by environmental factors.[5] As dental pulp material is a good source for DNA analysis, two vital teeth (canines/premolars) can be extracted and sent to the forensic DNA laboratories.[6,7,17,18] In any event, it is advisable to collect multiple samples from the outset, in order to avoid the time consuming work of collecting and labeling new samples at a later point in time.

In view of the possibility that victim identification may take considerable time, the issue of preservation of samples during storage arises.[2] Preservatives can be used to conserve soft tissue at room temperature. The use of preservatives in provisional morgue stations with limited cooling capacities is also recommended. Samples should not be preserved in formalin, as formalin will destroy DNA. Caputo could reliably and accurately type different genetic systems including autosomal STRs and mitochondrial and Y-chromosome haplogroups from DNA samples obtained from cadaver tissue stored in salt for up to 365 days. This can be cost efficient alternative for storage of human remains in mass disaster locations.[19]

DENTISTRY IN MASS DISASTER

Dental Record Comparison

The identification process is fundamentally the same as that in a routine comparative dental identification, but the inherent problems are magnified.[20] Problems of body fragmentation, mutilation, commingling and incineration, idiosyncratic dental records from numerous regions, poor working conditions and psychological stresses all confound the identification process.

Dental identification takes two main forms. Firstly, the most frequently performed examination is a comparative identification that is used to establish (to a high degree of certainty) that the remains of a decedent and person represented by antemortem dental records are the same individual. Information from the body or circumstances usually contains clues as to who has died. Secondly, in those cases where antemortem records are not available, and no clues to the possible identity exist, a postmortem dental profile is completed by the forensic dentist suggesting characteristics of the individual which will likely to narrow down the search for the antemortem materials.[21] Separate pictures should be taken of the upper and lower jaws and teeth in occlusal position.

Comparative Dental Identification

Many people are familiar with the concept of dental identification; it is frequently mentioned on television news. But the nuances and complexities of the process are rarely understood. The central dogma of dental identification is that postmortem dental remains can be compared only with antemortem dental records, including written notes, study casts and radiographs to confirm identity. The information that could be used to identify an individual may be lost if dental records are destroyed after certain periods of time as currently being practiced in certain jurisdictions. Clearly, individuals with numerous and complex dental treatments are often easier to identify than those individuals with little or no restorative treatment.

Once the postmortem record is complete, a comparison between the two records can be carried out. A methodical and systematic comparison is required, examining each tooth and surrounding structures in turn. While dental restorations figure significantly in the identification process, many other oral features are assessed. Such additional features play an increasingly important role in those individuals with minimal restorations. Because of the progressive decrease in dental caries, so-called nonrestorative cases are likely to become more common.

Additionally, the placing of name, serial number or some other unique marking on prostheses such as dentures greatly assist the identification process. These markings provide an initial point of inquiry to the practitioner or manufacturer that could then lead to identification of the deceased.

Similarities and discrepancies should be noted during the comparison process.[22] There are two types of discrepancy, those that can be explained and those that cannot. Explainable discrepancies normally relate to the time elapsed between the antemortem and postmortem records. Examples include teeth extracted or restorations placed or enlarged. If a discrepancy is unexplainable, for e.g., a tooth is not present on the antemortem record but is present on the postmortem record, then exclusion must be made. A range of conclusions can be reached when reporting a dental identification. The American Board of Forensic Odontology recommends that these be limited to the following four conclusions:[23]

1. *Positive identification:* The antemortem and postmortem data match in sufficient detail, with no unexplainable discrepancies to establish that they are from the same individual.

2. *Possible identification:* The antemortem and postmortem data have consistent features but because of the quality of either the postmortem remains or the antemortem evidence, it is not possible to establish identity positively.
3. *Insufficient evidence:* The available information is insufficient to form the basis for a conclusion.
4. *Exclusion:* The antemortem and postmortem data are clearly inconsistent.

It is important to note that there is no minimum number of concordant points or features that are required for a positive identification. In many cases, a single tooth can be used for identification if it contains sufficient unique features. Equally, a full-mouth series of radiographs may not reveal sufficient detail to render a positive conclusion.[24] The discretion of identification lies with the odontologist who must be prepared to justify the conclusions in court, surely the ultimate in peer-review. Notably, it has been recognized by the Interpol Disaster Victim Identification that if a positive match is found using dental identification, it can be relied on as a stand-alone identifier.

Postmortem Dental Profiling

When antemortem dental records are unavailable and other methods of identification are not possible, the forensic odontologist can assist in limiting the population pool to which the deceased is likely to belong and thus increase the likelihood of locating antemortem dental records. This process is known as postmortem dental profiling. The information from this process will enable a more focused search for antemortem records. A postmortem dental profile will typically provide information on the deceased's age, ancestral background, sex and socio-economic status. In some instances, it is possible to provide additional information regarding occupation, dietary habits, habitual behaviors and occasionally on dental or systemic diseases.

If the postmortem profile does not elicit the tentative identity of the deceased, it may be necessary to reconstruct the individual's appearance during life. This is the responsibility of forensic artists who use the dental profile to help with the facial reproduction.

OTHER METHODS OF IDENTIFICATION

a. **Restoration of facial features:** When a dead body is unrecognizable due to decomposition, skeltalization or mutilation, a craniofacial reconstruction (CFR) should be considered. The goal of CFR is to recreate a likeness with the face of missing individuals immediately prior to their death. This reconstructed face may help to identify the missing person. Several 3-D manual methods for CFR are currently being used. One of these consists of physically modeling a face on a skull replica (the target skull) with clay or plasticine. However, this method requires a high degree of anatomical and sculptural expertise and hence, remains difficult and subjective. The progress in computer and the improvement of medical imaging technologies during recent years have lead to the development of software for computer based CFR methods. By this method, automated creation of multiple reconstructions from the same skull using different modeling assumptions (like age, BMI, ancestry, gender) is possible. As a result, the computer generated CFR process becomes accessible to a wide range of people without the need for extensive expertise.[6]

b. In **superimposition photography**, the skull of the deceased is X-rayed. The photographs of the front and side view of the head of the deceased taken while he was alive are enlarged to same size and are superimposed on the negatives of skull to tally contours of the face and skull which may help in identification.
c. **Virtual autopsy (Virtopsy)** is a bloodless and minimally invasive procedure to examine a body for cause of death. It utilizes imaging techniques (CT and MRI), photogrammetry and 3-D optical measuring techniques to get a reliable, accurate geometric presentation of all findings (the body surface as well as the interior). During the Victorian Bushfire in 2009, CT scanning proved to be very useful in the victim identification process. This technique also helps improve quality assurance through digital data archiving and transfer. Because of its minimal invasiveness to the body, it can also be introduced in cultures with low autopsy acceptance. In some cases, physical examination should still be performed in addition to the virtopsy to provide more physical and external information of the victims.[6]
d. **Frontal sinus comparison** can be done as this is thought to be unique between individuals. If a person has had a radiograph taken of this part of the skull during life, a postmortem radiograph of the same area can be compared for anatomical similarity. The comparison of antemortem and postmortem radiographs for identification has come under scrutiny, since the uniqueness of these anatomical structures has not been stringently tested.

This is not an exhaustive list of victim identification methods, but it represents the most commonly used methods, especially in cases of mass disasters. Finally, it must also be remembered that identification by exclusion may also be useful.

ADVANCEMENT IN INDIA

The key to successful mass disaster identification is preparedness. In this respect, the authorities evacuated about 800,000 people, one of the largest such evacuations in India's history before the powerful cyclone Phailin crashed into India's eastern coast in October 2013. The effective evacuation in Odisha ahead of cyclone will be highlighted as a global example in the World Conference on Disaster Risk Reduction, in 2015.The Head of the UN Office for Disaster Risk Reduction (UNISDR) lauded Odisha for its 'landmark success' actions in limiting the number of deaths directly caused by the cyclone to 21. More than 10,000 people were killed 14 years ago when a powerful cyclone came in roughly the same area, and more than 300,000 were killed in 1970 when a storm hit Bangladesh.[25]

Recently, the Department of Forensic Medicine and Toxicology at Goa Medical College in Bambolim has established the country's first mass disaster medical infrastructure with a capacity to accommodate 150 bodies from a calamity site and a live forensic autopsy auditorium.

RECOMMENDATIONS IN INDIAN SETUP

At Site

i. Digital photography of the victims at the site of occurrence during the process of recovery and during PM examination.[26,27]

ii. Single and definitive numbering system for each unidentified body, preferably by laminated papers, tied to the body part (other means may be by covering the numbered paper with plastic or putting it inside the gloves and tying it to the body part).[7] Number 6 and 9, wherever present must be written in words.[26,27]
iii. Early transportation to the Morgue.

At Mortuary

i. Preservation of the bodies in the cooling chambers with body numbers written outside the door.
ii. Fresh numbering of the bodies during PM (as in most of the cases the bodies are sent in a haphazard manner) in the same manner as mentioned earlier, and keeping the old number as a reference. Body parts should be separately numbered as A, B, C etc. or by any other unique system.[26,27]
iii. Conducting the medicolegal examinations as close to the disaster site as possible. This helps to avoid destruction or loss of evidence caused by body transport (loss of teeth or particular bones that could be useful in criminal investigations, such as the hyoid bone).[7]

Operational

i. Contact information of relevant authority dealing with emergency situations.
ii. Mobilizing man power at the autopsy site especially the dissectors, autopsy technicians and people who can carry the bodies.[26,27]
iii. Onsite presence of an autopsy room manager, supervising all examination activities of the different teams as well as managing the arrival of new bodies. He/she should also enforce the SOPs and take necessary actions, should problems occur. A DNA manager should be present for the DNA sampling.[7]
iv. Separate X-ray room where radiological examination of the body would help in locating the presence of foreign bodies (for e.g., osteosynthesis, prosthesis, tubar clips, vascular stents or pacemakers) and bony abnormalities. The presence of suitable dental X-ray equipment, portable and handheld digital dental X-ray units are also desirable.[6] Radiology could be complementary to the limited internal autopsy which may provide very little information as to validly evaluate anatomical characteristics under these difficult conditions.[7,15,26,27]
v. Training exercises to familiarize the team with SOPs and to be better prepared for any kind of eventuality. Attempts should be made during training exercises to demonstrate the complex challenges using simulations and mock disaster scenarios, and by studying previous responses and events.[6,28,29]

CONCLUSION

The identification of large numbers of casualties in mass disasters is complex and fraught with hazards, both physically and emotionally. The identification of human remains is an area that is constantly being re-evaluated in the light of new developments. The multidisciplinary approach to the identification process is vital to the successful outcome of a mass disaster incident. Early body examinations, unique numbering system and taking photographs at the scene of death before body removal and during examination will all improve the chances of a positive identification. However, the final identification result depends on the presence of quality antemortem data and in particular availability of physical evidence such as antemortem X-rays, fingerprints, dental records and DNA.

One of the most important factors in DVI is the timely collection of samples and data. The collection of samples for fingerprints and DNA should also occur in a timely manner to prevent decay or loss of comparative material. Timely collection of records of suspected missing persons should be done in order to prevent destruction of records before identification is complete.

Adequate victim identification management goes through strict methodology and protocols. This requires adopting and applying SOPs, in agreement with the Interpol DVI Standing Committee guidelines. Any mass fatality response plan of India must incorporate these guidelines. If planned and implemented properly, the problem of dead body identification would be solved in a much better way and will help the community in the most befitting manner. The availability of experienced investigation and forensic teams, technical infrastructure and preparation will produce markedly different results.

India is equipped with many of the scientific resources necessary for good disaster management. The problem is a lack of collaboration between knowledge-creating and policy-making bodies. There is a great paucity of any organized plans for identification of mass disaster causalities. Mostly, identification is relied upon the nonprofessional approach. Therefore, there is great need for professional approach as it is being currently undertaken in other parts of the world.

REFERENCES

1. Disasters and emergencies. WHO/EHA Pan-African emergency training center, Addis Ababa.2002. p. 3. Available from: http://www.who.int/disasters/repo/7656.pdf.
2. DVI guide. Interpol 2009. p. 1-55. Available from: http://www.interpol.int/Public/Disaster Victim.
3. International strategy for disaster reduction. Disaster, technology, basic terms of disaster risk reduction. Available from: http://www.unisdr.org/library/lib-terminology-eng%20home.htm.
4. Khan H, Vasilescu LG, Khan A. Disaster management cycle—a theoretical approach. *J Management Marketing* 2008; 6: 43-50.
5. Ziętkiewicz E, Witt M, Daca P, Żebracka-Gala J, Goniewicz M, Jarząb B, et al. Current genetic methodologies in the identification of disaster victims and in forensic analysis. *J Appl Genetics* 2012; 53: 41-60.
6. Pittayapat P, Jacobs R, Valck ED, Vandermeulen D, Willems G. Forensic odontology in the disaster victim identification process. *J Forensic Odontostomartol* 2012; 30: 1-12.
7. Beauthier JP, Valck ED, Lefevre P, Winne JD. Mass disaster victim identification: the Tsunami experience. *Forensic Sci J* 2009; 2: 54-62.
8. Jones DG. Odontology often is final piece to grim puzzle. *J Calif Dent Assoc* 1998; 26: 650-51.
9. Disaster category classification and peril terminology for operational purposes. Available from: http://www.cred.be/publication/disaster-category-classification-and-peril-terminology-operational-purposes.
10. Shultz PW, Nolan JM, Cialdini RB, Goldstein NJ, Griskevicius V. The constructive, destructive and reconstructive social power of norms. *Psychological Science* 2007; 18: 429-34.

11. Disaster Statistics - India - Asia - Countries and Regions. Available from: http://www.preventionweb.net/english/countries/statistics/?cid=79.
12. National Policy on Disaster Management, National Institute of Disaster Management; 2009. p. 8-9. Available from: http://ndmindia.nic.in/NPDM-101209.pdf.
13. Simpson EK, Byard RW. Unique characteristics at autopsy that may be useful in identifying human remains. In: Tsokos M (ed). Forensic pathology reviews. Vol. 5. Totowa, NJ: Humana Press; 2008. p. 175-96.
14. Gonzales AR, Henke TA, Hart SV. Mass fatality incidents: a guide for human forensic identification. US Department of Justice, 2005. Available from: http://www.ojp.usdoj.gov/nij.
15. Kahana T, Ravioli J, Urroz C, Hiss J. Radiographic identification of fragmentary human remains from a mass disaster. *Am J Forensic Med Pathol* 1997; 18: 40-44.
16. Biswas G. Identification I and II. Review of forensic medicine and toxicology. 2nd ed. New Delhi: Jaypee Brothers; 2012. p. 45-82.
17. Schwartz TR, Schwartz EA, Mieszerski L, McNally L, Kobilinsky L. Characterization of deoxyribonucleic acid (DNA) obtained from teeth subjected to various environmental conditions. *J Forensic Sci* 1991; 36: 979-90.
18. Sweet D, Hildebrand D. Recovery of DNA from human teeth by cryogenic grinding. *J Forensic Sci* 1998; 43: 1199-02.
19. Caputo M, Bosio LA, Corach D. Long-term room temperature preservation of corpse soft tissue: an approach for tissue sample storage. *Investigative Genetics* 2011; 2: 17-22.
20. Morlang WM. Mass disaster management update. *CDAJ* 1986; 14: 49-57.
21. Sweet D, DiZinno JA. Personal identification through dental evidence-tooth fragments to DNA. *J Calif Dent Assoc* 1996; 24: 35-42.
22. Silverstein H. Comparison of antemortem and postmortem findings. In: Bowers CM, Bell G (eds). Manual of forensic odontology. 3rd edn. Ontario: Manticore. 1997. p. 31-35.
23. Saukko P, Knight B. Mass disasters—the role of the pathologist. Knight's forensic pathology. 3rd edn. London: Arnold; 2004. p. 41-51.
24. American Board of Forensic Odontology. Body identification guidelines. *J Am Dent Assoc* 1994; 125: 1244-54.
25. India: Cyclone evacuation to become a global example. Available from: http://www.preventionweb.net/english/professional/news/v.php?id=35964.
26. Trengrove H. Operation earthquake: Christchurch earthquake disaster victim identification. *J Forensic Odontostomartol* 2011; 29: 1-7.
27. Das S, Pandey SK, Chakraborty P. An approach for identification of individuals in a mass disaster in Indian set up. *J Indian Acad Forensic Med* 2011; 33: 161-62.
28. Pretty IA, Webb DA, Sweet D. The design and assessment of mock mass disasters for dental personnel. *J Forensic Sci* 2001; 46: 74-79.
29. Woodward JD. Identification of victims following a mass disaster. *Ky Dent J* 1982; 34: 37-41.

FORENSIC PATHOLOGY

Judicial Hanging

Gautam Biswas

'Judicial execution can never cancel or remove the atrocity it seeks to punish: it can only add a second atrocity to the original one.'
Auberon Waugh (English journalist)

ABSTRACT

Hanging is one of the oldest methods for capital punishment in most countries with India being no exception. The procedure of execution has largely remained unchanged over the centuries. Some modifications to its process were introduced in the late 19th century to make it more humane, quick and painless, and without decapitation. But still death in most cases were due to strangulation causing delayed deaths and not the intended fracture of cervical column which would cause instantaneous death. After autopsy examination of many cases of judicial hanging, researchers proposed that for instant death, the position of the knot should be submental and the 'drop' length should be based upon the weight of the condemned person.

The other concern is the involvement of doctors in the process of execution which is considered against the Hippocratic Oath. Over the years, doctors have helped the state to devise newer methods of execution. They are actively involved in preparing the condemned person, checking on their health with the purpose of supervising their death, prescription of the lethal cocktails, putting in of intravenous lines, pronunciation of death, and some are also involved in removal of their organs. The Medical Council of India should strongly oppose to doctors taking part in execution process. Ethical practice guidelines should be framed in lines similar to American Medical Association. Actions which are at the most acceptable are providing sedative to calm anxiety at the prisoner's request and certification of death after another person had pronounced it.

Keywords: Death penalty, short drop, standard drop, long drop, hood, knot, pinioning, hangman's fracture, ethical practice in capital sentence.

INTRODUCTION

Death penalty has been a mode of punishment since time immemorial and hanging has been and remains one of the oldest and most commonly used methods of execution.[1,2] Some of the early methods involved torture like burning at the stake, breaking on the wheel, drawing, hanging and quartering, crushing under elephant's feet, boiling in the oil and stoning to death. The Chinese also devised a number of ingenious ways, including the 'Death of a Thousand Cuts', 'Death of a Thousand Drips' and 'Five Pains'.[3] With the advances of civilization, the modes of death punishment have also witnessed significant changes in many countries—from more humane methods to total abolition. Although many countries have abolished capital punishment, India, China, United States (US) and Indonesia continue with death penalty where over 60% of the world's population lives.[4] An estimated 85–90% of world's executions take place in Asia.

Besides India, hanging remains the standard method of capital punishment in many countries—Pakistan, Bangladesh, Japan, Singapore, Malaysia, South Korea, Botswana, Zimbabwe, Iran, Iraq, Egypt, Jordan, Kuwait, Lebanon, Syria and in most Caribbean states. Hanging is very common in Afghanistan, Bangladesh, Botswana, Iraq, Japan, Pakistan, Singapore, St. Kitts and Nevis and Sudan.[2,4-6]

In 2011, 430 hangings were recorded in nine countries and 238 in six countries during 2010.[5] In India, the last execution took place in February 2013 (57th person to be executed since independence) and before that in November 2012.[7,8] According to a December 2012 report, 477 people were on death row in India. Based on the official statistics of the National Crimes Records Bureau, between 2001 and 2011, an average of 132 death sentences were handed down each year.[7] In a recent judgment by a fast track court, death sentence was awarded to the four convicts in the December 2012 Delhi rape-and-murder case.

In United Kingdom (UK), the Royal Commission in its report on capital punishment (1949–1953) stated that while executing the death sentence, it should be quick and less painful, and there should be least mutilation of the body. The Law Commission in India also in its report concluded that a method which is certain, humane, quick and decent should be adopted.[2,3,8,9]

Judicial hanging is neither a quick and simple nor a decent method of execution, as it involves immense pain and sometimes mutilation of the body. There have been several case reports where hanging has not resulted in immediate death. Deaths in such cases were due to asphyxia or strangulation which caused lingering and painful death of the condemned person. The standard of human decency is also progressively evolving to higher levels. Punishment which was regarded as legitimate, reasonable and proportionate few decades back may now be regarded as inhuman, barbaric and disproportionate. For this reason, hanging has been abolished in some of the developing countries and most of the developed countries. It has been substituted by electrocution, gas chamber or lethal injection which is considered being more acceptable, civilized and humane. These modes are considered to be less painful and cause less suffering to the convict undergoing the death sentence.

Many people have criticized the death penalty in general, saying that 'two wrongs do not make a right' and the concept of 'an eye for an eye' cannot be grounds for death penalty. A number of commentators including a former Supreme Court Chief Justice and human rights groups such as Amnesty International have pointed out that the Indian judicial system, and the death penalty in particular, is generally biased against the poor, the illiterate and the marginalized. The European Union (EU) also called on India to stop and abolish capital punishment. Moreover, there is no convincing proof that the death penalty has a deterrent effect on heinous crimes.[3,4,10]

This chapter is not an attempt either to justify or condemn death penalty, but focuses on how the death penalty was carried out over the centuries, how hanging has evolved over the years, and autopsy findings in judicial hanging along with a discussion on ethical aspects of death penalty.

DEFINITIONS

Some definitions which the reader ought to be familiar with:[4,11]

- **Capital punishment (death penalty)** is a legal process whereby a person is put to death by the State as a punishment for certain crimes. The term originates from the Latin word '*capitalis*', which literally means 'regarding the head'. As history would prove, capital punishment usually meant decapitation, the severing of one's head.
- **Hanging:** The suspension of a person by a ligature, usually with a noose or cord tied around the neck, causing death. The *Oxford Dictionary* defines hanging as 'the practice of hanging condemned people as a form of capital punishment'.
- **Drawing:** The act of dragging or drawn to the place of execution on a hurdle (a wooden frame). The term was also used synonymously with 'disembowelment'.
- **Disembowelment:** The act of removing some or all of the vital organs usually from the abdomen (bowels or viscera).
- **Quartering:** The act of severing of the trunk into four parts (quarters).
- **Gallows (gibbet):** It is an instrument of execution consisting of a wooden frame from which the condemned person is executed by hanging.
- **Lynching:** Putting a person to death, often by hanging, carried out by a mob for an alleged offence without a legal trial in order to punish an alleged transgressor, or to intimidate, control, or manipulate the people.

HISTORY

Hanging as a method of execution is contemplated to have originated approximately about 2,500 years ago in the Persian Empire (Iran). It is also mentioned in the 22nd book of Homer's *Odyssey* composed near the end of the 8th century BC. It described the hanging of 12 disloyal servants by Odysseus's son Telemachus, as this was considered worse than being hacked to pieces (which was the common method of execution during that time). However, it was the Anglo-Saxon tribes from Germany who introduced hanging as a method of execution during their invasions of the Roman Empire and UK in the 5th century. This was meant for male criminals only, while women were strangled at the stake (hanging was considered indecent for females).[5,11,12]

Hanging rapidly become a popular execution method in Europe and was adopted as a punishment for many crimes—treason, robbery, murder and piracy. During this period, this was not restricted to men only, but women and children were also hanged quite frequently. It was considered ideal because it was the simplest method to carry out. The equipment was easy to come by and did not give the condemned person a particularly cruel death. At that time, executions were regularly held in public squares and attracted massive, unruly crowds eager to take part in a communal ritual of punishment. This event was also used by the people for a family picnic. The modern phrase 'gala day' is derived from the Anglo-Saxon 'gallows day'. This was used to demonstrate the state's power and to embarrass the convict's family.[12]

The technique and method of hanging remained mostly unchanged over the next 15 centuries. The earliest form of gallows was a tree, with prisoners being hauled up manually by the hangman or pulled off a ladder or a wagon. Drawing and quartering was also a part of the penalty in England till 1867, when it was abolished. To be hanged, drawn and quartered, first the convicts were fastened to a hurdle, or wooden panel, and drawn by horse to the place of execution, and then they were hanged (usually not to the death), disemboweled, quartered and beheaded. Quartering usually was done by tying each of the four limbs to a different horse and driving them in different directions. The punishment was given in the conviction to prevent the ascension to heaven, since it was believed that bodies had to be kept whole, so they could rise at the second coming. Support for public executions began to diminish in the late 19th century. In the past century, capital punishment was carried out behind prison walls and witnessed by only a select few.[11,12]

In 1846, Michigan became the first state in the world to abolish capital punishment. In UK, the last execution by hanging took place in 1964 before being abolished in 1965. In 2004, the 13th Protocol to the European Convention on Human Rights became binding on UK, prohibiting the restoration of the death penalty for being a signatory to the Convention. The last execution by hanging in the US was in 1996 in Delaware and only the states of New Hampshire and Washington presently allow hanging as an option.[5,13] Since 2003, 10th of October is celebrated as World Day against the death penalty. In 2013, the 11th World Day against the death penalty was dedicated to the Greater Caribbean where some executions still takes place.

In India, not much has changed on the issue of mode of execution of death sentence. The Criminal Procedure Code dictates that hanging should be the mode of execution. In 1980, in Bachan Singh vs. State of Punjab (AIR 1982 SC 1325), the validity of death sentence was upheld by the Constitutional Bench of the Supreme Court by majority of 4:1 and reiterated that hanging did not constitute an 'unreasonable, cruel or unusual punishment'. Similar views were expressed in Deena vs. Union of India (1983)4 SCC 645. In the judgment, the court also upheld the constitutional validity of Sec. 354(5) of Code of Criminal Procedure (CrPC) of 1973 for carrying out of death sentence by hanging by neck till he is dead as the best available method in India to electric chair, shooting or lethal injection.[1,3,9]

In a recent judgment, a Bangladeshi court sentenced 152 people to death on 5th November 2013 for a mutiny in Dhaka in 2009.

METHODS OF EXECUTION

The death penalty was executed by various modes and methods. Some of these methods are mentioned below:[3]

i. **Burning at the stake** dates back to the Christian era as popular means of torture and method of execution. This was used mostly for witches, heretics and suspicious women. The last legal execution by this method took place at end of the Spanish Inquisition in 1834.

ii. **Crucifixion** involves nailing a person to a wooden cross and leaving him there till he is dead. This cruel but popular method of executing death sentence was prevalent during the Christian era (Jesus Christ was crucified in this manner).

iii. **The wheel** as a method of torture and execution involved attaching the condemned person to the outer rim of the wheel and then rolled over sharp spikes, or down a hill, to his death. The wheel could also be used like a turntable, with the person tied to it. The people would take turns beating the person with iron rods, breaking his bones and ultimately death. This method was used throughout Europe, especially during the middle ages.

iv. **Sicilian bull or Brazen bull** was particularly used by the Greeks and Romans. It was bronze or brass cast in the shape of a bull which was hollow from inside. The person was forced inside through the door and then placed over an open flame. This would slowly burn him to death. They were supposedly used at banquets and feasts as a sort of entertainment, and the smell was considered to be an aphrodisiac.

v. **Headman's axe** was a popular form of execution in Germany and England during the 16th-17th centuries, since decapitation was thought to be the most humane form of capital punishment. An executioner, usually hooded, would chop off the person's head with an axe or sword. The last beheading took place in 1747 in England.

vi. **Mazzatello** was similar to beheading and used in Italy. The setup was much like a beheading since there was a victim, block, executioner and drawing and quartering sometimes followed. However, instead of an axe, the executioner used a large square-headed mallet or hammer to crush the skull.

vii. **Guillotine** was a device used for carrying out executions by decapitation. It consists of a tall upright frame from which a heavy blade is suspended. The blade is raised with a rope and then allowed to drop, severing the victim's head from their body. This was a popular form of execution in France, particularly, during the French Revolution. The last public execution by this method was carried out in 1939, and the last use was in 1977.

viii. **Garotte** was also a common method of torture and execution, and was similar to hanging. Strangulation is caused by compression of the neck by an iron collar which was tightened by a screw known as *Spanish windlass.* This resulted in sudden loss of consciousness and collapse. Garroting was practiced in Spain, Portugal and Turkey.

ix. **Hanging** was and still is a very common method for execution among the various methods available. The prisoner could simply be hanged with a noose. However, if torture was also intended, then the person would be drawn, hanged and then quartered.

x. **Firing squad** as a form of execution is carried out in the state of Utah, Afghanistan, Belarus, Ethiopia, Indonesia, North Korea, Nigeria, Yemen, Vietnam and China. This is also permitted in India when a death sentence is given by court marshal. Usually, the condemned person is tied to the pole or a chair and is blindfolded, and a cloth patch is put on heart. A team of five executioners aims at the person's heart. In few countries, some of the rifles are loaded with blank bullets so that the true identity of the executioner is not known.

xi. **Gas chamber** is authorized in few states of the US as an alternative to lethal injection. The condemned person is restrained in a metal chair and sealed in an airtight chamber. A long stethoscope is also affixed to the person's chest so that a doctor sitting outside can monitor the heart beat and pronounce death. Beneath the chair is a bowl filled with sulphuric acid mixed with distilled water, and sodium cyanide pellets suspended in a gauze bag just above it. The executioner in a separate room operates a lever that releases the cyanide into the liquid resulting in formation of hydrocyanic gas fumes.

Prisoners are advised to take deep breath after the gas is released, as this will shorten their suffering. Unconsciousness takes place very rapidly, although the heart continues to beat for 10–20 min. Convulsion may occur if the prisoner holds his breath and death can be delayed.

xii. **Electrocution** as a method of execution is used in some of the states of US and the Philippines. In a typical execution, condemned person is strapped to a specially built chair. The head and body is shaved to provide better contact with the moistened copper electrodes that the executioner attaches. Usually, three or more executioners' are involved in pushing the buttons, but only one is connected to the actual electrical source so the real executioner is not known. An alternating current is used and the voltage varies in power in different jurisdictions, and is also determined by the convict's body weight.

xiii. **Lethal injection** is the primary method of execution in several states of the US, and also used in the Philippines and Guatemala along with China experimenting with this method. In this procedure, intravenous injections of three drugs are used in sequence to bring death. The condemned person is secured on a wheeled stretcher with lined ankle and wrist restraints. A cardiac monitor and a stethoscope are attached, and two saline intravenous lines are started, one in each arm. The intravenous lines are turned off and sodium thiopental is injected, causing the person to fall into a deep sleep in about a minute. Then a muscle relaxant, pancuronium bromide is given which stops breathing due to paralyses of the diaphragm and respiratory muscles. Finally, potassium chloride is injected, which stops the heart.[6]

The present trend seems to be that of favoring execution by lethal injection. Of all the available methods, this appears to be the quickest, least painful and humane. However, even this method can result in cruel and unusual suffering with reported delayed deaths in many cases. Recently, in July 2014, in Arizona (US), execution process of the prisoner Joseph Wood took nearly two hours after injection, before being pronounced dead.

As per the report of the Law Commission of India, lethal injection is currently being contemplated by them as the method of execution. The recommendations are, however, not binding on the government.[3,8,9]

Some other forms of judicial punishments are also carried in some countries, especially in those whose legal system is based on Islamic law—caning; whipping, flogging and lashing; and mutilation, including eye gouging, chemical blinding, amputation of fingers, hands or other body parts. This may not result in death but there is severe physical injury and permanent scarring.

HANGING TECHNIQUES

The execution technique of hanging, introduced by the Angle, Saxon, and Jute Germanic tribes during their invasions of the Roman Empire and Britain in the 5th century, has remained largely unchanged over time. During this period, death by hanging was often prolonged and inconsistent, with many cases of decapitation or recovery recorded.

There are basically four methods to carry out a judicial hanging—the short drop, suspension hanging, the standard drop, and the long drop.[3-5,11,13,14] A modified form, the 'upright jerker', was also experimented with in the 19th century.

Short Drop

In short drop, the prisoner drops just a few inches. The suspended body weight and physical struggling causes the noose to tighten, causing death by strangulation or carotid or vagal reflex. This can be done by various means—by placing the condemned person on the back of a cart, horse or other vehicle with the noose around his neck. The carter is then moved away leaving the person dangling from the rope. Prior to 1850, it was the universal method used. This method is still used in Middle Eastern countries, particularly in Iran.

Suspension Hanging

Suspension hanging is similar to short drop, except the gallows themselves are movable. This method uses hydraulic mechanisms (for e.g., barrels of tanks and mobile crane jibs) for raising the condemned. It serves as both the gallows and the means of getting the prisoner suspended. This method is currently used in Iran and the Taliban controlled Afghanistan.

Standard Drop

In standard drop, the condemned person drops to a pre-determined height, typically 4–6 feet (1.2 to 1.8 meters). This was often equivalent to their height, and not based on the weight of the person. It was considered an improvement of the short drop since it was intended to cause fracture of the cervical spine and immediate death. However, a drop of this distance was often not sufficient to cause the intended fracture, and many died due to strangulation. In some cases, unconsciousness resulted by the force of the drop and by the impact of the heavy coiled knot against the side of the neck. Occasionally, they were decapitation when the drop was too long. This was the common method adopted in most Commonwealth countries and in the US in the late 19th and early 20th centuries.

Long Drop

The long drop or measured drop was introduced in 1872 by hangman William Marwood. This was considered a scientific improvement to the standard drop wherein the condemned person was falling to the same standard distance. In long drop, the person falls to a pre-determined distance based on his weight so as to ensure that the spine was fractured.[12]

Initially, the drop given was usually between 4 to 10 feet depending on the weight of the prisoner. In accordance with the recommendations of the Aberdare Committee in UK, from 1886 to 1892, the length of the drop was worked out by the formula 1,260 foot/pounds (5,600 N) divided by the body weight of the person in pounds = drop in feet. It was postulated that this force would fracture the neck, either at the 2nd and 3rd, or 4th and 5th cervical vertebrae.[12,15]

Cases of decapitation were reported with the use of the long drop. Between 1892 and 1913, the length of the drop was shortened, presumably to avoid the decapitation. After 1913, other factors were also taken into account and the drop was calculated to give a force of around 1,000 ft/lbs (4,400 N). From 1939, it became customary to add another nine inches to the drop calculated, to give a force of around 1100 ft/lbs.[12,15]

This method was adopted in India, Egypt, Singapore, Malaysia, Australia, Canada, Pakistan, Bangladesh and the Caribbean nations who desired to make executions more humane and was meant to make the person's suffering less traumatic. Even today, despite further refinements in technique and revised drop lengths, failures with hanging are still reported.

Hanging Debacle

Execution failures were caused by built of the condemned, position of the knot and the drop, or by hardware problems, or by factors related to the hangman himself. Sometimes, when death was not ensuing or the condemned is struggling, the hangman would intervene by pulling him by the legs, by lifting and jerking the body, or by sitting on the shoulders. This added more weight and pressure on the neck to ensure completion of the execution process. There are documented cases in which the executed convicts were revived, either at the hanging site, in the anatomy theater, or in the coffin while being transported on a wagon to the graveyard.[11,12]

Hardware issues included rope breakage and trapdoor malfunction. There are also reports of unsuccessful executions because the hangman was under the influence of alcohol or did not pay attention to details like the built of the convict, or unusual situations like the presence of a tracheotomy.[12]

EQUIPMENT

The equipment used in all of these methods are namely the gallows, noose, hood and pinioning.[5]

Gallows: Gallows ranged from a tree to an upright with a projecting beam to intentionally designed platforms with traps through which the condemned would fall. Some places also use cranes as gallows. Modern gallows in India, Australia, Singapore, Malaysia and other former British colonies typically have double trapdoors and operated by a lever on the platform with no steps.

Noose: The simplest type of noose is a slipknot. Variables include the length of or number of cords composing the rope. The traditional hangman's noose consisting of 5 to 13 coils is still used in the US, Iran and Iraq (Fig. 17.1). In the US, the coiled noose is prepared from 30 feet of 3/4-1" diameter Manila hemp rope, boiled to take out stretch and any tendency to coil. It is formed into six coils and then waxed, soaped or greased so that the knot slides easily.

Britain and most ex-Commonwealth countries use(d) a simple noose consisting of a loop worked into one end of the rope with the other end passed through it. This was improved in the 1890's by passing the free end of the rope through a brass eyelet instead of a loop of rope which made it more free running. This type of noose was supposed to cause a quicker death. Modern materials such as nylon have been tried in Iran for short drop/suspension hangings, but it is too elastic for long drop hangings.

Knot placement: The trend in the 19th century was to use a submental knot which resulted in death by strangulation. With the introduction of the long drop, the traditional submental knot was found to be unsuitable as it resulted in knot

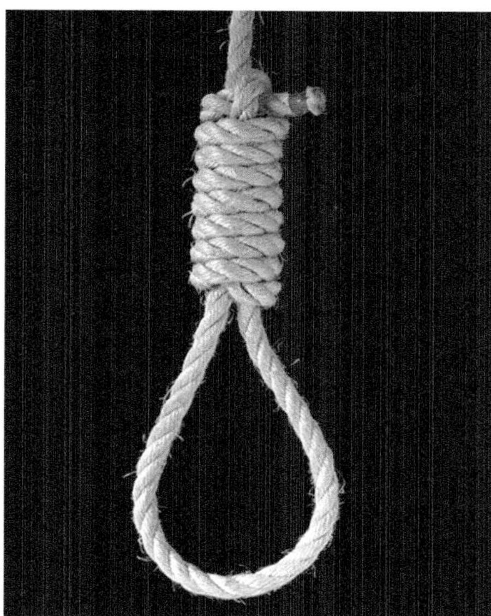

Fig. 17.1 Hangman's noose

slippage. Hangmen started using the subaural knot. However, the results with the subaural knot were not as effective and cases of decapitation were recorded. The cause of death was still strangulation, rather than the intended fracture of the cervical spine. Subaural knots could cause fracture of base of the skull; however, this was less ideal than fracture of the cervical spine.[11,12]

In 1886, after witnessing several hangings, de Zouche Marshall suggested that the submental knot was more effective than the subaural knot. In 1886-88, the Aberdare Committee also strongly advocated the use of submental knots. In 1913, Wood-Jones recommended substituting the subaural knot with a submental knot for effective and painless execution. However, in India and US, the recommended knot is still subaural in most of the manuals on execution.[11,12]

Hood: It is a convention to hood the prisoner before execution in most countries. Normally, a black cotton or denim hood is used. In some countries, particularly in UK, South Africa and Australia, a white linen or cotton hood was the norm. Typically, the prisoner is hooded before the noose is put around their neck. Iraq, Malaysia and Singapore hood the prisoner before leading them to the execution chamber. Some places such as Iran do not use a hood, although a blindfold may be used at some public executions. The possible reasons of hooding the prisoner are:

- To prevent alteration in the position of the noose—movement at the last moment in long drop hangings when the lever is being pulled may alter the knot which may cause a slower death.
- To minimise rope burn—the hood is generally put over the head before the noose which also prevents the hood being blown off by the updraft created by the body falling.
- It also ensures those witnessing the execution do not see the condemned person's face as they are about to die.

Pinioning: The prisoner's hands are pinioned usually behind their back or in front with either handcuffs or a leather strap. Some countries like Kuwait use additional straps for the arms or even leather harnesses for the arms and wrists. In long drop or standard drop hangings, the prisoner's legs are pinioned with a cord or strap around the ankles to prevent them getting their feet onto the sides of the trap when it opens. In the 20th century, an extra strap was placed round the lower thighs in UK, to prevent indecent exposure of women's underwear due to the short skirts worn by them during that period. For short drop and suspension hangings, the legs were usually left free.

EXECUTION PROCEDURE IN INDIA

The procedure of judicial hanging has remained unchanged for centuries before significant modifications to its process were introduced and applied in the last two centuries. Sec. 368(1) CrPC, 1898 provided for hanging by neck till death. This has not been amended in the Sec. 354(5) CrPC, 1973 which states that 'When any person is sentenced to death, the sentence shall direct that he be hanged by the neck till he is dead.'[1]

The jail manuals of various States provide for the method of execution of death sentence in India. Once death sentence is awarded and is confirmed after exhausting all the possible available remedies, the execution is carried out in accordance with Sec. 354(5) CrPC. It is also provided under The Air Force Act, 1950, The Army Act, 1950 and The Navy Act, 1957 that the execution has to be carried out either by hanging by neck till death or by being shot to death.[3] Chapter XXXI, Jail Manual of Punjab and Haryana, and in Chapter XI of 'Model prison manual for the superintendence and management of prisons in India' issued by Bureau of Police Research and Development (BPRD), Ministry of Home Affairs provides for the various steps leading to the execution of the death sentence.[3,16]

Rope

A well twisted and fully stretched cotton yarn/Manilla rope of 19 feet length and 1–1.5 inches (2.59 to 3.81 cm) diameter should be used for executions. It should be of equal thickness, capable of passing readily through the noose-ring and sufficiently strong to bear a strain of 280 lbs. with a 7 feet drop. It also recommends of keeping at least two such ropes at every jail where executions are likely to take place. The testing of the rope to be used for the execution should be done at least before a week from the date of the execution and on the evening before such execution is to take place. The method for testing such rope is by attaching the sack of clay or sand to one end which is equivalent to one and half times of the weight of the prisoner. The length of the drop to be kept same as required for the condemned prisoner. The 'drop' is the length of the rope from a point on the rope opposite the angle of the lower jaw of the condemned as he stands on the scaffold to the point where the rope is embraced in the noose after allowing for the constriction of the neck that takes place in hanging.

According to the BPRD manual, the height of the prisoner to the angle of the jaw below the left ear is to be measured and the height from the drop shutter (when fixed in position) to the lower portion of the ring in the beam to which the rope will be affixed is also measured. These two measurements will determine the distance when the prisoner is standing in position on the drop, from the point of the latter's jaw to the ring in the beam. The length of rope for any given drop should be the length of the drop plus the distance from the angle of the prisoner's jaw to the ring in the beam. The measurement of the prisoner's neck is also taken.[16]

Regulation of the drop: In the jail manual, the drop recommended for a prisoner < 100 lbs weight is 7 feet, < 120 lbs weight is 6 feet, < 140 lbs weight is 5.5 feet and < 160 lbs weight is 5 feet. The length of the drop as per the BPRD manual is given in Table 17.1. In the module prepared by the BPRD and the jail manual, it requires the medical officer to provide details of the drop based on the weight of the prisoner and his personal opinion.

Time of the execution: The time of the execution is recommended for the early hours of the day, but the exact time varies as per the season: from November–February: 8 AM; for March, April, September and October: 7 AM; and from May–August: 6 AM.

Procedure

The actual execution process is described briefly:

i. The officers usually present at the execution are the Superintendent and Medical officer of the jail, and the District Magistrate.
ii. The execution is carried out by the public executioner. If he is not available, then some trustworthy individual who is locally trained can be assigned this job.
iii. The condemned prisoner is marched to the scaffold by the Deputy Superintendent. After reaching at the scaffold, the warrant is read in the language of the convict.
iv. The warders holding the person places him under the direct beam to which rope is attached.
v. The executioner then strap his legs tightly together, place the hood over his head and face, and adjust the rope tightly around his neck. The BPRD manual recommends a cotton hood with flap to be put on the prisoners face just before he enters the gallows enclosures as he is not allowed to see the gallows.

Table 17.1 Recommended drop

Weight	*Drop*
<100 lbs (45 kg)	8 feet or 2.5 m
>100–133 lbs (45–60 kg)	7 feet 8 inches or 2.3 m
>133–166 lbs (60–75 kg)	7 feet or 2.2 m
>166–200 lbs (75–91 kg)	6 feet 6 inches or 2 m
> 200 lbs (>91 kg)	6 feet or 1.83 m

vi. The noose (knot or metal eye) is to be placed one and half inches to the right or left of the middle line and free from the flap of the cap so as to run up behind the ear when the prisoner falls and receives the jerk. The rope is adjusted so that the part to which the metal eye belongs should pass in front of the throat.
vii. The warders then withdraw their hands holding the person, and at the signal from the Superintendent, the executioner draws the bolt.
viii. The body of the executed person was to be kept hanging for half an hour till the medical officer declares the life extinct. However, in 1995, a two-Judge bench of the Supreme Court opined that it is an uncivilized act and ruled that 'a convict should remain hanged till he is declared dead by the medical officer'.[9]
ix. The Superintendent then returns the warrant with the endorsement that the sentence has been carried out.

PATHOPHYSIOLOGY

In spite of significant modifications in the technique, majority of those hanged in the 21st century is speculated to have died slowly and painfully by strangulation. Immediately after suspension, the person may exhibit signs of struggling for 1–3 min. After this, there is a quiescent phase which is followed by the convulsive phase that occurs after loss of consciousness. There may be spasmodic and uncoordinated movements of the limbs, legs may be drawn up and heaving of the chest may occur for some time. This may be due to the nervous and muscular reflexes, and does not indicate consciousness. Consciousness is usually lost in about 8–10 seconds or persists for longer to a minute. The heart may continue to beat for some period after the brain can no longer be resuscitated. It is thought that brain death occurs in about 6 min and the heart stops beating within 10–15 min. The time of death in such cases is a matter of convention and pronounced at cardiac arrest. Cases are also on record that the person died without any struggle or may have struggled for few seconds before dying.[3,5,8]

Any damage to the phrenic nerve which originates in the neck (C3-C5) and controls the diaphragm may cause cessation of breathing immediately, leading to asphyxia. Since the diameter of the noose usually reduces to 5–7 inches from its original diameter after the drop, it will constrict the jugular veins and carotid arteries too. Compression of the jugular veins and carotid arteries requires about 4.5 pounds/square inch and 11 pounds/square inch of pressure respectively. It may cause stoppage of the heart due to carotid/vagal reflex. The vertebrae protect the vertebral and spinal arteries which also supply blood to the brain. However, these arteries emerge out the 4th vertebrae which may result in obstruction if the pressure on the neck is high enough (about 40-50 pounds/square inch). It may also constrict the trachea which requires about 33 pounds/square inch of pressure to compress.[5]

Asphyxia may also result from the weight of the person's body forcing the larynx and the base of the tongue moving upwards, thus preventing breathing. Fractures of the hyoid bone and larynx may occur which can prove fatal if breathing is restricted or prevented.

Biomechanics of Hangman's Fracture

At the end of the drop, the body is still accelerating under the force of gravity but the head is constrained by the noose. If the eyelet is positioned under the left angle of the jaw it rotates the head backwards, which combined with the downward momentum of the body, fracture the cervical vertebra and ruptures the spinal cord. This causes deep unconsciousness and instant death. The later use of the brass eyelet in the noose was intended to fracture the vertebra with more certainty. It is only in the last six inches or so of the drop that the trauma to the neck and vertebrae occur, as the rope constricts the neck and the force is applied to the vertebrae. The duration of the process is between 0.02–0.03 seconds depending upon the length of drop given.[12,17]

In the 1950s and 1960s, several researchers observed cervical spine fractures following motor vehicle accidents. Gilbert Hamilton, an anatomist, noted the similarities between the cervical fractures seen following traffic accidents and those occurring following judicial hangings as reported by Wood-Jones. In 1965, Schneider and colleagues presented several cases of cervical fractures following motor vehicle accidents. The cervical injuries seen in car accidents resulted from a hyperextension-compression mechanism of injury. They also noted that the third cervical vertebra forms a fixed point between the craniocervical junction and the lower cervical spine. Forces acting downward from the skull through the atlanto-occipital and atlanto-axial joints divide in the frontal plane and are united in the axis body. These continue downward, turning 90°, and are distributed in three distinct lines, along the line of the vertebral bodies and discs medially, and along the line of the pre- and post-zygapophyses bilaterally. These three lines pass through the weakest part of the neural arch of the axis, which is prone to fracture, causing an avulsion fracture of the axis. During judicial hanging with a submental knot, a hyperextension-distraction effect is produced by the knot and the drop. This results in rupture of the ligament system, fixing the cervical spine ventrally, and leaning of the arch of the axis on the third cervical vertebra and, as a consequence, its fracture (Fig. 17.2).[5,12,17] The continuous longitudinal traction results in complete detachment of the cervical spine from the cervicocranial junction, and results in severe neurological consequences that are usually fatal. Schneider coined the term '*hangman's fracture*' based on the similarities of the cervical fractures observed following judicial hangings and those caused by motor vehicle accidents.

Cause of Death

Evaluations of the causes of death during judicial hanging have been based on autopsy and retrospective evaluations. Hanging can cause death by one or more of the following mechanisms: asphyxia, apoplexy and fracture dislocation of the cervical vertebra. If a judicial hanging is carried out in a textbook manner, it is expected to cause instantaneous death by the traumatic spondylolisthesis of C-2 (hangman's fracture), with accompanying contusion or transection of the spinal cord.[18] However, research has shown that 'hangman's fracture' is seen in only a few cases of judicial hangings and the cause of death can be attributed to a range of head and neck injuries, viz. compression or rupture of the vertebral and carotid

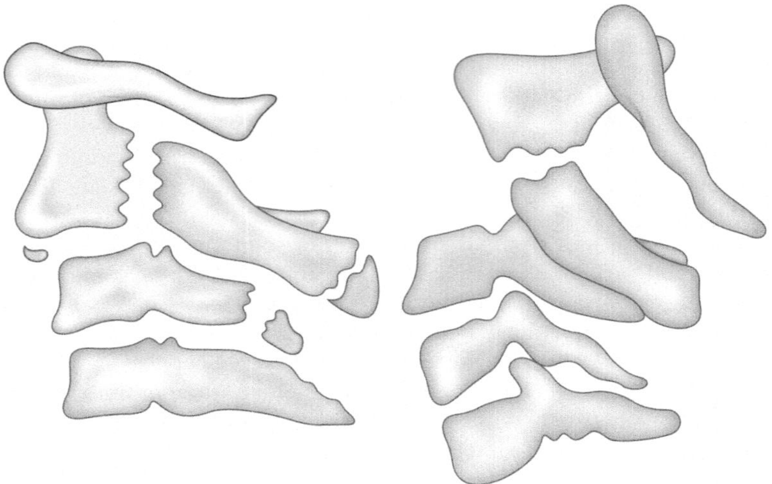

Fig. 17.2 Fracture of the posterior arch of the axis, which remained attached to the cervical spine below, whereas the anterior part of the axis and the atlas remained attached to the skull base

arteries leading to cerebral ischemia or a relatively slower death by asphyxiation (strangulation).

AUTOPSY FINDINGS

There are no autopsy studies of judicial hangings available in India since there is no provision for postmortem; it is not known whether death was caused by strangulation or by fracture dislocation of cervical vertebra. However, in UK postmortem was carried out during the 20th century on the executed person's to establish the exact cause of death.

The body will typically show inverted 'V' shaped ligature mark ('furrow') where the knot of the noose was situated and the neck gets flexed to the side opposite to the knot. The tongue may protrude out with dribbling of saliva from the angle of the mouth (depending on the position of the knot). In some cases, there may be involuntary discharge of fecal matter and urine. In males, there may be penile turgidity and involuntary discharge of semen. The opening of the sphincters may be due to an adrenaline rush which is common in circumstances of extreme fear. If the jugular veins are occluded before the carotid arteries, the face may become engorged and cyanosed, and there may be bleeding from eyes and nose due to impaired venous return and accumulation of blood. There may be petechiae on the face and in the eyes. If death has occurred through vagal reflex, the face will typically be pale and bluish in color and may not show any petechiae.[5,18]

Hangman's Fracture

Studies in late 19th and early 20th centuries suggested fracture of the cervical spine as the cause of death, and some even implicated a role of the odontoid process. In 1908, Wood-Jones examined 100 exhumed bodies of Nubian men who were hanged by the Roman Empire. He found fractures of the skull base that were the most likely cause of death. He also examined the cervical spines of five persons hanged using a submental knot and a long drop. He concluded that the odontoid process had no part in causing death. Instead, the common finding was a fracture of the posterior arch of the axis, which remained attached to the cervical spine below, whereas the anterior part of the axis and the atlas remained attached to the skull base (Fig. 17.2). This fracture was caused by a violent jerk, which threw the person's head backward and fractured the axis, causing injury to the spinal cord and resulting in instantaneous death. This type of cervical fracture had not been reported to occur when a subaural knot was used. Subaural knots were associated with basilar skull fractures without cervical spine injuries, whereas submental knots resulted in fracture or dislocation of the axis without basilar skull fracture.[11,12,15]

Hellier and Connolly examined the skeletal remains of George Kelly and found fracture of first cervical vertebra but no 'hangman's fracture'. No skeletal evidence of death by strangulation was found by them. It was speculated that unconsciousness and subsequent death, would probably have resulted due to vertebral artery damage due to the fracture of cervical vertebra.[14,19]

Spence and colleagues examined the skeletons of six persons executed by judicial hanging in two Canadian prisons. The injuries seen were fractures of the hyoid cornua, styloid processes, occipital bones, and cervical vertebral bodies (C2) and transverse processes (C1, C2, C3, and C5). The trauma to the skeletal structure and the cause of death varied among individuals although there was uniformity of the hanging technique with a subaural knot. It was concluded that this variation was probably due to minor differences in hanging practices and individual anatomic peculiarities of the victims.[20]

In 1992, James and Nasmyth-Jones analyzed 34 victims of judicial hangings and observed that fracture of the axis occurred in only six cases. The fractures were of two types—three were the traditional 'hangman's fracture' whilst three were of a type previously unreported. The pathologists opined that the long-drop method caused death due to strangulation or asphyxia, without the intended instantaneous death due by cervical fracture.[21]

Extensive study was done by Wallace and colleagues using modern imaging techniques such as computed tomography (CT) and magnetic resonance (MR) imaging on two judicial hanging cases. They found that in the first case (subaural knot was used) there were cervical spine ligamentous injury and partial disruption of the vertebral arteries without vertebral subluxation or injury to the cervical cord. Pathologic diagnosis was hanging by ligature with intervertebral ligamentous separation at C2-3 and C5-6 associated with small marginal avulsion fractures of the cervical vertebrae, extensive soft-tissue and paravertebral muscle hemorrhage with extension into the mediastinum, fractures of the left wing of the hyoid cartilage and midline of the thyroid cartilage, epidural cervical spinal cord hemorrhage with focal traumatic subarachnoid hemorrhage, and a prominent abrasion furrow of the neck. Angiography showed lacerations of both vertebral arteries, associated with subarachnoid hemorrhage at the base of the brain. Carotid arteries were intact. In the second case (submental knot was used) there was complete ligamentous disruption and subluxation at C2-3 with cord transection. Pathologic diagnosis was hanging by ligature with disruption of ligaments and transection of the spinal cord at C2-3, subarachnoid hemorrhage, fractures of the rightwing of the hyoid bone and thyroid cartilage, extensive soft-tissue injury to the posterior neck, mediastinal hematoma and intimal tears in both carotid arteries. In both cases, minimally displaced transverse process fractures were present, and CT and MR imaging of the head showed diffuse subarachnoid hemorrhage. It was inferred that in the first case, loss of consciousness probably resulted from subarachnoid hemorrhage or cerebral hypoxia, followed by death due to cerebral anoxia. In the second case, there was spinal cord injury at C2-3 with subarachnoid hemorrhage.[15]

Hence, the above studies indicate that the traditional hangman's fracture occurred in only a small proportion of cases of judicial hanging. The rapidity of loss of consciousness and type of injury is highly dependent on the positioning of the knot and the length of the drop.

SAMPLE POSTMORTEM REPORT

Ruth Ellis' was the last woman to be executed in the UK after being convicted of the murder of her lover, David Blakely. She was hanged at Holloway Prison, London, by Albert Pierrepoint. Her autopsy was carried out by one of the most eminent forensic pathologists, Professor Keith Simpson.[5] I have reproduced the autopsy report for the benefit and interest of the readers (Box 17.1).

LEGAL ASPECTS

In the Indian Penal Code (IPC) and several legislative Acts, the offences punishable by capital punishment are laid down. A death sentence may also be imposed for a number of offences committed by members of the armed forces. In Bachan Singh vs. State of Punjab, Supreme Court held that the death penalty was constitutional only when applied as an exceptional penalty in 'the rarest of the rare' cases. Courts may interpret Bachan Singh case as overriding other law when sentencing for offenses resulting in death. In a Supreme Court ruling in February 2012, it held that mandatory death sentence as unconstitutional in light of the judgments in Bachan Singh vs. State of Punjab and Mithu vs. State of Punjab.[1,9]

Offences Punishable by Death

The offender involved in the following offences can be sentenced to death:[1,7]

1. *Aggravated murder:* Murder is punishable by death under Sec. 302 IPC.
2. *Other offenses resulting in death*
    - If any member of a group commits murder in the course of committing an armed robbery.
    - Kidnapping for ransom in which the victim is killed.
    - Being a member of an association or promoting an association, while committing any act using unlicensed firearms or explosives that results in death.
    - Engaging in organized crime, if it results in death.
    - Committing, or assisting another person in committing sati (immolation of a widow) under The Commission of Sati (Prevention) Act, 1987.
    - *Calumniation:* To make maliciously or knowingly false statements by a witness in a capital case against a member of a scheduled caste or tribe, resulting in that person's conviction and execution under The Scheduled Castes and Scheduled Tribes (Prevention of Atrocities) Act, 1989.

Box 17.1 Postmortem examination report*

Name Ellis, Ruth **Apparent Age** 28 years. **At** H. M. Prison, Holloway **Date** July 13 1955.	
EXTERNAL EXAMINATION	Well nourished. Evidence of proper care and attention. Height 5 ft. 2 ins. Weight 103 lbs. Deep impressions around neck from noose with a suspension point about 1 inch in front of the angle of the left lower jaw. Vital changes locally and in the tissues beneath as a consequence of sudden constriction. No ecchymosis in the face or elsewhere. No marks of restraint.
How long dead	1 hour.
INTERNAL EXAMINATION	
Skull Basic meninges	Fracture—dislocation of the spine at C2 with a 2 inch gap and transverse separation of the spinal cord at the same level.
Mouth, tongue, esophagus	
Larynx, trachea	Fracture of both wings of the hyoid and right wing of the thyroid cartilage, larynx also fractured.
Lungs	Air passages clear and lungs free from disease or other change. No engorgement. No asphyxial changes.
Pericardium, heart and blood vessels	No organic changes. No petechiae or other evidence of organic change.
Stomach and contents	Small food residue and odor of brandy. No disease.
Peritoneum	Normal.
Intestines	Terminal congestion only.
Liver and gall bladder	Normal.
Spleen	
Kidneys and ureters	Slight terminal congestion only.
Bladder	
Generative organs	Lower abdominal operation scar for ectopic pregnancy, operation in L. tube, now healed. No pregnancy.
Other remarks	Deceased was a healthy subject at the time of death. Mark of suspension normally situated and injuries from judicial hanging—to the spinal column—must have caused instant death.
CAUSE OF DEATH	Injuries to the central nervous system consequent upon judicial hanging.

Signed Keith Simpson
M. D. Lond.
146, Harley St. W. 1 and Guy's Hospital (Pathologist)
Registrar in Forensic Medicine, London University

*With kind permission from Richard Clark (He is a well known historian whose research into capital punishment has spanned decades)

   - Assisting individuals who are under the age of 18, mentally ill, mentally disabled, or intoxicated in committing suicide.
   - Those found guilty of making and selling spurious liquor which causes death (only in Gujarat).
3. *Terrorism-related offenses resulting in death*
4. *Terrorism-related offenses not resulting in death* which may likely to endanger life or cause serious damage to property.
5. *Rape:* Under Sec. 376A IPC, rape is punishable by death if it leads to death or if it leaves the victim in a 'persistent vegetative state'. Under Sec. 376E IPC, repeat perpetrators may also get capital punishment.
6. *Kidnapping* not resulting in death or if the kidnapper threatens to kill or harm the victim or if the victim is actually harmed.
7. *Drug trafficking* not resulting in death: If an individual who has been convicted with offenses related to drug trafficking (for e.g., trafficking of cannabis and opium) commits another offense related to narcotic and psychotropic substances under The Narcotics, Drugs and Psychotropic Substances (Amendment) Act, 1988.
8. *Treason*: Waging or attempting to wage war against the government.
9. *Espionage (spying):* Obtaining secret or confidential information without the permission of the holder of the information.
10. *Military offenses* not resulting in death: Mutiny, desertion, cowardice, treacherous acts, dereliction of duty, aiding the enemy, imperiling Indian or allied military, air, or naval forces.
11. *Other offenses* not resulting in death
    - Being a party to a criminal conspiracy to commit a capital offence.
    - Attempts to murder by those sentenced to life imprisonment, if the attempt results in harm to the victim.

Offenders Excluded from the Death Penalty[7]

- **Age:** According to the Juvenile Justice (Care and Protection of Children) Act 2000, individuals who are less than 18 years of age at the time of commission crime cannot be given death penalty. In Bachan Singh vs. State of Punjab, advanced age was considered a mitigating factor in sentencing, although it does not have the same exclusionary effect as a minor does.
- **Conviction of a pregnant woman:** Sec. 416 CrPC states that if a woman sentenced to death is found to be pregnant, the High Court should order the execution of the sentence to be postponed and may, if it thinks fit commute the sentence to imprisonment for life. This is necessitated by the fact that if a pregnant woman is sentenced to death, it would result in killing of the fetus also. According to CrPC (Amendment) Act, 2008, if a pregnant woman is sentenced to death, the High Court should commute the sentence to imprisonment for life. Post delivery, if the mother is put to death, the child will be orphaned and punished for no fault of his/her.
- **Mentally ill and mentally retarded:** According to Sec. 84 IPC, individuals who were of unsound mind at the time of the crime and who did not understand the nature of the act or know that the act was wrong or contrary to the law cannot be held criminally liable. This could also be interpreted to exclude mentally retarded persons from the death penalty.

Appellate Process

In case death sentence was awarded by Session Court, the defendant has the right to appeal both the sentence and the conviction to a High Court, and if a case was originally tried before a High Court, then the defendant can appeal to the Supreme Court. The High Court is the first appellate court for capital cases, except for certain terrorism-related cases where the Supreme Court is the first court of appeal.[1,2,7]

In the High Court, trials are presided over by a bench composed of at least two Judges. The High Court can confirm a death sentence, commute the death sentence to another punishment, convict the defendant for another offense, order a new trial, or acquit the defendant. If a lower court does not impose a death sentence on an individual, the state can still appeal to the High Court to increase the penalty to a death sentence. There is no automatic right of appeal to the Supreme Court. However, in cases where the High Court increases a defendant's sentence to the death penalty after a lower trial court acquitted the defendant, the case may be appealed to the Supreme Court.[1,2,7]

In the military system, sentences passed by courts-martial under the Army, Navy or Air Force cannot be appealed to a higher court.

However, the Constitution gives the President and the Governor of a State the right to suspend, pardon or commute death sentences. With the advice of their cabinets, these executives can pardon or commute the death sentence of any offender to any other punishment provided by the Penal Code.

Judicial Discretion

It has been completely left upon the court's 'discretion' to decide whether a case falls under the category of '*rarest of rare case*' or not. However, the apex court laid down a few principles which were to be kept in mind while deciding the question of sentence. One of the important principles is regarding aggravating and mitigating circumstances. It has been the view of the court that while deciding the question of sentence, a balance sheet of aggravating and mitigating circumstances in that particular case has to be laid down. Full weightage should be given to the mitigating circumstances and even after that if the court feels that justice will not be done if any punishment less than the death sentence is awarded, then only death sentence should be imposed. The Supreme Court has also discussed such circumstances in many cases. Some of these circumstances are given in Box 17.2.[1,7]

Box 17.2 Aggravating circumstances

- Murder committed in an extremely brutal, grotesque, diabolical, revolting or dastardly manner so as to arouse intense and extreme indignation of the community.
- Murder for a motive which evinces total depravity and meanness.
- Murder of a scheduled caste or scheduled tribe, arousing social wrath (not for personal reasons).
- Bride burning/dowry death.
- Murderer in a dominating position, position of trust or in course of betrayal of the motherland.
- Where it is enormous in proportion.
- Victim was an innocent child, helpless woman, old or infirm person, public figure loved and respected by the community.

Mitigating Circumstances

The court may take into consideration the mitigating circumstances in the determination of sentence (Box 17.3).[7] On the basis of which, lesser punishment can be imposed.

If upon taking an overall view of all the circumstances and taking into account the answers to the question posed by way of the test of rarest of rare cases, the circumstances of the case are such that death penalty is warranted, the court would proceed to do so. In recent judgments, the Supreme Court bench headed by Chief Justice P. Sathasivam commuted the death sentence of Sushil Sharma to life imprisonment in the 1995 Naina Sahni murder case which they considered was committed by the accused due to strained personal relationship with his wife, and not a crime against society. This was a mitigating factor for commuting the death sentence to life imprisonment. The trial court had on November 2003 sentenced him to death for killing his wife on July 1995.[22] In another recent judgment, the Supreme Court commuted to life term the capital punishment awarded to a man for a triple murder in which they opined that brutality cannot be the sole criterion for considering a case under the rarest of rare categories. It also cautioned the courts to act with utmost responsibility when awarding death penalty, as it is the exception and life sentence is the rule. It can be said that death sentence can be inflicted in special cases only.[23]

Delay in Execution of the Death Sentence

Delay in execution of death sentence is a factor which may be taken into consideration for commuting the sentence of death to life imprisonment.

Unanimity of decision: The Global Position

It is fundamental that there should be unanimity among the Judges awarding the death penalty. Fair and reasonable procedure should be followed, and more so, where people are to be given capital punishment. A number of countries including the US and the Commonwealth that retain the Jury system and continue to award the death sentence require a unanimous verdict by all Judges.

Box 17.3 Mitigating circumstances

- Offence committed under extreme mental or emotional disturbance.
- Accused is young or old.
- Accused probably would not commit criminal acts of violence, as would constitute a continuing threat to society.
- Accused probably can be reformed and rehabilitated.
- State should provide evidence to prove that the accused does not satisfy the above two conditions.
- Accused believed that he was morally justified in committing the offence, based upon the facts and circumstances of the case.
- Accused acted under the duress of domination of another person.
- Accused was mentally defective which impaired his capacity to appreciate the criminality of his conduct.

In the case of a non-unanimous verdict, common law convention is to commute a death sentence to life imprisonment. It was decided that in criminal cases in the US that no person should be awarded the death sentence except by the unanimous verdict of a twelve member Jury. This law is binding in all the states that have retained the death penalty in criminal and federal cases. In US Martial and Military Tribunal Courts, the Uniform Code of Military Justice states that a death sentence can only be awarded with unanimity of opinion of a five member panel that tries the case.[1,2]

In India, Jury trials were abolished following a 1962 Supreme Court ruling. However, there are often differences of opinion among apex court bench Judges, and in spite of differences in their opinion, the death penalty is still being imposed.

ETHICAL ISSUES IN CAPITAL PUNISHMENT

Historically, medical personals have actively participated in designing execution methods, making existing methods more efficient and even carrying out the death penalty. The techniques used in hanging were perfected by early executioners only after consultation with medical professionals. In most of the countries, health professionals are involved in the process of capital punishment. In such cases, the line between a medical practitioner and an executioner is crossed.[2,3,6]

In the 18th century, Dr Antoine Louis designed and Dr Joseph-Ignac Guillotine advocated the decapitating machine ('guillotine') as less painful and a more humane method of execution. Dr Alfred Southwick, a dentist, helped design the electric chair that was considered 'more humane' for many years. In the US, Dr MacDonald and Dr Spitzka, supervised the first execution by the electric chair. Medical expertise also played an important role in the use of the gas chamber. Dr Deutsch, an anesthesiologist, proposed the lethal injection along the lines of intravenous induction of general anesthesia. Since 1982, doctors were required to administer the injection and as such they were directly involved in the execution. In 1993, in Washington, Westley Dodd was executed by hanging wherein the medical examiner calculated how far the condemned would have to fall to die instantly.[9,24-26]

There is also the dilemma faced by doctors attending failed executions. Sometimes, the person examined was found to be alive, but they were required by the State not to sustain his life. On the contrary, they were required to instruct the executioner that the man required continuation of the trauma to complete the execution. For example, in cases where execution is by hanging, the doctor must periodically examine the person after the hanging to look for signs of life. If the person is found alive, instead of resuscitating, the doctor is to ask the hangman to continue to hang till death. This seems to be in conflict with medical ethics. The doctors were deviating from what is permitted by the World Medical Association's (WMA) 1981 declaration that 'a physician's only role would be to certify death once the state had carried out the execution.'[27] Ethical dilemma is also faced by psychiatrists looking after condemned but psychotic patients. In most of the countries, it is unethical for insane prisoners to be executed. The psychiatrists are required to treat the mental illness so that with his mental health is restored and the condemned prisoner can be executed. The American

Psychiatric Association has condemned this as 'a perversion of medical ethics' and has opposed psychiatrists participating in capital punishment.[24-26]

The Hippocratic Oath and the principle of *primum non nocere* ('first, do no harm') require that medical professionals are intended to save and prolong life, not to bring an end to them. Internationally, many medical associations that have taken a position that forbid participation of medical and other health professionals in the procedure of capital punishment. In 1980, before the first scheduled execution by lethal injection, the American Medical Association (AMA) passed a resolution against physician participation in executions. In 1981, the WMA strongly opposed medical participation in the death penalty. The British Medical Association (BMA) held that it is opposed to any method of execution that would require the participation of a medical practitioner either in carrying out the actual process or in instructing others in the technique of that process. Brazil Medical Association and the medical associations of the Nordic countries (Denmark, Finland, Iceland, Norway, and Sweden) share the same view.[27] In 1992, the AMA came out with detailed guidelines on medical acts in the process of execution that do or do not violate medical ethics which was modified further (Box 17.4).[3,9,28]

In the US, rules were proposed for lethal injections, and mandated that at least one physician attend the execution and pronounce death. The AMA, American College of Physicians (ACP), the American Nurses Association, the American Public Health Association (APHA), the Society for Correctional Physicians, and the National Commission on Correctional Health Care all opposed this rule. As a result, in 1993, the Justice Department eliminated the mandatory presence of a doctor and his/her requirement to pronounce death. However, the Justice Department did not prohibit physician participation in executions. Medical associations from Europe, with the lead provided by the BMA, consistently opposed the death penalty and played an active role in ensuring its abolition from most European countries.[24-26]

However, there are no appropriate guidelines on the issue of capital punishment by the Medical Council of India or the Indian Medical Association and other organizations responsible for the ethical practice of medicine in this country. The 1995 court ruling that a medical officer monitor vital signs while the person is hanging compromises the medical ethics. Further, the Law Commission of India in its report recommended the use of a lethal injection. The day is not far off when the Supreme Court decides or Parliament enacts a law, and hanging is replaced by a lethal injection.[9]

In the past few decades, the law and judiciary have made systematic efforts to promote doctors' participation in the capital punishment. Some states in the US have responded to this conflict by adopting statutory mechanisms to encourage medical participation in capital punishments. Among these included 'safe harbor policies', which prohibit State Medical Boards from taking disciplinary action against licensed medical personnel, and granting anonymity and confidentiality to those who participate in executions. Moreover, some doctors felt an obligation not to abandon the condemn person in their dying moments. The attending doctors believe that they are helping to alleviate the pain of the person who is put to death.[25,29]

Box 17.4 AMA guidelines for medical practitioner participation in capital punishment

1. An individual's opinion on capital punishment is the personal moral decision of the individual. A physician, dedicated to preserving life, should not participate in a legally authorized execution.
2. Physician participation in execution is defined generally as actions which would:
   - Directly cause the death of the condemned;
   - Assist, supervise, or contribute to the ability of another individual to directly cause the death of the condemned;
   - Automatically cause an execution to be carried out on a condemned prisoner.
3. Physician participation in an execution includes the following actions:
   - Prescribing or administering tranquilizers and other psychotropic agents and medications that are part of the execution procedure;
   - Monitoring vital signs on site or remotely (including monitoring ECGs);
   - Attending or observing an execution as a physician; and rendering of technical advice regarding execution.
4. In the case where the method of execution is lethal injection, the following actions by the physician would also constitute participation:
   - Selecting injection sites;
   - Starting intravenous lines as a port for a lethal injection device;
   - Prescribing, preparing, administering, or supervising injection drugs or their doses or types; inspecting, testing, or maintaining lethal injection devices
   - Consulting with or supervising lethal injection personnel.
5. The following actions *do not* constitute physician participation in execution:
   - Testifying as to medical history and diagnoses or mental state as they relate to competence to stand trial, testifying as to relevant medical evidence during trial, testifying as to medical aspects of aggravating or mitigating circumstances during the penalty phase of a capital case, or testifying as to medical diagnoses as they relate to the legal assessment of competence for execution;
   - Certifying death, provided that the condemned has been declared dead by another person;
   - Witnessing an execution in a totally non-professional capacity;
   - Witnessing an execution at the specific voluntary request of the condemned person, provided that the physician observes the execution in a non-professional capacity; and
   - Relieving the acute suffering of a condemned person while awaiting execution, including providing tranquilizers at the voluntary request of the condemned person to help relieve pain or anxiety in anticipation of the execution.
6. Physicians should not determine legal competence to be executed. A physician's medical opinion should be merely one aspect of the information taken into account by a legal decision maker such as a Judge/Jury. When a condemned prisoner has been declared incompetent to be executed, physicians should not treat the prisoner for the purpose of restoring competence, unless a commutation order is issued before treatment begins. The task of re-evaluating the prisoner should be performed by an independent physician examiner. If the incompetent prisoner is undergoing extreme suffering as a result of psychosis or any other illness, medical intervention intended to mitigate the level of suffering is ethically permissible. The physician should not be compelled to participate in the process of establishing a prisoner's competence or be involved with treatment of an incompetent, condemned prisoner if it is contrary to the physician's personal beliefs. Under those circumstances, physicians should be permitted to transfer care of the prisoner to another physician.
7. Organ donation by condemned prisoners is permissible only if:
   - The decision to donate was made before the prisoner's conviction.
   - The donated tissue is harvested after the prisoner has been pronounced dead and the body removed from the death chamber.
   - Physicians do not provide advice on modifying the method of execution for any individual to facilitate donation.

CONCLUSION

The death penalty has existed since the beginning of recorded history. Hanging was the preferred method of execution in UK and other Commonwealth countries for centuries and was the method of execution in the US till the mid 20th century. In India, the provision of 'rarest of rare case' in awarding death sentence (sometimes non-unanimous) is defined not by objective criteria but subjective to Judges' discretion that is sometimes influenced by public opinion and media bias. As per the CrPC, the execution of the death penalty in India is being carried out with hanging by neck till death during the last over hundred years. It was emphasized that the punishment by way of death sentence should be swift and humane, and hanging is considered most humane of all the available methods.

The law also mandates the presence of medical officer during execution to declare death as determined by absence of heart sounds. Lethal injection has become the preferred method of execution in many countries because this appears to be less offensive to the public and more humane for the prisoner. Law Commission in India also recommended lethal injection so as to give a medical face to capital punishment. This is equivalent to active participation in capital punishment which is considered an unethical act in violation of the Hippocratic Oath.

Our medical associations and medical councils should come out with specific guidelines similar to AMA that must articulate and implement ethical codes related to capital punishments.

REFERENCES

1. Kumar RS. Death sentence - A compilation. Available from: http://www.goforthelaw.com/articles/fromlawstu/article19.htm.
2. Hiremath V. Law commission report proposes lethal injection for the death penalty. *Issues Med Ethics* 2003; 11: 93-94.
3. 187th Report of the Law Commission of India on 'Mode of Execution of Death Sentence and Incidental matters. Law Commission of India 2003. Available from: http://lawcommissionofindia.nic.in/reports/187th%20report.pdf.
4. Hanging. Available from: http://en.wikipedia.org/wiki/Hanging.
5. Clark R. Capital punishment UK. Available from: http://www.capitalpunishmentuk.org/contents.html.
6. Background—Human rights watch. Available from: http://www.hrw.org/reports/1994/usdp/ 5.htm.
7. Babcock S. Center for International Human Rights at Northwestern law school's Bluhm legal clinic. The death penalty in India - death penalty worldwide. Available from: http://www.deathpenaltyworldwide.org/country-search-post.cfm?country=India#f3-1.
8. Mudur GS. Death by hanging takes minutes New Delhi, Nov. 21. Available from: http://www.telegraphindia.com/1121122/jsp/nation/story_16226564.jsp#.Ug8fjn__neo.
9. Jesani A. Medicalisation of 'legal' killing: doctors' participation in the death penalty. *Indian J Med Ethics* 2004; 1: 104-5.
10. Kumara S. West Bengal carries out first hanging in India in a decade; 2004. 30 Sept. Available from: http://www.wsws.org/articles/2004/sep 2004/indi-s30.shtml.
11. Wood Jones F. The medico-legal aspect of judicial hanging. The Medico-legal Society of Victoria. 29th Aug. 1931. Available from: http://mlsv.org.au/files/1931-1933/TheMedico-Legal Aspect Of Judicial Hanging.pdf.

12. Rayes M, Mittal M, Rengachary SS, Mittal S. Hangman's fracture: a historical and biomechanical perspective: Historical vignette. *J Neurosurg Spine* 2011; 14: 198-208.
13. *Capital punishment* in the United Kingdom. Available from: http://en.wikipedia.org/wiki/Capital_punishment_in_the_United_Kingdom.
14. Jha MK, Majumder BC, Garg A, Aggarwal KK, Oberoi SS. Judicial hanging-cause of death. *J Punjab Acad Forensic Med Toxicol* 2012; 12: 96-98.
15. Wallace SK, Cohen WA, Stern EJ, Reay DT. Judicial hanging: Postmortem radiographic, CT, and MR imaging features with autopsy confirmation. *Radiology* 1994; 193: 263-67.
16. India. Prisoner sentenced to death. Chapter XI. Model prison manual for the superintendence and management of prisons in India. Bureau of Police Research and Development. Ministry of Home Affairs. Government of India New Delhi. 2003. p. 133-44. Available from: http://bprd.nic.in/writereaddata/.../1445424768-ContentChapters.pdf.
17. Nokes LD, Roberts A, James DS. Biomechanics of judicial hanging: a case report. *Med Sci Law* 1999; 39: 61-64.
18. Biswas G. Asphyxia. Review of forensic medicine and toxicology. 2nd edn. New Delhi: Jaypee brothers; 2012. p. 138-64.
19. Hellier C, Connolly R. Cause of death in judicial hanging: a review and case study. *Med Sci Law* 2009; 49: 18-26.
20. Spence MW, Shkrum MJ, Ariss A, Regan J. Craniocervical injuries in judicial hangings: an anthropologic analysis of six cases. *Am J Forensic Med Pathol* 1999; 20: 309-22.
21. James R, Nasmyth-Jones R. The occurrence of cervical fractures in victims of judicial hanging. *Forensic Sci Int* 1992; 54: 81-91.
22. Tandoor murder case: Supreme Court commutes death sentence of Sushil Sharma to life imprisonment. India Today Online. 2013 Oct 8. Available from: http://indiatoday.intoday.in/story/naina-sahni-tandoor-murder-case-sushil-sharma-supreme-court/1/313592.html.
23. Brutality can't be sole criteria for awarding death: Supreme Court. PTI 2013 Oct 14. Available form: http://articles.timesofindia.indiatimes.com/2013-10-14/india/43025779_1_capital-punishment-death-penalty-brutality.
24. Rix KJ. White coated healer or black coated executioner: Health professionals and capital punishment. *J Forensic Leg Med* 2013; 20: 659-66.
25. Sawicki NN. Doctors, discipline, and the death penalty: Professional implications of safe harbor statutes. Research paper 2008. University of Pennsylvania law school. Available from: http://papers.ssrn.com/abstract=1096545.
26. Zimmers TA, Lubarsky DA. Physician participation in lethal injection executions. *Curr Opin Anaesthesiol* 2007; 20: 147-51.
27. Clare AW. Doctors and the death penalty: an international issue. *BMJ* 1987; 294: 1180-81.
28. American Medical Association. Capital punishment: Opinion 2.06. Available from: http://www.ama-assn.org//ama/pub/physician-resources/medical-ethics/code-medical-ethics/opinion206.page.
29. Gawande A. When law and ethics collide - Why physicians participate in executions? *N Engl J Med* 2006; 354: 1221-29.

Dyadic Deaths

Nageshkumar G Rao

'Murder and suicide are interchangeable acts – suicide sometimes forestalling murder, and vice versa.'
Karl A. Menninger (Eminent psychiatrist)

ABSTRACT

Dyadic deaths are instances of homicide followed by suicide of the perpetrator, after the act of murder. They are the most tragic fatal violent acts involving most intimate partner or family members. Perpetrators are usually male and are of extremes of age group (18 to 60 years). Causes of dyadic death in India range from domestic quarrels due to strained relationship, broken love affair, infidelity (real or delusional), alcoholism to factors like psychiatric illness, physical ill health, financial crisis of the perpetrator, including *'dowry'* commitments. In dyadic deaths, a second victim acts in consort with, is associated with, or is killed by a person who, contemporaneous with the first death, then suicides. Dyadic deaths thus include both homicide-suicides and 'suicide pacts' where a partner has been coerced to commit suicide. Most such deaths are unwitnessed, occur in the bedrooms, and are more common in lower socio-economic groups. Although in western countries, this was found to be more in middle class groups. This chapter discusses the demographic characteristics and causative factors associated with dyadic deaths.

Keywords: Homicide-suicide; triadic deaths, murder-suicide; spousal dyadic death; consortial dyadic death; intimate violence; suicide pact, filicide-suicide, familicide-suicide, extrafamilial homicide-suicide.

INTRODUCTION

Case of Interest

Mystery of death of millionaire Christopher Foster and his family[1]

On August 2008, an extraordinary manor in Shorpshire, West Midlands region of England was burnt completely along with three family members living in it (a millionaire businessman Christopher Foster, 50, his wife Jillian, 49, and daughter Kirstie, 15). On investigating thoroughly in the ruins of the building, bodies of all the three were recovered.

A meticulous investigation of the case and also the closed circuit television (CCTV) recordings in the house, enabled police in reconstruction of events; resulting in solving the mystery. The millionaire businessman was believed to have first shot his wife and then his daughter. He killed them both, since his business had collapsed to such an extent that he could not surrender his family to an 'undignified' change in lifestyle. He then killed himself by setting fire to his mansion, burning himself, committing suicide. In other words, it's a case of homicide-suicide.

Although Christopher Foster appeared to be a successful businessman, actually he was in an extreme financial crisis, requiring a conversion of his family's life style. At the time of his death, he had assets of £3.1 million but also had debts of £4.4 million, including three mortgages on his house.

Homicide-suicides are rare unusual deaths with social importance. Homicide-suicide, murder-suicide and dyadic death all refer to an episode wherein a homicide is committed, followed by the suicide of the perpetrator.[1-3] Such incidences are mentioned in the histories of Ming dynasty in China and in Greek tragedies as well. *Dyadic deaths (homicide-suicide)* are thus conditions of violent event in which an individual kills another and subsequently commits suicide immediately or after some time.[1] In dyadic deaths, a second victim acts in consort with, is associated with, or is killed by a person who, contemporaneous with the first death, then suicides.

These are human tragedies in which the perpetrator, more often a male, kills one or more victims, typically his own wife and/or children and/or some other intimate ones from family, and then commits suicide within minutes or few hours. *Suicide pact* is also a form of dyadic death. This is highlighted in the case by Avis et al where a couple committed suicide by hanging, and the weight of one partner was necessary in executing the hanging.[1-3]

Further dyadic deaths are intriguing from several viewpoints. It is considered as the most tragic forms of violence, and although it is infrequent, can aggravate the family commotion, psychological trauma and a public concern.[4] Though this constitutes a significant portion of homicidal deaths, it has been studied less often than other forms of homicides.[5] Homicide-suicide cases are difficult to investigate because they rarely have legal consequences and official records simply lack in most countries. As far as the law enforcement or police, these cases are quickly solved; and for a pathologist, they offer the opportunity to match the wounds with positions of bodies at crime scene; and for a psychiatrist they present an opportunity to expound on the motives and psychodynamics of relations involved.[6,7] However, despite such interesting facts, there is a scarcity of reports on the phenomenon in the past as well as recent years. Paucity of incidences and scarcity in forensic literature merits compiling of this chapter.

DEFINITIONS

- **Dyadic death:** A fatal event in which one individual kills another, and subsequently commits suicide within a short time interval ranging from one hour to one week (some consider up to 3 months between the events).[2,3,8]
- **Suicide pact:** A condition, wherein, an agreement made between two or more people to commit suicide together at a given place and time, i.e. the members are coerced to commit suicide.[6,8]

In England and Wales, for epidemiological purposes, people who have committed suicide within three days of each other in the same registration subdistrict are considered potential victims of a suicide pact.[2,3,6] Berman also defined dyadic death as a terminology that encompasses both *suicide pacts* and *homicide-suicides.*[2,3,6,9] Dyadic deaths thus include both homicide-suicides and suicide pacts.

Synonyms: Some of the synonymous terminologies often used for the dyadic death are murder-suicide, homicide-suicide, filicide-suicide, familicide-suicide, extra-familial homicide-suicide, parents and siblings homicide suicide, spousal dyadic death and consortial dyadic death.

EPIDEMIOLOGY

Dyadic deaths are relatively rare when compared to separate incidences of homicide or suicide worldwide and related to demographic profiles of population. As observed from various case reports, demographic characteristic of perpetrator and victim are more or less same. Most incidents occurred at home, and perpetrator is usually a well-known intimate family member of the victim. Nonfamilial incidents are very rare.[10-14]

Murder-suicides rates are low with 0.2–0.3 per 1,00,000 populations found in some western studies.[8] An estimate states that dyadic deaths accounts for 5–10% and 5% of all homicidal deaths in England-Wales[15] and the United States (US)[16] respectively. The percentage of incidence has also been reported to vary from 3% to 60% in other countries.[14] Gillespie reported from Canada that 10% of all homicide offenders in his study series ended their life after committing homicide.[17] It is also observed that the variation in dyadic death rate is inversely related to the homicide incidence in a given region, and thus, the higher the homicide rate, lower is the percentage of homicide-suicide.[18] For example, incidence of dyadic deaths was reported as high as 42% in Denmark where homicide is less, compared to 4% in the US, where homicide rates are much higher.[8] In India, there is no such statistics and the National Crime Records Bureau gives no such information regarding incidences of dyadic deaths.[19]

Homicide-suicide incidence occurred two times more among 55 years and older individuals compared to those who are of less than 55 years age.[20] Likewise, according to yet another study by Eisofir and Cohen, the observations on homicide-suicide incidences doubled in the population of 55 years and older, while it remained the same among the younger age groups.[21] However, West reported that homicide-suicide incidences were more common among the old and sick, constituting 2% of all the suicidal deaths in his study.[22] According to a larger major study by Milroy, the sex incidence of the perpetrators as reported male: female ratio of 16:1, who killed their own near and dearer ones, especially their spouse and/or children.[23]

Recently, in India, various case reports of dyadic death were reported from different parts of the country. It was surprisingly noticed more commonly among the low socio-economic group of population, who are poor and hail from illiterate families, and included single or multiple victim incidences.[2-3,10-13,19] In several studies reported from Western countries, this phenomenon was predominantly found in middle-class groups.[8]

CLASSIFICATION

Currently, there is no classification system validated for this phenomenon. The homicide-suicide cases can be considered as:[24]

a. *'Standard cases'* involve individuals who are well-known to each other. Often, one spouse (most often male) may kill the other and then kill himself. Sometimes, a parent may kill one or more children and/or spouse before committing suicide.
b. *Homicide followed by delayed suicide* may occur with the arrest of the perpetrator who then commits suicide which may not be a part of the plan. There may be delay of days or months between the events.
c. *Random strikes against strangers* may be carried out by perpetrators carrying any weapon (gun, knives) who may kill people who are not known to them with apparent aim to kill as many people as possible. An interesting phenomenon is *run-amok* seen in chronic use or sudden consumption of cannabis. This is characterized by a peculiar homicidal mania. After intake, there is a period of depression, followed by excitation, confusion and a violent attempt to kill people (*impulse to murder*). The addict first kills a person against whom he may have real or imaginary enmity and then kills anyone who comes in his way, until the homicidal tendency lasts. The person may then commit suicide or surrender himself to the law enforcement authority.[25]
d. *Religious and/or politically motivated killings* are intended to kill as many people of a different faith/background. The suicide of the perpetrator may be an integral part of the plan. The Wisconsin gurudwara shooting which took place on 5th August 2012 can be considered as an example of this. The perpetrator shot six people dead and wounded four others in Oak Creek, Wisconsin. He then wounded an officer; after being shot in the stomach by another, he fatally shot himself in the head. Apart from the shooter, all the dead were members of the Sikh faith. The perpetrator was an American white supremacist and US Army veteran from Cudahy, Wisconsin.[26]

Mazruk et al have suggested a system of classification based on type of relationship between perpetrator and victim. Based on this, the dyadic deaths can be classified as spousal/consortial, familial and extra-familial type (Table 18.1).[8,11] The commonest form of dyadic death is spousal followed

Table 18.1 Classification of homicide-suicide

Spousal or consortial	*Familial*	*Extra-familial*
Perpetrator: spouse, consort	*Perpetrator:* mother, father, child (<16 years), other adult family member (>16 years)	• Amorous jealousy • Mercy killing • Altruistic or extended suicides • Family, financial or social stressors • Adversarial or retaliation • Other and unspecified
Type of homicide • Spouse-killing (uxoricide) • Murder of lover (consortial)	*Type of homicide* • Neonaticide (<24 hours) • Infanticide (1 day to 1 year) • Pedicide (1–16 years) • Adult family member (>16 years)	

by filicide-suicide.[1] Other rare forms of dyadic death are familicide-suicide, extrafamilial homicide-suicide and homicides involving parents and siblings.[1,2]

SPOUSAL HOMICIDE-SUICIDE

This is homicide-suicide observed among married couples. Determining the underlying reasons that lead to such deaths is difficult, but deterioration in relationships between spouses appears to be central.[27] The perpetrators were in age group of 18 to 60 years, who had made a unilateral decision to commit the act. He usually suffered from 'morbid jealousy' with history of suspicions, delusional or actual infidelity.[8,11] This individual appeared to have thought about the act of homicide-suicide for months or even years in advance, and the wife probably never knew about it. Killing of wife when she was asleep or a shot in the back of the head confirms this fact.[5,7,20-23,27] He may also murder the spouse's lover before committing suicide, which has been termed as *triadic death.*[8] When domestic violence occurred, the attack was noticed to be aggressive and violent, causing multiple fatal wounds to the victim.[7,20]

In an additional study, Cohen reported that in older spousal homicide-suicide, the mean age of the perpetrator and the victim was 65 and 50 years respectively.[28] Most of the perpetrators and victims in this age group were sick and had the tendency for physical violence, verbal discord and embroiled in law suits mutually. What motivates an elderly married man to commit a homicide-suicide rather than to kill himself is further analyzed in yet another study by Cohen.[29] He specified that most of the men who committed homicide-suicide were good caregivers, but had an evident decline in health, financial problems, social isolation and depression prior to the act. At times, she too may be a willing participant, in case the act was decided and planned in advance by both. Cohen characterized three types of spousal/consortial homicide-suicide among married couples.[20,28,29] They are:

i. Dependent-protective
ii. Aggressive
iii. Symbiotic

Dependent-Protective Type

This occurs in 50% of married couples and is more common among the elderly couples (age > 55 years). The couple is usually married for a long time, and they are highly dependent on each other. The man, who has been dominant in the relationship throughout, is now suspicious of losing control of his ability to take care or protect his wife. Even if the woman is not sick, a real or perceived change in the man's health, along with depression and multiple stresses can precipitate the process. A common variant is care given dependent homicide-suicide, where serious depression from years of care giving, coupled with increasing isolation produces despair in the male caregiver and triggers the act.

Aggressive Type

This occurs in 30% of married couples and is more common in young couples (age < 55 years), but it does occur among elderly couples (age > 55 years) as well.

There is a definite marital conflict of domestic violence in these couples. The perpetrator is usually much older than the victim. Pending or actual separation, issuances of a restraining order or threatening behavior are common precipitants to trigger the act.

Symbiotic Type

This occurs among 20% of the married couples and is more common among the elderly couples (age > 55 years). This is characterized by an extreme degree of inter-dependence in the couples. One of them or usually both are very sick (may be suffering from HIV or cancer), leading the husband to perform *mercy killing* of the wife and then to commit suicide.[8] The husband and wife are so enmeshed to each other that their individual characteristics are blurred. The male perpetrator is often the dominant personality and the female victim is frequently submissive.

Homicide-suicide in older couples may not be just acts of love or altruism, they are acts of depression as well. Majority of people were reported to be suffering from depression or other psychiatric problems including alcohol abuse. Some of them had also often talked about committing suicide and had actually attempted to commit suicide as well.[20]

FAMILIAL HOMICIDE-SUICIDE

Familial homicide-suicides involve a parent who kills their children and then commits suicide. Suicide following infanticide is rare in most countries with the exception of Japan, where about 500 cases are documented annually.[8] In homicide-suicides involving children, females are usually the perpetrators. This can be viewed as their action of killing the children an extension of suicide, and that the perpetrator is acting 'altruistically' to save her children from the dangers of the world.[8,30]

Sometimes, a dependent adult child suffering from significant physical or mental impairment is killed by a parent who feels incapable of providing the necessary care because of age, infirmity or financial problems. This has similar features with elderly spousal homicide-suicides and 'mercy killing'.[8]

EXTRA-FAMILIAL HOMICIDE-SUICIDE

These are homicide-suicides involving individuals outside the family. Extra-familial homicide-suicide includes not only mass murders, but also cases where the perpetrator is in a moral or emotional relationship with the victim such as a neighbor, landlord or employee.[1] The perpetrators can either be adults or adolescents, but adolescents are less likely to commit suicide following the homicide.[1,2] Extra-familial homicide-suicide can further be subdivided into:[8]

i. *Adversarial homicide-suicide:* In this, a dissatisfied employee or an ex-employee or a disgruntled student may seek revenge for real or perceived insults, harm or ill-handling. Failure to achieve promotion or attain monetary gain like increment/bonus in employment or termination of services may be predisposing factors. In the US, several high school shootings have occurred involving students who returned to school armed with firearms with the intention to kill their peers.

ii. *Pseudo-commando homicide-suicide:* In this, a number of bystanders ('secondary targets') may be killed and number of firearms may be used. This murder-suicide is further subdivided into 'indiscriminate' and 'pseudo-community' types. In the indiscriminate type, the perpetrator kills as many people as possible, their only common characteristic being proximity to the killer. In the pseudo-community subgroup, a perpetrator targets a specific group (like the Wisconsin gurudwara shooting discussed earlier).
iii. *Kamikaze homicide-suicide:* This consists of those involved in terrorist actions, where the perpetrator dies as a result of the device or action that he/she has used to kill a large number of people. Kamikaze was a suicide bombing method used by the Japanese in World War II. In recent years, the 11th September 2001 World Trade Center attacks involved the hijacking of passenger planes which were deliberately flown into the twin towers of World Trade Center in New York City and the Pentagon, killing everyone aboard the planes and thousands more in and around the targeted buildings. Similarly, former Prime Minister Rajiv Gandhi was assassinated by suicidal bombings on 21st May 1991 by a member of the LTTE.[31]

PERPETRATOR-VICTIM RELATIONSHIP

The Hanzlick and Koponen typology included demography and epidemiological features of individual cases.[8] Relationships are described as:

- Spouse by marriage, unmarried partner in relationship, extra-marital consort (lover), real or perceived rival lover
- Parent, offspring, sibling, grandparent, grandchild, niece/nephew, aunt/uncle, cousin
- Family member other than those listed
- Acquaintance or stranger
- Same or opposite gender as perpetrator
- Same or of different race as perpetrator
- Lives in same or in different household

METHODS USED

In contrast to female offenders, the methods used by male offenders tend to be more violent for committing both murder and suicide. Shooting is the most common form in homicide-suicide in the US, Switzerland and parts of England.[8,32] Certain studies indicate that strict gun control laws may be an important preventive factor of such events. Other weapons associated with homicide-suicide include knives, blunt objects, and other methods like strangling/asphyxiation, poisoning and physical assaults or vehicular accidents.

This contrasts with female offenders who were less likely to use firearms for the murder or the suicide. A more 'passive' mode of homicide-suicide consisting of poisoning, suffocation, hanging, burns and carbon monoxide exposure were favored by female offenders.[8,19]

In India, except for firearms, all other methods—knives, blunt objects, suffocation, hanging, strangulation, burns and poisoning are frequently used in dyadic deaths. Drowning is also a common method of killing, particularly children. Bardale and Dixit reported dyadic deaths with mother as assailant and the victims were her children, using the methods of hanging and drowning.[33]

PRECIPITATING FACTORS

Determining the underlying cause is quite complex and probably differ markedly from case to case. Studies by Milroy[5,15,34,35] and Copeland[6] are considered as some of the major study series reported till date in the literature. While Copeland's study comprised of data from the files of Medical Examiner office in Miami, Florida, US covering 7 years period consecutively extending from 1977 to 1983;[7] Milroy did his study by examination of the data available in literature, presenting actual international scenario on dyadic deaths.[15]

Milory has reported the cause for homicide-suicide episodes in one of his study as broken relationship with spouse (46%), mental illness (21%), physical ill health (11%) and financial stress (10%).[5,11,15,19,34,35] Graser in a study done in South Africa, identified a number of precipitating factors in perpetrators of familicide including marital and financial problems, unemployment, depression and social isolation, alcohol abuse, physical and mental illness. Victim precipitation in the form of behavior of spouse often provides a 'trigger' for the family murder.[19] The personalities of perpetrators and their victims, the prevailing circumstances and the manner in which latter are defined, interact, possibly ending in tragedy. Some of the common precipitating factors are summarized in Box 18.1.[8]

Psychiatric and psychological illness appears to play a dominant role in most of the categories mentioned above. Jealousy, marital discord over extra-marital, sexual or love affairs, rejection, threat of separation or actual separation from intimate partner or physical ill health are important factors seen in spousal homicide or in familial cases.[8,11] At times, depression may play a significant role in cases where a parent, usually a mother, murders her children.[30]

Stressful life events like financial or work-related problems, including loss of employment or nonpayment of salaries also may be contributory factors. Histories of domestic violence by the perpetrator towards the victim may be elicited.[8] The risk of child abuse and wife battering is greater among those who are poor and/or unemployed and among those who had low prestige jobs.[10,11,19,30]

Revenge may be a significant motive in cases of separated spouses, and also in cases of disgruntled employees and students. Those who kill a large number of persons are more likely to exhibit delusional or paranoid ideation with religious overtones. Some of them may be impulsive with poor control of aggressive impulses and antisocial personalities. Loss of self-esteem, frustration and low personal achievement has all been documented.[8]

Box 18.1 Predisposing factors

- Impending divorce or previously divorced
- Real or imaginary parting of nonmarital partner (girlfriend, lover)
- Retaliation or jealousy against a real or apparent rival lover
- Altruism (to save from 'evils of the world')
- Family stress or dysfunction including financial stressors
- Perpetrator intoxicated with alcohol and/or drug(s)
- Perpetrator had known history of psychiatric illness
- Mercy killing

There may be a history of previous suicide attempts and consultation with psychiatrist. Alcohol and drug abuse may also be aggravating factors in these cases, although drugs or alcohol are not always detected.[8]

In Indian context, financial loss/distress has been found to be a predominant factor for familicide-suicide. Moreover, financial burden and marital disharmony are the principle reasons for suicide in India.[11]

INVESTIGATIONS AND AUTOPSY

Since, homicide-suicides are uncommon events, they require careful investigations. The investigation in such cases is often difficult because in most cases all the family members may have died and relevant information of the incidence is lacking. Confusion of double homicides with homicide-suicide is possible. Therefore, characteristic features of homicide-suicide should be carefully looked for, both in the history and at the death scene.[24] Sometimes, crime scenes are staged to falsely suggest that the death is due to a suicide rather than homicide. In the investigations of such deaths, the forensic pathologist must view the autopsy with a high degree of suspicion. The doctor should first rule out homicide in such cases. Suspicion should arise in cases of married couples, in extreme age groups and belonging to low socio-economic strata. Evidence retrieved from crime scene should also be corroborated with the incident.[8]

Many perpetrators have histories of depression with possible treatment from a psychiatrist. Psychological autopsies with review of the medical records of the perpetrator and interviews with colleagues, friends and relatives may provide some insight into the events leading up to the fatal attack.[8]

CONCLUSION

Men commit the vast majority of domestic homicide-suicide, wherein a perpetrator kills their intimate partner (spouse) and/or family members (children) before taking their own life. Determining the underlying motives that can lead to such deaths is understandably not easy, but deterioration in relationships between spouses appears to be a crucial factor. The commonest reason for homicide-suicide episode is simple domestic quarrel, precipitated by factors such as sexual infidelity which may be real, imaginary or delusional. The male is usually depressed, paranoid or intoxicated. Financial stress, dowry commitments, worry about future and security of daughters could be other potential factors.

Legally, and for the police, these cases are not high profile cases since they just demands proper investigation and correct recording, and finally closure of the case, since the wrongdoer is already dead. However, in order to achieve health policies for the society, it is better to undertake proper social, psychological and psychiatric investigations in order to decrease or to stop such incidences. The phenomenon of homicide-suicide episodes is not just limited to the particular affected family, but it also has high impact on society. Though, these occur in lesser numbers, they are the vista to many of the unseen, unknown veracities of life. It is absolutely essential to establish national surveillance system for such episodes to know exact circumstances of each case.

REFERENCES

1. du Plessis M, Hlaise KK. Homicide-suicide (dyadic death)—a case study of double hanging. *Am J Forensic Med Pathol* 2012; 33: 262-64.
2. Rao NG, Menezes RG, Shetty SKB. Dyadic death in married couples—report of two cases. *IJFPR* 2012; 2: 73-76.
3. Rajagopal S. Suicide pacts and the internet complete strangers may make cyberspace pacts, *BMJ* 2004; 329: 1298-99.
4. Chan AY, Beh SL, Broadhurst RG. Homicide-suicide in Hong Kong 1989-97. A preliminary analysis. Paper presented at the *6th World Congress of police medical officers, Sydney*. 17-21, 2002.
5. Milroy CM, Magdalene D, Ranson DL. Homicide-suicide in Victoria, Australia. *Am J Forensic Med Pathol* 1997; 18: 369-73.
6. Brown M, Barraclough B. Epidemiology of suicide pacts in England and Wales, 1988-92. *BMJ* 1997; 315: 286-87.
7. Copeland AR. Dyadic death-revisited. *J For Sci* 1985; 25: 151-88.
8. Byard RW. Murder-suicide: An overview. In: Tsokos M (ed). Forensic pathology reviews. Vol. 3. Totowa, NJ: Humana Press Inc.; 2005. p. 337-50.
9. Berman AL. Dyadic death: a typology. *Suicide Life Threat Behav* 1996; 26: 342-50.
10. Gupta S, Vaishnav H. Dyadic diwali. *J Indian Acad Forensic Med* 2008; 30: 75-78.
11. Dhawane SG, Mukherjee AA, Bardale RV. Dyadic deaths: Analysis of homicide-suicide episodes. *Medicolegal Update* 2007; 7: 11-12.
12. Gupta BD, Jani CB, Patel BJ, and Shah PH. Homicide-suicide deaths (dyadic): Two case reports. *J Forensic Medicine Toxicol* 2000; 17: 31-37.
13. Gupta BD, Singh OG. A unique trend of murder-suicide in the Jamnagar region of Gujarat, India (A retrospective study of 5 years). *J Forensic Leg Med* 2008; 15: 250-55.
14. Comstock RD, Mallonee S, Kruger E, Rayno K, Vance A, Jordan F. Epidemiology of homicide suicide events Oklahoma, 1994–2001. *Am J Forensic Med Pathol* 2005; 26: 229-35.
15. Milroy CM. The epidemiology of homicide-suicide (dyadic death). *For Sci Int* 1995; 71: 117-22.
16. Marzuk P, Tardiff K, Hirsch CS. The epidemiology of murder-suicide. *JAMA* 1992; 267: 3179-83.
17. Gillespie M, Hearn V, Silverman RA. Suicide following homicide in Canada. *Homicide Studies* 1998; 1: 46-63.
18. Coid J. The epidemiology of abnormal homicide and murder followed by suicide. *Psychol Med* 1983; 13: 855-60.
19. Ghormade PS, Shrigiriwar MB. Dyadic deaths (homicide-suicide): three case reports. *Journal of Forensic Medicine, Science and Law.* http://www.mlam.in/pdf/dyadic deaths (homicide- suicide) - three case reports.pdf.
20. Cohen D, Llorente M, Eisdorfer C. Homicide-suicide in older persons. *Am J Psychiatry* 1998; 155: 390-96.
21. Eisdorfer D, Cohen D. Homicide suicide rates in older people. Presented at the 9th Congress of the *International Psychogeriatric Association*, Aug. 24; Vancouver, British Columbia, Canada, 1999.
22. West DJ. Murder followed by suicide (An enquiry carried out for the Institute of Criminology), London, Heinemann, 1965.
23. West DJ. Murder followed by suicide, Cambridge, Harvard University, 1966.
24. Wyatt JP, Squires T, Norfolk G, Payne-James J. Forensic aspects of death. Oxford Handbook of Forensic Medicine. 1st ed. New York: Oxford university press; 2011. p. 29-66.
25. Biswas G. Deliriants - Cannabis. Review of forensic medicine and toxicology. 2nd edn. New Delhi: Jaypee Brothers; 2012. p. 500.
26. Wisconsin Sikh temple shooting. Available from: http://en.wikipedia.org/wiki/Wisconsin_Sikh_temple_shooting.

27. Malphurs JE, Cohen D. A statewide case-control study of spousal homicide suicide in older persons. *Am J Geriatr Psychiatry* 2005; 13: 211-17.
28. Cohen D, Malphurs JE, Eisdorfer D. Homicide and dementia. *J Mental Health Aging* 1998; 4: 301-05.
29. Cohen D. Homicide-suicide in older people. *Psychiatric Times* 2000; 17: 1-7.
30. Types of homicide-suicide (dyadic death). Available from: http://tea-and-skeletons.tumblr.com/post/25116189740/types-of-homicide-suicide-standard-cases.
31. Suicide attack. Available from: http://en.wikipedia.org/wiki/Suicide_attack.
32. Grabherr S, Johner S, Dilitz C, Buck U, Killias M, Mangin P, Plattner T. Homicide-suicide cases in Switzerland and their impact on the Swiss weapon law. *Am J Forensic Med Pathol* 2010; 31: 1-16.
33. Bardale R, Dixit P. Mom you too! Case reports of dyadic deaths with mother as perpetrator. *JPAFMAT* 2010; 10: 45-47.
34. Milroy CM. Homicide followed by suicide (Dyadic Death) in Yorkshire and Humberside. *Med Sci Law* 1993; 33: 167-71.
35. Milroy CM. Reasons for homicide and suicide in episodes of dyadic death in Yorkshire and Humberside. *Med Sci Law* 1995; 35: 213-17.

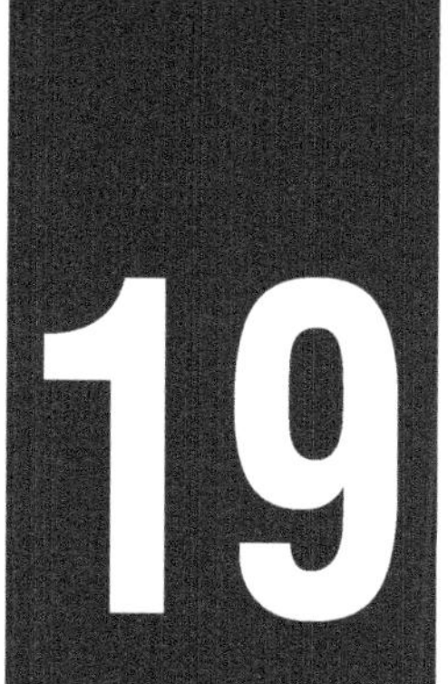

Fat Embolism

Prateek Rastogi

'Fat can be fatal, in whatever form it may be.'
Anonymous

ABSTRACT

Fat embolism is a dreaded complication of trauma, although, it is seen sometimes in non-traumatic cases also. Mobilized fat globules get deposited in pulmonary capillaries and systemic circulation. This complication can be seen within hours to days of triggering event (trauma or imbalance in fat metabolism). Fat embolism assumes medicolegal significance if a recovering hospitalized patient collapses suddenly, thereby arising suspicion and an allegation of negligence on part of doctor and his/her team. This chapter provides a brief overview of this potentially lethal and common complication of trauma.

Keywords: Sudden death, trauma, pulmonary fat embolism, systemic fat embolism.

INTRODUCTION

Fat embolism is a common sequelae of mechanical trauma to bone or fatty tissues of body resulting in fat mobilization from body fat deposits.[1,2] Post-traumatic fat can be demonstrated histologically in majority of cases of fractures or trauma to the fatty parts of the body.[1] According to Mason, fat can be seen in lung even in non-traumatic deaths, but amount will be less as compared to traumatic deaths.[3]

Primarily, after damage to fat containing tissues, fat globules are released to pulmonary circulation. Subsequently, after leaking to systemic circulation these globules can cause severe disability and even death, if impacted in vital organs.[1] This chapter introduces the concept of fat embolism with a case report. This is followed by a detailed review of its epidemiology, classification, etiology, pathophysiology, clinical features, investigations, postmortem findings and medicolegal issues.

DEFINITIONS

Fat embolism: It can be defined as the pathologic condition ensuing from the introduction of liquefied fat into the circulation and its transportation by the bloodstream to occlude the fine blood vessels in various parts of the body.[4] Mason described it as the presence of fat and/or marrow emboli in lungs and systemic circulation. It comprises of small, multiple emboli, mostly caused by fracture of long bone, soft tissues and burns.[3] If the obstruction in circulation is by fragments of adipose tissue, it is called fat-tissue embolism.[5]

Fat embolism syndrome (FES): It is characterized by pulmonary insufficiency, neurologic symptoms, anemia and thrombocytopenia. Symptoms appear 1–3 days after injury with sudden onset of tachypnea, dyspnea and tachycardia. The syndrome manifests more frequently in closed fractures of the pelvis or long bones. The petechial rash, which usually resolves in 5–7 days, is said to be pathognomonic for the syndrome, but occurs only in 20–50% of cases. The pathological marker of this entity is marked pulmonary edema.[1,6]

CASE REPORT

A 22-year-old male while walking on the road was hit by a jeep. He was admitted to the hospital immediately, but died after 15 days while on treatment. Conjunctivae, face and chest showed yellowish discoloration.

On postmortem examination, **external injuries** seen were:

1. Surgical sutures, present on the right hand in the 4th webspace.
2. A tracheotomy wound, measuring 2 × 2 cm, present on the front of neck in the midline.
3. A contusion, purplish black in color, measuring 6 × 5 cm, present on the front of right leg in its middle one-third with underlying fracture of shaft of tibia and fibula.
4. A surgical incision, measuring 3 × 0.5 cm, subcutaneous deep, present on the front of right ankle.

No other external injuries were present on the body.

Internally, undersurface of scalp and meninges, kidneys, liver, heart, thoracic walls, ribs, cartilages, intestines, mesentery and abdominal fat showed yellowish discoloration (Fig. 19.1). Brain showed petechial hemorrhages (Fig. 19.2), lungs were congested and edematous, and spleen was congested.

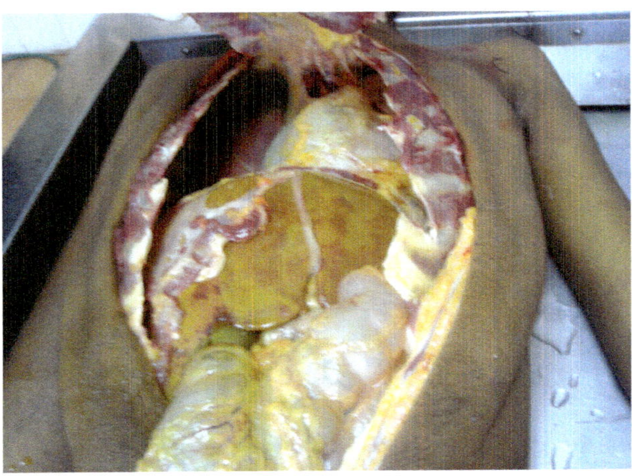

Fig. 19.1 Contents of abdomen showing yellowish discoloration

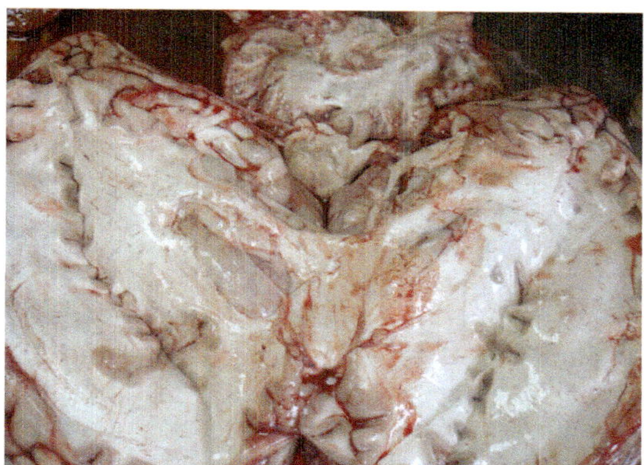

Fig. 19.2 Brain showing petechial hemorrhages

One piece of each lung, one piece of liver, one piece of each kidney were preserved for histopathological examination.

Histopathology report showed congestion of kidney and liver. Lungs showed features of edema, congestion, hematopoietic foci in blood vessels, foci of pneumonic consolidation and compensatory emphysema. The findings were suggestive of fat embolism from bone marrow. Clinically, hospital records documented death as a result of cardiorespiratory arrest due to fat embolism. Final opinion of cause of death was given as fat embolism due to complication of fracture of right tibia and fibula.

HISTORY

Fat embolism at autopsy was first described by Zenker in 1862 as natural post-traumatic embolism in lungs of victim of crush injury to chest and abdomen, while clinically it was diagnosed for the first time in 1873 by Von Bergmann.[7,8]

EPIDEMIOLOGY

Fat embolism is a clinical diagnosis; its frequency is estimated to be 3–4% with a mortality rate of 10–20%. Fat emboli occur in about 90% of all cases with severe skeletal trauma, of which only 10% are symptomatic. The risk of FES can be reduced by early immobilization of fractures, early operative correction and steroid prophylaxis of high-risk patients. Patients with increased age, multiple underlying medical problems, and/or decreased physiologic reserves have worse outcomes. The mortality rate of FES is approximately 10–20%.[6,8]

CLASSIFICATION

The classification of fat embolism is based on various criteria:

Based on site

i. **Pulmonary fat embolism:** Impaction of fat globules in pulmonary circulation resulting in pulmonary insufficiency.

ii. **Systemic fat embolism:** Impaction of fat globules in organ system after passing pulmonary circulation. The brain, kidneys and myocardium are the most vulnerable organs. Death is most likely if emboli gets impacted in brainstem capillaries.[1]

Based on etiology[4]

i. **Traumatic fat embolism:** It results from trauma to bones and fatty tissues. Fat is mechanically liberated from the bone marrow fat cells and enters the veins of Haversian system which communicates freely with intramedullary sinusoidal blood channels. Since marrow fat is insufficient in children, fat embolism is rare in this age group.
ii. **Non-traumatic fat embolism:** It results from chemical imbalance in fat metabolism, burns or fatty liver. This phenomenon is produced by alteration in suspension ability of endogenous serum fat, resulting in conversion of chylomicrons into fat emboli. It has been documented that fat embolism can occur in 50% of deaths from natural causes.

Based on origin[7]

i. **Exogenous:** This type of emboli have their origin outside the body, for e.g., oily abortifacients or intravenously induced oily preparations.
ii. **Endogenous:** This type occurs when fat which originates within body forms emboli, for e.g., injury or trauma to bones or soft tissues or changes in fat metabolism.

Based on clinical presentation[4]

i. **Sub-clinical:** Amount of fat is so small that no clinical signs or symptoms are elicited.
ii. **Clinical:** Definite signs and symptoms are manifested.
iii. **Fatal:** Extreme stage with severe symptoms.

ETIOLOGY

The cause of fat embolism are multiple:[4,7,8]

i. **Trauma related:** Blunt trauma especially fractures, burns, decompression sickness or barotrauma, soft tissue injuries or injury to pelvic fatty tissues during childbirth.
ii. **Disease related:** Acute pancreatitis, diabetes mellitus, sickle cell crisis, pathologic fractures, osteomyelitis, fatty liver, pneumonia or *Clostridium welchii* infection.
iii. **Treatment related:** Joint reconstruction, orthopedic surgical procedures, liposuction, cardiopulmonary bypass, parenteral lipid infusion, steroid therapy or surgical procedures on fatty tissues (for e.g., mastectomy).
iv. **Poisoning related:** Carbon tetrachloride, phosphorous, sodium and ammonium hydroxide poisoning or alcohol toxicity.

PATHOPHYSIOLOGY AND PATHOGENESIS

Researchers have proposed various therories to explain the pathogenesis of embolism:[4,6,8,9]

a. **Mechanical theory:** After trauma, large fat droplets are released into the venous system and get deposited in the pulmonary capillary beds, resulting in pulmonary fat embolism. Subsequently, these droplets pass the arteriovenous shunt; enter the systemic circulation and lodges in target organs resulting in local ischemia and inflammation, causing concomitant release of inflammatory mediators, vasoactive amines and platelet aggregation. Another thought relates to transportation of fat droplets to lungs via lymphatic system and innominate vein in place of bloodstream.
b. **Biochemical theory:** Trauma and/or sepsis causes hormonal changes which in turn induce systemic release of free fatty acids like chylomicrons, acute-phase reactants such as C-reactive proteins, resulting in aggregation of chylomicrons causing local ischemia and inflammation, with concomitant release of inflammatory mediators, vasoactive amines and platelet aggregation.

It is also thought that several mechanisms together or singly may be involved in pathogenesis of fat embolism.[5,10]

i. *Mechanical:* Mobilization of fat following trauma.
ii. *Emulsion instability:* Fat embolus formed by aggregation of plasma lipids (chylomicrons and fatty acids) due to disturbances in emulsification of fat.
iii. *Intravascular coagulation:* This results from disseminated intravascular coagulation (DIC).
iv. *Toxic injury:* Blood vessels injury due to free fatty acid, resulting in increased vascular permeability and pulmonary edema.

Biochemical changes occurring in the blood plasma during shock can disrupt the lipid suspension system resulting in formation of fatty acids and free fat. Under stress (traumatic or non-traumatic), fats gets mobilized, as they are the richest source of energy, resulting in fat embolism.[4]

Presenting History

The patient usually presents with a history of trauma to long bone or pelvis, orthopedic procedures, parenteral lipid infusion or recent corticosteroid administration.[8]

CLINICAL FEATURES

An asymptomatic latent period of about 12–48 hours precedes the clinical manifestations (Table 19.1).[1,4,8] The fulminant form presents as acute cor pulmonale, respiratory failure and/or embolic phenomena leading to death within a few hours of injury. Unlike emboli that arise from thrombi (blood clots), fat emboli are small and multiple, and thus have widespread effects. The clinical manifestations depend upon the quantum of fat reaching the pulmonary and subsequently the systemic circulation. If the patient survives, the affected organ may show infarct.

Table 19.1 Clinical features in fat embolism

System	*Features*
Cardiopulmonary	Early persistent tachycardia, tachypnea, dyspnea, hypoxia, hypocapnia occuring 12–72 hours after injury, fever with high-spiking temperatures.
Dermatologic	Reddish-brown non-palpable petechiae over the upper anterior portion of body including chest, neck, upper arm, axilla, shoulder, oral mucosa and conjunctivae which are pathognomonic. They appear within 24–36 hours of insult or injury, and disappear within hours (results from occlusion of capillaries by fat and increasing the capillary fragility).
Eyes	Retinal hemorrhages with intra-arterial fat globules on fundoscopy, and paracentral scotomas.
Neurologic	Confusion, decerebrate rigidity, agitated delirium, aphasia, hemiparesis, seizures, stupor, and unresponsive coma.

INVESTIGATIONS

Following investigations may be done to evaluate the patient, depending on facilities available in the set-up:

- **Arterial blood gas:** Unexplained increase in pulmonary shunt fraction alveolar-to-arterial oxygen tension difference, especially if it occurs within 24–48 hours of a sentinel event associated with FES is strongly suggestive of the syndrome. Hypoxemia is present in nearly all patients with FES, often to a PaO_2 of well below 60 mm Hg.[8]
- **Blood studies:** Thrombocytopenia, anemia, and hypofibrinogenemia are indicative of FES. Hypocalcemia can be seen as free fatty acids have an affinity to calcium ions.[4,8]
- **Urine studies:** Urinary fat stains are not felt to be sensitive or specific enough for diagnosing fat embolism or for detecting a risk of it. Fat globules in the urine are common after trauma.[8]
- **Chest radiography:** Serial radiographs reveal increasing diffuse bilateral pulmonary infiltrates within 24–48 hours of onset of clinical findings.[8] In later stages, chest X-ray may show evenly distributed, fleck-like pulmonary shadows (snowstorm appearance), increased pulmonary markings and dilatation of the right side of the heart.[1]
- **Non-contrast CT head:** It may reveal diffuse white-matter petechial hemorrhages consistent with microvascular injury.[8]
- **Nuclear medicine ventilation/perfusion imaging of the lungs:** It may demonstrate subsegmental perfusion defects.[8]
- **Helical chest CT:** Parenchymal changes consistent with lung contusion, acute lung injury, or adult respiratory distress syndrome (ARDS) may be evident. Nodular or ground glass opacities in the setting of trauma suggest fat embolism.[11]
- **MRI:** Multiple, non-confluent, hyperintense lesions seen on proton density and T2-weighted images.[12]

- **Transcranial doppler sonography:** Cerebral microembolic signals can be detected as long as 4 days after injury.[8]
- **Transesophageal echocardiography (TEE):** TEE may be of use in evaluating intraoperative release of marrow contents into the bloodstream during intramedullary reaming and nailing. The density of the echogenic material passing through the right side of the heart correlates with the degree of reduction in arterial oxygen saturation.[8]

DIAGNOSIS

A window period or lucid interval is seen between pulmonary and cerebral fat embolism, where the clinical presentation can be confused with development of extradural or subdural hematoma.[1]

- **Major criteria:** Respiratory symptoms, signs of radiologic disease, cerebral signs without other etiologies, and petechial rash.
- **Minor criteria:** Pulse > 110 per minute, fever > 38.5°C, retinal changes of fat globules or petechiae, renal dysfunction, jaundice, acute drop in hemoglobin and/or platelets, and elevated sedimentation rate.

One major and four minor criteria, plus fat microglobulinemia must be present to formally diagnose FES. Diagnosis of FES may be difficult because, except for the petechiae, there are no pathognomonic signs.[4,8]

Laboratory tests are mostly non-specific:

- Serum lipase level increases in bone trauma.
- Cytologic examination of urine, blood and sputum with Sudan or oil red O staining may detect fat globules that are either free or in macrophages.
- Decreased hematocrit occurs within 24–48 hours. Alteration in coagulation (thrombogenesis) and thrombocytopenia.
- Presence of bone marrow particles and bony spicules in lungs following bony trauma.

Biopsy: Biopsy of petechiae shows sudanophillic material in the lumina of dermal vessels.

DIFFERENTIAL DIAGNOSES

1. **Pulmonary embolism:** It can present a picture similar to cardiopulmonary manifestations of fat embolism.
2. **Thrombotic thrombocytopenic purpura (TTP):** There is fall in platelet count and petechiae on skin.

In both these cases, detailed history, clinical examination and investigations can clinch the diagnosis.

TREATMENT

Medical Care

To check shock, in addition to balanced electrolyte solution, albumin can be used as it not only restores blood volume but also binds fatty acids, and may decrease the extent of lung injury.[6]

Medical care for fat embolism is supportive and includes maintenance of adequate oxygenation and ventilation, stable hemodynamics, hydration, prophylaxis of deep venous thrombosis and stress-related gastrointestinal bleeding, and nutrition. Continuous pulse oximetry monitoring in at-risk patients, early oxygen therapy and possibly steroids decreases the chances of hypoxic insult and possible systemic complications of FES.[13]

Surgical Care

Reaming or nailing the marrow reduces volume of fat embolization. Inferior vena cava filters reduces volume of fat reaching the heart.[8]

COMPLICATIONS

Pulmonary fat embolism: Widespread obstruction causes sudden death. Fat emboli may cause cor pulmonale if adequate compensatory pulmonary vasodilation does not occur. Circulating free fatty acids are directly toxic to pneumocytes and capillary endothelium in the lung, causing interstitial hemorrhage, edema and chemical pneumonitis.[6]

Systemic fat embolism: These may get lodged in capillaries of organs like brain, kidney or skin causing minute hemorrhage and microinfarcts.[6]

PROGNOSIS

Pulmonary sequelae usually resolve almost completely within 1 year but residual subclinical diffusion capacity deficits may exist. Residual neurologic deficits may range from non-existent to subtle personality changes, memory and cognitive dysfunction to long-term focal deficits.[8]

Prevention

The most effective prophylactic measure is reduction of long bone fractures at the earliest. Methyl prednisolone is the preferred drug for prophylaxis of FES.[4,8]

Death scene findings: Not specific, crime scene is undisturbed.

CAUSE OF DEATH

Cause of death is confirmed histopathologically and is usually opined as fat embolism as a complication of trauma/natural disease process.

POSTMORTEM CHANGES

On autopsy, following findings may be seen:

- **External findings:** Petechial hemorrhages (caused by impaction of fat in venules) on skin especially over the front of chest, face and eyelids.[1]
- **Internal findings:** Petechial hemorrhages in white matter of brain (cerebrum, cerebellum and brainstem) and leptomeninges. Besides lungs, fat emboli is common in kidneys followed by brain.[2,5]

- **Microscopy:** Microinfracts of brain, edema and hemorrhages are seen.[5] Cerebral petechiae will show central fat globule surrounded by hemorrhage, while others will be visible without any hemorrhage. There may be fat in the retina and in the optic nerve. Fat may be seen in interfibre capillaries in myocardium and glomeruli of kidneys.[1] Microscopic sections of lungs show massive intravascular fat droplets, as well as free fat in the alveoli. In addition, lungs show hyperemia, edema, petechial hemorrhages and changes of ARDS.[2,5] If patient has survived for more than 4 hours after trauma, the number of emboli found at autopsy will decrease.[1] Diagnosis at microscopy is confirmed by frozen section using Sudan dyes, oil red O and osmic acid.[5]

DISCUSSION

The amount of free fat capable of causing death in human beings ranges from 12–120 ml. The speed of entry of these fat particles in circulatory system plays a major role in the outcome.[1] Three conditions are necessary for pulmonary and systemic fat embolism to occur following fracture:[7]

- Disruption of adipose tissue in marrow space.
- Traumatic opening of venous channels.
- Transient rise in bone marrow pressure above the venous pressure.

Post-traumatic fat globules enter the circulation by rupture of marrow sinusoids or venules. As discussed earlier, pathogenesis of fat embolism involves both mechanical obstruction and chemical injury. Globuli causes obstruction while free fatty acids cause toxic injury to endothelium. Petechial rash is consequent to thrombocytopenia resulting due to removal of platelets adhered to fat globules.[10]

Coagulation abnormalities are manifested by fall in hematocrit, erythrocyte aggregation, increased platelet adhesiveness, relative thrombocytopenia, elevation of fibrin degradation products, prolonged prothrombin and partial thromboplastin times, increase in haptoglobin and alpha -1- antitrypsin.[7] One case is reported in literature, where a 55-year-old woman died of massive fat embolism after developing pancreatitis due to endoscopic retrograde cholangiopancreatography (ERCP).[14]

Pulmonary circulation attempts to compensate capillary blockage, so moderate degree of occlusion is accommodated by slight rise in vascular resistance. If this compensatory mechanism fails, cor pulmonale follows.[7] Mason devised a scale to assess the histological severity of embolism in frozen sections of lungs using oil red O stain (Table 19.2).[1]

Table 19.2 Grading of severity of embolism

Grade	*Findings*
Grade 0	No emboli seen.
Grade 1	Emboli found after some searching.
Grade 2	Emboli easily seen.
Grade 3	Emboli present in large numbers.
Grade 4	Emboli present in potentially fatal numbers.

Histopathologically, fat emboli appear as round, oval or elliptical optically clear, well defined areas within the lumina of small arteries and arterioles. Since, the presence of occasional fat droplets may be artefactual, it is necessary to observe deformation of emboli as proof of their antemortem origin. In long standing cases of fat embolism, intra-alveolar edema, hemorrhage, hyaline membrane formation and bronchopneumonia results.[7]

During Mount Erabus investigations, fat and bone marrow emboli were noticed in lungs of decapitated victims. It is postulated that even in cases of instantaneous death, the effects of decompression shock at high altitude might have resulted in embolism.[3] Fat embolism usually occurs within seconds of injury, even few heartbeats are sufficient to bring the fat, not only to lungs, but also to systemic circulation. Thus, it can be seen even in instantaneous deaths, although the amount will be small, as the quantum is directly related to the period of survival following trauma.[2]

MEDICOLEGAL ASPECTS

Widespread obstruction of pulmonary circulation due to extensive pulmonary embolism can result in sudden death.[5] Sudden death in a post-traumatic/post-operative patient within hours to days of precipitating event can raise complex medicolegal issues related to quality and competency of doctor, nursing team and hospital authorities.

Evidence of pulmonary fat embolism is dependent upon the time for which circulation continued after injury. This concept is useful in determining the duration of survival or time of death after an accident where there are multiple fatalities involving members of the same family. This can be important in civil cases wherein life insurance policies and the disposal of the estate may have to be decided. This opinion is expressed on the assumption that no external cardiac massage has been attempted. Since, resuscitation may cause rib fractures, and if an effective circulation has been established, the finding of pulmonary fat emboli should be considered as an artifact.[15]

CONCLUSION

Fat embolism is an underdiagnosed condition—both clinically and in autopsy. In suspected cases, it should be sought diligently. In fat embolism, fat microglobules impair small vessel perfusion, causes endothelial damage in pulmonary capillaries leading to ventilation/perfusion mismatch, vascular congestion, interstitial hemorrhage, alveolar wall damage and airway collapse. Resulting clinical manifestation is a life threatening impairment of pulmonary gas exchange.[7] Mild to moderate degrees of pulmonary fat embolism with any systemic overspill must not be given as cause of death, unless there are clinical findings suggestive of such an event.

REFERENCES

1. Knight B. Complications of injury. Forensic pathology. 2nd edn. London: Arnold; 1996. p. 337-39.
2. Di Maio DJ, Di Maio VJ. Emboli due to air, fat and amniotic fluid. Forensic pathology. New York: Elsevier; 1989. p. 410.

3. Mason JK, Herdson PB. The role of pathology in mass disasters. In: Mason JK, Purdue BN (eds). The pathology of trauma. 3rd edn. London: Arnold; 2000. p. 45.
4. Tedeschi LG, Hechtman HB. Post-traumatic embolism. In: Tedeschi CG, Eckert WG, Tedeschi LG (eds). Forensic medicine. Philadelphia: WB Saunders Company; 1977. p. 406-22.
5. Mohan H. Body fluids and circulatory disturbances. Textbook of pathology. 3rd edn. Bangalore: Jaypee Brothers; 1998. p. 123-4.
6. Fat embolism. Available from: http://en.wikipedia.org/wiki/Fat_embolism.
7. Gordon I, Shapiro HA, Berson SD. Regional injuries of medicolegal importance. Forensic medicine: a guide to principles. 3rd ed. Edinburgh: Churchill Livingstone; 1988. p. 328-32.
8. Kirkland L. Fat embolism. Available from: http://emedicine.medscape.com/article/460524-overview.
9. Schnaid E, Lamprey JM, Viljoen MJ, Joffe BI, Seftel HC. The early biochemical and hormonal profile of patients with long bone fractures at risk of fat embolism syndrome. *J Trauma* 1987; 27: 309-11.
10. Mitchell RN, Kumar V. Hemodynamic disorders, Thrombosis and shock. In: Kumar V, Cotran RS, Robbins SL (ed). Basic Pathology. 6th ed. Bangalore: Prism Books; 1997. p. 60-80.
11. Gallardo X, Castener E, Mata JM. Nodular pattern at lung computed tomography in fat embolism syndrome: A helpful finding. *J Computer Assisted Tomography* 2006; 30: 254-57.
12. Stoegar A, Daniaux M, Felber S, Stockhammer G, Aichner F, Zurnudden D. MRI findings in cerebral fat embolism. *Eur Radiol* 1998; 8: 1590-93.
13. Wong MW, Tsui HF, Yung SH, Chan KM, Cheng JC. Continuous pulse oximeter monitoring for inapparent hypoxemia after long bone fractures. *J Trauma* 2004; 56: 356-62.
14. Kanen BL, Loffeld RJLF. Pancreatitis with an unusual fatal complication following endoscopic retrograde cholangiopancreaticography: a case report. *J Medical Case Reports* 2008; 2: 215.
15. Sarvesvaran R. Medicolegal aspects of embolism with a case illustration. *Malaysian J Pathol* 1991; 13: 89-100.

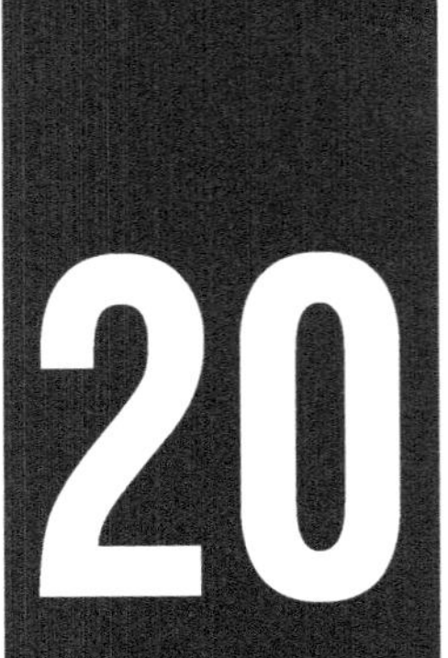

Tattoo: Historical, Social and Psychological Aspects

Prabhas Chandra Chakraborty, Abhishek Das

'Show me a man with a tattoo and I'll show you a man with an interesting past.'
Jack London (American novelist, journalist, and short-story writer)

ABSTRACT

Tattoos are permanent marks or patterns on the skin. They are most personal and intimate art form that alters a person's identity and appearance, either temporarily or permanently for the lifetime. Tattoo, as a decorative purpose was in vogue in most of the communities throughout the world for thousands of years.

Tattoos are either accidentally or intentionally obtained. They can be amateur, such as prison or gang tattoos, while others are professionally applied. Aspects of a decedent's history may also be deduced from certain tattoos. It may give an indication of life style, status, mentality, habits, and medical and addiction history. In tribal communities, extensive tattooing rituals elaborating over almost whole of the body have been associated with rites of passage into adulthood. Many subculture groups of population used tattoo as a mean to differentiate from the homogeneity of general crowd. For example, commemorative military tattoos are most often found in war veterans, rudimentary tattoos in the form of lines with antisocial and anti-police messages were indicative of previous imprisonment, and sometimes depiction of marijuana leaves or different forms of mushrooms or 'ecstasy' are suggestive of drug usage. Some tattoos may also be applied for medical reasons, for e.g., as markers for radiotherapy and laparoscopic surgery. From forensic aspects, tattoos have been considered extremely useful data for identification. If there is superficial burn from fire, tattoos can still be visualized from the dermis of a person's skin. Tattoos are even visible in decomposed cases, and can persist for considerable time after immersion in water. Tattoos are one of the features that is specifically searched for in decomposed unidentifiable bodies of victims in mass disaster situation. The various aspects of tattooing including historical, cultural, social, psychological and forensic issues have been discussed.

Keywords: Art form, identification, lifestyles tattoos, decorative tattoos, erotic tattoos, religious tattoos, medical tattoos, complications of tattoos.

INTRODUCTION

Case of Interest

Policeman's Tattoo helps Reunite Mumbai Family

The policeman was separated from his parents in 1989, aged just six, when they were boarding a train. He ended up on his own in Mumbai, where he was taken care of by a fisherman and then at two orphanages. A car accident later left him unconscious for four months, struggling to remember details of his family or home. He spent years searching through missing person records at police stations—before joining the force himself in 2011. He continued on with his search for finding his family using the only clue he had: a tattoo of his mother's name on his right arm. To add more to the piece of the puzzle, which was forgotten after his car crash, came from records at his first orphanage where he had given his home place as 'Mama Bhanja', a forested area in a district neighbouring Mumbai. When he went back to his native area with his police colleagues, upon asking his said mother searched for an identification mark in the form of tattoo (Fig. 20.1). Ultimately, they were re-united after a long 24 years.[1]

Similar case was encountered while doing medicolegal autopsy at the authors' institution wherein an unknown person received burn injury. The burnt out superficial epidermal layer on his hand, when cleared and examined, revealed a tattoo depicting a Hindu religious symbol which ultimately helped in identification of the victim (Fig. 20.2).

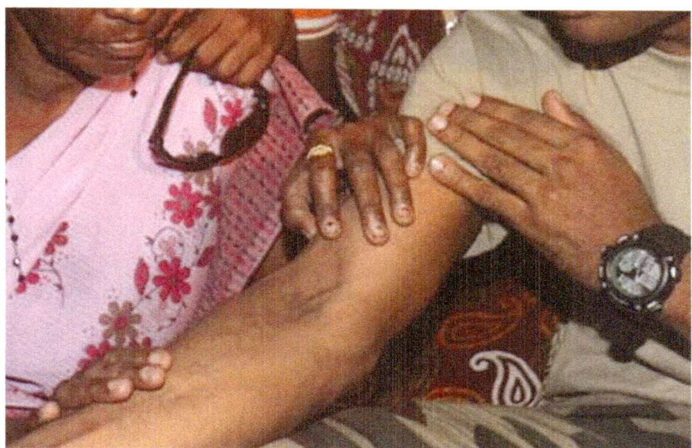

Fig. 20.1 Identification tattoo in hand

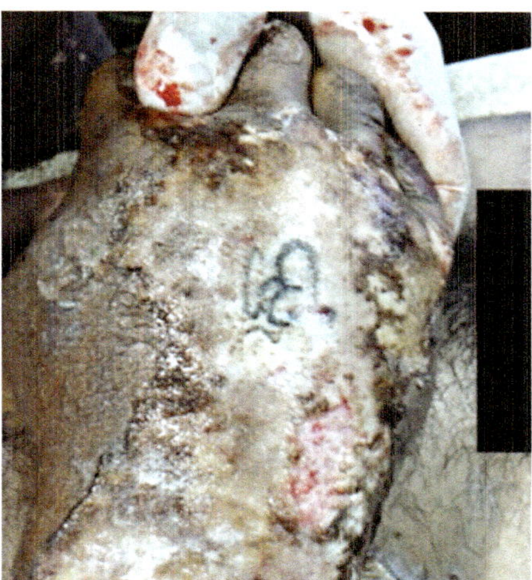

Fig. 20.2 Burnt out epidermis clears out a tattoo

Earlier, vision of a young girl walking down the street with tattoos over her body was a bit rare in civilized society. The very first thought that used to come to mind on encountering such a scene was 'this girl is a tramp' or 'she looks scary' or 'she must be a sexually explicit one'.[2] Parry discussed a rape case wherein the prosecutor, the Jury and the Judge decided that the men accused could not be convicted because the girl had been guilty of 'contributory negligence' because she had a meaningful provoking tattoo. As an inference, she was characterized as misleading men to think that she can be stamped as 'loose character'.[3] In the 21st century, people all over the world have different views, ideas and beliefs about tattoos. Even though some groups of people who oppose these views (for e.g., Bedouins are never tattooed almost),[4] there are also many who support this. There has been somewhat of a renaissance in Western, as well as in the developing countries over the past three decades regarding tattoos. Atkinson described this modern Western culture as 'a culture of body modificationists'.[5] They have gained popularity as a fashion statement, promoted by celebrities. Tattoos can now be found on any type of person, not just in sailors, pirates, prisoners, soldiers and prostitutes or lower-class men, as was previously asserted.[6] Hence, assumptions and opinions about the particulars of tattooed individual have to be guarded and should be given cautiously.

Tattoos may be very useful in assisting with body identification, if facial features or fingers have been damaged or removed. As with scars, tattoos are often remembered by friends or relatives. It may give some indication of social as well as cultural background.[7] This chapter is an overview on tattoos from historical, cultural, social and psychological aspects which may help provide some clues about certain aspects of the individual's life that may help in identification where antemortem data is unavailable.

DEFINITIONS

- *Tattoos:* Designs imprinted by causing multiple punctures on the skin surface with the help of needles dipped in coloring matter.[2,8,9] The term came from *'ta tau'* (Polynesia) or arguably *'tattow'* (Tahiti). The root *ta* means 'drawing', and the word in its entirety means 'a drawing in the skin'. The word *tattow* first appeared in Captain Cook journal in July 1769 after his visit to Tahiti, and has since passed virtually unchanged into the European languages.[10-12]
- *Tattoo machine:* A hand-held, usually electricity driven device used to create a tattoo. Tattoo artists generally use the term 'machine', or even 'iron' to refer to their equipment. The word 'gun' is often used, but many tattoo professionals dislike it.[10]
- *Tattoo enthusiast:* A person who has a personal and/or cultural fascination with tattoos, and at some point in his/her life decided to become tattooed (by Atkinson).
- *Tattooist:* A person who applies tattoos. This term has numerous interchangeable forms used to describe these people including *tattoo artist* and *tattooer*. A slang term, as a negative form is *scratcher* as it is meant to denote a person with little or no artistic skill.[2]
- *UV tattoos/ Black light tattoos:* Tattoos made with a special ink that is visible under an ultraviolet light (black light). Depending upon the ink, they can be hardly visible or even invisible in non-UV environments.

HISTORY

Tattooing has been practiced for centuries throughout the world. The earliest tattooing is evident from the archeological articles recovered in Europe from the upper Paleolithic era (38,000–10,000 BC) or at least the Neolithic era. It had skin puncturing tools and pigment reserves along with small, decorated figurines engraved with tattoos.[13] Mummies from the 11th dynasty of ancient Egypt in the 2nd millennium BC (mummy of Amunet) have revealed tattoos that depicted dancing girls. Many mummified and preserved remains of Bronze Age have been discovered bearing a large number of tattoos. These have added much to our understanding of the historical significance of this body art practice.[11]

Therapeutic practice: Tattoos were probably used in ancient medicine as part of the treatment of the patient. In 1898, Dr Daniel Fouquet wrote an article on 'medical tattooing' practices in ancient Egypt, in which he speculated that the tattooed markings on the female mummies found at the Deir el-Bahari site may have served a medicinal or therapeutic purpose: 'The examination of these scars, some white, others blue, leaves in no doubt that they are not, in essence, ornament, but an established treatment for a condition of the pelvis, very probably chronic pelvic peritonitis'.[14] A Bronze Age warrior, named Otzi (or Oetzae) the Iceman, dating from the 5th to 4th millennium BC, was found in the Ötz valley in the Alps had some 57 carbon tattoos. A series of parallel lines over the lower back, mainly at lumbar spine and ankle, over medial and lateral malleoli and a cross on the medial aspect of one knee seemed to correspond to underlying arthritic disease or rheumatologic complications for which he was treated indigenously.[6,9,14-16]

Identification tattoos have been used as a symbol of royalty, nobility and status in some cultures but have also been used to mark slaves and prisoners, and for a long time represented a symbol of outcast or criminality.[10] In ancient Greece, tattoos were regarded as the mark of an 'outsider' as an effort to distinguish clearly between civilised peoples (Greeks) and barbarians (Celts, Scythians and Germanic tribes).[9,17] At that time, any person with tattoos was poorly regarded. Romans used both tattoos and branding to stigmatise slaves and criminals in addition to the identifying features. The Latin word for 'tattoo' was 'stigma', hence the English word 'stigmatise'.[18] Later, tattoos were also used by military men and traders as a specification of their occupations. Roman soldiers were required by law to have identifying tattoos on their hands in order to make it difficult to hide, if they deserted. It was a common practice to tattoo 'Stop me, I'm a runaway' on the foreheads of slaves. Emperor Constantine I banned tattooing the face around AD 330.[18] It was at this time that the Christian tattoos appeared. Christianity was both an unofficial and outlawed religion, followers of this religion used tattoos as a covert method of recognition. This practice increased until a verdict from Pope Hadrian (Second Council of Nicaea, 787 AD) banned tattoos in the Christian community.[9,17,18] In Britain, in 1717, tattooing replaced branding as a method of marking the deserters from the military community. It continued till 1879, when deserters were tattooed with a 'D'. From 1832, French civilization used tattoos to identify the convicts sentenced to forced labour.[6,9,17]

A long history of tattooing dating back to the 5th century BC can be encountered among the Japanese. As with other subgroups and subcultures, tattoos were considered as an indicator of 'outside normal society'.[9]

The most enduring set of tattoos were displayed by the people of South Pacific island. Each group has its individualistic designs and, as with the Scythians and other groups, tattoos were mostly reserved for the warriors of mainly the upper classes. *Moko,* practiced mostly among the Maori people consisted of facial tattoos combined with scarification. Another type of tattooing called *Pe'a* which was seen in Samoans mainly from the waist to the knees.[18,19] These types of tattoos are unique in that they have significance as a traditional form even to this day (Fig. 20.3).

Tattoos as fashion statement: The acceptability of tattoos as a marker of fashion statement was a debatable issue. In medieval Europe, crusaders and pilgrims to the Holy Land often tattooed their bodies with Christian symbols, such as the Cross of Jerusalem, and a shrine in Loreto offered tattoos to its pilgrims.[6] In the 19th century, tattoos were considered fashionable among female members of European and English aristocrat society. For example, Lady Randolph Churchill sported a tattoo of a snake around her wrist which was very much popular.[9]

The evolution of tattoo's cultural status crossed several domains from an antisocial activity in 1960s to that of a trendy fashion statement in the 1990s.

Not all cultures of the world used tattooing for body modification, for e.g., the Tasmanians rely on elaborate scarification instead of tattooing.[19] Extensive scarification is still found among certain African tribal groups also.

EPIDEMIOLOGY

In the United States, an estimated 7–20 million people have at least one tattoo. Information regarding the prevalence of tattooing among adolescents and young adults continues to be published, and the numbers show a progressively increasing trend of body art, which has become mainstream among individuals aged 16–25 years.[11] It is estimated that 10–16% of adolescents have tattoos compared to 3–9% of the general population.[20] In one cross-sectional study of 2101 adolescents in European countries in 1995, 10% of the study population was found to have tattoos. Data from surveys of high school and college students

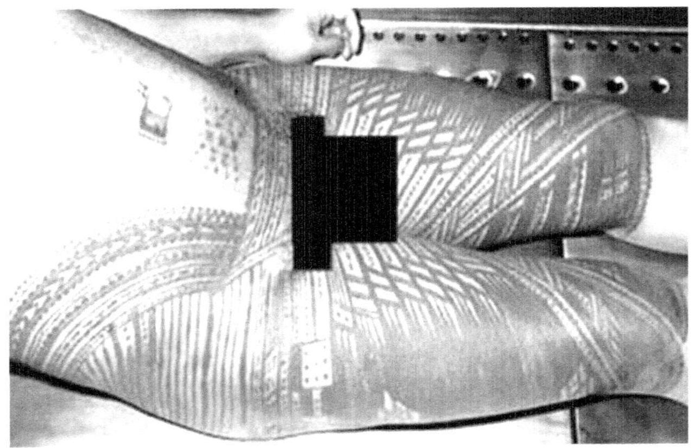

Fig. 20.3 Tribal tattoo

(13–25 years of age) indicate a prevalence of 15–25% for tattooing and 24% of Americans between ages of 18–50 years have at least one tattoo.[11,12] In a secondary analysis of survey data in 2002 from a representative sample (spread nationwide) of 6702 adolescents (11 to 21 years of age) in developed countries, 4.5% were found to have permanent tattoos. A 2003 survey of 1010 people conducted by Ohio University revealed that one in every seven adults has a tattoo, with young adults about 10 times more likely to have one, compared with their parents.[21]

Findings from a recent study in the US (2012) suggested that one in five adults have at least one tattoo (21%) which is up from the 16% and 14% who reported having a tattoo when this question was asked in 2003 and 2008, respectively. Adults aged 30–39 are most likely to have a tattoo (38%), compared to both those younger (30% of those 25–29 and 22% of those 18–24) and older (27% of those 40–49, 11% of those 50–64 and just 5% of those 65 and older) individuals.[22] Satisfying data in India regarding the prevalence of tattoo is still to be obtained on an authentic basis.

CLASSIFICATION OF TATTOO

Tattoos can be divided into following groups depending on type and depth of pigments:[10,11,23]

a. *Nonpermanent or temporary tattoo* is a non-permanent image on the skin resembling a real tattoo that last for few days to weeks. They can be drawn, painted or airbrushed, as a form of body painting, but usually these tattoos are transferred to the skin. Temporary tattoos are used for numerous purposes including self-expression and identification. Mehndi or henna tattoos is the application of a temporary form of skin decoration which is practiced mainly in the Indian subcontinent (particularly in India, Nepal, Pakistan, Bangladesh and Maldives), Middle East and North Africa.
b. *Semi-permanent tattoos* such as permanent makeup used for cosmetic purpose may last for few years. These are applied using a tattoo gun and are supposed to gradually fade away over time, leaving no trace. Some tattoo artists claim that the inks are inserted closer to the surface, allowing them to gradually slough off, while others claim to use special inks that naturally disperse over time.
c. *Permanent tattoos* meant to persist during whole life. Permanent tattoos have been used as cultural symbols among many tribal populations, as well as the caste-based Hindu population of India.[14] It was very common in southern India especially in Tamilnadu before 1980's where they are called '*pachakutharathu*'. In northern India, permanent tattoos are called '*godna*'.

Classification of tattoos can be based on color (single or multicolored) or style (professional, amateur, medical, cosmetic, traumatic). The American Academy of Dermatology distinguishes five types of tattoos:[9,10,18,21]

i. Traumatic tattoos (also called 'natural tattoos' resulting from injuries, especially from road injuries or pencil lead); these are unintentional and unwanted tattoos.
ii. Amateur tattoos.
iii. Professional tattoos (using both traditional methods and modern tattoo machines).

iv. Cosmetic tattoos (also known as 'permanent makeup').
v. Medical tattoos.

Traumatic Tattoos

Tattoos are usually the intentional deposit of pigment into the skin. However, some tattoos are not always intentional. An entity named 'non-intentional tattoo' or 'unintentional tattoo' can be seen in coal miners where deposition of carbon particles under the skin takes the form of a tattoo. Similarly, accidental dermabrasion in road traffic accidents can result in a traumatic tattoo when substance such as asphalt is rubbed into a wound. These are particularly difficult to remove as they tend to be spread across several different layers of skin, and scarring or permanent discoloration is almost unavoidable depending on the location. Another form in this category is seen in close range firearm injury (Fig. 20.4). The unburnt gunpowder gets deposited on the superficial layers of skin around the wound of entry, having evidence of multiple punctured marks. This can also be due to an explosion, or accidental implantation of graphite pencil points or ink punctures. Amalgam tattoos of the oral mucosa following dental filling is another example of non-intentional tattooing.[8,10,12,18,24]

Amateur and Professional Tattoos

An amateur tattoo can be applied by anyone, at home, using a needle and a bottle of India ink. They often mention love names, heart and arrow symbols. A professional tattoo is created by a trained tattoo artist at a salon or tattoo parlour which involves endless symbols, figures, animals or flowers. The main difference is in the number of colors used and level of penetration. An amateur tattoo often uses single color carbon based ink, whereas professional tattoos contain several colors. A professional tattoo is applied uniformly beneath the skin as opposed to an amateur tattoo which is applied at varying depths. Amateur tattoos are much easier to remove compared to more complicated designs in professional

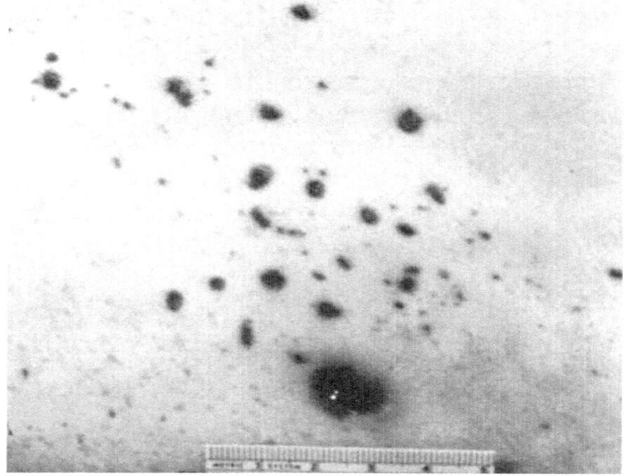

Fig. 20.4 Gunshot tattooing (non-intentional)

tattoos, where there is shading and the appearance of three dimensional forms with greater quantities of ink and variety of colored pigments which saturate the lower layers of the skin.[10,12,18]

Cosmetic Tattoos

Cosmetic tattoos have been used for centuries. They include permanent makeup, camouflaging skin discolorations, such as birthmarks (hemangiomas) or scars, or tattooing 'hair follicles' into bald areas. In this procedure, tattoos are also used to enhance eyebrows, lips, eyes (liner), and even moles, usually with natural colors, as the designs are intended to resemble makeup. The therapeutic variant is known as dermatography which is often used for scar correction and camouflaging bald areas. Tattooing is used to repigment the skin in conditions that cause hypopigmentation or hyperpigmentation, including burns, and micropigmentation of the lips and fingertips in patients having vitiligo. Corneal tattooing is done in perforating injury, measles keratitis and other conditions that result in cosmetically disfiguring discoloration of the cornea.[9,10,18,25]

Medical Tattoos

A medical tattoo is used for indicating a medically relevant condition or body location. Medical tattoos can be encountered in the following situations:[25,26]

a. *Medical alert tattooing:* Medical practitioners, at times, may encounter tattooed messages of instructional or advisory in nature. These tattoos may be seen in elderly patients or in those with chronic medical condition, like insulin-dependent diabetes mellitus or drug allergy or previous treatments that are not to be repeated (Fig. 20.5). They should be considered as a guide to treatment decisions.[9]

   Tattoos may sometimes be in the form of advance directives, such as do-not-resuscitate (DNR) directives or not to prolong life by using feeding

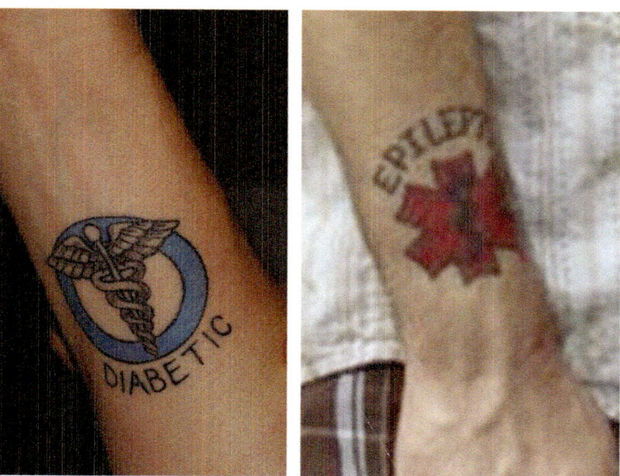

Fig. 20.5 Medical alert tattoos

gastrostomy (PEG) tubes.[9] These types of tattoos pose practical and ethical problems: to follow the advice of the tattoo without a verbal instruction from the unconscious patient or to follow normal resuscitation procedures. Tattoos that state an advance directive for health care are not recognized as meeting the legal requirements for advance directives. They may not reflect a person's current wishes, and they may have even been applied as a joke.

b. *Blood group tattooing* was used in a few states in the US in the early 1950s as part of a program to provide a 'walking blood bank'. However, the practice fell out of favor as doctors questioned the reliability of tattoos for medical information. Military personnel may also have their blood groups tattooed on their upper arms to assist medical personnel with resuscitative efforts.

c. *Reconstruction surgery:* During breast reconstruction after mastectomy or breast reduction surgery, tattooing of the nipple-areola complex is usually done by the surgeon.

d. *Delineation in radiotherapy:* Tattoos are often applied to delineate the radiation field in order to minimize damage to surrounding tissues. The radiotherapist put black tattoos with India ink 1–2 mm in size on the body that can aid in adjusting the beam properly for subsequent treatment.[24]

e. *Endoscopic tattooing* is commonly used for directing endoscopic procedures. Tattooing of the segment to be resected helps in proper visualization of diseased bowel segments which otherwise may result in resecting the wrong segment of bowel during laparoscopic surgery. Endoscopic tattooing is also used to facilitate identification of subtle mucosal lesions at the time of subsequent endoscopy. For example, tattooing is done at the site of colonic polyp removal, and for follow-up of Barrett esophagus.

- *Therapeutic procedures:* In certain cultural groups in West Africa, traditional healers utilise tattoos and scarification as therapeutic tools. For example, a thin line on the forehead is drawn to treat epilepsy, and tattoos are systematically drawn on the hands and legs for treating peripheral neuropathy.[9] However, its benefits are doubtful.

In cases where there is little information on the medical history, these types of tattoos may help to identify possible underlying conditions.

TATTOO STYLES

Despite considerable variation in styles, researchers have categorized tattoos into several defined categories as given in Table 20.1.[9,27-29]

Table 20.1 Various tattoo styles

a. Traditional western	a. Abstract	a. Black and gray
b. Contemporary western	b. Naturalistic	b. Color
c. Traditional eastern	c. Gang	c. Portrait and fine-line
d. Traditional tribal	d. Tribal	d. Tribal
e. Contemporary tribal	e. Dedication and Memorial	e. Freehand custom
f. Gang and prison	f. Simplification	f. Cover-up, touch-up, and rework
	g. Complex	

Traditional western (old school) is the older style of tattoo which includes designs, such as mermaids, ships, anchors, banners, sparrows, hearts, roses, daggers, animals and names of family members. They were often found among sailors or ex-navy personnel and sometimes had specific meanings. Most people nowadays who have these tattoos are unaware of the symbolism associated with them and have usually chosen the design for aesthetic reasons. Swallow tattoos were popular among sailors. A sailor tattooed with one swallow had travelled over 5,000 nautical miles (9,260 km); a sailor with two swallows had travelled 10,000 nautical miles (18,520 km). People tattooed cobwebs to symbolize a lengthy term in prison. The symbolism of the cobweb is the association with spiders trapping prey, and criminals being trapped behind bars. Cobweb tattoos are popular these days with people who were never convicts. Playing cards or suits of the deck commonly indicate an inmate who likes to gamble. However, if tattoo is colored, it is probably not a prison tattoo, since they rarely have access to colored ink.

Contemporary western (new school) encompasses fine line styles and detailed photorealistic work that is produced in either grayscale or color, with new shades such as vibrant purples, and advances in shading techniques. It is basically combining multiple styles of tattooing into one piece.

Traditional eastern designs are usually intricate and colorful, depicting complex scenes that often tell a story. The style is said to have originated when peasants, who were forbidden to wear colorful clothing, tattooed a 'suit' of vibrant designs onto their bodies. Asian themed tattoos frequently use Koi fish, cherry blossom, Buddha, lotus, dragon, samurai or geisha.

Traditional tribal originated from various old tribes like those from Borneo, Haida, Native Americans, Celtic, Maori and other Polynesian tribes. The shapes and motifs of these tribal tattoos are deeply rooted in the tribe's mythology and view of the world. The designs have specific meanings, and usually represent a transition in status. They also reflected the social and religious values of the tribe, such as the rituals of the tribe, the ancestors, the origins of the world and the relationship with the gods. These tattoos are customarily produced by expert tribesmen using traditional tools, and are monochromatic (produced in black ink only). Haida is a design of the Eskimo and the Native Americans wherein animal, birds and totems are popular subjects.

Contemporary tribal tattoos are usually monochromatic, although occasionally some color is used. The style is defined by sweeping solid curves and sharp points, with untattooed spaces left in between to form intricate designs. The modern versions of Polynesian tribal tattoos are popular amongst celebrities (for e.g., the design on Mike Tyson's face is a Maori-inspired design) and are responsible for the resurgence of interest in tattoos in the West. Modern tribal designs do not generally have any symbolic meanings, and are simple body decorations for those who are unsure of what kind of picture they could live with. Celtic designs, gangland style lettering and Japanese characters all come under this description in modern tattooing.

Gang and prison tattoos consists mostly symbols of skulls, serpents, tombstones and grim reaper which are often crude, and highlighting death and violence.

Black and gray tattoos are basically done with use of degrees of black to gray shading. They are typically used to create a 3-D effect without using color. This type of tattoo is particularly suited to darker skin tone which does not accept color well, and also to those who are regularly go out in the sun.

Color tattoos are full color designs lined with black and also shaded.

Fine-line is mostly used for portrait work. It can be used for high detail and definition in larger tattoos.

Abstract tattoos are modern style of art, and usually without any outline or artwork. They are mostly derived from ancient styles of tattooing and include tribal and Celtic styles, old English lettering and Chinese symbols. These tattoos are mostly done in shades of black and gray, and are commonly made around the navel, chest and calves, though the arms and upper back are also emerging as a popular choice.

Naturalistic tattoos involve portraying of minute details, shading and perspective in such a way that imparts a realistic style, often in the 'natural' form. The designs comprises of faces of celebrity, political and religious leaders.

Dedication tattoos are commonly known as 'pledges'. It involves the use of the sailor-based designs, like the anchor with a ship name, and the insignia of a military regiment.

Memorial tattoos can be images representing a person's life in some way. It may be a religious image, crosses, banners, praying hands, poems, flowers, or sometimes, a portrait. The tattoos incorporate items that had meaning or significance to the deceased and or their family. Often this type of tattoo is accompanied by lettering with the person's name and date of birth and/or death.

Simplification tattoos do not have any limiting boundaries in terms of the designs. Almost any, and every shape and size can be included in this type, as long as it is done by the tattoo artist. The range of designs is quite wide—from action figurines and animals to flowers and hearts. Panthers, lions, dragons and zodiac signs are also popular designs.

Complex tattoos (combination tattoos) comprise of a mixture of various tattoos, making them much more impressive than other types of designs. The most popular are the traditional Japanese body suits and combinations of unrelated images.

Freehand tattoos are drawn directly onto the body area without use of a stencil or pre-prepared drawing. The advantage is that the tattoo can be better fitted to the body, since it makes use of the body shape so as to give the image more movement. Freehand is also used for cover-up tattoos, to allow a more direct fitting of the new image over the old by making use of the existing shape and lines.

Rework includes some bad tattoos which are restored to a proper version of the original design, but the majority are usually saveable through cover-ups, and may be limited on the choice of design.

REASONS AND IMPLICATIONS OF TATTOOING

Being Tattooed

Before being tattooed, a person goes through a series of psychological process which includes the following four specific stages of events:[2]

i. Deciding to be tattooed
ii. Locating a tattooist

iii. Choosing a meaningful design
iv. Locating the specific desired body part where the tattoo to be inscribed.

The reasons for selection of design may be varied (Table 20.2).[9,11,23]

Decorative

Decorative tattoos which are an expression of individual taste and style are by far the most common. They are, nowadays, accepted as fashion statement in all social classes with little or no symbolic significance.[10,24] Customised tattoos, often designed by the wearer to reflect personal taste and content are becoming more popular, and may be used to celebrate a special occasion, such as the birth of a child, the beginning or end of a relationship or other significant life achievements.[9] Sometimes, tattoos are applied due to peer pressure or as a memorial for loved ones who have died.

Voluntary Group Membership

Some individuals are tattooed to reflect membership of a group or gang, most commonly paramilitary, street or motorcycle groups. Military personnel use tattoos to denote membership of specific platoons or involvement in specific fields of combat.

Members of the military have their vital information tattooed to them, usually on the rib cage below the armpit which is referred to as 'meat tags'. Tattoos designed to reflect sexual orientation like the flying blue bird on the dorsum of the hand between thumb and index finger serves as business card among homosexuals. Other designs, such as the rainbow flag may also reflect a gay lifestyle.[9]

'La Eme' or 'The M' is the symbol of the Mexican mafia. Yakuza or 'Japanese mafia' have a full body or 'suit' of highly colored and intricate tattoos with complicated designs (Fig. 20.6).[9,10,29] The Aryan Brotherhood, a white supremacist gang in the US prison have tattoos of shamrocks and/or the letters 'AB', as well as nazi symbols such as the swastika and SS bolts. In the Russian prison system, a tattoo on the chest symbolizes a 'Prince of Thieves'.

Involuntary Group Membership

Tattoos were used for identification wherein people have been forcibly tattooed. Inmates of Nazi concentration camps in World War II had identification numbers tattooed on their arms, a practice reminiscent of Roman methods of identifying slaves and criminals. Nowadays, grandchildren of inmates sometimes have the number tattooed on their forearms as a commemorative (Fig. 20.7).[9,18]

Table 20.2 Reasons for tattoo application

Decorative/ ornamental	Religious and political
Involuntary group membership	Voluntary group membership
Cosmetic and medical	Advertising and marketing
Psychological	Veterinary

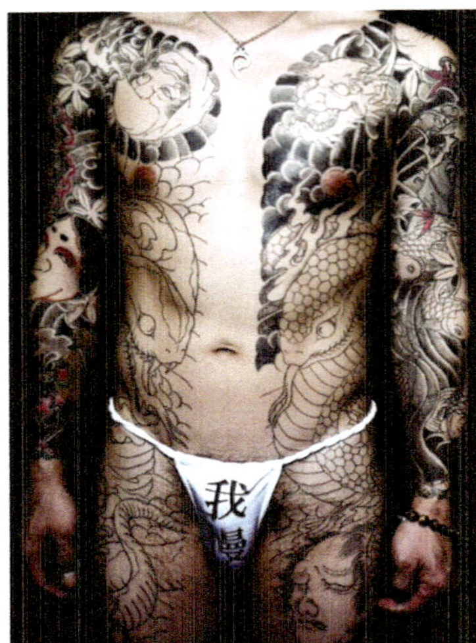

Fig. 20.6 Full body tattoo

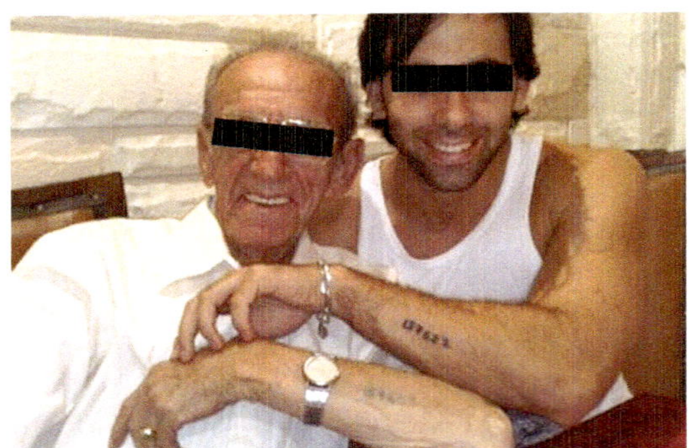

Fig. 20.7 Identification tattoo on a survivor of concentration camp

Religious and Political

Tattoos have always been an expression of culture, religion and political affiliation. Tattoos depicting religious themes are a method for people to advertise their religion. In Hindu religion, tattoos are seen as a normal expression of faith, and are used to ensure fertility and to ward off the evil eye. In contrast, both the Bible and the Koran forbids this practice. Tattoos may also be used to exhibit political or ideological values, the most common of these being fascist or racist symbols and images adopted by neo-nazis and white supremacists. Patriotic symbols such as flags and emblems are also common.[9,10,12,27]

Cosmetic and Medical

Tattoos have been used cosmetically for centuries. As discussed earlier, the most common being the 'derma-pigmentation' or 'permanent makeup' and tattoos to cover birthmarks or scars. Tattoos are also seen in elderly patients or in those with a chronic medical condition, who for metal allergy, are unable to wear medical alert bracelets.[25]

Advertising and Marketing

Tattoos, nowadays, are also used in marketing and advertising. The companies are paying people to have logos of brands like HBO, Red Bull and Sailor Jerry's rum tattooed in their bodies. This practice is known as 'skinvertising'.[23] Skinvertising gained popularity in the early 2000s when online casino GoldenPalace.com secured a tattoo on boxer Bernard Hopkins's back. Tattoos are being used as 'walking billboards', and people are paid for sporting advertisements.

Psychological Issues

It is often believed that in adolescence body piercing and tattooing are manifestations of rebellion, and can be considered as indicators of mental illness and high-risk behavior. It has been suggested that tattoos can be used as a diagnostic indicator for psychiatric problems, such as alcohol and drug abuse, anti-social personality disorder, schizophrenia, borderline personality disorders, fetishism and paraphilias. For example, there are often strong links between adolescents who are tattooed or pierced at a young age (<13 years) and high-risk behaviors, such as drug abuse, gang membership and violence. In contrast, individuals tattooed and pierced after the age of 20 years do not appear to engage in these behaviors to the same degree as younger individuals.[9]

Veterinary

Tattoos are also placed on animals, though rarely for decorative reasons. Pets, show animals, thoroughbred horses and livestock are sometimes tattooed with identification and other marks through which their owners can be identified. Tattooing for identification purposes also occurs in laboratory animals.[9,18]

TECHNIQUES OF TATTOOING

Techniques used in tattooing have evolved over the centuries. Traditional tattoos were produced by incising or puncturing the skin and rubbing in soot or other forms of carbon or pigments. The dyes of these earlier forms of tattoo were mostly of natural origin. The instruments were of metallic or plant origin. The Inuit used relatively crude instruments such as a bone needle coated in soot and a procedure resembling weaving technique of present day.[17] The Shan tribes in Myanmar used heavy metal tipped awls to pierce the skin.[30] Other cultures used sticks, bones, shells and animal teeth to make instruments with sharp and/or pointed ends that were capable of fine work.[30]

Tattoo Machines

Nowadays, tattoo machines are universally used by professional tattooist. Tattoo machines contain electromagnetic coils to move an armature bar up and down (Fig. 20.8). Connected to the armature bar is a needle assembly that delivers the

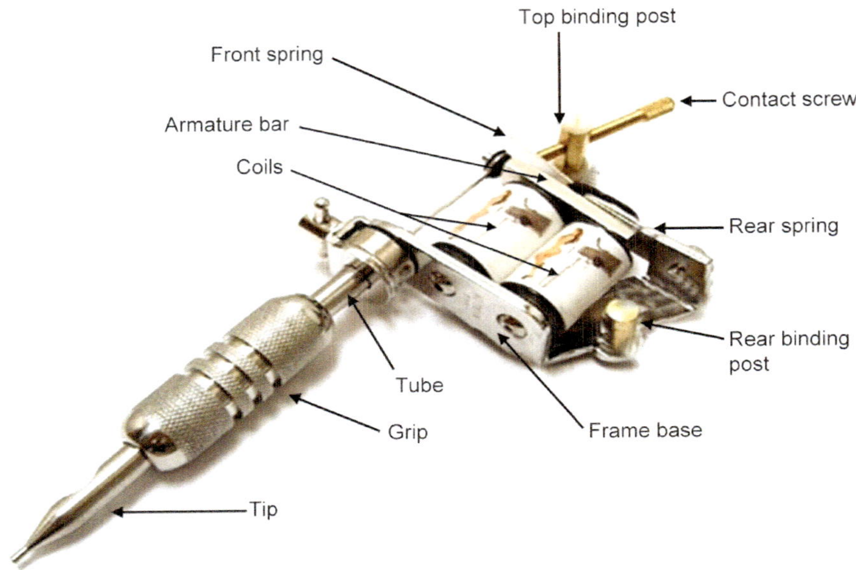

Fig. 20.8 Tattoo machine

dye into the skin. Besides 'coiled' tattoo machine, there is also 'rotary' tattoo machine which is powered by regulated motors rather than electromagnetic coils. Most of the modern forms of tattoos are produced using tattoo machine with multiple needles that rotates or moves to and fro between 50 to 300 times per minute. Dyes are picked up by the composite needles from reservoirs and injected into the superficial layer of the dermis.[31]

Actually, there is little change from the machine that Thomas Edison designed for making embroidery patterns, and patented under the title *Stencil-pens* in New Jersey, US in 1876.[16,17] In 1891, Samuel O'Reilly modified the device to introduce ink into the skin, and later patented a tube and needle system to provide an ink reservoir.[9] Most modern tattoo machines can minutely control needle depth, speed, force of application and area of delivery of dyes. Various improvisations in this field over time have allowed tattooing to become a very precise art form.

There are many types of tattoo machines. Of these, liners and shaders are the commoner varieties of machines from a technical standpoint. Machines are usually categorized into long stroke and short stroke varieties. The longer-stroked machines are good for coloring and shading, as well as sculpting lines, while doing less damage to skin. Shorter-stroke machines are commonly used for lining in a single pass style, and also in a shader setup to achieve a more subtle gradation of black, such as in portraits.[31]

The techniques and complexity of tattoos have changed significantly over the last 15 years in Western cultures. Earlier, tattoos were mostly black and white, lacking intricate detailing—the 'traditional western' tattoos. The introduction of the 'fine line' style has allowed a complex and more colorful designs with detailed depiction of symbols and images, sometimes exactly like photographs. Since studies and epidemiological researches reveal that most people acquire their first tattoos in their late teens to early 20s, the differentiation between new, fine line tattoos and those of the older thick outline style may help to establish the approximate age of a tattooed individual.[9]

Tattoo Inks or Dyes

The composition of the ink used for tattooing purposes is complex. In general, the ink consists of one or more colorants, a carrier and some additives.[10] The components of various dyes have remained relatively unchanged for many years and include India ink, mercuric sulphide (cinnabar), cadmium, chromium and cobalt salts (Table 20.3).[11,32]

Since the most common color used in the tattoos is black, most tattoo inks are made of carbon based pigments. They are colored using a variety of natural and man-made components that make the colors stay in one place under the skin and prevent fading, smudging, soaking and blurring over time. These inks are usually non-toxic. Several natural pigments are in use, such as the ones originated from tropical wood (*Pterocarpus santalinus* or *Santilin* from India or *Caesalpinia echinata* from Brazil). The use of heavy metals such as mercury, cadmium and lead has been banned for cosmetic purposes, and it is rare to find these elements in the tattoo inks nowadays in the US and most European countries. Many inks may contain impurities because they are originally developed and produced for industrial purposes, like printing ink and motorcar paint.[10]

Another type of tattoo ink uses nitrogen based azo dyes, and are often found in artists' paints. These compounds are less common and not many tattoo artists use them because they have not been as extensively researched as the carbon based pigments. Another interesting (but not practically very common) tattoo ink is Chameleon tattoo inks which are UV light sensitive, and only appear when they are exposed to black light. These inks can be used to create an entirely invisible tattoo design or to supplement a more traditional tattoo with an intriguing glow. They are very popular for supplementing images like lizard tattoos and other animal tattoos that can be easily accented. However, these dyes also are somewhat controversial, since they have not been on the market for very long, and some users' report that the inks spread and blur relatively quickly, leaving a black light sensitive smudge area on the skin rather than a detailed design.[32]

Table 20.3 Ingredients of tattoo pigments

Dye color	*Dye content*
Black	Carbon
Red	Mercury sulfide
Blue	Cobalt aluminate
Purple	Manganese
Brown	Hydrated iron oxide
Green	Chromium oxide
Lilac	Magnesium
White	Titinium oxide
Yellow	Cadmium sulfide

Finally, there are completely unconventional tattoo dyes, such as those used in prison tattoos. These can be made of anything from ashes to clay, just like the materials used for thousands of years by indigenous tribes. In fact, many of these are more often made of ink from pens or even melted checkers. These inks are very risky because they are not sterilized. Furthermore, these tattoos are very unsafe because they often are made using shared needles or makeshift needles that also are not sterilized. This can lead to spread diseases and infections, like hepatitis or HIV among an entire prison population.[30,32]

UV Tattoo or Black-Light Tattoo

UV tattoos or black-light tattoos are made with a special ink that is visible specifically under ultraviolet light (commonly called as 'black-light'). Depending upon the ink, they can be very faint or even invisible in non-UV environments, thus a popular consideration for people seeking a subtler tattoo. Although, these tattoos may appear invisible in normal light, scarring during the inscription of tattoo may remain. A UV tattoo becomes visible under black-light, when it glows in colors ranging from white to blue to purple, depending on the specific dye used (Fig. 20.9). Colored ink is also available where the ink is visible in normal light (as with a regular tattoo), but the ink will glow vividly under UV light. However, some UV inks are not as bright under normal light as normal tattoo ink and are considered not as vibrant. UV tattoo ink is also many times more expensive than regular tattoo inks. In time, it may also not glow in black lighting. Blue UV inks are known to turn yellow or slightly brown with sun exposure. Color/black UV inks are known to become colored in all lighting. Therefore, it might permanently appear as a regular tattoo.[33] The effect of these dyes becomes dull if regular dye is used on top of them.[33]

The composition of UV inks has been improved over last few years. For this reason, there is little or no reaction these days. These tattoos are suitable for those who restrict their choice of tattoo show off and placement (because of their profession or any other obligation or choice).

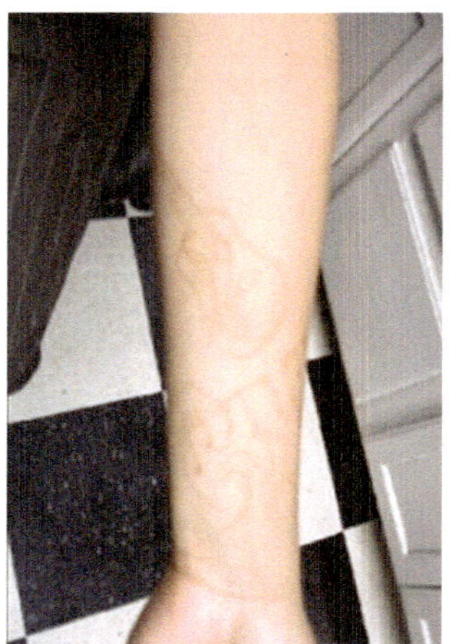
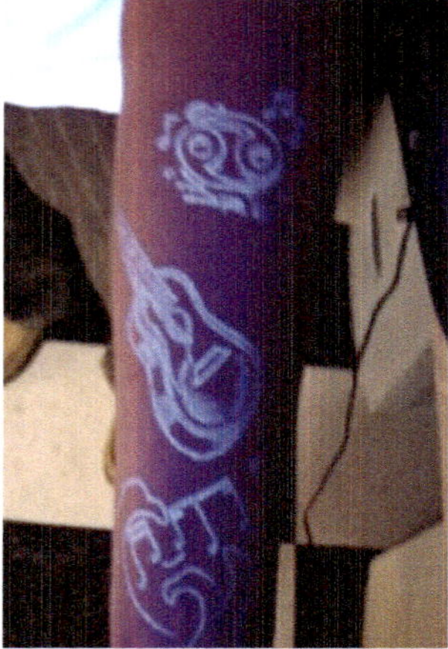

Fig. 20.9 Black-light tattoo (visible under UV ray)

Tattoo Shading

Without shading, a tattoo looks unexciting and old fashioned. Shading gives tattoo an artistic and more realistic look. With shading, a tattoo acquires depth and converts a flat, 2-dimensional drawing to a 3-dimensional image form. Tattoo shading is an advanced skill and one of the biggest challenges for a tattoo artist. Shaded tattoo gives an idea of expertise and calibre of the tattoo artist.[34]

According to some historians, black and gray tattoos are traditional style of tattoos which originated in prisons in the 19th century. Because colored pigments were not available in prisons, techniques were developed to add interest to designs created with black ink. These techniques included tattoo shading in many occasions which was accomplished by varying the intensity of the pigment, from dark black to different shades of gray. The depth of injection was also a matter of consideration to create dark and light areas within the tattoo design.[34]

Today, the most effective type of tattoo shading is done with tattoo machine since the depth of the puncture can be precisely controlled—an important requirement for tattoo shading. Designs that feature portraits are well-suited for shading. Other examples are images of skulls, animals, flowers and landscapes. Fantasy creatures like dragons are also good subjects for tattoo shading.

LOCAL TISSUE CHANGES IN A TATTOO

Tattoos undergo a sequence of changes due to tissue responses to different injected pigments. The first reaction seen is erythema and swelling, followed by sloughing of the epidermis, usually without any blistering. After 5-7 days, the tattoo is indurated with crusting of the surface. Healing occurs after about 14 days.[9] In histological sections, tattoos appear as aggregates of pigment material (commonly black) within the interstitium, and macrophages within the dermis. The presence of inflammatory reaction is usually insignificant. Aggregated pigment may also be revealed at adjacent regional lymph nodes.

LONGEVITY OF TATTOO

The rate of fading depends mainly upon the composition of pigment, depth of penetration and sites where it is tattooed. The process of tattooing is also a matter of consideration. Body parts receiving frequent friction and sunrays erase a tattoo overlying it after a few years. Parts protected by clothing and not subjected to constant friction will retain the design for a longer period.[4,35]

Duration of persistence of a tattoo also depends on the depth at which the pigment materials used has been impregnated. In order for the tattoo to be permanent, pigments are injected in papillary and reticular dermis, i.e. the superficial layer of dermis upto a depth of 1–2 mm under the skin (Fig. 20.10). A plane superficial or deep to it gives a tattoo a shorter duration of persistence. Pigments injected at the epidermis gradually fade out with time due to sloughing off and normal turnover of the keratinized cell layer (Fig. 20.11). Pigments put in the deep dermis are taken up by macrophages or the lymphatics, and the tattoo disappears within a few months.[11,12]

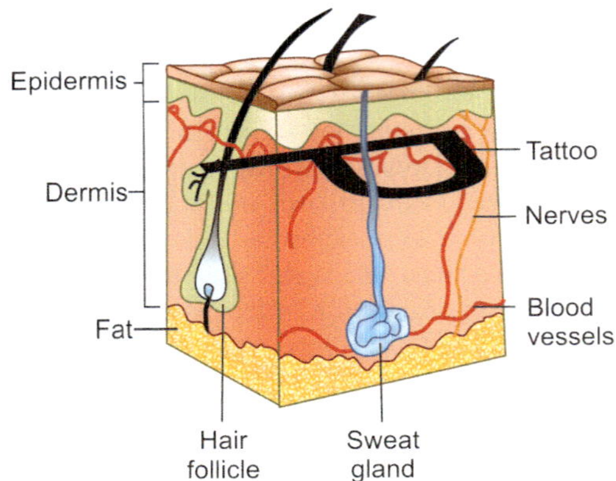

Fig. 20.10 Level of pigment for permanent tattooing ('P')

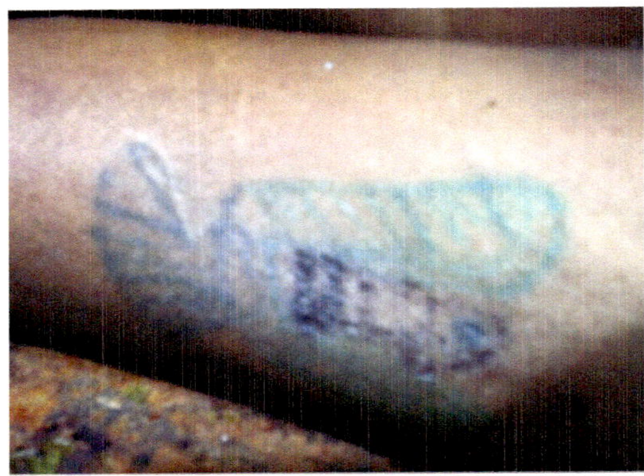

Fig. 20.11 Faded green tattoo

COMPLICATIONS OF TATTOO

Complications may be acute, secondary to a physical injury from the injection of pigments or may occur after months or years (Table 20.4).[10,24]

Tattoo Associated Dermatoses

It can be classified under three categories:[9,36-39]

1. Allergic (mostly to the untoward response to dye particles).
2. Granulomatous (chronic inflammatory reactions to tattoo pigment granules).
3. Lichenoid reactions (delayed type hypersensitivity simulating a graft vs host response).

Allergic reactions: Various reactions to the salts, inorganic compounds and organic preparations have been reported. In these cases, the most common reactions are allergic contact dermatitis and lichenoid dermatitis mainly due to the red pigment (mercury). Reactions to mercury-based inks include swelling,

Table 20.4 Complications of tattooing

Allergic reactions	*Infections*	*Miscellaneous*
Urticaria Eczematous dermatitis Photosensitivity Foreign body reaction Lichenoid reaction Granulomatous hypersensitivity reaction Vasculitis Erythema nodosum	*Bacterial infections* Pyogenic (Streptococci, Staphylococci, and *Pseudomonas*) *Mycobacterium tuberculosis*, atypical mycobacteriae Syphilis *Leishmania* *Fungal infections* Sporotrichosis Candidiasis Zygomycosis *Viral infections* Hepatitis A, B, C, D and HIV Herpes simplex-zoster Papilloma virus, poxvirus	Koebner effect Migration of pigments to lymphatic ganglia Malignant skin neoplasias Pseudoepitheliomatous epidermal hyperplasia Sarcoidosis Postsurgical complications/scars/keloids MRI complications

erythema and pruritus. In recent years, alternatives to the mercury-based red inks have been developed which include sienna/red ochre (ferric hydrate), cadmium red (cadmium selenide) and organic vegetable dyes such as sandalwood and Brazilwood with fewer incidences of sensitivity and reactions.[10,12,24,25] Photoinduced reactions are mostly associated with yellow pigments and present as erythematous, pruriginous nodules that appear following sun exposure.[24]

Granulomatous reaction is a foreign body reaction to the pigment. It is associated with the use of mercury, chrome, cobalt and manganese containing dyes. It is generally limited to the colors of the tattoo and reflects a localized hypersensitivity reaction to the components of the pigments.[9,24]

Sarcoidal reactions are rare in tattoos. They generally occur as a reaction to the ochre dye, mostly with silica-rich pigments and may represent a nonspecific finding or a manifestation of systemic sarcoidosis. Pseudolymphomatous reaction presents as hardened erythematous nodules or violaceous plaques that appear on the tattoo. This type of reaction is more commonly associated with red, green and blue pigments.[10,24]

Other cutaneous conditions that localize in tattooed areas include vaccinia, verruca vulgaris, herpes simplex, herpes zoster, psoriasis, lichen planus, keratosis follicularis (Darier disease), chronic discoid lupus erythematosus and keratoacanthoma. Other possible conditions include keloid, erythema multiforme, localized scleroderma and lymphadenopathy.[25]

Infections

The risk of tattoo-related infections depends on the conditions under which the procedure was carried out and the expertise of the tattooist. The possibility and the incidence of the transfer of diseases via professionally-produced tattoos are very low. However, materials can be contaminated and devices are often difficult to sterilize. Concerns are more when tattoos are produced by amateurs in an unsterile condition, such as those found in prisons or other lower social set up.[9,25]

The most frequent are local bacterial infections at the site of the tattoo. They are often caused by common pathogens such as *Streptococcus pyogenes* and *Staphylococcus aureus*. Secondary infections reported are erysipelas, cellulitis, furunculosis, sepsis and spinal abcesses, either due to *Streptococcus pyogenes, Staphylococcus aureus* or *Pseudomonas* species.[10,12,25]

Potential transmissions of blood borne diseases are possible due to lack of sterilized equipments. Among various possibilities, incidence of tuberculosis and hepatitis C is high. There is chance of transmission of human immunodeficiency virus (HIV), though specific epidemiological data regarding incidence is not available. Other transmissible infections include syphilis, leprosy, tuberculosis cutis, rubella, chancroid, tetanus and molluscum contagiosum.[10,12,25,40]

Contemporary tattoos which are created with sharp instruments and inks are often found in individuals in lower socio-economic class or in prisoners. As these are very often created using unsterile instruments, a great deal of concern regarding possibility of infectious diseases such as hepatitis C or HIV should be kept in mind in the mortuary environment, especially while doing the autopsy dissections or dealing with body fluids.[9]

Malignancy

Malignancies associated with tattoos include squamous cell carcinoma, basal cell carcinoma, malignant melanoma, leiomyosarcoma, primary non-Hodgkin lymphoma and dermatofibrosarcoma protuberans. These malignancies may be considered coincidental, but carcinogenicity of the tattooing colorants is a concern to be addressed.[2,25,41,42]

MRI Complications

The metallic ferric acid pigments used in tattoos can conduct heat on the skin during MRI, resulting in traumatic burns. This has also been reported to occur with tattoos with nonferrous pigments. Patients should be asked before MRI if they have tattoos, so that this complication can be avoided.[25]

Complications with UV Tattoo

Some people may have reactions to ingredients in the UV tattoo ink, ranging from minor itching to dermatitis. Several UV inks are suspected carcinogens and allergens but till date no research has been conducted regarding the side effects of long term exposure to these dyes. Many people who have received UV tattoos have had physical effects on the skin which can be a result of not protecting the tattoo from UV rays within three months of receiving the tattoo, or by using scented creams or lotions on the tattoo area.

VISIBILITY OF A TATTOO

An apparently invisible tattoo can be made visible in a number of ways:[2]

i. Causing vesication by applying a little heat (applied on the area for some time and then by rubbing the area).

ii. By treating the area with 3% H_2O_2 (which removes the product of decomposition temporarily).
iii. Under ultra-violet lamp.
iv. By using infra-red light and photography.
v. Sometimes, burnt out superficial epidermis reveals the underlying tattoo more prominently, since the pigments reside in the superficial dermis in case of a permanent tattoo (refer to Fig. 20.2).
vi. Peeling of epidermis by rubbing the area in a decomposed body (Fig. 20.12).

REMOVAL OF TATTOO

Approximately 28% of people who get tattoos regret the decision within the first month. Although the minimum age to obtain a tattoo is 18 years in the US, such age bar is not strictly adhere to and 71% of people requesting tattoo removal have had applied when they were under the minimum age.[11] The number of tattoo removal procedures in the US reached 45,224 in 2013 compared to 40,801 procedures in 2011 with females accounting for 32,888 (72.7%) of procedures.[43] The most common reason to seek tattoo removal was to enhance self-esteem by freeing oneself from the stigmatizing lesion that was the source of many years of regret. In addition, tattoo owners felt their marks were socially discrediting, perceived pressure by family members to remove them, and believed improvement in employment opportunities would result after removal.[11,12] Similarly, a European study has shown that intermingling of a complex psychology works behind a person's decision of deliberate removal of tattoo—just decided to remove it (58%), suffering from embarrassment (57%), lowering of body image (38%), achieves new career (38%), conflicts with wardrobe (37%), experiencing stigma (25%) and marking an occasion (21%).[9]

The first evidence of tattoo removal attempts was found in Egyptian mummies, dated 4000 BC. Ancient Greek writings describe tattoo removal with salt abrasion

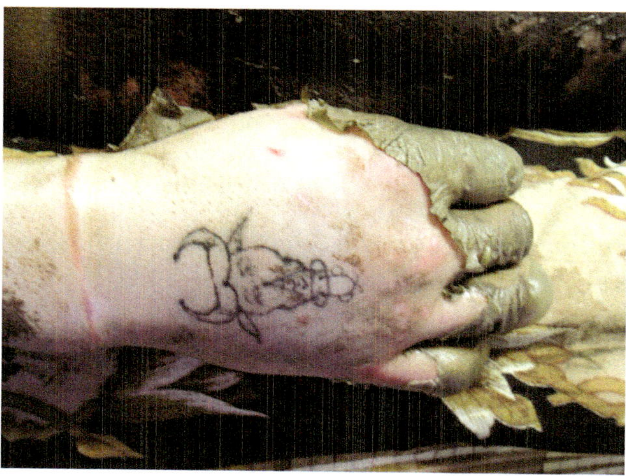

Fig. 20.12 Tattoo visible after removal of epidermis

or with a paste containing cloves of white garlic mixed with Alexandrian cantharidin.[12] Early removal methods used mechanical destruction, such as dermabrasion, chemical peels and continuous-wave lasers. These methods left patients with unsatisfactory results, and were associated with suboptimal removal and scarring.[11]

Alternatively, a larger tattoo may be superimposed over another in an attempt to either disguise or obliterate the previous work.[13] Chronic eczema may also make a tattoo invisible in the long run.

The various methods that are currently in use are:[11]

Dermabrasion: The tattoo is gradually removed via exfoliation of the surface and middle layer of pigments by machines, laser or salt. The upper layer of skin is abraded or sanded, and the underline of skin replace the damaged layers, allowing the pigment to leach out of the skin. In some cases, rubbing the skin is followed by the application of caustic chemicals, for e.g., tannic acid, silver nitrate (*Variot's method*) or trichloroacetic acid (chemical peels). Other methods like 'salt abrasion' wherein salts like zinc chloride are applied, and hot flames may also be used. Rarely electrolysis is the measure.

Surgical excision/resection: The tattoo is cut out, and either sutured or allowed to heal depending on size, and putting a skin graft on it. The efficacy of this technique is dependent upon the individual surgeon, the size of the area to be resected, the tension of the skin in the area and the individual's tendency toward scarring or developing a keloid.

Laser surgery: Currently, laser surgery is probably the most common form of tattoo removal. The tattoo is removed by targeting selective pigments with the high intensity laser beam which break the pigment into tiny fragments. The body's own defense mechanism then clears away the fragmented ink and the tattoo fades over time. The most common lasers currently used for tattoo removal are Q-switched Nd: YAG, Q-switched Ruby, Q-switched Alexandrite and Pico Sure.[12] The type of laser is generally dependent upon the color to be removed. This modality offer highly effective approach with minimal side effects. At best, using the laser can remove up to 95% of a tattoo at once (Fig. 20.13). Most of the methods of removal result in scarring. For correction, skin grafting is done thereafter.

Intense Pulsed Light Therapy (IPL): Intense pulsed light therapy is the newest dimension added in the perspective of tattoo removal. It is a dermal enhancer currently being used in some spas and tattoo parlours. It uses high intensity light (instead of laser light) in nearly same manner. This method is said to be less painful and more effective than traditional laser therapy, but there are many tattoo removal experts who contradicts the applicability of IPL.

Frequently, the clinicians are confronted with complications and side effects of tattoo removals that were performed by non-professionals. Hence, an ethical question is 'who should be allowed to use laser devices for the removal of tattoos?' In most European countries, well trained dermatologist or healthcare professionals with clinical knowledge and adequate training in laser device are involved in this. However, laser tattoo removal is being done by non-physicians not only in India, but in developed countries like the US as well.[44]

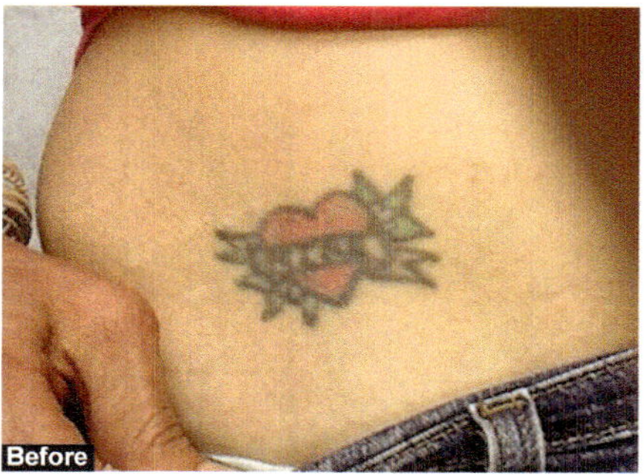

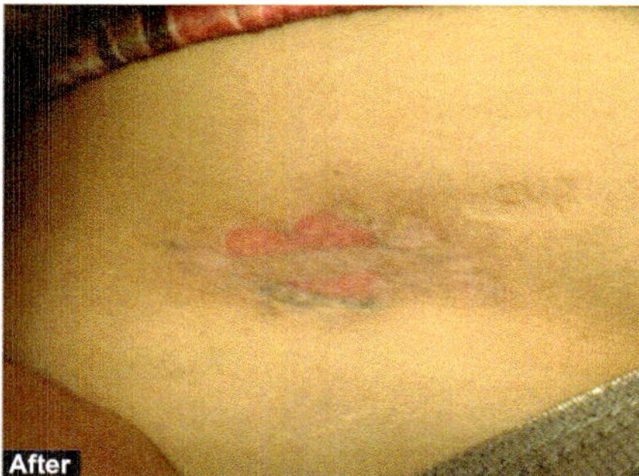

Fig. 20.13 PicoSure removal of tattoo (with permission from Lynne Brownell, Newport Beach, CA)

DIAGNOSTIC DIFFICULTY

Diagnostic difficulty might arise is misinterpretation of the significance of the tattoo, if the antecedent's details are not known. Due to changing trends and styles, tattoos can no longer be used to identify specific cultural groups, precisely as 'traditional tribal' style. To add more to the confusion, calligraphy in tattoos including the language used can now be found on persons with no connection to the cultural or ethnic groups from which the style has originated.

Pigmented lesions in decorative tattoos cause diagnostic difficulties at a clinical and dermoscopic level. In cases of laser removal of tattoos, hidden suspicious naevi may be revealed gradually. Many a times, tattooing is a method to conceal the puncture marks of intravenous drug abusers, especially over cubital fossa, anterior abdominal wall and other accessible parts of the body. It demands special attention during autopsy and may create difficulty in identifying the addicts.[8,35]

CONCLUSION

Tattoos may provide information, both in living and dead, regarding possible occupation, particular association or affiliation, drug or addiction habits, previous military service, names of family members or the loved ones (Fig. 20.14A), medical conditions, previous travel destinations, religious and cultural background (Fig. 20.14B), hobbies (Fig. 20.14C), preferences and many more.[9] Certain tattoos typical of individuals with prison records and when found usually indicate that the deceased will in all likelihood have previous police record.[9]

Tattoos may be useful in identifying individuals, as dermal pigments remain almost intact even after the putrefaction or loss of superficial skin layers due to burn injuries. So coming across a tattoo during autopsy in the mortuary or during examination of a living person always claims proper documentation in terms of all the details, i.e. size, shape, location, words or letters inscribed in it. A photographic documentation maintaining the precautions is appreciable.

Many governments insist that anyone who receives a tattoo must wait a minimum of six months before they are allowed to donate blood. Most stores in Japan deny entry if a person enters with a full body tattoo, since full body tattoos are considered to be of a typical criminal gang symbol.

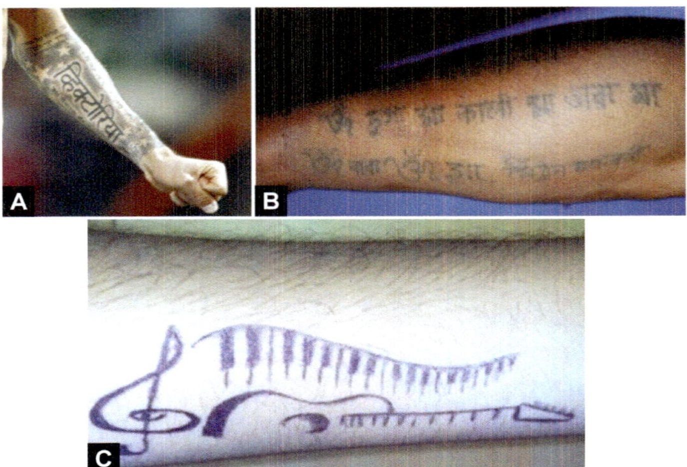

Figs 20.14A to C (A) Tattoo on forearm of David Beckham; (B) Religious tattoo; (C) Profession and hobby tattoo

Though tattoos are not well accepted in the higher profession and association in many countries including India, still it can be said that it helps people to express their views, how they see themselves, and has become an integral part of the civilized population.

REFERENCES

1. Tattoo helps Ganesh Raghunath Dhangade find his mum in India after 24 years. Source: AFP. 2013 October 16. Available from: http://www.news.com.au/lifestyle/relationships/tattoo-helps-ganesh-raghunath-dhangade-find-his-mum-in-india-after-24-years/story-fnet0he2-1226742038815.
2. Adams MD. Constructing one's self: becoming a tattooed person [Undergraduate senior honors thesis]. Muncie, Indiana: Balls State University; 2001.
3. Parry A. Tattoo: secrets of a strange art practiced by the natives of the United States. New York: Literary licensing, LLC; 2011.
4. Karmakar RN. Wet specimen. Forensic medicine and toxicology. 4th ed. Kolkata: Academic publishers; 2013. p. 129-31.
5. Atkinson M. Tattoo as body modification. Tattooed: the sociogenesis of a body art. Toronto, Canada: University of Toronto Press; 2003. p. 3-22.
6. Caplan J. Speaking scars: the tattoo in popular practice and medicolegal debate in nineteenth-century Europe. *Hist Workshop J* 1997; 44: 107-42.
7. Kuczkowski KM. Diagnostic tattoo in a parturient with ecstasy use. *Anaesthesia* 2003; 58: 1251-52.
8. Mukherjee JB. Identification. In: Karmakar RN (ed). JB Mukherjee's forensic medicine and toxicology. 4th edn. Kolkata: Academic publishers; 2011. p. 89-90.
9. Cains GE, Byard RW. The forensic and cultural implications of tattooing. In: Tsokos M (ed). Forensic pathology reviews. Vol. 5. Totowa, US: Humana press; 2008. p. 197-220.
10. Cotapos ML, de Cuyper C, Cossio L. Tattooing and scarring: Technique and complications. In: de Cuyper C, Cotapos ML (eds). Dermatologic complications with body art: Tattoos, piercings and permanent make-up. London: Springer; 2009. p. 29-42.

11. Vejjabhinanta V, Caperton CV, Wong C, Charoensawad R, Nouri K. Laser treatment of tattoos. In: Nouri K (ed). Lasers in dermatology and medicine. London: Springer-Verlag; 2011. p. 83-91.
12. Adatto MA, Halachmi S, Lapidoth M. Tattoo removal. Allemann IJ, Goldberg DJ (eds). Basics in dermatological laser applications. *Curr Probl Dermatol* 2011; 42: 97-110.
13. Green T. The tattoo encyclopaedia, a guide to choosing your tattoo. New York: Simon and Schuster; 2003.
14. History of tattooing. Available from: http://en.wikipedia.org/wiki/History_of_tattooing.
15. Murphy WA, Nedden D, Gostner P, Knapp R, Recheis W, Seidler H. The iceman: discovery and imaging. *Radiology* 2003; 226: 614-29.
16. Swift B. Body art and modification. In: Rutty GN (ed). Essentials of autopsy practice: recent advances, topics and developments. London: Springer; 2004. p. 159-86.
17. Sperry K. Tattoos and tattooing. Part 1. History and methodology. *Am J Forensic Med Path* 1991; 12: 313-19.
18. Types of tattoos - The missing ink - Tattoo and piercing. Available from: http://themissinginktattoo.weebly.com/types-of-tattoos.html.
19. Pe'a. Wikipedia [Internet]. Available from: http://en.wikipedia.org/wiki/Pea.
20. Roberts TA, Ryan SA. Tattooing and high risk behaviours in adolescents. *Pediatrics* 2002; 110: 1058-63.
21. Schmidt RM, Armstrong ML. Tattooing in adolescents and adults. Up to date. Wolters Kluwer health [Internet]. 2013 August 29. Available from: http://www.uptodate.com/contents/tattooing-in-adolescents-and-adults.
22. One in five US adults now has a tattoo. Available from: http://www.harrisinteractive.com/News Room/HarrisPolls/tabid/447/mid/1508/articleId/970/ctl/ReadCustom-Default/Default.aspx.
23. Tattoo. Wikipedia [Internet]. 2013 December 03. Available from: http://en.wikipedia.org/wiki/Tattoo.
24. Cruz FAM; Lage D; Frigério RM; Zaniboni MC; Fávaro Arruda LHF. Reactions to the different pigments in tattoos: a report of two cases. *An Bras Dermatol* 2010; 85: 708-11.
25. Glassy CM, Glassy MS, Aldasouqi S. Tattooing: Medical uses and problems. *Cleve Clin J Med* 2012; 79: 761-70.
26. Medical tattoo. Available from: http://en. wikipedia.org/wiki/Medical_tattoo.
27. Tattoo styles. Available from: http://www.sinonskin.ca/tattoo-styles.html.
28. Beginner's guide to tattoos. Available from: http://tattoos.wikia.com/wiki/Beginner's_Guide_to_Tattoos.
29. Types of tattoos. Available from: http://uniqueinktattoo.com/tattoos/types-of-tattoos/
30. Byard RW. Tattoos: forensic considerations. *Forensic Sci Med Pathol* 2013; 9: 534-42.
31. Jordan CR. Basic fundamentals of modern tattoo. Jordan Y (ed). Phoenix Arizona: Tattoo books online LLC; 2009. Available from: http://en.wikipedia.org/wiki/Tattoo_machine.
32. Tattoo inks: Types and methods of tattooing. Tattoo Johny [Internet]. 2009 March 12. Available from: http://www.tattoojohnny.com/wiki/tattoo_inks%3A_types_and_methods_of_tattooing.
33. Think before you ink: Are tattoos safe? US food and drug administration [Internet]. 2009 February 23. Available from: http://en. wikipedia.org/wiki/UV_tattoo.
34. Tattoo shading techniques. Knotan's blog [Internet]. 2010 October 17. Available from: http://knotan.wordpress.com/2010/10/17/tattoo-shading-techniques/.
35. Nandy A. Identification. Principles of forensic medicine including toxicology. 3rd edn. Kolkata: New central book agency; 2010. p. 154-57.
36. Jacob C. Tattoo-associated dermatoses: a case report and review of the literature. *Dermatol Surg* 2002; 28: 962-65.

37. Leggiadro RJ, Boscamp JR, Sapadin AN. Temporary tattoo dermatitis. *J Pediatrics* 2003; 142: 586.
38. Mortimer NJ, Chave TA, Johnston GA. Red tattoo reactions. *Clin Exper Dermatol* 2003; 28: 508-10.
39. Papageorgiou PP, Hongcharu W, Chu AC. Systemic sarcoidosis presenting with multiple tattoo granulomas and an extra-tattoo cutaneous granuloma. *J Eur Acad Dermatol Venereol* 1999; 12: 51-53.
40. Ghorpade A. Inoculation (tattoo) leprosy: a report of 31 cases. *J Eur Dermatol Venereol* 2002; 16: 494-99.
41. Shmerling R. Tattoos, moles and melanoma. Harvard health publications. Harvard Medical School [Internet]. 2013 August 05. Available from: http://www.health.harvard.edu/blog/tattoos-moles-and-melanoma-201308056578.
42. Friedman T, Westreich M, Mozes SN, Dorenbaum A, Herman O. Tattoo pigment in lymph nodes mimicking metastatic malignant melanoma. *Plast Reconstr Surg* 2003; 111: 2120-22.
43. Caba J. Tattoo regret: Why the majority of middle-aged Americans are deciding to blast away their ink? Available from: http://www.medicaldaily.com/tattoo-regret-why-majority-middle-aged-americans-are-deciding-blast-away-their-ink-274428.
44. Karsai S, Krieger G, Raulin C. Tattoo removal by non-professionals-medical and forensic considerations. *J Eur Acad Dermatol Venereol* 2010; 24: 756-62.

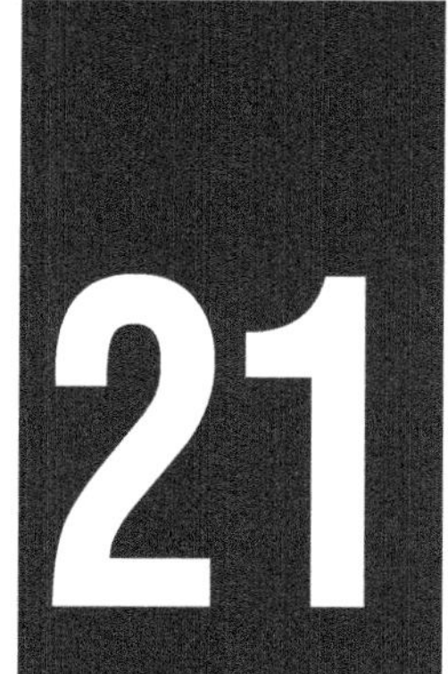

Sudden Infant Death Syndrome

Tapas Kumar Bose, Shouvanik Adhya

'Petechiae are never present on the conjunctiva, eyelids or on or in other soft tissues of the head or neck in SIDS.'

John MN Hilton (Pediatric forensic pathologist)

ABSTRACT

Sudden infant death syndrome (SIDS) is unexpected death of an infant without any medical history and remains inexplicable even after a thorough autopsy and meticulous death scene investigation. Cot death or crib death is synonymous to SIDS as most cases are discovered at bed during sleep. SIDS was the 3rd leading cause of infant mortality in the US in 2011. Centres for Disease Control and Prevention show that the incidences of SIDS have been waning since 1988. The exact basis of SIDS is unidentified, but some factors related with this have been recognized. The Triple-Risk Model describes three fundamental issues—an underlying biological factor, critical developmental age and an external trigger. SIDS avoidance strategies consist of: putting the infant to sleep on supine posture, a separate firm mattress which is close to parents, no loose bedding, cool comfortable environment and prevention of exposure to tobacco smoke. Infanticide and child abuse cases may be misinterpreted as SIDS and vice versa due to improper investigation, and caregivers of infant are sometimes wrongly accused or actual offenders are falsely acquitted. Accidental suffocations are also at times misdiagnosed as SIDS. This chapter is a critical review of the demographic characteristics and the mechanism of SIDS.

Keywords: Death, infant, unanticipated death, cot death, bed sharing, autopsy

INTRODUCTION

Sudden infant death syndrome (SIDS), cot death or crib death is the term that is used when a previously healthy infant is found unpredictably dead after sleeping, with no reason for the death being recognized.[1] While a majority of incidences of unanticipated infant death have been attributed to SIDS, it remains a debatable issue with opinion for and against it as a distinct 'diagnostic entity'. Major problems exist due to the deficiency of pathognomonic characteristics at autopsy.

After the discovery of specific environmental risk factors, community awareness campaigns were undertaken that have resulted in deaths from SIDS declining abruptly in many communities.[2] For example, the number of SIDS deaths per year in California, US, has reduced from 110.5/100,000 live births in 1990 to 47.2/100,000 live births in 1998,[3] and the number of SIDS deaths nationally in Australia has diminished from over 500 annually in 1988 to just 134 per year in 1999.[4] Research has clarified probable mechanisms of death, with the 'triple risk' or 'fatal triangle' models being projected to incorporate multifaceted individual susceptibilities with developmental stages and environmental factors.[5]

In spite of these great successes, however, problems still persist. Infant deaths are investigated poorly till date in many jurisdictions, with deaths being ascribed to SIDS without satisfying the requirements of recognized definitions or following established protocols for autopsy and death scene survey. Infants whose deaths are now accredited to SIDS also often appear from socially underprivileged groups, who may be hard to scrutinize and counsel.[6] This chapter discusses the various aspects of SIDS and the current theories of its pathophysiology as of today.

DEFINITION

In 1969, at the Second International Conference on causes of sudden death in infants, SIDS was defined as 'the sudden death of any infant or young child which is unexpected by history and in which a thorough postmortem examination fails to demonstrate an adequate cause for death'.[7]

More recently in the United States, the National Institute of Child Health and Human Development (NICHD) group revised the definition as 'the sudden death of an infant under one year of age which remains unexplained after a thorough case investigation, including performance of a complete autopsy, examination of the death scene and review of the clinical history'.[8] Although one of the concerns with the NICHD definition is the cut-off point of one year of age, SIDS is a condition of early infancy, with unforeseen deaths after the first year being atypical.

HISTORICAL BACKGROUND

Sudden infant death syndrome (SIDS) is not a new entity, having been heard for many thousands of years to be caused by a sleeping parent lying over an infant in a shared bed. It is notified in the Bible, where the Judgment of Solomon (1 Kings 3: 19) reads '. . . and this woman's child died in the night because she overlaid it'.

Given the poor level of investigation of unexpected infant deaths in the past, it is not possible to determine the epidemiology of infant deaths and the number of SIDS deaths in previous centuries with any accuracy. Charles Templeman (1892),[9] a Scottish police surgeon in the second half of the 19th century, who was a staunch follower of overlaying as a major basis of infant death, proposed that it should be banned for infants and young children to sleep in bed with their parents. He also suggested that parents who had slept in an inebriated condition with their children should be prosecuted. Nearly 100 years later, sleeping in an intoxicated state in the same bed as that of an infant, who was afterwards found dead was still considered to be unlawful under the *Children and Young Persons Act of Great Britain.*[10]

The unduly high number of infant deaths on Saturday nights in Victorian Dundee gave some credibility to Templeman's theories. His conclusion was that 'the prime factors producing this great mortality from overlaying are ignorance and carelessness of mothers, drunkenness and overcrowding.' Though overlaying is diagnosed less often nowadays, it still may be unfeasible to rule out as a cause of death if an infant is found dead in bed with a sleeping adult, more commonly if the adult is obese or in intoxicated state.[11]

One of the most primitive alternate theories to imply that sudden infant death may be caused by factors other than overlaying was *mors thymica,* described by Plater in 1614, and repopularized in 1830 by Kopp as 'thymic asthma'. This suggested that tracheal occlusion occurred in susceptible infants due to pressure from a hypertrophied thymus gland.[12]

A slightly less strange theory was that of Paultauf's *Status Thymicolymphaticus*; infants who were victim of SIDS were thought to have had grossly enlarged thymus glands connected with widespread lymphadenopathy, and arterial and adrenal hypoplasia. Death was thought to happen from airway compression or pressure on neighboring nerves, or ill-defined metabolic disbalances.[12]

EPIDEMIOLOGY

Each year in the United States, about 4,000 infants die suddenly of no immediately, obvious cause. About half of these sudden unexpected deaths of infancy (SUDI) are due to SIDS, the leading cause of SUDI and of all deaths among infants aged 1–12 months.

The occurrence of SIDS, once greater than 6 deaths/1000 live births/year in certain communities, has recently diminished to less than 1 death/1000 live births annually in areas where risk campaigns have been already undertaken.[13] Despite the fact that SIDS is a sporadic happening, it remains the most frequent cause of unexpected death in infants aged between one week and one year of life in Western countries, and has ranged from the seventh to the eighth most important cause of death in the US in terms of years of potential life lost (YPLL) before the age of 65.[14]

Statistics taken from SIDS autopsies in South Australia over a 10-year period display the factors of young age, male predominance and high winter rates that are found again and again, as well as the inconsistency in incidence from year to year.[15]

INFANT CHARACTERISTICS

Male infants are affected more often than females, and there may be a history of prematurity, even if this has not always been established. Low birth weights and prolonged stay in hospital have been noted, with the most common age at death being between 2 and 4 months. There may be a history of meagre prenatal care. Although, infants are most frequently found dead in their cribs after sleeping, death due to SIDS can happen at any time of the day. A rise in deaths has occurred at weekends.

ENVIRONMENTAL FACTORS

Prone Sleeping

The relationship of infant death with sleeping posture was reported many years back by Abramson (1944). He suggested that 'the routine nursing practice of placing infants in the prone position be avoided, except during such times as the babies are constantly attended' and that 'the practice should, furthermore, be entirely done away with at night'.

Infants who sleep on their sides also have an enhanced threat of SIDS, as they may turn on to their abdomens, and infants who sleep prone for the first time (so-called 'unaccustomed prone') are in a higher-risk cluster. Postulated mechanisms have incorporated diaphragmatic splinting/fatigue, rebreathing of carbon dioxide, reflex lowering of vasomotor tone with tachycardia, blunting of arousal responses together with decreased cardiac response to auditory stimulation, modification of sleep patterns, compromise of cerebral blood flow, upper airway obstruction from deformation of nasal cartilages, posterior dislodgment of the mandible, soft bedding, nasopharyngeal bacterial overgrowth, and overheating. It is also probable that prone position in infants may lead to unfavorable ventilation/perfusion ratios.[16-20]

Cigarette Smoke Exposure

In spite of conflicting proof, it is now acknowledged that infants who have been exposed to cigarette smoke toxins, before and after delivery, have an enhanced risk of SIDS of up to five times.[21] The accurate mechanism is doubtful, but it has been recommended that smoking may be liable for reduction in body and placental size in SIDS infants compared with matched controls, as an indicator for unfavorable *in-utero* factors. A current study has shown that poor postnatal weight gain increases the danger of SIDS.[22] Impaired arousal has also been established in infants exposed to tobacco smoke.[23]

Hyperthermia

Infants who have died of SIDS may have had a history of elevated temperatures or copious night sweats.[24] Intrathoracic petechiae reported in infants dying from environmental hyperthermia may propose a connection between SIDS and overheating.[25] Elevated temperatures in SIDS infants may be endogenous from infections or increased amounts of brown adipose tissue or may result from external factors, such as increased room heating or too much clothing.[26] As the comparatively larger head in infants radiates a significant amount of generated heat, the wearing of a bonnet or covering the head with blankets in an infant sleeping prone with a large part of the face against the mattress interferes with usual heat exchange.[27] This is exacerbated when the ambient temperature is raised. The probable role played by an increase in body temperature in causing unexpected death is not well understood. However, various mechanisms have been proposed. These consist of vagally mediated cerebral ischemia, surfactant denaturation, enhancement of the laryngeal closure reflex, overlooked convulsions, apnea, collapse of respiratory control and respiratory chemoreceptor dysfunction.[28]

Bed Sharing

There is escalating proof that infants who sleep in close proximity to their parents will have a reduced possibility of SIDS, probably due to increased arousals.[29] It has been revealed, however, that the risk of infant death doubles if an infant shares a bed with a mother who smokes, though the mechanisms of this association remain uncertain. Some present-day practices are accountable for making bed sharing unsafe, for instance placing infants between obese, sedated or intoxicated parents on a yielding mattress.[30]

Maternal Characteristics

Mothers of SIDS infants have a tendency to be young (< 20 years of age), of lower socioeconomic position and have had a number of children over a comparatively short period of time.[31]

The probable defensive role of breastfeeding has been debated enthusiastically, with studies showing a lower frequency of SIDS in breastfed infants being challenged over a failure to control for social class and smoking practice. The finding of lower levels of docosohexaenoic acid (DHA) in the brain tissue of formula-fed infants compared with breastfed controls offered a probable mechanism to clarify the increased rates of SIDS in this group, as DHA is essential for neural maturation.[32]

Maternal smoking during and after pregnancy is linked with an increased risk of SIDS. Infants of mothers who have used cocaine, appear to have unusual cardio-respiratory and electrocardiographic patterns, with a elevated risk of sudden death.[33] Maternal abuse of opiates also enhances the risk of infant death,[34] and breastfed infants exposed to opioids in breast milk have increased risks of apnea. Serious postnatal ingestion of alcohol has been related with an increased threat of infant death.[35]

Geographic and Climatic Factors

The occurrence of SIDS varies between diverse geographic areas, being usually more common in colder northern and southern climates.[36] SIDS has a winter preponderance and a link with low temperatures.

Racial Differences

A number of researches have shown a low prevalence of SIDS in oriental groups, but this may be due partly to local diagnostic practices, with deaths being accredited to suffocation rather than to SIDS.[37] Certain native populations and African-American groups do have elevated rates of infant death.[38]

Sibling Deaths

The reported higher rate of SIDS of between two and 10 times in infants who have had a sibling or twin death. While it is usually accepted that any increase in incidence is due almost certainly to exposure to the same environmental risk factors rather than to heritability, genetic factor cannot be excluded in the etiology of SIDS. This includes the likelihood of an inborn metabolic disease in some cases. Characteristics that should be considered in the occurrence of concurrent SIDS deaths in siblings are carbon monoxide exposure, poisoning, overheating and mechanical obstruction of the airways.[39]

Families where SIDS deaths have a tendency to occur now have been termed 'chaotic' due to social nuisance, including substandard housing, domestic cruelty, joblessness and illegitimate drug use.[40]

The epidemiologic features as understood are given in Box 21.1.

DIAGNOSIS

The opinion of sudden infant death syndrome (SIDS) can be considered only after other causes of sudden death have been sought meticulously, and if unusual autopsy findings have been interpreted perfectly, given that the established present definition of SIDS is one of exclusion. There are, therefore, a number of complications that may confront a pathologist when dealing with a 'typical' case of SIDS, predominantly as the presenting history and autopsy findings are frequently characteristic but are in no way diagnostic of the entity.[42] The diagnosis of SIDS does not depend on the demonstration of any particular pathognomonic characteristics.

In some countries, an infant death may be ascribed to SIDS without doing a postmortem examination. For instance, in the Netherlands, in the past, only 50–60% of children dying within the first year of life were autopsied, and in Belgium, the autopsy rate was less than 25%. It is important, therefore, that epidemiologic and tissue research results from regions where autopsies are not a compulsory part of the diagnostic procedure are interpreted with care.

INVESTIGATION INTO SUDDEN INFANT DEATH SYNDROME

Death Scene Investigation

The revised definition given by the NICHD group emphasizes that 'a complete postmortem examination must include an investigation of the scene of death'.[8] Diagnosis of SIDS cannot be done or defended if there has not been an examination of the death scene by skilled persons who are competent to deal sympathetically with bereaved parents while at the same time inspecting for proof of accidental or nonaccidental injury.[43]

The Sudden Unexplained Infant Death Investigation Report Form (SUIDIRF) formulated by the Centers for Disease Control outlines model steps that should

Box 21.1 Epidemiologic features of sudden infant death syndrome (SIDS)[41]

Age 2–4 months	Male	Premature
Low birth weight	High birth order	Multiple birth
Prone sleeper	Short inter-pregnancy interval	Lower socioeconomic family
Young parents (<20 years)	Previous premature deliveries	Cigarette smoke exposure
Maternal drug abuse	Infection during pregnancy	Illiteracy

be undertaken in the investigation of unforeseen infant death. The information necessary to obtain from death scene is given in Table 21.1.[41]

Medical History Review

Review of the dead infant's medical history is an obligatory part of the autopsy. This consists of details of pregnancy and delivery, growth and development parameters, type of feeding, immunization status, previous illnesses, recent fevers, respiratory infections, gastrointestinal upsets, recent medications. Family history of sudden death (particularly infants and young children), and any major parental illness and addiction.[41]

It may provide hints to the likelihood of a potentially fatal medical condition that should be checked for, such as a congenital cardiac anomaly. The immediate antemortem history may be noteworthy, like presence of a fever over several days may be a clue to the existence of fatal sepsis.

Pathological Features

The International Standardized Autopsy Protocol (ISAP) was devised for a all-inclusive autopsy by SIDS International and the NICHD.[44] All stages of the autopsy that are precise in protocols, including external examination, radiology, internal examination, histology, microbiology, toxicology, electrolyte/metabolic studies and molecular/genetic studies have been shown to have investigative values.

Macroscopic autopsy findings

The morphologic features in infants who are afterwards considered to have died of SIDS are not definite, although there are a number of findings that are typically present.[45] Pulmonary edema fluid may be seen as frothy white fluid exuding from the nostrils or mouth; sometimes it may be blood-tinged or fill the trachea.[46] It most probably represents terminal left ventricular failure. Purulent mucus in this fluid may confirm the presence of antemortem upper respiratory tract infection. Frank blood around the mouth and nares is a concern and raises the chance of asphyxia, if cardiopulmonary resuscitation has not been attempted.[47] On opening the pleural cavity, the lungs are usually bulky, edematous and congested. Intrathoracic petechial hemorrhages are often found plenty in the

Table 21.1 Information to obtain from death scene

Child	Age of child, details of sleeping arrangements, for e.g. shared or not, and previous medical history. Time and circumstances of death, position of body, details concerning discovery of the body and subsequent resuscitation attempts, evidence of injury to body.
Family	Medical history, including previous infant/child deaths. Details concerning household activity over the preceding 24 hours.
Environment	Type of crib/bed, mattress size (size relative to crib), type of room heating, type of clothing and bedding, presence of plastic coverings. Any unusual features at death scene.

thymus, over the epicardium and over the pleural surfaces of the lungs, and have been observed in 68–95% of SIDS victims (Beckwith, 1989). The presence of petechiae on the skin of the face, neck or conjunctivae indicates asphyxia from chest or neck compression, unless there is proof of generalized petechiae from other conditions, such as meningococcal disease, hematological disease, or a history of forceful vomiting or coughing from pertussis.[48]

Dysmorphic lesions, such as pectus excavatum, polydactyly and talipes, and lesions such as hemangiomas and nevi may occur in SIDS infants,[49] but are in no way definite to this group of infants, and are generally absent.

Microscopic features

Histological sections from intrathoracic organs, specifically the thymus and lungs, will substantiate the presence of petechial hemorrhages. Petechiae have a tendency to be found in greater numbers in infants dying of SIDS than in infants dying of asphyxia, drowning or recognizable diseases.[50] The alveoli are filled with eosinophilic proteinaceous fluid, extravasated erythrocytes and scattered macrophages. Intra-alveolar hemorrhage has been proposed as a indicator of airway obstruction from overlaying or smothering.[51] Subpleural aggregates of hemosiderin-containing macrophages demons-trating areas of previous interstitial hemorrhage have been proposed as histologic markers of prior anoxia. Focal collection of submucosal chronic inflammatory cells are often found within the upper airways, extending sometime to the alveolar septae. No importance is attributed to a variety of other reported histologic changes, such as fibrinoid necrosis of the vocal cords, cardiac myocytolysis and pulmonary lymphatic dilation, although it was hypothesized that the vocal cord changes may be a indicator of gastric reflux.

MECHANISM OF SUDDEN INFANT DEATH SYNDROME

Sudden infant death syndrome is the common endpoint for a variety of mechanisms that signify a complex mix of precipitating factors, environmental stresses and underlying vulnerabilities (Table 21.2).

Respiratory Theories

The apparent plausibility of airway occlusion, underlying defects in respiratory control and malfunction of arousal in early infancy has postulated a number of hypotheses implicating respiratory failure in the causation of SIDS.[52] These proposals have been positioned into the categories of obstructive, central, mixed and expiratory apneas.

Obstructive apnea is characterized by failure of inspiratory airflow, despite continued respiratory efforts. An usual example occurs with foreign body impaction in a major airway. Anatomical abnormalities that have been reported in SIDS infants include narrowed nasal passages, shallow temporomandibular joints, retroposition of the maxillae, short mandibular rami and close proximity of the soft palate to pharyngeal walls.[53] A high position of the larynx in infants with relatively short necks also predisposes to airway blockage when the tongue and mandible displace backwards. At autopsy, the narrowness of the normal infant upper aerodigestive tract is striking, and it is easy to realize how further narrowing

Table 21.2 Possible mechanisms responsible for SIDS[41]

System	*Possible causes*
Respiratory	Defective brainstem respiratory or peripheral pulmonary receptors. Abnormal surfactant, pulmonary immunologic abnormalities, intrinsic upper airway obstruction, laryngomalacia or laryngospasm. Extrinsic upper airway obstruction, rebreathing/toxic gas inhalation, overlaying, positional asphyxia or smothering.
Cardiovascular	Defective brainstem cardiac control centers, aberrant conduction pathways, prolongation of the QT interval, intrapulmonary venous shunting, vertebral artery compression or cardiac chamber compression.
Central and peripheral nervous system	Defective autonomic control, abnormal brainstem nuclei, vagal or chemoreceptor dysfunction, arousal/ sleep state disturbance, hyperpyrexia, abnormality of neurotransmitters or pineal gland, maturational imbalance, increased neuronal degeneration or activation of diving reflex.
Gastrointestinal	Gastric aspiration or gastroesophageal reflux.
Microbiologic	Viral or bacterial infections, or phospholipase A2 producing bacteria
Immunologic	Anaphylaxis, immunologic incompetence or sequel to immunization.
Metabolic	Congenital enzyme deficiencies.
Endocrine	Adrenal insufficiency, disturbed calcium metabolism or hyperthyroidism.
Nutritional	Vitamin or trace metals deficiencies.
Environmental	Toxin exposure, hyperthermia or sleeping position.

might occur with sleep-related pharyngeal hypotonia. This could be exacerbated by increased secretions and submucosal edema from nasopharyngitis or by tonsillar and adenoidal hyperplasia. Greater compliance of the nasal cartilages in infancy has been liable for nasal obstruction due to downward pressure from the head in infants who are sleeping prone. It has also been suggested that the tongue is anatomically larger in SIDS infants, probably predisposing to upper airway obstruction.[54] Proliferation of dendritic cells within bronchioles of victims of SIDS has been proposed as a marker for peripheral airway narrowing, with consequent reduction in airflow.[55] Formation of petechiae are from the interaction of an array of factors, including severe hypoxia with sustained blood flow, terminal left ventricular failure and unsuccessful gasping respiratory efforts, and that this may be exacerbated by the presence of infection.[48,56]

Functional immaturity in autonomic control of the larynx has been considered as a possible cause of fatal laryngospasm in infancy based partly on the results of animal experiments. It has been suggested that a deficiency of neurons within the hypoglossal nucleus may contribute to upper aerodigestive tract obstruction by causing impaired movement of the tongue. It is also hypothesised that fatal laryngospasm due to compression of the left recurrent laryngeal nerve by the pulmonary artery may occur in SIDS due to left-to-right shunting of blood.

Reduction in postpalatal pressure causing suction of the tongue into the pharynx has been demonstrated in infants with partial nasal occlusion. This may combine with an absence of positive distending pressures within the infantile pharynx preventing reopening of the airway once blockage has occurred and exacerbated by mucosal adhesive forces. As relaxation of the pharyngeal musculature is known to occur during rapid eye movement (REM) sleep, this may signify a predominantly vulnerable time for obstruction.[57]

Central apnea is characterized by failure of both airflow and respiratory efforts. Vulnerable infants show breathing abnormalities that are also found in premature infants, in patients with seizures, and normally during REM sleep. A particularly vulnerable time for central apnea occurs during REM sleep, when lowered hypercapnic respiratory drive in combination with reduced intercostal muscle tone and relative underinflation of the lungs predisposes to hypoxemia.

The final group of infants who have shown abnormal respiratory patterns, demonstrated marked hypoxemia with continued expiratory efforts and no inspiratory flow, the so-called '*apnea braking syndrome*'. The mechanism may be sudden alveolar collapse with intrapulmonary shunting of venous blood.[58] A causative factor to alveolar collapse may be qualitative or quantitative abnormalities of surfactant which is a complex phospholipid produced by type II pneumocytes, for reduction of surface tension within alveoli and thus assists in lung inflation by decreasing compliance. Surfactant may also be modified secondarily, and it has been postulated that both phospholipase A2 (PLA2) producing bacteria[59] and denaturation of surfactant due to overheating may diminish the levels of active phospholipid in SIDS cases.

In support of antemortem hypoxia, Naeye has claimed that there are a number of slight morphologic changes in infants who have died of SIDS. These are pulmonary arteriolar thickening, right ventricular hypertrophy, altered carotid body volume, bone marrow erythroid hyperplasia, increased extramedullary hematopoiesis in the liver, increased amounts of periadrenal brown fat and brainstem gliosis.[60]

Bronchopulmonary dysplasia is a chronic lung disease characterized pathologically by emphysema and interstitial fibrosis with squamous metaplasia and smooth muscle hypertrophy of bronchioles. There is a seven fold increase in the risk of SIDS in infants who leave hospital with this condition.

Studies have shown a reduction in the number and increase in the size of type 1 fibers in the diaphragm of SIDS infants. This might render the diaphragm vulnerable to early fatigue, particularly in the prone position.[61]

Cardiovascular Theories

Defective brainstem cardiac control centers, autonomic imbalance and aberrant conduction pathways have all been involved in causing SIDS, with the suggested terminal event being arrhythmia rather than apnea. Other entities such as the prolonged QT interval syndromes, congenital heart block and Wolff-Parkinson-White syndrome in which abnormalities of cardiac conduction have also been related to an increased risk of sudden infant death.

Problems arising in attempting to establish a cardiac basis of SIDS include deficiency of antemortem ECG tracings in the majority of infants who die of SIDS, the apparent insensitivity of routine light microscopy in assessing central cardiac control pathways, and the complexity in relating mechanisms of death to morphologic findings. The discovery of an apparent anatomic abnormality in the heart, such as intimal thickening of the nodal arteries, lymphocytic infiltrates or accessory pathways, may be to some extent coincidental to the cause of death. Even though hearts from SIDS infants often show septal fiber disarray reminiscent of hypertrophic cardiomyopathy, the absence of septal and individual myocyte hypertrophy indicates that this is part of normal postnatal maturation. As endocardial fibroelastosis is well-known to be related to sudden death, the discovery of considerable amounts precludes the diagnosis of SIDS.

A number of physiologic studies have confirmed apparent cardiac abnormalities, such as prolongation of the QT interval in infants who afterwards die of SIDS or in relatives of SIDS infants.

Other rhythm disturbances found in infants who consequently die of SIDS include elevation and variation in mean heart rate, diminished heart rate variability in the waking state, and reduced variation in cardiac rate during REM and quiet sleep.[62] There have also been sporadic reports of prospective links between heart block and junctional escape, and with Wolff-Parkinson-White syndrome.

Unsuitable activation of the diving reflex has also been considered as a possible physiologic process linking bradycardia with apnea.[63] Other probable mechanisms include intrinsic vagal dysfunction as a cause of bradycardia in certain infants at enhanced risk of sudden death.

Central and Peripheral Nervous System Theories

Central and peripheral nervous system malfunction is considered to be the root cause for a number of the above cardiorespiratory abnormalities seen in infants who have afterwards died of SIDS.[64]

Brainstem gliosis has been reported in a number of researches, and is found most notably in the tegmental region of the medulla, involving the dorsal nucleus of the vagus, the inferior olivary nucleus, the solitary nucleus and the reticular nuclei.

Enhanced numbers of dendritic spines in brainstem reticular neurons have been described in SIDS infants.[65] This may be due to developmental postponement in neuronal function, with the likelihood of consequent effects on control of cardiorespiratory function. A further finding that reflects more chaotic than delayed maturation of neurons is the display of increased neuronal degeneration in SIDS infants based on enhanced staining of neurons using the monoclonal antibody ALZ-50. This antibody was elevated against extracts from brains of patients with Alzheimer's disease.[66]

Alterations have been described in the white matter of SIDS infants, consisting of leukomalacia in the periventricular and subcortical regions. It has been proposed that an apparent delay in central nervous system myelination in SIDS infants may be an expression of a related developmental disorder.[67]

Another theory suggests that an increase in brain endorphin levels may lead to respiratory depression and bradycardia in at-risk infants. Elevated β-endorphin levels have also been seen in the cerebrospinal fluid (CSF) of infants who have suffered considerable apneas. Elevated CSF β-endorphin levels have also been correlated with increased hypoxanthine levels in vitreous humor and brainstem gliosis, suggesting previous hypoxic episodes.[68]

More recently, abnormalities have been identified within the arcuate nucleus of the ventral medulla in SIDS victims. Kinney et al have demonstrated defects in the medullary serotonergic network, including the arcuate nucleus, with reduced muscarinic, kainate and serotonergic receptor binding. These receptors are implicated in responses to carbon dioxide and may play a critical role in hypoxic or hypercapnic states.[69]

Disturbed vagal function could cause respiratory abnormalities due to hypoventilation, with loss of the typical response to hypercarbia, Hering-Breuer or cough reflexes. Some studies have shown abnormalities in the structure of the vagus. Although the mean number of myelinated fibers in the vagus nerve appears normal, a considerable decrease has been noted in the number of fibers of less than 2 μm in diameter in SIDS infants.[41]

Derangement of the essential homeostatis by the carotid body and peripheral chemoreceptors in monitoring blood pH and oxygen levels with direct feedback to brainstem autonomic centers are liable for defective mechanisms in SIDS infants.

The sleep states on their own may increase susceptibility to sudden death by modifying the interaction between suprapontine structures and cardiorespiratory control centers in vulnerable infants or by acting through the brainstem reticular formation. It has also been demonstrated that siblings of SIDS infants have a diminished arousal response to partial nasal obstruction during quiet sleep.

Gastrointestinal Theories

Cases of death owing to massive aspiration of gastric material into the lungs are quite exceptional in infants. The most probable explanation for stomach contents to be found in the peripheral airways is agonal aspiration secondary to the terminal event or just to postmortem drainage of fluid subsequent to movement of the body.

Reflux of gastric contents into the upper aerodigestive tract has also been implicated as a cause of SIDS, with a variety of diverse mechanisms being thought. The increased prevalence of reflux reported during active sleep. Mechanisms by which reflux could lead to sudden death other than filling of peripheral airways with gastric contents entail stimulation of peripheral esophageal receptors by acid stomach contents, resulting in vagally mediated fatal apnea or bradycardia.[70] Certain infants who are at risk of SIDS may be strangely responsive to laryngeal stimulation. It is likely, therefore, that laryngeal receptors are more susceptible to the effects of acid than are those within the esophagus. Reflux of cow's milk protein into the airways may also result in lethal anaphylaxis and that acid damage to type II pneumocytes may compromise surfactant production causing alveolar collapse.

Microbiological Theories

Numerous factors give plausibility to a likely microbiological etiology in SIDS. These consist of increased occurrence in winter, the presence of upper respiratory infections in many infants dying of SIDS, the link of obstructive apnea with upper respiratory infections, histories of antemortem pyrexia, and the known occurrence of sudden infant death in a wide variety of infectious diseases. A range of viruses and bacteria have been implicated as potential agents liable for SIDS, including respiratory syncytial virus (RSV), cytomegalovirus (CMV) and *Bordetella pertussis*.[71] Occasionally, routine postmortem bacteriology detects a previously unsuspected infectious agent, but this happens comparatively infrequently and normal C-reactive protein levels in the sera of SIDS infants suggests that significant bacterial sepsis is improbable in most cases.[72] According to some other workers, toxins from commonly occurring bacteria may be involved in SIDS pathogenesis in infants at the time period between waning of maternal immunoglobulin levels and the development of acquired immunity.[73]

Immunologic Theories

The diminished immunoglobulin levels in premature infants and in infants of mothers who have smoked during pregnancy have led to the implication that these infants are immunologically incompetent. It has also been observed that mothers with short inter-pregnancy intervals may be protein-deficient.

An alternate approach proposes that SIDS infants are immunologically 'too' competent, and that allergic responses to a large number of materials are accountable for their unanticipated deaths. Many substances, including a variety of intrauterine pathogens, fungal organisms, house dust mite (*Dermatophagoides pteronyssinus*) and cow's milk protein have been suggested.[74] Elevated levels of IgG, IgM and IgA have been reported in pulmonary lavage fluid taken from a series of SIDS victims, along with an increase in immunohistochemical staining for immunoglobulins in lung sections. That particular group in the past reported a difference in cellular phenotype of pulmonary lavage fluid cells, with noticeably reduced expression of macrophage antigenic sites that mark with CD14A antibodies. Elevated levels of interleukin-6 in CSF in SIDS infants have been suggested as a indicator of immune activation causing respiratory depression.[75] Different studies confirmed realistically that immunization is not linked causally with SIDS.

Metabolic Theories

The most frequently recognized defect is a dearth of medium-chain acyl-coenzyme A dehydrogenase (MCAD). This enzyme catalyzes the breakdown of C16–20 fatty acids in the beta-oxidation pathway. Disruption to the pathway renders an individual vulnerable to hypoglycemia, as substitute glycogen reserves are much smaller than fat stores. The chance of a metabolic defect should be considered mostly in infants presenting with SIDS who have a family history of similar episode.[41]

Endocrine Theories

An elevated level of serum tri-iodothyronine in SIDS infants suggests thyroid dysfunction.

Nutritional Theories

Deficiency of normal levels of trace elements, particularly magnesium, has been claimed as a cause of SIDS. A wide range of vitamin deficiencies have been implicated in the etiology of SIDS, including a lack of vitamins A, C, D and E, biotin and thiamine, but none appears noteworthy.

Environmental Theories

The likelihood of accumulated toxins causing sudden death in infancy has been investigated comprehensively. One study established that lung lead concentrations were elevated, and an additional study reported elevated levels of lead in serum from SIDS cases. The possibility of carbon monoxide poisoning due to faulty domestic heating and ventilation should also be well thought-out in multiple home deaths, but it is not an issue in the pathogenesis of SIDS.

According to Richardson, a fungus, *Scopulariopsis brevicaulis,* metabolizes antimony-, arsenic-, and phosphorous-based fire-retardant chemicals within mattresses and/or their PVC coverings, producing fatal quantity of highly toxic trihydride gases, stibine, arsine and phosphine, and sleeping infants exposed to these gases die.[76]

MEDICOLEGAL ISSUES

Regrettably, SIDS is not so much a 'diagnosis' as a conclusion that is reached by a process of exclusion. As a result, there is undoubtedly no hesitation that cases of infanticide and fatal accidents have been, and will continue to be, misdiagnosed as SIDS.[30,77]

A number of years ago, John Emery created a certain amount of debate by asking whether the diagnosis of SIDS was being made too enthusiastically, resulting in a 'diagnostic dustbin' into which a broad array of disorders were hurriedly placed. More recently, Meadow has asked whether the diagnosis of SIDS should be interrupted, given the number of misdiagnosed cases of homicide that were primarily placed under the SIDS banner.[78]

Dealing with cases of unexpected infant deaths in the court adds yet another dimension of difficulty. As many of these cases may have no, or only trivial pathological findings, it may be complicated to support or disprove a diagnosis based entirely on pathological findings.[79] Inconvenience may occur when theoretical links to underlying findings in certain SIDS infants, such as inflammatory mediators like cytokines,[80] are given too much weight and used as proof in court that a particular infant death must be due to SIDS. It is important to distinguish that such hypotheses are theoretical and unproven and cannot, therefore, be used as confirmatory 'evidence' for a cause of death.

Different problems also occur in different countries. For example, infant caregivers in certain jurisdictions have been charged with manslaughter when infants in their care have died while sleeping face down. The hypothesis has been made that there has been negligence in leaving such infants in a position where they are at risk of asphyxiation. The basis for this is, however, incorrect. As the majority of infants who sleep face down do not die, the mechanism of death is not simple asphyxia in most circumstances. Death cannot, therefore, be credited to suffocation entirely on the grounds of an infant being found in the prone position.[79]

Other problems arise in cases of unexpected infant death when untrained forensic experts become involved in cases. For example, in a recent widely revealed case in the United Kingdom, retinal congestion was mistaken for antemortem retinal hemorrhage, leading to an erroneous diagnosis of shaken infant syndrome. In the same case, lacerations to the brain caused by postmortem removal were mistaken for inflicted antemortem trauma. Finally, isolation of the bacteria *Staphylococcus aureus* in pure growth from multiple sites, including the CSF, was not regarded as significant. These errors led to a mother being convicted of the murder of two of her infants. The conviction was eventually overturned upon special review.[79]

The submission of proficient judgment by individuals who are not skilful in pediatric forensic pathology often leads to perplexing and inconsistent information. Courts attempt to deal with masses of incongruous information by simplifying, which regrettably often does not work. Attempting to summarize and classify these extremely complex cases into a sequence of questions with yes/no answers is analogous to producing a one-page synopsis of a big novel. Although, no one would combat that the fundamentals of the idea could be captured by such an exercise, there is no uncertainty that important nuances assigning the true meaning and conclusions would be nowhere to be found. An illustration of wrong expert judgment in the past has been the declaration that the majority of cases ascribed to SIDS have been homicides. This has been shown to be incorrect following the remarkable fall in numbers of SIDS deaths following 'reducing the risk' campaigns.[79] Without a doubt, some cases of homicide have been misdiagnosed as SIDS; however, these definitely represent a small percentage of overall cases of infant death.

CONCLUSION

One of the purposes of this text is to aid in the separation of cases of sudden infant death in which a cause is found from cases in which no sufficient justification for death can be determined. It is the latter group that represents those physiologically compromised infants who beyond doubt deserve the label of SIDS.

In one category are found those entities in which the clinical presentation may be indistinguishable from SIDS, in that a previously apparently well infant was found dead in his or her crib. However, at autopsy, a lesion or disease is found that has caused death. In the next group are found those infants with no diseases or lesions found at autopsy to whom the term SIDS can actually be applied. In the final category are those infants in whom the autopsy discovers an aberration that appears to be significant but whose exact role in the terminal episode is hard to conclude.

REFERENCES

1. Beckwith JB. Discussion of terminology and definition of the sudden infant death syndrome. Sudden infant death syndrome. In: Bergman AB, Beckwith JB, Ray CG (eds). Seattle: University of Washington press; 1970. p. 14-22.

2. Henderson-Smart DJ, Ponsonby AL, Murphy E. Reducing the risk of sudden infant death syndrome: a review of the scientific literature. *J Paediatr Child Health* 1998; 34: 213-19.
3. Byard RW, Krous HF. Sudden infant death syndrome–an overview and update. *Pediatr Dev Pathol* 2003; 6: 112-27.
4. Byard RW. Inaccurate classification of infant deaths in Australia: a persistent and pervasive problem. *Med J Aust* 2001; 175: 5-7.
5. Filiano JJ, Kinney HC. A perspective on neuropathologic findings in victims of the sudden infant death syndrome: the triple risk model. *Biol Neonate* 1994; 65: 194-97.
6. Willinger M, Ko CW, Hoffman HJ, Kessler RC, Corwin MJ. Factors associated with caregivers' choice of infant sleep position, 1994-1998: the national infant sleep position study. *JAMA* 2000; 283: 2135-42.
7. Beckwith JB. The sudden infant death syndrome. *Curr Prob Paediatr* 1973; 3: 1-36.
8. Willinger M, James LS, Catz C. Defining the sudden infant death syndrome (SIDS): deliberations of an expert panel convened by the National Institute of Child Health and Human Development. *Pediatric Pathology* 1991; 11: 677-84.
9. Templeman C. Two hundred and fifty-eight cases of suffocation of infants. *Edinburgh Med J* 1892; 38: 322-29.
10. Russell-Jones DL. Sudden infant death in history and literature. *Arch Dis Child* 1985; 60: 278-81.
11. Gilbert-Barness E, Hegstrand L, Chandra S, Emery JL, Barness LA, Franciosi R et al. Hazards of mattresses, beds and bedding in deaths of infants. *Am J Forensic Med Pathol* 1991; 12: 27-32.
12. Kraus JF, Greenland S, Bulterys M. Risk factors for sudden infant death syndrome in the US collaborative perinatal project. *Int J Epidemiol* 1989; 18: 113-20.
13. Hauck FR. Changing epidemiology. In: Byard RW, Krous HF (eds). Sudden infant death syndrome. Problems, progress and possibilities. London: Arnold; 2001. p. 31-57.
14. Centers for Disease Control and Prevention. Sudden infant death syndrome–United States, 1980-88. Morbidity and Mortality Weekly Report 1992; 41: 515-7.
15. Douglas AS, Allan TM, Helms PJ. Seasonality and the sudden infant death syndrome during 1987-9 and 1991-3 in Australia and Britain. *BMJ* 1996; 312: 1381-83.
16. Chong A, Murphy N, Matthews T. Effect of prone sleeping on circulatory control in infants. *Arch Dis Child* 2000; 82: 253-56.
17. Franco P, Groswasser J, Sottiaux M, Broadfield E, Kahn A. Decreased cardiac responses to auditory stimulation during prone sleep. *Pediatrics* 1996: 97: 174-78.
18. Galland BC, Taylor BJ, Bolton DPG. Prone verses supine sleep position: a review of physiological studies in SIDS research. *J Paediatr Child* Health 2002; 38: 332-38.
19. Kemp JS, Livne M, White DK, Arfken CL. Softness and potential to cause re-breathing: differences in bedding used by infants at high and low risk for sudden infant death syndrome. *J Pediatr* 1998; 132: 234-39.
20. Myers MM, Fifer WP, Schaeffer L, Sahni R, Ohira-Kist K, Stark RI et al. Effects of sleeping position and time after feeding on the organization of sleep/wake states in prematurely born infants. *Sleep* 1998; 21: 343-49.
21. Blair PS, Fleming PJ, Bensley D, Smith I, Bacon C, Taylor E et al. Smoking and the sudden infant death syndrome: results from 1993-5 case-control study for confidential inquiry into stillbirths and deaths in infancy. *BMJ* 1996; 313: 195-98.
22. Blair PS, Nadin P, Cole TJ, Fleming PJ, Smith IJ, Ward Platt M et al . Weight gain and sudden infant death syndrome: changes in weight z scores may identify infants at increased risk. *Arch Dis Child* 2000; 82: 462-69.
23. Horne RSC, Ferens D, Watts AM, Vitkovic J, Lacey B, Andrew S et al. Effects of maternal tobacco smoking, sleeping position, and sleep state on arousal in healthy term infants. *Arch Dis Child Fetal Neonatal Ed* 2002; 87: F100-05.

24. Taylor BJ, Williams SM, Mitchell EA, Ford RPK. Symptoms, sweating and reactivity of infants who die of SIDS compared with community controls. *J Paediatr Child Health* 1996; 32: 316-22.
25. Krous HF, Nadeau JM, Fukumoto RI, Blackbourne BD, Byard RW. Environmental hyperthermic infant and early childhood death. Circumstances, pathologic changes, and manner of death. *Am J Forensic Med Pathol* 2001; 22: 374-82.
26. Kleemann WJ, Schlaud M, Poets CF, Rothamel T, Troger HD. Hyperthermia in sudden infant death. *Int J Legal Med* 1996; 109: 139-42.
27. Guntheroth WG, Spiers PS. Thermal stress in sudden infant death: is there an ambiguity with the rebreathing hypothesis? *Pediatrics* 2001; 107: 693-98.
28. Fleming PJ, Levine MR, Azaz Y, Wigfield R, Stewart AJ. Interactions between thermoregulation and the control of respiration in infants: possible relationship to sudden infant death. *Acta Paediatrica* 1993; 389: 57-59.
29. McKenna JJ, Mosko S. Mother-infant co-sleeping: toward a new scientific beginning. In: Byard RW, Krous HF (eds). Sudden infant death syndrome. Problems, progress and possibilities. London: Arnold, 2001. p. 258-74.
30. Byard RW, Hilton J. Overlaying, accidental suffocation, and sudden infant death. *J SIDS Infant Mortality* 1997; 2: 161-65.
31. Daltveit AK, Irgens LM, Oyen N, Skjaerven R, Markestad T, Alm B et al. Sociodemographic risk factors for sudden infant death syndrome: associations with other risk factors. The Nordic epidemiologic SIDS study. *Acta Paediatrica* 1998; 87: 284-90.
32. Byard RW, Makrides M, Need M, Neumann MA, Gibson RA. Sudden infant death syndrome: effect of breast and formula feeding on frontal cortex and brainstem lipid levels. *J Paediatr Child Health* 1995; 31: 14-16.
33. Davidson Ward SL, Keens TG. Prenatal substance abuse. *Clin Perinatol* 1992;19:849-60.
34. Kandall SR, Gaines J, Habel L, Davidson G, Jessop D. Relationship of maternal substance abuse to subsequent sudden infant death syndrome in offspring. *J Pediatr* 1993; 123: 120-26.
35. Alm B, Wennergren G, Norvenius G, Skjarven R, Oyen N, Helweg-Larsen K et al. Caffeine and alcohol as risk factors for sudden infant death syndrome. *Arch Dis Child* 1999; 81: 107-11.
36. Vege A, Rognum TO, Opdal SH. SIDS – changes in the epidemiological pattern in Eastern Norway 1984–1996. *Forensic Sci Int* 1998; 93: 155-66.
37. Knobel HH, Yang WS, Chen CJ. Risk factors of sudden infant death in Chinese babies. *Am J Epidemiol* 1996; 144: 1070-73.
38. Read AW. What are the national rates for sudden infant death syndrome for Aboriginal and Torres Strait Islander infants? *J Paediatr Child Health* 2002; 38: 122-23.
39. Koehler SA, Ladham S, Shakir A, Wecht CH. Simultaneous sudden infant death syndrome. A proposed definition and worldwide review of cases. *Am J Forensic Med Pathol* 2001; 22: 23-32.
40. Mitchell E, Krous HF, Donald T, Byard RW. Changing trends in the diagnosis of sudden infant death. *Am J Forensic Med Pathol* 2000; 21: 311-14.
41. Byard RW. Sudden death in infancy, childhood and adolescence. 2nd. New York: Cambridge University Press; 2004. p. 490-575.
42. Sturner WQ. Sudden infant death syndrome–the medical examiner's viewpoint. *Perspect Pediatr Pathol* 1995; 19: 76-86.
43. Hanzlick R. Death scene investigation. In: Byard RW, Krous HF (eds). Sudden infant death syndrome. Problems, progress and possibilities. London: Arnold; 2001. p. 58-65.
44. Krous HF. The International standardised autopsy protocol for sudden unexpected infant death. In: Rognum TO (ed). Sudden infant death syndrome. New trends in the nineties. Oslo: Scandinavian university press; 1995. p. 81-95.

45. Rognum TO. Definition and pathologic features. In: Byard RW, Krous HF (eds). Sudden infant death syndrome. Problems, progress and possibilities. London: Arnold; 2001. p. 4-30.
46. Byard RW, Krous HF. Sudden infant death syndrome-definition and diagnostic trends. *J Jpn SIDS Res Soc* 2003; 3: 11-16.
47. Krous HF, Nadeau JM, Byard RW, Blackbourne BD. Oronasal blood in sudden infant death. *Am J Foren Med Path* 2001; 22: 346-51.
48. Byard RW, Krous HF. Petechial hemorrhages and unexpected infant death. *Legal Med* 1999; 1: 193-97.
49. Molz G, Brodzinowski A, Bar W, Vonlanthen B. Morphologic variations in 180 cases of sudden infant death and 180 controls. *Am J Foren Med Path* 1992; 13: 186-90.
50. Byard RW, Moore L. Can thymic petechiae be used to separate SIDS infants from controls? *Pathology* 1993; 25: 7.
51. Yukawa N, Carter N, Rutty G, Green MA. Intra-alveolar hemorrhage in sudden infant death syndrome: a cause for concern? *J Clin Pathol* 1999; 52: 581-87.
52. Keens TG, Davidson Ward SL. Respiratory mechanisms and hypoxia. In: Byard RW, Krous HF (eds). Sudden infant death syndrome. Problems, progress and possibilities. London: Arnold; 2001. p. 66-82.
53. Rees K, Wright A, Keeling JW, Douglas NJ. Facial structure in the sudden infant death syndrome: case-control study. *BMJ* 1998; 317: 179-80.
54. Siebert JR, Haas JE. Enlargement of the tongue in sudden infant death syndrome. *Pediatr Pathol* 1991; 11: 813-26.
55. Haque AK, Mancuso MG. Proliferation of dendritic cells in the bronchioles of sudden infant death syndrome victims. *Modern Pathol* 1993; 6: 360-70.
56. Poets CF, Meny RG, Chobanian MR, Bonofiglo RE. Gasping and other cardiorespiratory patterns during sudden infant deaths. *Pediatr Res* 1999; 45: 350-54.
57. Franco P, Szliwowski H, Dramaix M, Kahn A. Decreased autonomic responses to obstructive sleep events in future victims of sudden infant death syndrome. *Pediatr Res* 1999; 46: 33-39.
58. Southall DP, Samuels MP, Talbert DG. Recurrent cyanotic episodes with severe arterial hypoxaemia and intrapulmonary shunting: a mechanism for sudden death. *Arch Dis Child* 1990; 65: 953-61.
59. James D, Berry PJ, Fleming P, Hathaway M. Surfactant abnormality and the sudden infant death syndrome—a primary or secondary phenomenon? *Arch Dis Child* 1990; 65: 774-78.
60. Naeye RL. The sudden infant death syndrome. In: Thurlbeck WM, Abell MR (eds). The lung: structure, function and disease. Baltimore: Williams and Wilkins; 1978. p. 262-70.
61. Tennyson SA, Pereyra PM, Becker LE. The development of the diaphragm in infants with sudden infant death syndrome. *Early Hum Dev* 1994; 37: 1-8.
62. Pincus SM, Cummins TR, Haddad GG. Heart rate control in normal and aborted-SIDS infants. *Am J Physiol* 1993; 264: R638-46.
63. Lobban CDR. The human dive reflex as a primary cause of SIDS. A review of the literature. *Med J Aust* 1991; 155: 561-63.
64. Hunt CE. The cardiorespiratory control hypothesis for sudden infant death syndrome. *Clin Perinatol* 1992; 19: 757-71.
65. Takashima S, Yamanouchi H, Becker LE. Development of catecholaminergic neurons and substance P-positive nerve fibres in the brainstem of victims of sudden infant death syndrome. In: Togawa K, Katayama S, Hishikawa Y, Ohta Y, Horie T (eds). Sleep apnea and rhonchopathy. Basel: Karger; 1993. p. 13-18.
66. Sparks DL, Hunsaker JC 3rd. Increased ALZ-50- reactive neurons in the brains of SIDS infants: an indicator of greater neuronal death? *J Child Neurol* 1991; 6: 123-27.
67. Kinney HC, Brody BA, Finkelstein DM, Vawter GF, Mandell F, Gilles FH. Delayed central nervous system myelination in the sudden infant death syndrome. *J Neuropath Exp Neur* 1991; 50: 29-48.

68. Storm H, Rognum TO, Saugstad OD, Skullerud K, Reichelt KL. Beta-endorphin immunoreactivity in spinal fluid and hypoxanthine in vitreous humour related to brainstem gliosis in sudden infant death victims. *Eur J Pediatr* 1994; 153: 675-81.
69. Kinney HC, Filiano JJ, Assmann SF, Mandell F, Valdes-Dapena M, Krous HF, et al. Tritiatednaloxone binding to brainstem opioid receptors in the sudden infant death syndrome. *J Auton Nerv Syst* 1998; 69: 156-63.
70. De Bethmann O, Couchard M, de Ajuriaguerra M, Lucet V, Cheron G, Guillon G, et al. Role of gastro-oesophageal reflux and vagal overactivity in apparent life-threatening events: 160 cases. *Acta Paediatr* 1993; 389: 102-04.
71. Variend S. Infant mortality, microglial nodules and parotid CMV-type inclusions. *Early Hum Dev* 1990; 21: 31-40.
72. Benjamin DR, Siebert JR. C-reactive protein and prealbumin in suspected sudden infant death syndrome. *Pediatr Pathol* 1990; 10: 503-7.
73. McKendrick N, Drucker DB, Morris JA, Telford DR, Barson AJ, Oppenheim BA. Bacterial toxins: a possible cause of cot death. *J Clin Pathol* 1992; 45: 49-53.
74. Coombs, RRA, McLaughlan P. The modified anaphylactic hypothesis for sudden infant death syndrome. In: Tildon JA, Roeder LM, Steinschneider A (eds). Sudden infant death syndrome. New York: Academic press; 1983. p. 531-38.
75. Vege A. Clues to understanding the death mechanism in sudden infant death syndrome (SIDS). Oslo: University of Oslo press; 1998.
76. Richardson BA. Cot mattress bio-deterioration and SIDS. *Lancet* 1990; 335: 670.
77. Byard R, Krous H. Suffocation, shaking or sudden infant death syndrome: can we tell the difference? *J Paediatr Child Health* 1999; 35: 432-33.
78. Meadow R. Unnatural sudden infant death. *Arch Dis Child* 1999; 80: 7-14.
79. Byard R, Krous H. Diagnostic and medico-legal problems with sudden infant death syndrome. In: Toskos M (ed). Forensic pathology review. Vol 1. New Jersey: Humana press; 2004. p. 189-98.
80. Blackwell CC, Weir DM, Busuttil A, Saadi AT, Essery SD, Raza MW et al. Infection, inflammation, and the developmental stage of infants: a new hypothesis for the aetiology of SIDS. In: Rognum TO (ed). Sudden infant death syndrome: new trends in the nineties. Oslo: Scandinavian University press; 1995. p. 189-98.

Post-autopsy Reconstruction

N Srinivasa Ragavan

'It takes less time to do things right than to explain why you did it wrong.'
Henry Wadsworth Longfellow (American poet and educator)

ABSTRACT

After completion of autopsy, the postmortem technical assistant or attendant is required to reconstruct the body with a high level of skill and care. It is restored to the best possible cosmetic appearance with the consideration that the deceased may be viewed by relatives following the autopsy.[1] All the organs are placed back into the body, except for the specimens kept as evidence or to assist to determine the cause of death.[1,2] The skull and body cavities viz. abdominal and chest are filled with wadding. All the organs and viscera are placed in a clear plastic bag to prevent fluid leakage and returned to the body cavity. The chest flaps are then closed and sewn back tightly with twine using the technique of 'under-stitching', whereby the skin is sewn from below. The skull cap also is sewed back in place. The dead body is then washed and dressed in a clean cover and then handed over to the police constable/investigating officer.[1,3] This chapter discusses the various visceral containment methods and sutural techniques so as to ensure that the persons handling the dead body do not come in direct contact with any of the biologically hazardous agents.

Keywords: Under-stitching, postmortem needle, biohazard bags, postmortem reconstruction, base-ball stitch, fetal reconstruction.

INTRODUCTION

Reconstruction plays a key role in the presentation of the dead to the relatives. The body may be viewed by the relatives for the purpose of identification after the autopsy and before the last rites. However, in line with the 'diminishing marginal utility theory of economics', many forensic pathologists nowadays, are not bothered about proper reconstruction of the body after postmortem, and this aspect of work is often overlooked. This theory states that when any work is repeatedly done in a monotonous way, there is always a possibility of the quality of work getting compromised due to over workload or due to oversight. In most of the facilities where autopsy is being conducted routinely, reconstruction techniques after the procedure are either rushed through and/or poorly executed.

There is also a possibility of slippage of the skull cap or sternal plate after suturing, which renders a poor cosmetic look for the body. Hence, one should consider how the body is going to be reconstructed afterwards and what will be the final cosmetic appearance. Poor reconstruction or rough handling can lead to unnecessary distress and potential grievances by surviving family members.[3,4]

The techniques used by these semi-skilled personnel do not adequately support the professional expertise provided by the facility. To achieve a satisfactory reconstruction, the autopsy procedure should be of highest standard and the forensic pathologist should reasonably be well versed in this procedure.[4] This chapter discusses methodologies to present an aesthetically pleasant reconstructed body, and also ensure a leak proof and contaminant-free construction technique.

CURRENT METHODOLOGY

Autopsy refers to the systematic examination of a dead person for medical, legal and/or scientific purposes. It is of three types:[5]

a. *Academic* dissection is carried out by students of anatomy.
b. *Pathological, hospital or clinical autopsy* is done by pathologists to diagnose the cause of death or to confirm a diagnosis. Physicians cannot order these autopsies without the consent signed by the next of kin.
c. *Medicolegal autopsy* is carried out under the laws of the State for the protection of rights of citizens. The basic purpose of this autopsy is to establish the cause and manner of death.

Brief description of autopsy procedure is given below:[5,6]

The autopsy is carried out by a registered medical practitioner. The doctor usually removes the organs himself. The postmortem technician or attendant assists the doctor as required, such as evisceration, sawing the skull cap and reconstructing the body. Earlier, the person responsible for handling, moving and cleaning the body was called a *diener* (German, servant).

All three major cavities of the body, i.e. skull, thorax and abdomen are opened and examined as a routine. The most common skin incisions is the *I-shaped incision* extending from the chin straight down to the symphysis pubis and avoiding the umbilicus (because the dense fibrous tissue is difficult to penetrate with a needle, when the body is stitched after autopsy). *Modified Y-shaped incision* is made in midline from suprasternal notch to symphysis pubis. The incision extends from suprasternal notch over the clavicle to its center on both sides and then passes upwards over the neck behind the ears. It is used when a detailed study of neck organs is required, for e.g., in hanging or strangulation. *Y-shaped incision* is rarely used.

Abdomen and Pelvis

After the skin incision, the rectus abdominis muscles are incised upto 5 cm above the symphysis pubis. A small nick is made in the fascia to admit the left index and middle fingers with palmar surfaces up, to protect the underlying structures, and the peritoneum is cut up to the xiphoid. The skin and muscles of the chest are dissected sidewise and carried back to the midaxillary line, down to the costal margin and up over the clavicles. The chest is opened by cutting the costal cartilages close to the costochondral junctions and starting from the upper border of the second cartilage with a cartilage knife. Then, disarticulation of the sternoclavicular joint is done on each side by inserting the point of knife into the semicircular joint.

This method of evisceration commonly followed is the *Virchow's,* which is simply removal of individual organs one by one with subsequent dissection of that isolated organ. Sometimes, the *en masse* method developed by Letulle or *en bloc removal* developed by Ghon may be used based on individual preferences.

The Skull

A coronal incision is made in the scalp, which starts from one mastoid to the opposite mastoid process just behind the ear and is continued over the vertex of the scalp. The scalp is reflected forwards to the superciliary ridges and backwards to a point just below the occipital protuberance. The temporal and masseter muscles are incised on either side, for sawing the skull. Triangular or V-shaped notches at an angle of 120° are placed laterally in the skull cap to facilitate realignment for postmortem reconstruction. Others use a 'step cut' or angled cut based on their personal or institutional preference. The saw-line is just above the superciliary ridges in front, to the base of the mastoid process on either side and just above the occipital protuberance behind.

After the postmortem and collection of tissues and body fluids samples for analysis, the remaining portions of organs are put inside the body cavity (mostly abdominal cavity) after removing as much as body fluids as possible. Next, the sternal plate is replaced in its position. The dissected skin flaps are brought close together and then sutured at or near a location where these skin flaps converge with a traditional running suture (zigzag or continuous) by using twine and needle. The skull is filled with remaining portion of the brain and the skull cap fitted in place. The scalp is pulled back over the vault and stitched with strong twine. The body is then washed with water, dried and covered with clothes and handed over to the police constable accompanying it or to the relatives.

However, with the above mentioned procedure there are chances of leakage of potential biohazard fluids through body openings or sutured surface. In most establishments, no wadding is used to soak up the remaining body fluids or blood that remains in the cavities. The attendant usually applies primitive suturing technique. And in many situations, the reconstruction of the body is also of a very poor quality from the cosmetic angle.

The very purpose of reconstructing the body after postmortem is not to improve the antemortem appearance of the individual, for e.g., if a patient has undergone a limb amputation or orchidectomy, the limb or the scrotum should not be reconstructed to simulate its presence. The aim is to prevent spilling of biologically hazardous agents so that it does not come in direct contact with individuals handling the dead body and to produce an esthetically pleasing end result for viewing by relatives of the deceased post-autopsy.[4,7]

The following procedure as described below should be undertaken to ensure a leak proof and contaminant-free reconstruction technique. It is albeit not possible for a properly reconstituted body to obscure the fact that there has been an autopsy, but the facial features and preferably the hands and feet should be readily viewable by relatives after the autopsy.[2]

REMOVAL OF ACCUMULATED FLUIDS

After evisceration of organs from the thoracic, abdominal and pelvic cavities, there will be residual fluids, tissues and bowel contents within it. It may be blood, ascitic or pleural fluid, serosanguineous fluids or fecal matter. All the remaining fluids should be aspirated, removed and dried to prevent leakage. This is to prevent any splashing or welling up of any serosanguineous fluids when placing the viscera back into the thoraco-abdominal cavities.[4,7-10]

With the use of scoop and jug, fluids are removed and disposed off into a basin which is connected to a drainage system. Any tissue left in the cavities is removed by hand or other appropriate method and returned to the body along with other body tissues.[4,7-10]

WADDING

Once the cavities are dry, the thoraco-abdominal cavities including the pelvic cavity are lined with adequate wadding or cotton wool to soak up any remaining body fluids or fluids that might continue to leak following the reconstruction. This ensures that no fluid leaks from the body after reconstruction. The materials used for wadding are cotton or wool, or materials like towel, cloth, saw dust or even newspaper can be substituted. Alternative materials such as incontinence pads, waste bags or refuse bags are not recommended. Some advanced institutions use action embalming crystals (absorbent crystals) which soaks up excess fluid.[3,4,7]

VISCERA CONTAINMENT

Post-autopsy, the forensic pathologist will have a large amount of unused viscera, since a very small amount of the tissues are required for evaluation in case of inconclusive diagnosis (histopathology and toxicology). All organs and viscera must be returned to the body unless prior consent for retention has been obtained. These should not be placed free into the body cavities. All these unused organs and tissues are placed in biohazard bags or clear plastic bags (Fig. 22.1). These bags are then placed into the cavities on top of the wadding (Fig. 22.2). The use of such bags will ensure the proper containment of these unused and discarded visceral tissues. This will also prevent the leakage from the body. Any excess air is removed by expressing and compressing the residual air from them after being placed within these cavities and then sealed. This will allow those bags to fit snugly within the thoraco-abdominal cavities. If these bags contain any air, then it will become difficult to fit them within this very limited space. The reason of sealing within the cavities is that new volume of air is not introduced during this containment. Once the placement of these biohazard bags have been completed within these cavities, more wadding is placed over it (Fig. 22.3).[3,4,7-10]

However, any foreign objects, for e.g., gloves, aprons, universal containers, blood tube sets, syringes or needles should be disposed off in appropriate separate waste bin. They should not be placed inside the body. If the body contained sharp objects, such as inferior vena cava filters, glass or needles, these

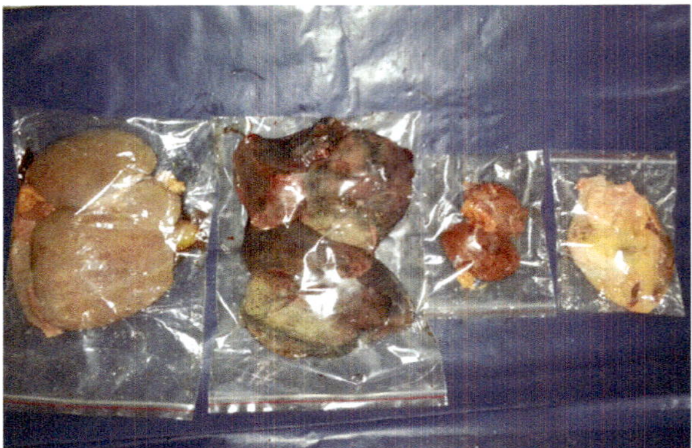

Fig. 22.1 Organs packed in plastic covers

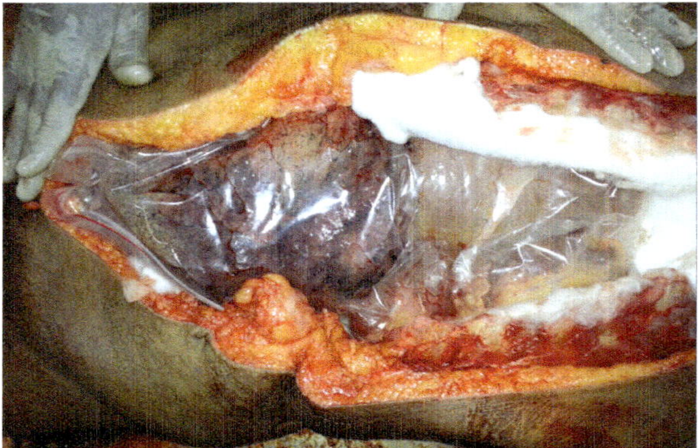

Fig. 22.2 Organs packed and sealed in plastic covers *in situ*

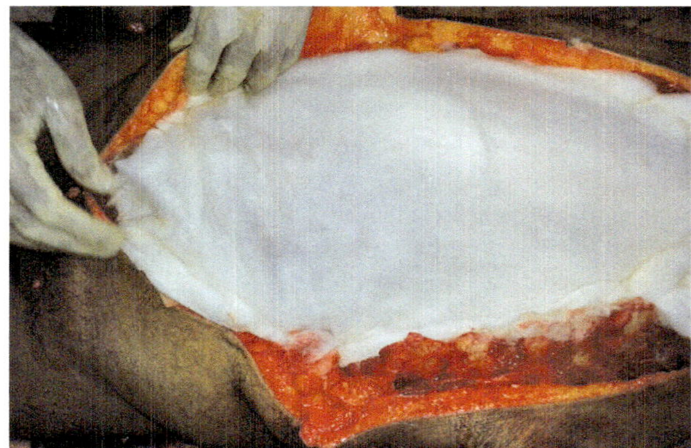

Fig. 22.3 Overlaying with cotton wadding after placing the organs

should be disposed off into a sharp bin. Under any circumstances, body parts not from the body in question should be placed into in any of these bags.[7-10]

SUTURING

The suturing process is a skill that most attendants develop over time with repeated use, and perform expeditiously. The first step in this suturing process is to get an autopsy suture needle that can be held comfortably in one hand. The second step is to put approximately an eight to ten feet length of autopsy suture and thread its length through the eye of this needle. Suturing is usually done using single good-quality mattress twine attached to a long cutting needle; straight, curved (Hagedorn needle) or serpentine depending on availability. This type of twine has now been replaced by suture twine supplied for this specific purpose.[4,9]

The suturing may start from above (chin) or below (mons pubis) depending on the individual's preference. In case of I-shaped incision, the preferred site for the initiation of suturing process is usually the mons pubis for it helps to approximate the abdominal skin evenly along the entire length of those incised margins of the abdomen. This suturing process is always initiated with a downward stroke for safety's sake. One should pull on the thread and not the needle when tightening the suture, since pulling on the needle weakens the thread.[4,9]

Postmortem Needles

In general, postmortem needles are larger and heavier than standard needles used for suturing. They are designed to match a heavier type of thread that is strong and durable for suturing large incisions through the chest and abdomen after autopsy is complete. With different sizes and curvature on the needles, the technician can choose the right needle for the incision size and the number of sutures that have to be completed. With new advances in forensic medicine, even the postmortem needle has advanced in its design, construction material, and even in the ways in which it is used. Cutting needles provide the option to have a stainless steel bland mounted in the thicker handle or grip part of the device. The specific design of postmortem needles has increased the lifetime use of the needles themselves.

Half curve or double curved postmortem needles come in a variety of sizes. These needles typically have a standard eye to insert the suture as well as a cutting edge on the needle itself. Additional features that can make using the needle much easier include a series of ridges on the curve of the needle that enhance finger grip without bulking up the needle diameter. Double curve needles make a flattened S shape and come in sizes 1 through 8. Half curve needles have the straight shank with a curve on the tip, allowing for easy and consistent suturing (Fig. 22.4).[11]

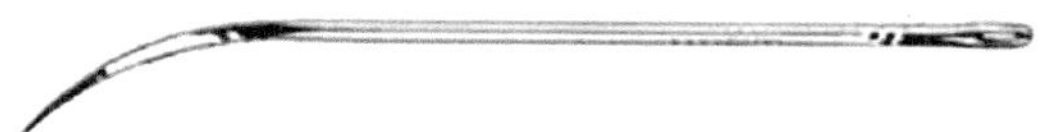

Fig. 22.4 Curved postmortem needle

Suturing Techniques

The various types of suturing techniques are: individual (bridge) sutures; baseball suture; single intradermal (hidden) suture; double intradermal suture; inversion (worm) suture; interlocking suture and continuous suture ('whip stitch'). Continuous suture is normally used by autopsy technicians to close long incisions (Fig. 22.5).

The following suturing techniques are recommended for the post-autopsy reconstruction:[4,7,12]

a. **Under-stitching:** In this technique, a knot is placed at the end of the suture to locate and secure the start. Suturing is done in such a way that the skin is sewn from below ('under-stitching'). Preference is given to this method as it produces a flatter cosmetic result, and much of the suturing is hidden from view. The stitches should be tight and placed approximately, 1 cm apart and 5 mm away from the incision edge. In average bodies, suture depths more than 5 mm are not appropriate, as they may draw fat up into the suture line producing poor cosmetic result. Care must also be taken not to catch cotton wool in the sutures, especially when closing the neck (Figs 22.6A and B).
b. **Running baseball** stitch is another suturing technique that is also frequently used in many facilities. The running suture is initiated by placing a simple interrupted suture at one end of the I-shaped incison that is tied but not cut. Simple suture passes are then placed down the length of the wound as a 'baseball suture', until the end of the suture line is reached. At this point, it is tied off with a simple knot created by the last loop of suture. It is an easy and rapid method of closing incisions (Fig. 22.7).
c. **Mattress suture:** Another type of suturing that can be used is the mattress suture. It is an interrupted stitch, which means that each stitch is tied off before creating the next stitch. It is strong and can be used to close the large incisions. There are two basic variations: the vertical and the horizontal (Fig. 22.8).

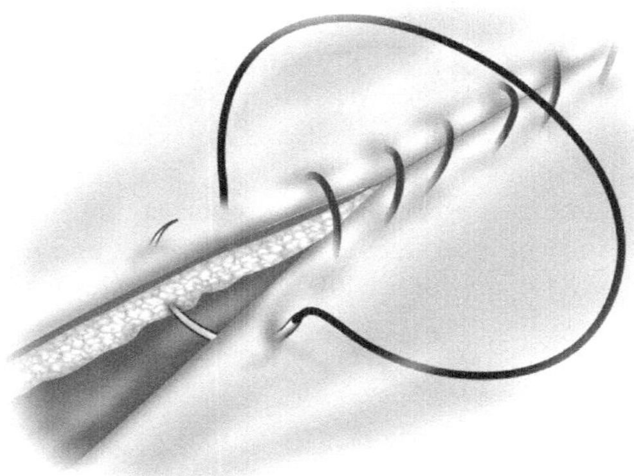

Fig. 22.5 Continuous suture

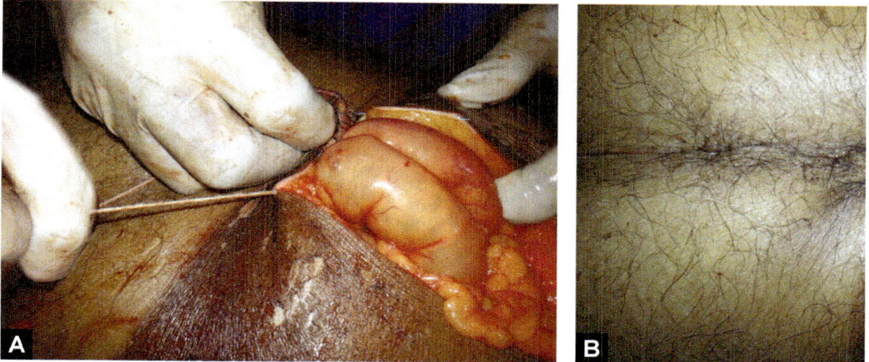

Figs 22.6A and B (A) Under-stitching; (B) Appearance of skin incision after under-stitching

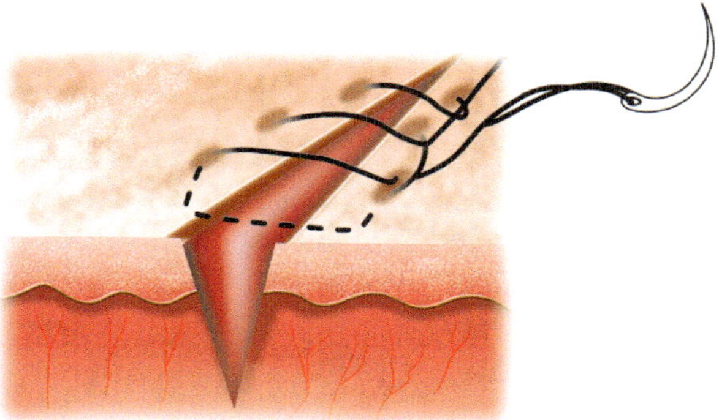

Fig. 22.7 Baseball suture

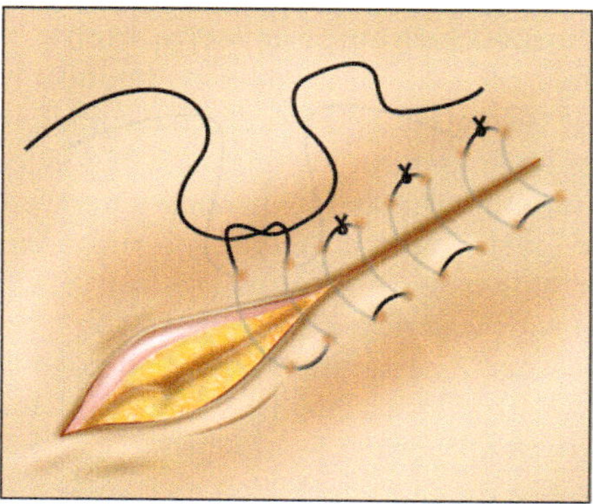

Fig. 22.8 Mattress suture

Sutures

The choice of suture is important. Lesser quality materials, for e.g., string or polythene twine, may cause knotting and/or suture breakdown. Sutures must be durable enough to hold tissue securely but flexible enough to be knotted. Nonabsorbable sutures made of special silk or synthetic polypropylene, polyester and nylon are available for use. Nylon should be used to close the body cavities and suture it.

Following are some of the common sutures available for use:[12,13]

- **Nylon suture** has high tensile strength. It is available as either a single monofilament or multiple braided filaments, both of which tend to pass through tissue easily. However, it has a tendency to return to its original state, a feature called *memory* which may cause the suture to coil, and the knots to unwind and become loose. Extra ties must be passed with this suture for the security of interrupted suture ties.
- **Silk** suture has been important in skin closures in living persons for many years and set apart as the standard for skin closure. This braided suture is easy to handle and tie but does have a significant amount of tissue drag. Because the suture is braided, it is comfortable to use and used frequently.
- **Cotton:** It is twisted, with low memory and good handling. Because of its cost-effectiveness, cotton is commonly used in most of the places for suturing in postmortem reconstruction.
- **Polypropylene** (prolene suture) is a synthetic compound created as a monofilament suture with a tensile strength equivalent to nylon. It is easier to handle than nylon because of an intrinsic stretching ability as it passes through tissue easily and ties well. However, it also has memory which can create slippage and knots to untie.
- **Polyester** sutures are made from tightly braided multifilamental fibers which have been shown to last indefinitely in the body surface. These sutures are easy to handle with good knot tying ability and little problems with recoil or memory. However, it is quite expensive.

THE NECK

When modified 'Y' shaped incision is made to expose the neck structures, the three points of the neck and chest skin incision must first be joined with a securing stitch, sewing several centimeters down the midline chest incision. The neck suture can then begin behind the ear on either side by under-stitching. The hiding of the suture line is aided by making a neck incision as posteriorly as possible when opening the body. Then the suturing is continued downwards from ear until the midline is reached. Any false teeth are replaced and mouth and neck are packed with wadding which should reach the line of incision to avoid any potential leakage. The suture is then continued upwards to the other ear, packing the neck as one proceeds. During sewing, the shape of the neck is adjusted properly so that it resembles the living neck as far as possible. Any excess packing will make the body look bloated. When the ear is reached, the suture is tied off, burying the knot in the process.[7]

THORAX AND ABDOMEN

As discussed earlier, adequate wadding is applied to the posterior surface of the cavities. Then the plastic bag containing the organs is kept with proper sealing. Wadding placed on top of the bag helps in stoppage of leak and is also helpful in reconstructing the original shape of the chest (Fig. 22.9). The sternal plate is placed on top of that in such a way that the cut end of ribs meet in close apposition. Few stay sutures are applied at the intercostals muscles to keep the sternal plate in position. Then the thorax and abdomen can be closed. The suturing proceeds where one left off from the start of the neck reconstruction. Same under-stitching method is adopted up to the supra-pubic region where it is tied off and buried.[3,7]

HEAD

When the skull is opened, consideration should be given as how to stop any movement of the skull after reconstruction. The chances of slippage of skull cap after replacement can be minimized by placing a triangular or square notch in the midline of the frontal bone incision (Figs 22.10 and 22.11). A second notch is placed on either side of the squamous temporal bones (Fig. 22.12). The posterior skull incision should be angled at approximately 60° to the incision in the squamous temporal bones. This will ensure appropriate relocation and minimal movement of the skull cap (Fig. 22.13).[7]

Any bone like orbital plate or middle ear, if not sampled for histology, are placed back in their respective sites. Sufficient wadding is placed inside the cavity to soak up any fluid (Fig. 22.14). This also helps to prevent the skull-cap from moving. The stripped dura and the brain are placed into the plastic bag and returned to the cranial cavity (Fig. 22.15). The brain should be placed back inside the cranial cavity whenever possible to retain a natural feel. The skull-cap is now replaced.[4,7]

To further stabilize the skull, the temporalis muscle on either side is sutured with periosteum. Otherwise, both side temporalis muscle are tied together with

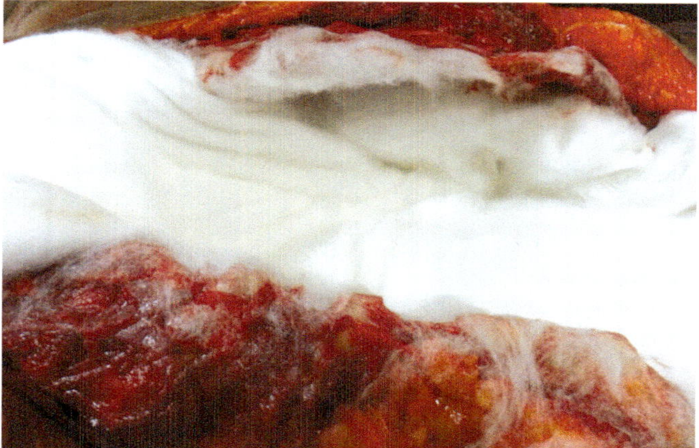

Fig. 22.9 Wadding with cotton placed in thoracic and abdominal cavity

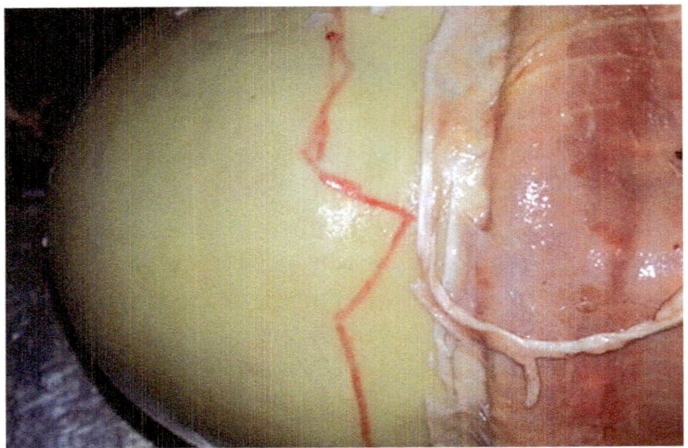

Fig. 22.10 Line drawing to show the wedged incision in frontal bone

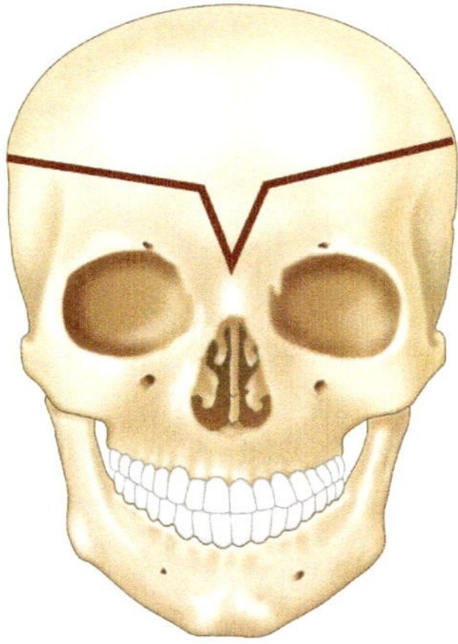

Fig. 22.11 Wedge shaped incision of cranial vault—frontal region

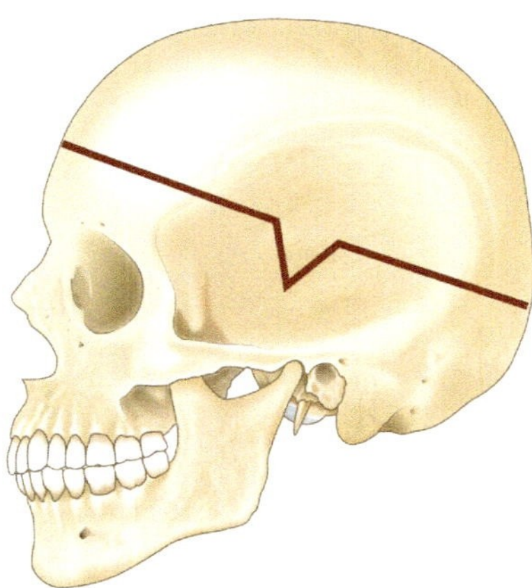

Fig. 22.12 Wedge shaped incision of cranial vault—temporal region

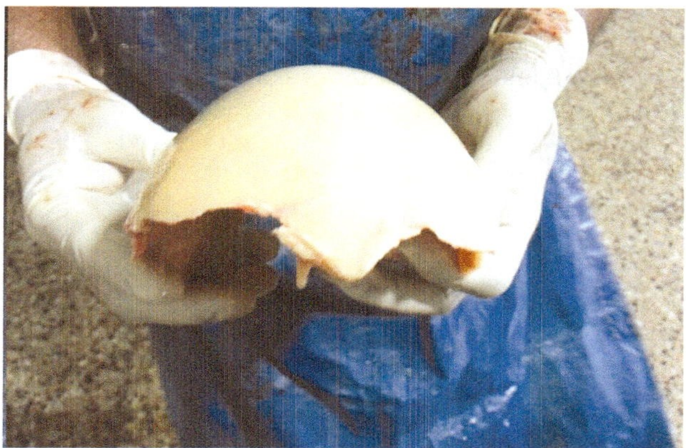

Fig. 22.13 Shape of cranial cap after removal

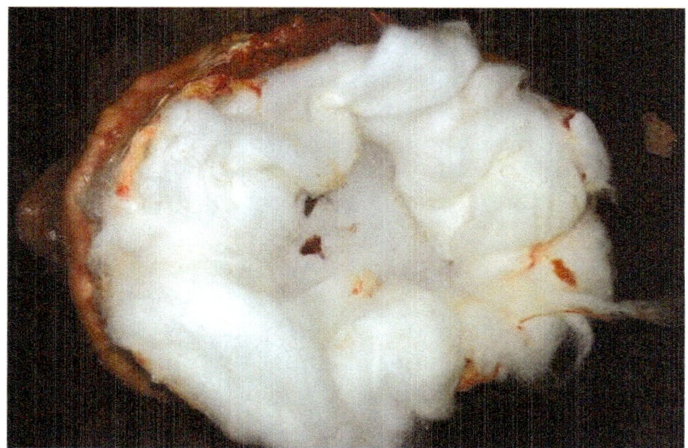

Fig. 22.14 Wadding of skull base

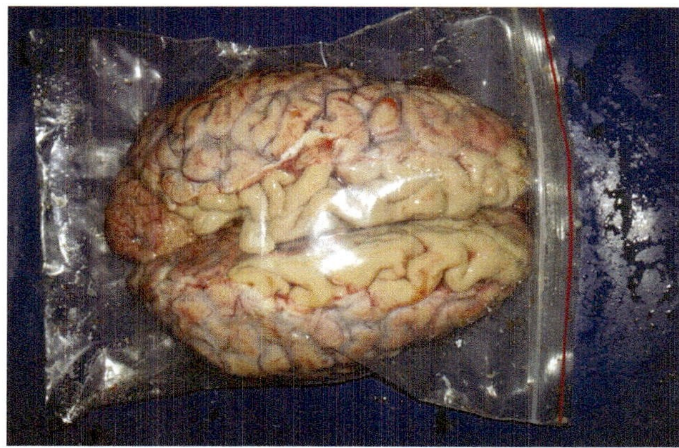

Fig. 22.15 Brain packed in sealed plastic cover

a length of suture that goes over the vertex of the skull. During removal of the scalp, the skin may stretch, and when the two halves are brought back together, it may overlap. To approximate this, posterior skin flap can be trimmed. The excess scalp tissue is placed into the plastic bag. The scalp tissue is closed by 'under-stitching' method from ear to ear after proper combing or brushing to avoid hair becoming entangled in the twine. After reaching the other ear, the suture is tied off, burying the knot in the process.[4,7]

WASHING

After reconstruction, the entire body must be cleaned of any residual bodily fluid or stains. Hot water should be avoided as it may cause dermal damage (abrasion or contusion)—may cause confusion in case of second autopsy. Detergents containing disinfectant may be used along with water to assist washing process. The back of the body and hair must also be washed. Then the body and tray are rinsed with warm water and dried with clean dry sponges. The whole body including the back and hair must be dried.[6,7,9,10]

Then, by keeping the head block under the neck, the hair is combed properly to recreate the original antemortem style. Finally, the body is dressed properly ensuring that all the identification labels are clearly accessible and visible. A wrist band or toe-tag may be placed on the body, before returning the body to cold-chamber (if not handed over to the police constable).[6,7,9,10]

SPECIAL CIRCUMSTANCES

The Eye

If only the vitreous has been removed during autopsy, then an equal volume of water is injected in the posterior chamber using the same needle, syringe and hole until it is re-inflated. In case of removal of eyeball, the orbit must be reconstructed. Wet cotton wool is packed at the back of orbit. Then dry cotton wool is added on top of this to mimic an eye globe. To get a better cosmetic look, the pupil is drawn on the globe with black marker pen. A transparent eye shield is placed over cotton wool; lids closed and sealed shut with fast drying adhesive glue applied to the undersurface of eyelid. Choosing a good quality adhesive is important, since many fast-drying adhesives are colorless when wet and turns white when it dries up.[7]

Wound and Incision

Sometimes, it is necessary to open the limbs during an autopsy, when seeking the presence of subcutaneous and muscular injuries, deep vein thromboses or fractures. Incisions into the limbs should be placed on their extensor surfaces wherever possible. At the end of the examination, the incision is packed with cotton wadding. The incision can then be closed using the 'under-stitching' method. Where the shoulders and buttocks have been examined, care must be taken during reconstruction not to cause distortion of the local anatomy.[4,7]

If there is any wound or surgical incisions on the body, they are closed with suturing only when second autopsy is not going to be performed. In case of homicide and other extraordinary situations, these wounds can be closed only after the opportunity for second autopsy has occurred. Small lacerations and incised wounds can be closed with tissue glue (if available).[7]

Emaciated Dead Body

Reconstruction of an emaciated cadaver is difficult. Satisfactory reconstruction can be achieved by adding additional absorbent material to the thoraco-abdominal cavity or by rotating the sternal plate by 180° from its normal anatomical position so that it can bridge the thoracic void. With the viscera and the chest plate in their respective positions, the attendant can now proceed with the suturing of the incision.[4]

Pelvic Dissection

In cases where the genital tract has been removed *en bloc*, the pelvic bone wedge is replaced to reconstruct the pelvic ring. A series of strong, deep sutures starting at the most posterior aspect and working anteriorly will reconstruct this area.[4,7]

Removal of any Member/Limb

Occasionally, when a long bone like femur has to be removed and retained at autopsy, a good cosmetic reconstruction can be achieved by using plastic rods or simple wood dowels of equivalent length. This is then covered by wadding, placed in the space of long bone to maintain the shape and also to soak up any fluid discharge. In infants, one can use smaller pieces of wood or plaster of Paris. Then the limb is sutured like any other place.[7,14]

If spinal cord has been removed, the space is lined by wadding and vertebral column replaced.

Decomposed Body

If the body has decomposed, the level of reconstruction will be determined by the state of the body. Sutures may need to be wider apart and placed deeper into the tissue (or other suturing techniques used) to enable the body cavities to be sealed without the tissue tearing.[7] The body is then placed into plastic sheet or an equivalent body bag and sealed.

High-risk Dead Body

There are certain circumstances in which, assuming an examination has occurred in the first place, the body should not be reconstructed. Bodies exposed to pathogens such as Lassa, Ebola, Marburg and CCHF (Crimean-Congo hemorrhagic fever), and some instances of chemical and radiological contaminated bodies fall into this category. These bodies would simply be placed in a purpose-designed body bag and disposed off as per guidelines.[7]

FETAL AND PEDIATRIC RECONSTRUCTION

The basic principles are same as an adult with the aim being to produce good cosmetic result. The choice of suture material may be different due to the size of the body. White cotton sutures are adequate; thick, black sutures should be avoided. In fetal autopsy, the fragility of the skin makes the suturing an unsuitable method of reconstruction. The body is dried with absorbent paper towels and loosely packed with cotton wool or any other suitable wadding. If available, the skin and soft tissues are reunited with fast acting tissue adhesives such as 2-octylcyanoacrylate (Dermabond) or 'Histo-acryl Blue'. Usage of excess glue or adhesives should be avoided, as it may produce an exothermic reaction on the body.[7,15]

The running baseball stitch can be used for children and with the additional sutured approximation of the subcutaneous tissues. The stitching of these tenacious dermal layers of skin are enough to ensure the static placement of this autopsy suture.

CONCLUSION

The post-autopsy restoration procedure is undertaken to ensure that the dead body is respectfully restored and cleaned before its release to the authorities or relatives. This process will also ensure that the person or persons handling the dead body after autopsy do not come in direct contact with any of the biologically hazardous agents that are universally present. In doing so, the authorities and the families will have much more respect for the professionalism of the medical institution and those responsible for conducting the postmortem examinations.

REFERENCES

1. Autopsy. Available from: http://en.wikipedia.org/wiki/Autopsy.
2. The Royal College of Pathologists of Australia. Autopsies and the use of tissues removed from autopsies. 2011 [Internet]. Available from: http://www.rcpa.edu.au/Library/College-Policies/Policies/Autopsies-and-the-Use-of-Tissues-Removed-from-Auto.
3. Petts G, Lloyd K, Osborn M. Observing an autopsy: Seeing a post mortem will make it easier to recommend one to patients and their relatives? Student BMJ. Available from: http://www.medscape.com/viewarticle/778850_5.
4. Ferguson WR. Postmortem cadaveric restoration. Technician's guide for postmortem examinations. United States: Xlibris Corp; 2010. p. 123-29.
5. Biswas G. Medicolegal autopsy. In: Review of forensic medicine and toxicology. 2nd ed. New Delhi: Jaypee brothers; 2012. p. 83-103.
6. Finkbeiner WE, Ursell PC, Davis RL. Basic postmortem examination. In: Autopsy pathology: A manual and atlas. 2nd edn. Philadelphia: Saunders Elsevier; 2009. p. 35-55.
7. Donlon S, Rutty GN. Reconstruction of the body. In: Burton JL, Rutty GN (eds). The Hospital Autopsy: A manual of fundamental autopsy practice. 3rd edn. New York: CRC press; 2010. p. 308-14.
8. Hoggarth P, Poole B. A pathologist guide to embalming. In: Rutty GN (ed). Essentials in autopsy practice. London: Springer-Verlag; 2001. p. 23-42.
9. Gresham GA, Turner AF. Reconstruction of the body after postmortem examination. Postmortem procedures: An illustrated text book. London: Wolfe Medical Publications; 1979. p. 131-32.

10. Polson CJ, Brittain RP, Marshall TK. The disposal of the dead. 2nd edn. London: English universities press. Hodder and Stonghton Educational; 1962.
11. The science behind postmortem needles. Available from: http://surgical-instruments-supplies.medical-supplies-equipment-company.com/post-mortem-needles-799.htm.
12. Kudur MH, Pai SB, Sripathi H, Prabhu S. Sutures and suturing techniques in skin closure. *Indian J Dermatol Venereol Leprol* 2009; 75: 425-34. Available from: http://emedicine.medscape.com/article/2044501-overview
13. Monheit GD. Wound healing and post-operative care: Laser resurfacing [Internet]. Available from: http://www.totalskinandbeauty.com/about-us-our-doctors-wound-closure-suture-technique.shtml.
14. Finkbeiner WE, Ursell PC, Davis RL. Special dissection procedures. Autopsy pathology: A manual and atlas. 2nd edn. Philadelphia: Saunders Elsevier; 2009. p. 67-79.
15. Gau GS, Napier K, Bhundia J. Use of tissue adhesive to repair fetal bodies after dissection. *J Clin Pathol* 1991; 44: 759-60.

Index

Page numbers followed by *f* refer to figure and *t* refer to table.

A

B

C

D

E

F

G

H

R

S

U

V

W

Z